Oxford Medical Publications

**Women's Health**

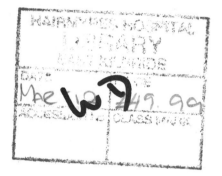

Whilst every effort has been made to ensure that the contents of this book are as complete, accurate, and up to date as possible at the time of writing, Oxford University Press is not able to give any guarantee or assurance that such is the case. Readers are urged to take appropriately qualified medical advice in all cases. The information in this book is intended to be useful to the general reader, but should not be used as a means of self-diagnosis or for the prescription of medication.

# Women's Health
## Fifth Edition

Edited by
### Deborah Waller
*General Practitioner, Oxford*

and

### Ann McPherson
*General Practitioner, Oxford*

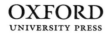
OXFORD
UNIVERSITY PRESS

*This book has been printed digitally and produced in a standard specification
in order to ensure its continuing availability*

# OXFORD
UNIVERSITY PRESS

Great Clarendon Street, Oxford OX2 6DP
United Kingdom

Oxford University Press is a department of the University of Oxford.
It furthers the University's objective of excellence in research, scholarship,
and education by publishing worldwide. Oxford is a registered trade mark of
Oxford University Press in the UK and in certain other countries

© Oxford University Press, 2003

The moral rights of the author have been asserted

Fourth edition published 1997 (reprinted 1998 with corrections)
Fifth edition published 2003
Reprinted 2012

British Library Cataloguing in Publication Data
Data available

Library of Congress Cataloging in Publication Data
Data available

ISBN 978-0-19-263286-9

# Preface

Welcome to the fifth edition of *Women's Health*. Rather than simply updating existing chapters we have tried to approach the subject matter afresh. To this end, there are many new authors giving new perspectives on subjects such as premenstrual syndrome, the menopause, urinary incontinence, breast disorders, sexual problems, and promoting the health of women. There are new chapters on vulval disorders, familial cancers, and domestic violence. The subject of cancer screening has been broadened to include cervical, breast, and ovarian screening, all of which are now brought together in a single chapter. All authors have been carefully chosen for their expertise in the field and continue to be GPs or to have an understanding of the particular needs of primary care. Certain elements from previous editions do not appear in this edition to keep the book to manageable size.

Just as space in the book is a problem for the editors, time limitation during the consultation is an issue for most women visiting their GPs. We have included examples of model ten-minute consultations throughout the book. The idea is to try and distil the salient points in the history and examination as well as the key issues to be discussed with the patient. Of course in practice we know that patients often come back for follow-up consultations and that there is no single right way of dealing with a problem. We hope that GPs will find the consultations helpful as a guide to how they might best use the time available when seeing patients.

Increasingly, within the field of women's health, there isn't one straightforward, correct answer to many of the questions women bring to us. The controversy surrounding hormone replacement therapy, discussed in the menopause chapter, is a good example of this. Choice and information have become the buzz-words of the last few years. Evidence-based medicine is vital to direct doctors and empower patients but at the same time health professionals should not abdicate responsibility by forcing decisions on patients when there is no right or wrong answer.

To help with some of these issues, authors have been asked where possible, to identify common questions that patients ask ('Frequently asked questions') and to respond thus making the book more patient-centred.

Although the internet is now used by both patients and health practitioners as a source of health information, we feel there is still room for a good book and hope that doctors, nurses, and patients alike will enjoy using this fifth edition of *Women's Health*.

*Oxford*                                                                          A.M and D.W
*May 2003*

# Acknowledgements

Ann McPherson and Deborah Waller are editing a series of ten minute consultations in the *British Medical Journal*. They would like to thank the *British Medical Journal* for allowing them to include some of these, relevant to women's health, in this book.

# Contents

List of Contributors  *xi*

**1** Menstrual problems  *1*
Margaret C P Rees

**2** Premenstrual syndrome  *46*
Fiona Blake

**3** The menopause and hormone replacement therapy  *73*
Elizabeth Barrett-Connor

**4** Contraception  *112*
John Guillebaud

**5** Unwanted pregnancy and abortion  *229*
Lis Davidson and Joanne Reeve

**6** Infertility and early pregnancy loss  *262*
Gillian M Lockwood

**7** Cystitis  *297*
Sally Hope and Ian Bowler

**8** Management of urinary incontinence in women  *322*
Ranee Thakar, Stuart Stanton and Judy Kane

**9** Vaginal discharge and sexually transmitted infections  *351*
Pippa Oakeshott

**10** Vulval disorders  *374*
Lois Eva

**11** Chronic pelvic pain  *399*
Stephen Kennedy and Jane Moore

**12** Breast disorders  *421*
Danielle Power and Jane Maher

**13** Women's cancer screening: cervical, breast,
and ovarian screening  *466*
Clare Bankhead and Joan Austoker

**14** Familial cancers and women's health *489*
*Anneke Lucassen and Eila Watson*

**15** Eating disorders *519*
*Deborah Waller and Christopher Fairburn*

**16** Sexual problems *552*
*Margaret Denman*

**17** Domestic violence *579*
*Iona Heath*

**18** Promoting the health of women in primary care *597*
*Sandra Nicholson and Yvonne Carter*

**19** Complementary medicine and women's health *619*
*Christine A'Court, Chi Keong Ong, and Jacqueline Wootton*

Index *671*

# Contributors

**Christine A'Court** is GP in Oxfordshire, and has various local and national roles concerned with the modernization of medical care, and information management, with particular reference to cardiovascular medicine. This may seem at odds with the subject area, complementary medicine, covered in her chapter. However, both fields explore different facets of patient-centred medicine. With improved service design and information management, clinicians may have more time to devote to the patient's agenda and to maximize the potential for a 'therapeutic interaction'.

**Joan Austoker** is the Director of the Cancer Research UK Primary Care Education Research Group, University of Oxford. She conducts research in screening for breast and cervical cancer, particularly relating to the acceptability of screening and provision of information to enable informed participation. She has also produced several evidence-based educational materials for primary care about screening for breast and cervical cancer and recently has been involved in producing an information pack for primary care regarding prostate cancer testing.

**Clare Bankhead** is a Research Fellow in the Primary Care Education Research Group, University of Oxford. Her research interests include breast and cervical cancer screening, and she has recently been involved in developing new patient materials to facilitate informed participation in screening. She is also investigating ways in which the processes of early diagnosis of ovarian cancer may be optimized.

**Elizabeth Barrett-Connor** is Professor and Division Chief of Epidemiology in the Department of Family and Preventive Medicine at the University of California, San Diego School of Medicine. Her research concerns healthy ageing with a particular focus on gender differences and women's health. Her pioneering work spans many areas, including cardiovascular disease, diabetes, cancer, osteoporosis, memory loss, and exogenous and endogenous hormones. She is founder and director of the Rancho Bernardo Heart and Chronic Disease Study, now in its 30th year, and has authored more than 500 publications.

**Fiona Blake** is a Consultant Psychiatrist in Cambridge. She has an interest in women's health and until 1999 ran a service in Oxford for women with mental health problems associated with their reproductive biology. She has been involved in teaching and research concerning premenstrual syndrome, psychological aspects of the menopause and postnatal depression.

**Ian Bowler** trained in general internal medicine, infectious diseases, and microbiology. He is a Consultant Microbiologist and Infection Control Doctor for the Oxford Radcliffe Hospitals NHS Trust and an Honorary Senior Clinical Lecturer in the University of Oxford. His interests are the prevention of hospital-acquired infection and the development of guidelines for the appropriate use of microbiological tests in hospital and general practice settings.

**Yvonne Carter** is Professor of General Practice and Primary Care at Barts and The London, Queen Mary's School of Medicine and Dentistry, University of London. She is also a part-time GP in Tower Hamlets. She is an elected Member of the Council of the Royal College of General Practitioners. She has a long-standing research interest in the prevention of injuries, both unintentional (accidents to children and older people) and intentional (child protection, domestic violence and aggression, and violence to primary health-care teams). She is the editor of many books, articles, reports, and training packs. She is committed to increasing the research capacity in primary care and is particularly interested in the accreditation of research practices and the development of primary care research networks.

**Chi Keong Ong** is the current holder of the Research Fellowship in Community and Complementary Medicine at Mansfield College, University of Oxford. He trained originally as a molecular biologist at King's College, London, and then developed an interest in complementary medicine whilst reading for a master's degree in medical geography at Oxford. Other research interests include the need for whole person care within modern biomedicine and the impact of spirituality on health and well-being. He is currently a consultant to the World Health Organization, mapping complementary medicine use throughout the 51 member nations of the WHO Euro zone.

**Lis Davidson** has been a GP in Liverpool since 1986. She also works at Liverpool Brook and is a Family Planning Instructor and a GP Trainer. She was perceived by her fellow author as a 'key informant' when Joanne undertook a review of local TOP services for Liverpool Health Authority. This fortunately coincided with the need to update this chapter.

**Margaret Denman** is a GP with a special interest in psychosexual medicine. She is a member of the Institute of Psychosexual Medicine (IPM). She leads training seminars for doctors in this field and is an examiner for the IPM.

**Lois Eva** is a Specialist Registrar in obstetrics and gynaecology in North East Thames. She has a special interest in vulval disorders.

**Christopher Fairburn** is Wellcome Principal Research Fellow and Professor of Psychiatry at Oxford University. He specializes in research on the nature and treatment of eating disorders. He has a particular interest in the development and evaluation of psychological treatments and is especially well known for his work evaluating the effectiveness of cognitive behaviour therapy, guided self-help, and interpersonal psychotherapy in the treatment of eating disorders. He has had research grants both in Britain and the United States, and he has published extensively in the area. Professor Fairburn was awarded the 'Outstanding Researcher Award' by the Academy for Eating Disorders in 2002. He has edited four books on eating disorders and has written a self-help book for people with binge eating problems.

**John Guillebaud** is Professor Emeritus at University College, London, having been given the world's first Chair of Family Planning and Reproductive Health in 1992. In 2002 he retired as Medical Director of the Margaret Pyke Centre, in order to focus on population, sustainable development, and conservation of the natural world: 'issues which must, for the sake of all our grandchildren, be brought fully into the "mainstream" of public life'. He is based in Oxford and continues in part-time practice. He is author or co-author of seven books and more than 300 other publications on birth control and related subjects, for both medical and lay readership. He considers himself an ex-GP, having worked during his training as a locum in a variety of practices from Barnsley, South Yorkshire to Eltham in South London.

**Iona Heath** has been a GP in London since 1977. She is a long-standing Member of the Council of the Royal College of General Practitioners; she is the Chairman of both the Health Inequalities Group and the Committee of Medical Ethics of the RCGP. She has written a booklet on *Domestic violence: the general practitioner's role* for the RCGP.

**Sally Hope** is a GP in Woodstock with a special interest in women's health. She is a founder member of the 'Primary Care Group in Gynaecology', deputy editor of the *Journal of the British Menopause Society*, and an honorary Lecturer in the Department of Public Health and Primary Care, University of Oxford.

**Judy Kane** has been a GP in Kingston for nearly 30 years. She is also Honorary Research Fellow at the National Heart and Lung Institute of Imperial College, London. Over the years in general practice she has developed a special interest in incontinence through dealing with so many women patients.

**Stephen Kennedy** is Clinical Reader in Obstetrics and Gynaecology at the University of Oxford and Honorary Consultant Gynaecologist at the John Radcliffe Hospital, Oxford. He is a graduate of Keble College, Oxford and Guy's

Hospital, London. He jointly heads an international group researching the genetics of endometriosis, which aims to identify genes that predispose women to develop the disease. He is also involved in health services research, studying the medical consultation and patients' attitudes towards diagnostic processes in chronic pelvic pain.

**Gill Lockwood** is Medical Director of Midland Fertility Services, at Aldridge in the West Midlands. Her first degree was in Philosophy, Politics and Economics and she initially worked in the Cabinet Office as a government statistician. A career change, inspired by a medical documentary, took her back to Oxford to read Medicine and she qualified in 1986. Her research doctorate was in reproductive endocrinology and her major research interests are polycystic ovarian syndrome and male factor infertility. She is Chair of the British Fertility Society Ethics Committee and lectures and broadcasts on ethical aspects of fertility treatment.

**Anneke Lucassen** is Consultant/Senior Lecturer in Clinical Genetics at the Wessex Clinical Genetics Service in Southampton. She has research interests in cancer genetics and in the ethical issues raised within clinical genetics. She has co-authored another book in the Oxford General Practice series: *Practical genetics for primary care.*

**Ann McPherson,** CBE, has been a GP in Oxford since 1979. She is also a part time Research Lecturer in the Department of General Practice, Oxford University, and a Fellow of Green College, Oxford. She has edited the *Women's Health Book* for Oxford University Press since the first edition in 1987. She researches and writes on the health of women and adolescents and is co-author of several books for teenagers and their parents, including the *Teenage Health Freak* series. As Medical Director of DIPEx she heads the research team producing the www.dipex.org website which presents patients' experiences for use by patients themselves and as a teaching resource. She sits on various government committees including the Independent Advisory Group on Teenage Pregnancy.

**Jane Maher** trained at Westminster Medical School; her training also included stints at the Royal Marsden Hospital, Harvard Medical School and the Kalahari Desert! She was voted Oncologist of the Year by Hospital Doctor in 1995. She currently works as a Consultant Clinical Oncologist at Mount Vernon Cancer Centre, with a particular interest in breast cancer, and Senior Clinical Lecturer at University College, London. She is Chief Medical Officer of Macmillan Cancer Relief and founder and Medical Director of the Lynda Jackson Macmillan Cancer Support and Information Centre and leads a research team with a particular interest in supportive oncology.

**Jane Moore** works as a gynaecology registrar at the John Radcliffe Hospital in Oxford. She has maintained an interest in pelvic pain and endometriosis including its surgical management in her general training. In 2000 she was awarded an MSc in clinical medicine for research into women's views about pelvic pain and its investigation. She is a member of the International Pelvic Pain Society.

**Sandra Nicholson** is a GP and Senior Clinical Lecturer in the Department of General Practice and Primary Care at Queen Mary's School of Medicine and Dentistry, University of London. Her main interests lie with the medical undergraduate curriculum. She has been responsible for the development of a community-based obstetric and gynaecology module in primary care that introduces all aspects of health promotion for women to students. This has involved working with all members of the primary health-care team to ensure that an appropriate educational environment for students is maintained.

**Pippa Oakeshott** trained at Cambridge and is a Senior Lecturer in General Practice at St George's Hospital Medical School and a GP in an inner London practice. Her main research interests are in sexual health and the management of hypertension in primary care.

**Danielle Power** qualified from UMDS of Guy's and St Thomas's Hospitals and is a Specialist Registrar on the Pan-Thames Rotation in Clinical Oncology, currently based at Charing Cross Hospital. She trained in general medicine and oncology in London and Sydney, Australia, and has a particular interest in breast cancer management and palliative care.

**Margaret Rees** is a Reader in Reproductive Medicine at the Nuffield Department of Obstetrics and Gynaecology, University of Oxford and Honorary Consultant in Medical Gynaecology. She is also a Supernumerary Fellow at St Hilda's College, Oxford. Her clinical and research publications focus on menopause, menstrual disorders, uterine angiogenesis, and neoplasia. She is the Editor-in-Chief of the *Journal of the British Menopause Society* and authors and edits books on the menopause.

**Joanne Reeve** trained as a GP in Liverpool. She is now a Specialist Registrar in Public Health Medicine.

**Stuart Stanton** is Professor of Reconstructive Pelvic Surgery and Urogynaecology at St George's Hospital Medical School. He has an Honorary Fellowship of the Royal Australia and New Zealand College of Obstetrics and Gynaecology. His Department is involved in the care and management of women with urogynaecological disorders. He has authored or co-authored more than 190 papers on gynaecology and urogynaecology, and authored or co-authored 13 textbooks. Outside medicine, his main interests are his family, modern ceramics, and photography.

**Ranee Thakar** is currently a Consultant Obstetrician and Gynaecologist and a Urogynaecology Subspecialist working at Mayday University Hospital, Croydon. She trained as a Subspeciality Trainee with Professor Stanton. Her main areas of interest are incontinence, prolapse, childbirth injuries, and hysterectomy and she has published extensively on these topics.

**Deborah Waller** is a GP working with Ann McPherson in a group practice in Oxford. She has particular interests in women's health and eating disorders. She is currently a member of the eating disorders guideline development group for the National Institute for Clinical Excellence.

**Eila Watson** is Deputy Director of the Cancer Research UK Primary Care Education Research Group, Department of Primary Health Care, University of Oxford. Her main research interests are cancer screening, informed decision-making, and primary care genetics.

**Jacqueline Wootton** is President of the Alternative Medicine Foundation, Potomac, MD, and director of 'HerbMed', the interactive herbal database project. She directs the Informatics project at the Rosenthal Centre, Columbia University College of Physicians and Surgeons, and has published widely on alternative medicine research information, women's health research, electronic databases, and the Internet. In 2001, she was an invited panel speaker on the Publication of Peer-Reviewed CAM Research for the White House Commission on Complementary and Alternative Medicine Policy.

# Introduction

## Ann McPherson and Deborah Waller

As far as health is concerned—the 'battle of the sexes' is over. The major challenge we face in the 21st century is how best to deal with the chronic diseases which affect our quality of life (whatever our gender) in middle and later years. We may need to accept an increase in the medicalization of our lives, along with unforeseen health outcomes, many uncertainties, and changes in our lifestyles. In dealing with these problems there will be some issues that are similar for both women and men. In this book we have tried to concentrate on those illnesses that are either unique to women or affect women in a different way to men, particularly those that make a significant contribution to the work of general practice.

## Historical perspective

It is clear that the general health of both women and men has improved dramatically since the 1800s. In 1841, life expectancy at birth was 41 years for males and 43 for females in England and Wales and by the end of the 20th century it had risen to 75 for males and 80 for women. However, life expectancy does not take into account the actual *quality* of this extended life. Healthy life expectancy, defined as 'expected years of life in good or fairly good self-assessed general health', has also improved but it has not risen as much as actual life expectancy. It has been calculated that women born in 1997 can expect 68.7 years of life in good or fairly good health whilst for men it is the slightly lower figure of 66.9 years. Because overall women live for approximately five years longer then men, these 'extra' years for women are more likely to be of 'poor quality'.

Data on the reporting of morbidity, defined in the General Household Survey as 'restriction in activity in the 14 days prior to being interviewed', show that in 1970, 8% of females and 7% of males in Great Britain reported some restricted activity, whereas in the late 1990s these figures had risen to 16% of females and 14% of males. This rise, not surprisingly, is most notable in the older age group.

From the early part of the 20th century reproductive processes have been the major concern for women's health—a concern mainly dealt with by improvements in overall hygiene, followed by the introduction of antibiotics. More recently there has been a steep rise in medical 'interference' in childbirth, demonstrated by rising Caesarean rates. This has been challenged by the 'natural childbirth' movement, instigated by women themselves. These opposing changes have occurred alongside an emphasis on women's health in general, associated with changes in the socio-economic status of women and the practice of evidence-based medicine. The term 'women's health' now encompasses a different range of conditions to that of a hundred years ago and even to that of twenty years ago when the first edition of this book was published.

## What makes women sick?

The main threats to women's health include cancer, coronary heart disease, mental illness, and unwanted teenage pregnancy. These problems, as well as the uptake of screening programmes and preventative medicines, are affected by social and economic conditions, lifestyle factors, and the availability of health care.

With an ageing population the incidence of **cancer** is on the increase. A third of the female population develop a cancer at some point in their lives and it is responsible for about a quarter of their deaths. Lung cancer in women has just now overtaken breast cancer as the main cause of death from cancer in the UK, even though the incidence of breast cancer has continued to rise over the last twenty years. This is because deaths from breast cancer have declined in the UK, partly as a result of improved treatment and partly as a result of population breast screening, though the exact role played by the latter is still seen as controversial on both sides of the Atlantic.

**Coronary heart disease** remains a major cause of mortality and morbidity in both sexes, even if it is not always perceived as a serious threat by women themselves or their doctors. There is, however, some evidence that women are not having their coronary heart disease recognized and treated as early or efficiently as men.

**Mental health problems** continue to be more prevalent in women than men, with a marked socio-economic bias. For example, over the period 1994–98, 77 out of every 1000 female patients living in industrial deprived areas in Britain were treated for depression, compared with 55 per 1000 female patients living in suburban areas, whilst for men the figures were 34 and 21 respectively.

**Contraception and pregnancy** are often 'considered' to be female health issues. Certainly the effects of unplanned or even planned teenage pregnancy are greater on the girl than on the boy involved in the actual act of conception. The UK still has the highest teenage pregnancy rates in Europe. A further 'side effect' of sex is the acquisition of **Sexually Transmitted Infections**. Although more men than women are diagnosed with gonorrhoea, the rise in incidence has occurred in both genders. There was an 80% rise in women diagnosed with genital chlamydia in 1999 compared to the previous five years. HIV infection has also increased among women due to heterosexual transmission and drug use.

## Changing lifestyles and changing environment

Women are more likely than men to be aware of the relationship between lifestyle and health and to modify aspects of their lifestyles. The consumption of fruit and vegetables has risen steadily since the mid 1980s, with more women than men eating the recommended five portions a day. However women do not necessarily have a healthier attitude to **food** in general. Even at the age of 15, at least 16% of girls are dieting to lose weight compared to 3% of boys. Anorexia nervosa and bulimia nervosa are much commoner in girls than boys, while at the other extreme 21% of women over the age of 16 are obese, with a BMI of over 30 compared to 19% of boys.

The role that **alcohol** plays in society from a health point of view is complicated. Women are advised to drink no more than three units per day. Two-fifths of women between 16 and 24 consume more than this amount, though this is not the case for older women. A recent review tried to calculate the overall mortality rate associated with alcohol consumption at different ages. It concluded that non-drinkers and heavy drinkers both had higher all cause mortality rates than light drinkers. These results reflect the fact that at a certain level of consumption the protection that alcohol provides against coronary heart disease outweighs the increased risks associated with alcohol of death from injury, cancer of the colon, cancer of the oesophagus, liver disease, and breast cancer. The 'best alcohol intake buy' for women using these health indicators is to drink no alcohol at all for the under 35s, rising to three units a week for the over 65s.

Doctors recognize that no food or drink is consumed merely for perceived health benefits. What advice we should be giving as health professionals gets more complicated almost by the day as new 'evidence' is published. To great fanfare, a recent paper in the *British Journal of Cancer* investigated the links between alcohol, tobacco, and breast cancer. No relationship was found between breast cancer risk and smoking habits, but an increased lifetime risk of breast cancer from 8.8% to 9.3% was found for women who drank more then one unit of alcohol a day and there appeared to be a linear increase in risk with alcohol consumption.

A major influence on women's health is **smoking**. In 1950 British women smoked half as many cigarettes as their male contemporaries, whilst in 1980 they smoked nearly as many. By the 1990s in younger age groups women were smoking more then men. The rate of lung cancer in women has soared and now exceeds that of breast cancer. Smoking in both men and women is higher amongst those from lower or unskilled backgrounds. Health education programmes have made attempts to aim messages specifically at women, particularly women who are pregnant. They have had a measure of success. Between 1985 and 1995 smoking amongst pregnant women fell from 30 to 24%, although the social class gradient remained. Meanwhile the tobacco companies have continued to promote certain brands of cigarettes to young women. Little attention has been paid to why there have been changes to the smoking patterns in men and women and how best to tailor anti-smoking advice to different groups within the community.

**Exercise** is another area in which men and women behave differently. Though there are signs in the General Household Survey that more women are taking part in sports and other physical activities than in previous years, it still remains inadequately low. In 1998, three-fifths of women aged 16–24 did less then one hour's sport or exercise a week and only 1 in 20 women did more then seven hours of exercise per week. For men the story was slightly better with almost a fifth saying they did seven or more hours of sport or exercise a week in 1998. By the age of 45 the gender difference had almost disappeared, though not because women had caught up: 64% of both men and women over the age of 45 took no exercise.

## Emerging morbidities

There are emerging morbidities that have been present as threats to women's health for many years, but are only now being fully recognized. There are also new areas of concern which have not been present in the past. Domestic violence, probably around for decades but unquantified, is now showing itself to be much more widespread across all social classes than was previously thought. But, as with many other societal threats to health, there still remains doubt as to what role the medical profession can usefully play in its recognition and management. As the proportion of women undertaking work outside the home increases we do appear to be seeing a more 'male pattern' of disease emerging amongst women. In 2001, 69% of women aged 16–59 were working, with 39% working full time and 30% part time. Comparative figures for men showed that 79% of men aged 16–64 were working with 73% engaged in full time work and 7% doing a part time occupation. Despite the changing culture of who does what in the home, most women still have the primary responsibility for children and the household, and have to juggle both roles. Women still earn less than men despite the advances of equal opportunities. What is unclear is to what extent these social pressures contribute to women's health problems in the current age.

## What women worry about

It is known that more women suffer from depression and anxiety than men but there has been little research into what women actually worry about. A survey by the popular Radio 4 programme 'Woman's Hour' in 1994 sheds some light on this. A random sample of over 500 women above the age of 16 were interviewed at home about their anxieties and attitudes to health. Only 1 in 10 women described their health as excellent, but nearly 50% said their health was very good. 10% thought they were not in control of their lives and 73% of this sample said they suffered from 'stressful nerves' compared with 46% of the whole sample. Breast cancer dominated women's fears at all ages, whilst for younger women aged 16–24, cervical cancer followed by stress about weight and their appearance were top worries. By the age of 45, reduced mobility, senility, and breast cancer scored the highest and these concerns continued into old age.

## The influence of health fashions

The increased medicalization of areas such as child birth, sex, relationship problems, and disease prevention may be in part responsible for the relatively high rate at which women attend GP's surgeries. These changes have lead to the emergence of 'health fashions', which are based to a variable degree on new scientific evidence. Attitudes towards the menopause, premenstrual tension, eating disorders, and faddish diets have been influenced by fashion and social pressures, as, to a lesser extent, have demands for counselling, alternative therapies, and anti-depressants. Exaggerated claims and inaccurate reporting in the general media and women's magazines have directed patients' thinking. Most recently it is claimed that 'research' shows that over 50% of women have sexual problems that would be improved by taking a drug like Viagra!

Attitudes to the menopause by women and the medical profession have changed over the years. Although there is very little direct reference to such risqué areas in Victorian literature it is possible that some characters, Mrs Nicholby for instance, were menopausal. However the lack of references to the menopause in literature may not have only been due to prudery and denial of women's problems, but to the fact that far fewer women succeeded in living long enough to experience it.

Doctors were slow to accept menopausal symptoms as a problem to which they could offer any contribution until patients and the media forced them to take notice. In this atmosphere of increased awareness the drug companies succeeded in producing and marketing suitable hormone replacement therapy. The interdependence of medical, pharmaceutical, and lay interests has encouraged the view that symptoms of the menopause are pathological. Nevertheless, permanent cessation of menstruation is something that happens to all women who survive beyond middle age and cannot therefore in itself be classified as a disease, though it likely that some women will have symptoms which can be effectively treated.

As always in medicine, symptoms have to be balanced against side effects of the therapy. Prevention of osteoporosis and heart disease and prolongation of an active sexual life by the use of hormone replacement therapy (HRT) has been presented by the drug companies and some doctors as the only way forward for women in their middle years. This attitude has been challenged by others who, having anxieties about the increase in breast cancer and possible other side effects, could not believe it normal for all women to need HRT. These views were ignored or down played for many years, until a recent study in the USA confirmed that HRT did not only appear to have no preventive role in heart disease but, in fact, women on HRT seemed to have a slightly increased risk of morbidity and mortality from heart disease, as well as confirming the association of HRT with breast cancer. The arguments have been polarized with the ever print-worthy Germaine Greer almost labelling women on HRT as 'HRT wimps', while some doctors suggested that taking HRT was analogous to 'wearing glasses' for age onset presbyopia, describing the menopause as 'nature's mistake'. Now there does at least seem to be more of a dialogue with agreement that some women will undoubtedly benefit from HRT whilst others will suffer more than they gain.

Uncertainty in health is something that women of all ages will increasingly have to face. Pill scares occur with monotonous frequency. The so-called user-friendly (third generation) oral contraceptive pills saw their market share cut from 80% to 5% because of the reported small increase in thrombo-embolic disease. However, although the scientific community has accepted this increased risk, a recent legal judgement proclaimed that there was no such risk. There have also been accusations that the promotion of second generation rather than third generation contraceptive pills was a cost cutting exercise of the government, whilst promoting the third generation pills was driven by the profit motives of the drug companies. Scientific truth, information for GPs and choices for women are often obscured by the media angst. What is certain is the uncertainty that remains both for this issue and many other health and illness decisions.

## Why do women go to their doctor?

GPs in England and Wales see more women patients then men and give them more medicine. In 1998 there were 157 million consultations by women and 107 million by men. Overall each person saw their GP on average four times per year but for females it was nearer five times and men less than four. Why is this? Who are these women? What illnesses do they have, and what medicines do they take?

There are, of course, more women then men in the community as a whole and the slightly larger number of men up to the age of 45 is more than offset by the longevity of women. The diseases of ageing, such as dementia and cancer, affect more women. Although it is true that women consult their doctors more often than men from the crude figures, many of the diseases are gender related. Once consultations which are not for illness are excluded, such as pregnancy and childbirth and diseases of the male and female genito-urinary system, the difference virtually disappears. But consultation rates are hardly an accurate reflection of illness and are complicated by the fact that men and women consult in different ways. Men for example are more likely to go to a genito-urinary clinic or an A&E department, whereas women are more likely to see their GP as a source of information. Much consultation goes on in an informal way prior to anyone going to see the doctor: women tend to talk more to their friends about health matters, they read more magazines with high health content than men. Women also have opportunities to consult on issues to do with their own health when bringing their children to child health clinics.

## Self-help and information sources

Self-help is nothing new and in the past it may have come from an impetus similar to the contemporary movement. There is a manuscript dating from 1500 that was re-issued in 1980 under the title '*Medieval Women's Guide to Health*'. This was produced, as the editor comments, 'because women were dissatisfied with their treatment at the hands of male physicians and were endeavouring to instruct one another as to how to help themselves with their gynaecological problems'.

The publication of '*Our bodies ourselves*' as a modern counterpart, by a group of non-medical women in Boston in 1971, produced a focus for women on the possibilities that self-help might offer them. The book was probably the first to challenge the idea that help in health matters was exclusively the prerogative of the medical profession—the authors all having experienced 'frustration and anger towards different doctors and the medical maze in general'; and the basic aim was 'learning to understand, accept, and be responsible for our physical selves'.

In today's world litigation is on the increase, there are frequent articles about medical mistakes in the media and there is a general air of dissatisfaction with the way in which the medical profession communicates. The IT revolution has enabled men and women as well as the self-help movement to get ever better informed. The Internet has revolutionized the way in which we gain access to what was previously often hidden health information. Not only do people want to be better informed and make health decisions with their doctor as a 'partnership' but in recent years the government has also backed this up, encouraging people to take responsibility for their own health. The establishment of NHS Direct and NHS Direct On Line are part of this movement.

## Women doctors

Women are not only the main users of the health service, but are also, as nurses, midwives, health visitors, hospital ancillary staff, radiographers, physiotherapists, etc. to a large extent the providers. Of all NHS and community health service staff employed in 1999, 76% were women and 24% were men.

Until recently the majority of doctors were also men but in 1991, for the first time, over 50% of the medical student intake throughout the country were women and in some medical schools now the intake is well over this. The national figures for the intake in 2002/3 were 2123 men and 3172 women.

Despite this, at consultant level in all hospital specialties only 15% are women: a much lower figure than might be expected from the previous percentage of female medical graduates.

There were 36 000 GP principals in the UK in 2002. The percentage of women principals in general practice has shown a steady increase from 19% in 1985 to 36% in 2001. 75% of women GPs are principals compared to 93% of male GPs. With the introduction of the new GP Contract in 2003, the change in the organization of general practice is likely to bring about a definitive shift in the male/female ratio. General practice is likely to become increasingly female dominated, with many women working part time at some stage in their career.

Various studies have looked at women's preference of the sex of their doctor and they all show that some, especially younger, women want to see a woman doctor for certain conditions, e.g. gynaecological and maternity. However these surveys always show variations dependent on the way the data was collected. There are anxieties that if the profession becomes too female dominated both women and men patients will be given less choice as to which doctor they can see.

Several factors now point to an increasingly fragmented service in primary care for the future: the reorganization of out-of-hours services in the new GP Contract, the European employment regulations restricting the number of hours a doctor can work at a stretch, the introduction of a salaried service for GPs, and the limited way in which women doctors (and some men) with young families want to work. As a consequence we may see a widening gulf between the service provided and what patients want in terms of increased access, continuity of care, and more choice.

## Conclusion

This introduction presents some ideas influencing women's health in general and those which specifically relate to general practice. Just as it has traditionally been necessary to be aware of the female/male differences in the anatomy, so it is important to consider the subtler female/male differences in psychological attitudes to disease during general practice training.

A major challenge for the future is how best to manage chronic diseases in the context of an ageing population. Evidence-based medicine has been the revolution of the last decade but with evidence-based medicine comes uncertainty. How to interpret the thousands of research papers on women's health produced each year, how to communicate uncertainties in the consultation, and how to avoid unnecessary medicalization of women's lives are some of the issues facing doctors, nurses, and women today.

## Sources used

BBC Broadcasting Research Survey on Women's Health (1994) for *Woman's Hour*. Personal communication.

Brown, G. and Harris, T. (1978). *Social origins of depression*. Tavistock Publications, London.

General Household Survey Annual Reports (2001). HMSO.

Logan, W.P.D. Illness, incapacity and medical attention among adults, 1947–1949. *Lancet*, **i**, 773–6.

OPCS. (2000). *Mortality statistics—general*, 2000.

Rowland, B. (ed.) (1981). *Medieval guide to health*. Croom Helm, London.

The Boston Women's Collective (1971). *Our bodies ourselves.* Simon and Schuster, New York.

Statistics for General Medical Practitioners in England: 1991–2001. Bulletin 2002/03.

Women in the labour market: results from the spring 2001 Labour Force Survey. Labour Market Trends, Vol. 110, no 3, ISSN: 1361–4819.

*British Medical Journal* (2002). **325**(7), 357–65.

*British Journal of Cancer* (2002). **87**, 1234–45.

Social Trends 32 2002 edition, office of National Statistics.

Chapter 1

# Menstrual problems
Margaret C P Rees

## Introduction

Disorders of menstruation form a significant part of the general practitioner's work. This is not surprising since women will each experience about 400 menstruations between the menarche and the menopause.

In a national community survey undertaken by MORI in 1990, 31% of women reported heavy periods. Of these, one-third had consulted a doctor within the past 4 months. The Fourth National Morbidity Survey in General Practice (1991–1992) (the latest figures since this survey is undertaken every 10 years) showed that for women aged 25–44 the consultation rates for menorrhagia were 65 per 1000 person-years at risk: and 5% women aged 30–49 consult their general practitioner for menorrhagia in one year. Menorrhagia is the main presenting complaint in women referred to gynaecologists and accounts for two-thirds of all hysterectomies, and nearly all endoscopic endometrial destructive surgery.

When it comes to hospital referral, menstrual disorders are the second most common cause of all referrals for all ages and both sexes. Menorrhagia is the main presenting complaint in women referred to gynaecologists and is a common indication for surgery. Management has changed with the use of new therapeutic options. In the mid-1980s therapeutic endoscopic endometrial destructive operations and in 1995 the levonorgestrel-releasing intrauterine device were introduced in the UK. In 1988 in NHS hospitals in England 78 043 hysterectomies and 649 endometrial destructive operations were performed. In 2000/01 there was a reduction in the number of hysterectomies (47 052) and an increase in endometrial destructive techniques (17 298).

An inverse social gradient in hysterectomy has been observed in several studies. Hysterectomies for menstrual bleeding have been shown to be inversely related to social class and education and have become more common at younger ages. It has recently been shown that the social differentials in hysterectomy are greater at younger rather than older ages, which may reflect different indications for surgery (Marshall *et al.* 2000).

The importance of menorrhagia led the Royal College of Obstetricians and Gynaecologists to publish two guidelines in 1998 and 1999 on its management in both primary and secondary care. However, uptake of the recommendations in primary care has not been uniform throughout the UK and substantial differences in management still exist between practices when investigating and prescribing for menorrhagia (Grant *et al.* 2000; Turner *et al.* 2000).

## Menstrual complaints

At any one time women might complain that their periods are: too short; too long; too frequent; too infrequent; too light; too heavy; too painful; too irregular; too early (menarche); too late (menarche); too early (menopause); too late (menopause); or too awful!

This is excluding the complaint that it is unfair that they should have them at all and men are remarkably lucky.

Menstruation has had magical and mythical connotations since ancient times. In many prehistoric cultures and up to the Middle Ages, the uterus was considered as a separate creature with autonomous rights. It was regarded by some as a type of wild beast roaming through the woman's body and endangering her life. Pliny noted that while menstrual blood cured epilepsy, gout, malaria and boils, it also caused iron to rust and copper to turn green. Menstruation has been considered to be a taboo subject. The word 'tabu' comes from the Polynesian where it means menstruation as well as things that are both sacred and unclean. In various cultures, women have been prohibited from preparing food, tending plants and having any contact with men; and have been banished to menstrual huts. In our own society, mothers may still tell their daughters not to bath, wash their hair or undertake physical exercise during menstruation. These attitudes have no doubt contributed to the relatively recent development of effective sanitary protection, with commercial tampons only being introduced in the 1920s.

As a result of these myths, it is not surprising that it can be difficult for women to distinguish between normal and abnormal menstruation. The purpose of this chapter is to try and suggest which symptomatology, as usually presented to the general practitioner, might indicate the need for further appropriate investigation and treatment either at a primary care level or by the specialist.

It is probably best when discussing menstrual disorders with patients to use simple descriptive English terms such as heavy or painful periods rather than take refuge behind school-boy classical Greek. For instance polymenometrorrhagia literally means frequent month womb rushing out rather than frequent heavy irregular periods.

This chapter first discusses the normal menstrual cycle and then its problems, whether excessive, painful or absent.

## The normal menstrual cycle

### Endocrine changes

The sequence of hormone events occurring in the menstrual cycle during which ovulation takes place is shown in Fig 1.1. At menstruation, plasma levels of the anterior pituitary hormone, follicle-stimulating hormone (FSH), are already rising, stimulating the growth of several Graafian follicles within the ovary. In general, the end result of this follicular development is (usually) one mature follicle and ovum. The developing follicle produces increasing amounts of oestrogens, notably oestradiol. As levels of oestradiol begin to rise early in the follicular phase of the cycle, production of FSH is suppressed

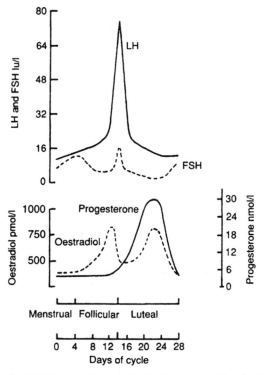

**Fig 1.1** Hormone changes during the menstrual cycle, showing fluctuating levels of the pituitary hormones, luteinizing hormone (LH) and follicle-stimulating hormone (FSH), and of the ovarian hormones, oestradiol and progesterone.

by negative feedback but oestradiol levels continue to increase over the next few days until a critical level is reached. Here, by positive feedback it triggers the anterior pituitary to release about 24 hours later a surge of luteinizing hormone (LH) with levels up to 50 IU/l and to a lesser extent FSH with levels up to 15 IU/l; such levels only occur for one day. Ovulation follows the onset of the LH surge within about 34–36 hours and the ruptured ovarian follicle develops into the corpus luteum which secretes both oestradiol and progesterone in the second half or luteal phase of the cycle. Levels of both oestradiol and progesterone therefore rise after ovulation, reaching peak levels between days 18 and 22 of a 28-day cycle. In the last few days of the cycle, if pregnancy has not occurred, the corpus luteum degenerates and oestradiol and progesterone levels fall before menstruation ensues. Plasma levels of progesterone can be measured to assess ovulation and levels greater than 16 nmol/l on days 18–22 are indicatory. The time period from the LH surge to menses is consistently close to 14 days but may vary normally from 12 to 17 days. However, variability in cycle length among women is principally due to varying number of days required for follicular growth and development in the follicular phase. Menstrual bleeding can occur both in ovulatory and anovulatory cycles. In the latter the ovary produces enough oestrogen to stimulate endometrial growth and bleeding occurs when oestrogen levels fall. Bleeding in anovulatory cycles tends to be irregular, painless and heavy. In the past decade it has been found that ovarian follicles also produce peptide hormones such as inhibin and activin, which inhibit and stimulate FSH production, respectively. While these peptides are not measured routinely, they may be in specialized centres.

## Endometrial events

The process of menstruation is poorly understood and it is not really known why women should bleed at all since it does not seem to fulfil any biological function. It only occurs in a restricted number of species: humans and most subhuman primates. Consequently, scientific understanding of the physiological mechanisms involved in the process of menstruation is based on animal as well as human data. Endometrium undergoes growth, degeneration and regression prior to menstruation and bleeding occurs from endometrial blood vessels, especially spiral arterioles. In most species that menstruate, endometrial arterioles are unusual in that they are profusely coiled as they run through the endometrium and also change throughout the menstrual cycle. Endometrial vessels have the unique property of undergoing benign angiogenesis (growth) during each menstrual cycle; otherwise this process is restricted to neoplasia and tissue injury. While this process is clearly under the control of ovarian steroids, endometrial endothelium lacks steroid receptors. These are present on endometrial epithelium and stromal cells, which produce angiogenic polypeptides, which then act on the endothelium. These arterioles undergo profound vasoconstriction which starts 4–24 hours before menstruation and lasts until the end of menstrual bleeding. Bleeding results from relaxation of individual blood vessels and then ceases as they constrict. If constriction did not occur, it could not unreasonably be expected that women would bleed to death at the menarche.

Another phenomenon that occurs during menstruation is myometrial contraction. The myometrium contracts throughout the menstrual cycle and there is increased activity during menstruation especially in women with primary dysmenorrhoea.

Of the pathways thought to play a major role in abnormal menstruation, the evidence for altered eicosanoid biosynthesis is compelling. Prostaglandins have the capacity to affect both haemostasis and myometrial contractility. Very high levels of prostaglandins are found in uterine tissues and menstrual blood. Prostaglandin levels are further increased in women with menorrhagia and dysmenorrhoea and clinically inhibitors of prostaglandin biosynthesis are effective in these disorders. In menorrhagia there is also additional evidence of an altered responsiveness to the vasodilator prostaglandin E2. Increased concentrations of prostaglandin E2 receptors are present in myometrium collected from women with excessive bleeding. In dysmenorrhoea the leukotriene pathway allied to prostaglandins has also been implicated in that higher levels of leukotrienes are present in endometrium of dysmenorrhoeic women. Finally, increased endometrial fibrinolysis has been implicated in menorrhagia leading to the use of antifibrinolytic agents.

## Variation in menstrual blood loss

The amount of blood loss at each menstruation has been measured in several population studies. In several hundred women not complaining of any menstrual problems, objective measurement of menstrual blood loss (MBL) shows a skewed distribution with the mean of about 35 ml and the 90th percentile of 80 ml. MBL is considered excessive if greater than 80 ml: without treatment, such a loss leads to iron deficiency anaemia and constitutes objective menorrhagia (Fig 1.2). Blood losses up to 1600 ml have been measured in some women. Despite variation in the total amount of blood lost, 90% is lost within the first 3 days, fitting in with patients' description of a tap being turned on and off.

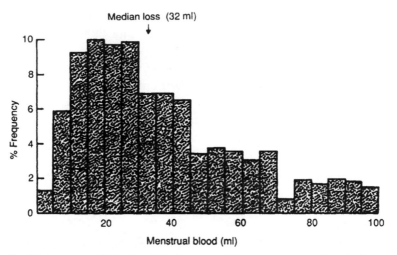

**Fig 1.2** Frequency distribution (%) of menstrual blood loss in several hundred women in Oxford before insertion of a intrauterine device. Mean menstrual loss is 33 ml; median loss is 32 ml. (From unpublished data of J Guillebaud, with permission).

## Variation in cycle length and duration of menstruation

Cyclical vaginal bleeding is known to occur at well defined intervals from the menarche to the menopause. Since ancient times it was shown that the length of the menstrual cycle, i.e. from day 1 of one period to day 1 of the next, approximated to the phases of the moon. The Greek 'men' means month. Women in many cultures refer to their periods as the moon and some women believe they are actually caused by the moon! Not surprisingly, the 28-day cycle has become the symbol of health and normality in relation to reproductive function and women begin to worry that something is wrong if their menstrual cycle deviates from this 28-day 'norm'. Furthermore, medications to induce artificial cycles, such as the oral contraceptive and hormone replacement, are also generally geared to producing 28-day 'ideal' cycles. It therefore leads to women seeking medical treatment to regulate periods if cycles become either short or long.

It is important that women should be informed that there is a large degree of variability in cycle length that is compatible with good health. Variability in cycle length was best evaluated in the classical study of Vollman (1977). The famous 28-day cycle happens to be the commonest cycle length recorded (Fig 1.3), but only just, and then in only 12.4% of cycles documented. Cycle length changes with age, forming a U-shaped curve from the menarche to the menopause. Mean cycle length drops from 35 days at age 12 to a minimum of 27 days at age 43, rising to 52 days at age 55 years with an enormous range of cycle length.

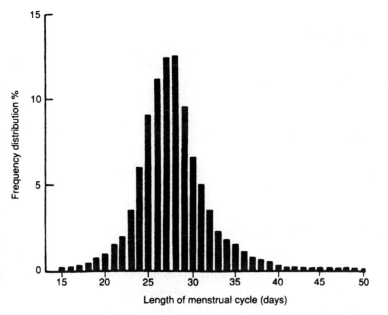

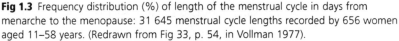

**Fig 1.3** Frequency distribution (%) of length of the menstrual cycle in days from menarche to the menopause: 31 645 menstrual cycle lengths recorded by 656 women aged 11–58 years. (Redrawn from Fig 33, p. 54, in Vollman 1977).

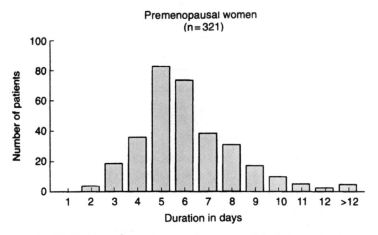

**Fig 1.4** Duration of menstruation. (Rees, unpublished observations).

Clearly, there is a wide variation in normal cycle length, especially in the first few years after the menarche and in the years preceding the menopause. It is important that normal biological variation be recognized by both women and their doctors so that they do not become obsessed by the 28-day 'ideal'.

Similarly, there are also misconceptions about duration of menstruation. In a series of 321 women in Oxford, average duration of menstruation was found to be 5–6 days (Fig 1.4, from Rees, unpublished observations). Furthermore, there was no difference in duration of menstruation between women with normal blood loss and objective menorrhagia.

## The abnormal menstrual cycle

In this chapter menstrual cycle problems, ways of dealing with them in general practice and indications for referral are presented.

### Menorrhagia (heavy blood loss)

Menorrhagia comes from the Greek 'men', month, and 'rhegynai', to rush out. It is a complaint of heavy cyclical menstrual blood loss over several consecutive cycles without any intermenstrual or postcoital bleeding. In objective terms it is a blood loss greater than 80 ml per period. Whilst various pathologies have been implicated in menorrhagia, in 50% of cases of objective menorrhagia no pathology is found at hysterectomy. Although 'unexplained' menorrhagia is a very appropriate term, this state is often labelled less clearly as dysfunctional uterine bleeding which implies endocrine abnormalities. It must be emphasized that most cases of menorrhagia are associated with regular ovulatory cycles and anovular cycles tend mainly to occur soon after the menarche or close to the menopause. In ovulatory cycles, excessive menstrual loss has been ascribed to abnormal uterine levels of prostaglandins with increased concentrations of receptors to the vasodilator prostaglandin E, and elevated levels of the fibrinolytic enzyme plasminogen activator.

### Assessment of menstrual blood loss

A common presentation of a patient with menorrhagia is a complaint of increased menstrual loss requiring more sanitary protection or the passage of clots and flooding. While soaking of bed sheets and staining of clothes is suggestive of a heavy period, women find it very difficult to assess accurately the amount of blood loss. Thus some women who are losing several hundred millilitres consider their flow to be normal while others losing only a few millilitres complain bitterly of menorrhagia. Furthermore, numbers of pads and tampons as well as degree of staining, parameters often used by doctors, do not give reliable estimates. Women with true menorrhagia may not necessarily have a drop in their haemoglobin concentration; losses of 800–1000 ml can occur without anaemia. Conversely, the presence of a hypochromic microcytic anaemia in a woman who menstruates should alert the general practitioner to the possibility that she might have menorrhagia. At present it has been estimated in hospital practice that only 40% of women complaining of menorrhagia have measured losses greater than 80 ml.

Although not available routinely, objective measurement of menstrual blood loss is a valuable investigation in the assessment of heavy periods. Menstrual blood loss can be easily measured using the non-invasive alkaline haematin method, where sanitary devices are soaked in 5% sodium hydroxide to convert the blood to alkaline haematin whose optical density is then measured. In order to get a semiquantitative measurement of the MBL, better suited to general practice or non-research gynaecological out-patient settings, a pictorial blood loss assessment chart (PBAC) was developed. However, the results of studies correlating PBAC scores and menstrual blood loss are conflicting (Reid *et al.* 2000).

## Causes of menorrhagia

A diagnosis of unexplained menorrhagia depends on exclusion of pathology. Menorrhagia may be due to systemic or pelvic pathology, or iatrogenic causes. However, this widespread view perpetrated by many gynaecological textbooks is based on clinical impression without essential objective menstrual blood loss measurement. Disorders of haemostasis such as von Willebrand's disease and deficiencies of factors V, VII, X, and XI and idiopathic thrombocytopenic purpura are thought to increase menstrual loss, but blood loss has only rarely been measured. In two studies where it was measured, menorrhagia since menarche was noted in a higher proportion of women with von Willebrand's disease and factor XI deficiency than those without a bleeding disorder.

With regard to pelvic pathology, fibroids (leiomyomas), endometriosis, pelvic inflammatory disease, and endometrial polyps are thought to cause menorrhagia. Again, there is a paucity of data with objective MBL measurement. The few studies where it has been measured show that these lesions are associated with objective menorrhagia in only about half to two-thirds of cases. While iatrogenic causes such as intrauterine contraceptive devices have been shown objectively to increase menstrual blood loss, there are no such data for anticoagulants. Women who have undergone tubal sterilization are no more likely than other women to have menstrual abnormalities (Peterson *et al.* 2000).

# 10-Minute consultation on menorrhagia

The patient, aged 32, has two children and her periods have become increasingly heavy. Her husband had a vasectomy a year ago.

## What should you ask?

- For how long have periods been heavy?
- Has there been any change?
- Is there flooding or passage of clots?
- How long do periods last and how often do they occur?
- Is there any intermenstrual bleeding or postcoital bleeding?
- Is there pelvic pain or dyspareunia?
- What contraception is being used?
- Are cervical smears up to date?

## What should you do?

- Arrange pelvic examination and cervical smear if due
- Check full blood count
- If menstruation regular with no abnormal bleeding and examination normal and no need for hormonal contraception, prescribe either mefenamic acid or tranexamic acid for 3 months and oral iron if anaemic and arrange follow-up appointment
- The above can also be prescribed for women using a non-hormonal intrauterine contraceptive device
- If hormonal contraception is required, consider the combined oral contraceptive pill, depot progestogens or the levonorgestrel-releasing intrauterine contraceptive device
- If irregular or intermenstrual/postcoital bleeding, or uterus greater than 10 week size, refer.

## Frequently asked questions

- Why have I got heavy periods?
- Do I have cancer?
- How do the tablets work?
- When do I need to take them?
- What are the side effects of the tablets?
- How long do I need to take them for?
- Do I need a hysterectomy?
- How good is the gynaecologist you are sending me to?
- What are the risks of surgery?

History-taking and general physical and pelvic examination should allow the general practitioner to reach a diagnosis and decide whether hospital referral is necessary. The length and interval of periods and duration of excessive bleeding as well as any intermenstrual or postcoital bleeding should be ascertained. The method of contraception should also be noted since intrauterine contraceptive devices are associated with increased menstrual blood loss. General examination, including bimanual and pelvic examination, should be performed. A cervical smear should be obtained if it is due. A particular search should be made for polyps protruding through the cervical os and for enlargement or tenderness of the uterus or adnexae.

## Investigations

A routine full blood count should be performed to check for anaemia in all women complaining of menorrhagia, since it is a common cause for anaemia. However, not all women with objective menorrhagia are anaemic. Ferritin is not recommended as a routine test in women complaining of menorrhagia. Testing for bleeding disorders should only be undertaken if clinically indicated, e.g. menorrhagia since the menarche and a history of bleeding after dental extractions and childbirth. Thyroid function tests should only be undertaken if clinically indicated. No other endocrine investigations are warranted.

The next step is to decide whether endometrial assessment is required. The incidence of endometrial hyperplasia and carcinoma is low under the age of 40 and increases significantly thereafter. However, there is insufficient evidence to perform an endometrial biopsy in everyone over the age of 40 complaining of menorrhagia, and it is controversial whether one should have an arbitrary age cut-off. Rather, the risk factors for endometrial neoplasia should be ascertained in all women. Thus if the bleeding is severe, does not respond to treatment, or is associated with intermenstrual bleeding and the woman is at increased risk of endometrial cancer (polycystic ovary syndrome, obesity, tamoxifen), endometrial assessment needs to be considered. However, in women with regular periods and no risk factors, a trial of a prostaglandin synthetase inhibitor or an antifibrinolytic agent could be used first since blood loss reduction tends not to occur in the presence of pathology.

The reasons for referral can therefore be for management of pelvic pathology, endometrial assessment or help with clinical findings if these are uncertain.

## Methods of endometrial assessment

The main methods of assessment are vaginal ultrasound, endometrial biopsy, and hysteroscopy. Women with menorrhagia who have not responded to initial medical management, whatever their age, are more likely to have intrauterine pathology such as endometrial polyps and submucosal fibroids.

Further investigation to assess the uterine cavity is needed and this may be performed using transvaginal ultrasound (TVS) and/or hysteroscopy. Whether transvaginal ultrasound or hysteroscopy are used in a particular hospital depends on the facilities available. A 'one-stop' menstrual problem clinic using out-patient hysteroscopy and transvaginal ultrasound within secondary care has been described. The cost-effectiveness of this approach still needs to be evaluated. The RCOG guidelines state that where possible, TVS should be used as an initial investigation, in order to select out the women with a normal cavity that do not need hysteroscopy. TVS can rule out any coexisting ovarian pathology.

### Transvaginal ultrasound

A thickened endometrium or a cavity filled with fluid is suggestive of malignancy or other pathology (hyperplasia, polyps). An endometrial thickness of 10–12 mm should be used as the cut-off point for endometrial hyperplasia and carcinoma on a TVS. Ideally, it should be performed after menstruation in the follicular phase of the menstrual cycle. Ultrasound can sometimes miss small polyps, particularly when performed in the late secretory phase when the endometrium is thicker. Detection of endometrial polyps can be enhanced by instillation of contrast medium into the uterine cavity. It is debated whether vaginal ultrasound can replace endometrial biopsy. However, it must be remembered that ultrasound does not give a histological diagnosis and cannot replace biopsy, but it is a useful adjunct.

### Endometrial biopsy

**Dilation and curettage**   The classic method of obtaining endometrium is by D&C. This technique was first described by Recamier in 1843; he described the use of a small scoop attached to a long handle for removing intrauterine fungal growths and called this method curettage. This instrument was controversial until antiseptics were available. Recamier reported three deaths from its use as a result of perforation and subsequent peritonitis. D&C is being increasingly replaced by out-patient procedures that avoid general anaesthesia and are also less costly. D&C is not without risk. Complications include perforation, haemorrhage, cervical laceration and even death. Despite having been considered a 'gold standard', D&C does not sample the whole of the endometrium. A study where curettage was performed pre-hysterectomy found that in 60% less than a half of the cavity was curetted and in 16% less than one-quarter. Since D&C is essentially a blind procedure, it can miss lesions such as polyps, submucous fibroids, hyperplasia and carcinoma.

For many years D&C has erroneously been considered to be a therapeutic as well as a diagnostic procedure. The reason is that traditionally follow-up after any gynaecological procedure is at 6 weeks when most women will have only had one postoperative period. Objective menstrual blood loss measurement has shown that whilst the first period after D&C is lighter than previous ones, subsequent ones are no different.

*Aspiration curettage*   Vacuum or aspiration curettage was introduced in 1970. The first instrument was a 3 mm diameter stainless steel cannula with a curved tip and a wide slit on the concave surface attached to a plastic aspiration chamber and a vacuum (Vabra). Since then, various types have been used with a plastic cannula (Rockett), which has either a 3 or 4 mm cannula. Suction can be generated either mechanically or electrically. More recently, internal piston suction devices have been devised (Pipelle, Wallach). They consist of a 3 mm plastic tube with an internal piston; its withdrawal after insertion into the uterine cavity generates suction, pulling in tissue into the cannula as it is rotated. The advantage of aspiration curettage is that it avoids general anaesthesia and has fewer complications than D&C. The technical skills required for out-patient endometrial biopsy are similar to those needed to fit an intrauterine contraceptive device and there is an argument in favour if its use in general practice after suitable training.

There have been many comparative studies of the different methods that support the use of out-patient aspiration curettage. Comparisons of Vabra, Pipelle and D&C show equal accuracy. However, a comparison of Pipelle and Vabra as measured by endometrial denudation in hysterectomy specimens showed that the Pipelle sampled significantly less of the endometrial surface than the Vabra. Conversely, Pipelle is less painful than Vabra curettage. In general, any discomfort is mild and lasts for about 10–15 seconds as the cannula is passed and the biopsy taken. Thus each tool has advantages and disadvantages.

## How to interpret endometrial biopsy reports

Proliferative and secretory changes are reported in endometrium removed from normal women. In the case of endometrial hyperplasia, the situation is more complicated because there have been several classifications over the years. The only important distinction in both prognostic and therapeutic terms is between hyperplasias that are associated with a significant risk of progressing into an endometrial adenocarcinoma and those devoid of such risk. The WHO classification has four categories:

1. simple hyperplasia;
2. complex hyperplasia;
3. simple atypical hyperplasia; and
4. complex atypical hyperplasia.

It is only hyperplasia with cytological atypia that has significant potential for malignant change. Kurman *et al.* (1985) reported that progression from hyperplasia to cancer occurred in only 1–3% of the patients with hyperplasia without atypia but occurred in 28% of those with atypical hyperplasia.

### Hysteroscopy

The hysteroscope provides direct visualization of the endometrial cavity and was introduced over a century ago. Hysteroscopy is indicated if the original TVS is abnormal. It allows the opportunity for blind or directed endometrial biopsy to be undertaken at the same time However, it has only recently been widely used. Flexible as well as rigid hysteroscopes are now available. Some women require paracervical blocks or intrauterine instillation of local anaesthetic for pain relief. It can be undertaken as an out-patient or in-patient procedure. Even hysteroscopy is not 100% accurate and, rarely, adenocarcinomas are missed on initial evaluation.

### Previous endometrial resection/ablation and endometrial assessment

We now see an increasing number of women who have had a previous endometrial resection or ablation. Here the endometrial cavity may be partially obliterated, and assessment of the endometrium extremely problematic.

### Who the general practitioner should treat and when to refer for specialist assessment

Women with otherwise uncomplicated regular heavy periods are extremely unlikely to have endometrial cancer or hyperplasia and referral for specialist opinion in the absence of clinically detectable pathology seems unnecessary. If there are no worrying signs such as a sudden increase in loss, blood-stained vaginal discharge, intermenstrual or postcoital bleeding, the general practitioner can use medical therapy to try and reduce blood loss if this is what the woman wishes. It must be remembered that there are two sorts of treatment failures:

1. those with extremely heavy periods and
2. those with a normal loss where therapy is only effective if the patient is rendered amenorrhoeic. Some women are prepared to put up with their heavy loss if it is not too debilitating or socially inconvenient, and fear the side effects of drug therapy in the long term. Anaemia should be looked for and corrected.

Young girls with heavy periods in the years after the menarche are very unlikely indeed to have any pelvic pathology. Probably all that is required is for the general practitioner to give reassurance by explaining to the girl and her mother that this type of menstrual upset usually settles with time. It is probably part of the maturation of the hypothalamic-pituitary–ovarian axis. General practitioners should be cautious about giving young girls hormonal treatment in the early years after the menarche because of possible long-term consequences. There are a very few young girls with persistent heavy irregular periods associated with anovular cycles. In these cases sustained unopposed oestrogen levels leads to endometrial hyperplasia, which may ultimately progress in later years to carcinoma. Specialist investigation is required in these young girls to consider the need for cyclical progestogens.

## Drug therapy

First-line treatment should be medical. A wide variety of options are now available. Each year about £7 million is spent on primary care prescribing for menorrhagia in the UK; 822 000 prescriptions were issued to 345 225 women for this condition in 1993 (Coulter *et al.* 1995). Medical therapy is indicated when there is no obvious pelvic abnormality and the women wishes to retain her fertility. Since menstrual loss, in the absence of pathology, does not change markedly, treatment is long term. Thus the drug regimen chosen must be effective, have few or mild side effects and must be acceptable to the patient.

The aims of therapy are to reduce blood loss, reduce the risk of anaemia and improve quality of life. Menorrhagia is the commonest cause of iron deficiency anaemia in Western women and thus iron therapy is often indicated as well as the options discussed below. It could be argued that blood loss should be reduced to be within the normal range (i.e. less than 80 ml per period). However, women who are keen to avoid surgery may accept a higher loss if they can cope with the flow and any anaemia is controlled with iron.

It is important to assess drug therapies in terms of reduction of measured menstrual blood loss, since there is poor correlation between objective and subjective assessment of menstrual blood loss. Well designed randomized,

**Table 1.1** Non-hormonal treatments for menorrhagia

| Non-steroidal anti-inflammatory drugs | Antifibrinolytics |
|---|---|
| Mefenamic acid | Tranexamic acid |
| Meclofenamic acid | Epsilon-amino caproic acid |
| Naproxen | Ethamsylate |
| Ibuprofen | |
| Flurbiprofen | |
| Diclofenac | |

controlled trials provide the best evidence of the efficacy of any intervention, as any differences between groups can be more confidently attributed to differences in treatment.

## Treatment options

Medical treatments for menorrhagia can be divided into two main classes: non-hormonal and hormonal. The former includes non-steroidal anti-inflammatory drugs and antifibrinolytics, and the latter progestogens, oral contraceptives, hormone replacement therapy, danazol, gestrinone and GnRH analogues. Non-hormonal treatment is taken during menstruation itself and should be a first line in general practice, using either mefenamic acid or tranexamic acid; both can be used together, but there are no good studies of the effect of the combination. Referral should be considered if neither inhibitors of prostaglandin synthesis nor antifibrinolytic agents are effective after 3 months of therapy.

### Non-hormonal

**Non-steroidal anti-inflammatory drugs**    Non-steroidal anti-inflammatory drugs (NSAIDs) can be chemically classified into five main groups: salicylates (aspirin), indoleacetic acid analogues (indometacin), aryl proprionic acid derivatives (naproxen, ibuprofen), fenamates (mefenamic acid, flufenamic acid, meclofenamic acid), and coxibs (celecoxib, rofecoxib). Of the five groups, the fenamates have been the most extensively studied for the treatment of menorrhagia.

The use of NSAIDs is based on the observations showing that prostaglandin (PG) biosynthesis is altered in menorrhagia. As well as inhibiting prostaglandin synthesis, the fenamates have the unique property of also binding to prostaglandin receptors: PGE (a vasodilator) receptor concentrations are significantly higher in women with menorrhagia. Also, fenamates are thought to improve endometrial haemostasis. Mefenamic acid reduces MBL by 29% (95% CI 27.9–30.2). The range of MBL reduction is 19–47% (Coulter *et al.* 1995). Mefenamic acid is given in a dose of 1.5 g/day during menstruation. The duration of menstruation was reduced in some studies, but not others. With regard to long-term therapy, follow-up 12–15 months after commencing treatment showed that mefenamic acid continued to be effective.

Reductions in menstrual loss have also been documented for other NSAIDs such as naproxen, ibuprofen, sodium diclofenac and flurbiprofen. The percentage reduction in blood loss varied from 25 to 47% depending on the agent and dose used. It has been reported that naproxen and ibuprofen were ineffective in women with leiomyomas. In general, NSAIDs are contraindicated in women with peptic ulceration, but otherwise have few side effects if taken for only a few days each cycle.

Thus NSAIDs should be considered as a first-line treatment in essential menorrhagia since they are well tolerated and suitable for long-term treatment. They are also effective in women with a copper or non-hormonal intrauterine contraceptive device. An added factor is that these drugs will also alleviate menstrual pain.

*Antifibrinolytics*   The use of antifibrinolytic agents is based on the observation of increased levels of fibrinolytic activity in endometrium in women with menorrhagia. Tranexamic acid reduces MBL by 46.7% (95% CI 45–46.7). The range of MBL reduction is 35–56% (Coulter *et al.* 1995). The recommended dose is 3 g/day.

Thus antifibrinolytics should be considered as a first-line treatment for menorrhagia. Symptoms of dysmenorrhoea were improved in some studies but not in others. Duration of menstruation is not reduced. Tranexamic acid is also effective in women with a copper or non-hormonal intrauterine contraceptive device. Side effects experienced during treatment are: nausea, vomiting, diarrhoea, headache, dizziness, weight gain and leg cramps in up to 60–80% of women taking this medication.

Serious side effects were originally suggested, including cerebral sinus thrombosis and central venous stasis retinopathy. However, over a 19-year time span and 238 000 woman-years of treatment with tranexamic acid from the late 1960s, no increase of thrombotic events over and above that of the general population of the same age was observed in Scandinavia.

*Ethamsylate*   Ethamsylate is thought to act by reducing capillary fragility, though the precise mechanisms are uncertain. Studies with objective MBL measurement using the currently recommended doses show that it is ineffective.

### Hormonal treatments
*Progestogens*   The use of progestogens is based on the concept that women with menorrhagia principally have anovulatory cycles and that a progestogen supplement is required. However, many studies have shown that most women with regular excessive menstrual bleeding have normal ovulatory cycles. Progestogens are the commonest prescription for women complaining of menorrhagia. The first report of its use was in 1960 in a study where menstrual blood loss was not measured, and the conclusions based on a subjective response. However, studies where MBL has been measured with luteal phase administration for 7 days of norethisterone 5 mg twice daily show either a decrease or even an increase in flow. Thus with current evidence the short-term use of norethisterone for ovulatory menorrhagia (i.e. regular heavy menstruation) cannot be justified. However, norethisterone 5 mg three times daily from

**Table 1.2** Hormonal treatments for menorrhagia

| | |
|---|---|
| Progestogens | Norethisterone |
| | Medroxyprogesterone acetate |
| | Dydrogesterone |
| Intrauterine progestogens | Levonorgestrel IUCD |
| | Progestasert IUCD |
| Combined oestrogen/progestogens | Oral contraceptives |
| | Hormone replacement therapy |
| Other | Danazol |
| | Gestrinone |
| | GnRH analogues |

day 5 to day 26 is effective. Oral progestogens can also be used to regularize irregular menstrual cycles, postpone periods or arrest a torrential bleed.

- *Regularizing irregular periods.* There are no good studies about the dose or duration of progestogen that should be used; but norethisterone 10 mg daily for 2–3 weeks out of 4 is usually effective.

- *How to postpone a period.* Sometimes women ask for something to postpone a period because of, for example, a special event such as wedding, an examination or a holiday. Periods can be postponed using a progestogen such as norethisterone 5 mg three times daily, starting 3 days before the anticipated period. An alternative, if given several months' warning, is to take the combined oral contraceptive pill continuously.

- *A torrential bleed.* Very large doses of progestogens such as 30 mg daily can be used to arrest a torrential bleed. This is usually effective within 24–48 hours, when the dose can be reduced and then finally stopped over the next few days when another, usually lighter, bleed will occur. Bleeding of this magnitude requires referral for specialist assessment, and may require emergency measures by the general practitioner.

Intrauterine progesterone or, more especially, levonorgestrel is much more successful than oral progestogens in reducing menstrual loss. With the levonorgestrel IUCD, reductions of MBL of 88 and 96% are found after 6 months and 12 months, respectively. The levonorgestrel IUCD also provides very effective contraception. It could now be considered to be a serious candidate as an alternative to both medical and surgical management of essential menorrhagia. Fertility is preserved and the cost is low when compared to surgery. However, it is important to emphasize the essential difference between the levonorgestrel IUCD and other IUCDS which can increase menstrual loss. Women also need to be counselled about irregular bleeding, which can occur in the first few months after insertion. The levonorgestrel IUCD can be fitted in a fibroid uterus but may be less effective or be expelled, especially if the lesions are submucous (but there is a paucity of data).

Continued use of long-acting progestogens renders most women amenorrhoeic and therefore could be considered for use in menorrhagia. Medroxyprogesterone acetate is available as a depot injection for contraception in the dosage of 150 mg administered every 3 months. It may cause unpredictable, irregular spotting and bleeding in the first few months of use and it can cause heavy bleeding in others, as well as other side effects such as weight gain and acne. However, with repeated administration, amenorrhoea becomes common and haemoglobin levels increase. Subdermal implants (e.g. Implanon®) that release etonorgestrel over several years are another way of administering long-acting progestogens for contraceptive purposes. Their efficacy needs to be assessed.

**Oestrogen/progestogen**   Combined oral contraceptive (COC) pills are often used clinically to reduce MBL. Their mode of action is unclear, and probably involves induction of endometrial atrophy. It seems clear that combined oral contraceptive preparations can reduce menstrual blood loss and, consequently, increase haemoglobin concentrations and reduce iron deficiency anaemia. Many of the studies cited used a higher dose than the 30–35 μg ethinyloestradiol of preparations currently in use. It is, therefore, less clear whether low-dose preparations are as effective in reducing MBL as the higher dosage preparations, and whether the particular progestogen used makes any difference. Although there is some indication that the frequency of menstrual disturbances, such as spotting and breakthrough bleeding, is less when the COC contains a relatively high dose of progestogen, no evidence is available to suggest that changing the progestogen influenced total MBL.

Monthly cyclical oestrogen/progestogen hormone replacement therapy is also used to treat menorrhagia in perimenopausal women. Although clinically it seems to work, there has been to date no randomized controlled trials. However, open studies of three preparations show that their measured withdrawal bleeds are not heavier than normal periods. Data on 3-monthly bleed regimens are awaited.

**Danazol**   Danazol is an isoxazol derivative of 17α-ethinyl-testosterone, which acts on the hypothalamic–pituitary–ovarian axis as well as on the endometrium to produce atrophy. Studies have shown MBL reductions ranging from 22 to 99%, which are directly related to dose and duration of treatment. However, the clinical use of danazol is limited by its androgenic side effects which include weight gain and skin rashes. The use of danazol is probably best restricted to women awaiting surgery. Women must be advised to use barrier methods of contraception because of potential virilization of a fetus if pregnancy occurs while on treatment.

*Gestrinone*   Gestrinone is a 19-nortestosterone derivative which has antiprogestogenic, antioestrogenic and androgenic activity. In a placebo-controlled study, gestrinone was given 2.5 mg twice weekly for 12 weeks to 19 women with proven menorrhagia. Ten women became amenorrhoeic and a marked reduction in MBL was seen in five; placebo had no effect. In three of the non-responders, submucous fibroids were found at subsequent hysterectomy. The therapy was well tolerated since all women completed the trial. However, gestrinone's androgenic side effects preclude long-term therapy and barrier contraception must be used.

*GnRH analogues*   These agents can be used to reduce MBL by pituitary downregulation and subsequent inhibition of ovarian activity resulting in amenorrhoea. However, the induced hypo-oestrogenic state with its adverse effects on bone metabolism limits its use beyond 6 months. GnRH analogues again should be considered as short-term treatment, perhaps while awaiting surgery or the natural menopause. When cyclical oestrogen/progestogen hormone replacement therapy has been used in conjunction with GnRH analogues, median MBL after 3 months' treatment in the women with objective menorrhagia was 74 ml. This treatment combination is expensive and should not be used as a first line. Specialist advice should be sought before using such regimens. Again barrier contraception should be used as contraception is not guaranteed.

### Treatment failures

Several options have to be considered when the patient says that the treatment has failed. First, her loss may be so excessive (e.g. (200 ml) that NSAIDs or tranexamic acid are insufficient to control it). Second, she may have a pre-treatment blood loss less than 80 ml and the perceived reduction in loss on therapy is not sufficient for her. This was illustrated in a study including women with normal MBL where therapy with mefenamic acid did not reduce loss and actually increased it. Last, the patient may have unsuspected uterine pathology such as a submucous fibroid or endometrial polyp, which makes medical treatment less effective or ineffective. It is unfortunate that many studies do not follow up their treatment failures with hysteroscopy to check for such pathology.

## Surgical treatment

Surgical treatment may be necessary to deal with pelvic abnormalities such as polyps, fibroids, chronic pelvic inflammatory disease or endometriotic masses. Operations should be as conservative as possible in women who wish to retain their fertility. Referral letters need to state what the problem is and what has been discussed with the patient. Surgical treatment is also indicated when medical treatment has failed. Surgical treatment includes removal of cervical or endometrial polyps, myomectomy and, ultimately, hysterectomy. Submucous fibroids or endometrial polyps should be removed hysteroscopically. Over recent years there has been increasing use of minimally invasive surgery options using laparoscopic or hysteroscopic approaches, which have the potential of shorter hospital stay and recovery times. These techniques will be discussed in some detail so that general practitioners can explain them to their patients (*Drug and Therapeutics Bulletin* 2000).

## Hysterectomy

Hysterectomy is offered more often to younger women whose families are complete because many are reluctant to take treatment for several years until the menopause. Although 100% effective, hysterectomy is accompanied by significant morbidity (pyrexia, haemorrhage, infection) but fortunately a low mortality rate. The perioperative mortality rate is 1 in 2000 in women under 50 years undergoing hysterectomy for non-malignant conditions. Short-term morbidity is high with complication rates of 25% for vaginal and 43% for abdominal hysterectomy. Febrile morbidity accounts for the majority of complications. Similarly, mortality for vaginal hysterectomy is half that of abdominal hysterectomy. The reason is unclear, but may reflect selection of healthier women for the vaginal operation.

Concern exists about the long-term sequelae, which may include premature onset of ovarian failure even when ovaries are conserved, psychosexual dysfunction, urinary tract and bowel symptoms. In general, hysterectomy has a beneficial effect on mental well-being. However, while some studies show increased sexual enjoyment, others show reduced libido. There is currently a vogue for subtotal hysterectomy, conserving the cervix, with the understanding that sexual function is better preserved than with total hysterectomy. The down side is that cervical smears have to be continued. Similarly, the evidence of the effects of total or subtotal hysterectomy on urinary tract and bowel function is conflicting.

## Ovaries and hysterectomy

Until relatively recently, it was naively thought that if ovaries were conserved at hysterectomy, they continued to function normally. There is conflicting evidence that ovarian function is compromised and the age of menopause is brought forward by several years. This increases the risk of developing cardio-vascular disease and osteoporosis. The diagnosis of ovarian failure is more difficult in the absence of menstrual function. It is important that women who have had a hysterectomy in their 30s are not told they are too young to be menopausal if they develop symptoms of ovarian failure a few years later, and undergo a premature menopause.

Oophorectomy is often performed prophylactically at the time of abdomi-nal hysterectomy in order to avoid the risk of ovarian cancer. Its use is highly debated in women not at risk of developing the disease, where it has been esti-mated that about 200 oophorectomies would need to be undertaken to avoid one case of ovarian cancer. Oophorectomy results in a surgical menopause with marked menopausal symptoms, and increased risk of cardiovascular disease and osteoporosis. It must be remembered that in Western societies cardiovascular disease is the major cause of death in women. Oophorectomy reduces average life expectancy in younger women by at least 5 years if they do not take oestrogen hormone replacement therapy. It is of concern that compliance with long-term hormone replacement therapy is low, with most women in the UK only taking it for a few months. Thus prophylactic oophorectomy in women at low risk of ovarian cancer cannot really be justified. In women with a family history of ovarian cancer who are considered to be at high risk, prophylactic oophorectomy is justifiable when their family is complete and after thorough counselling. It must be remembered, however, that familial ovarian cancer may be a more generalized disease in the peritoneal cavity and some doubt exists about the efficacy of oophorectomy, since cases of intra-abdominal carcinomatosis have been reported following surgery in which subsequent review of the ovarian specimen revealed a small focus of ovarian cancer.

### Laparoscopic hysterectomy

The laparoscope can be used in a variety of ways to assist in performing a hysterectomy. If the uterine vessels are defined and secured by laparoscopic techniques, the procedure is considered to be a true laparoscopic hysterectomy. If the laparoscopic portion of the operation is discontinued at any stage before the uterine vessels are secured, the procedure is described as a laparoscopically assisted vaginal hysterectomy. The uterine tissue is either removed from the abdominal cavity vaginally or through the umbilical port instruments. There is interest about retaining all or part of the cervix, or coring out the centre of the cervix including the transformation zone. Complication rates associated with laparoscopic techniques are similar to those found with standard vaginal hysterectomy approaches.

## Endometrial destructive techniques

The concept of endometrial destruction as a treatment for menorrhagia is based on the observation that destruction of the endometrium led to amenorrhoea and is called eponymously Asherman's syndrome. Because of the significant regenerative capacity of the endometrium, it is essential to destroy its basal layer for the techniques to be successful. The aim of the various methods is to remove or destroy all the endometrium and up to 3 mm thickness of myometrium. The methods employed include resection of the endometrium, or ablation of the endometrium by laser, rollerball diathermy, radiofrequency, cryoablation, microwaves and thermal balloons.

Like hysterectomy, these treatments should only be offered to women who desire no further children. Higher rates of amenorrhoea are achieved in older rather than younger women. However, although the risk of pregnancy is minimal, patients cannot be assured it is a sterilization procedure. Pregnancies, both intrauterine and ectopic, have been reported; there are also concerns about the potential risk of placenta accreta (where the placenta becomes embedded in the myometrium) in view of the altered endometrium. Some gynaecologists offer laparoscopic sterilization at the time of resection.

Many hysteroscopists recommend preoperative medical therapy to render the endometrium atrophic in order to simplify surgery and thus maximize the possibility of complete resection. The most frequently used agents are progestogens, danazol and GnRH analogues, with the last providing the most promising approach.

**Efficacy and complications**   Success of endometrial destruction has been generally measured in terms of induced amenorrhoea or significantly reduced menstrual flow. Endometrial destruction appears less likely to reduce menstrual loss in women aged 40 years or less, who have fibroids or who do not have objective menorrhagia (MBL <80 ml). In follow-up studies lasting up to 4 years, 38% women required repeat surgery. It has been suggested that endometrial destruction is not suitable where there is significant dysmenorrhoea or irregular cycles, but this has not been substantiated in clinical trials. However, premenstrual pelvic pain not related to excessive bleeding is considered to be a relative contraindication.

The most common complications are haemorrhage, perforation, need for emergency surgery and absorption of distending medium (radiofrequency induced thermal ablation, microwaves and thermal balloons do not use a distending medium). Perioperative complications occur in about 4–5% of women and mortality is 2–3 per 10 000. There is no difference in terms of perforation between the most widely used techniques (0.7–2.5% with combined resection and rollerball, resection alone or laser ablation). Whether endometrial destruction hinders the diagnosis of endometrial cancer is unknown. However, the need for emergency surgery is greater for resection alone (2.4%) when compared to the resection and rollerball (1.4%) or laser ablation (0.3%).

### Comparison of endometrial destruction with hysterectomy

Endometrial destruction cannot really be considered to replace hysterectomy since it does not render all women amenorrhoeic or sterile, but it can be considered as an alternative strategy. Furthermore, when hormone replacement therapy is given after endometrial destruction, the oestrogen must be opposed with progestogen to prevent development of hyperplasia and carcinoma in any remaining endometrium. Operating time, hospital stay, return to daily activities and work were shorter after destruction than after hysterectomy. On average, women return to work sooner following endometrial destruction (2–3 weeks) than following hysterectomy (6–12 weeks). While patient satisfaction is high after both approaches, it is higher after hysterectomy. Initially, endometrial resection appears to be less costly than hysterectomy; however, this advantage decreases with longer follow-up because of the need for repeat surgery. Further costs may not fall with increased use of endometrial destruction since availability of these techniques may mean that the threshold for surgery is lowered.

### Counselling, information and patient preferences

It is of concern that only 40% of women complaining of menorrhagia actually have objective menorrhagia. Thus the majority of women could be considered to have inappropriate treatment, and counselling would be a better option in these cases. A study of 17 women referred for hospital treatment for menorrhagia, in whom blood loss was less than 80 ml, showed that counselling is effective (Rees 1991). A 3-year follow-up of these women showed only one woman had opted for hysterectomy, two had taken drug therapy and the remainder had accepted the advice. The effectiveness of giving information and incorporating patient preferences into decision-making has recently been evaluated in a randomized controlled trial in 900 women in the UK. It significantly reduces the hysterectomy rate (Kennedy *et al.* 2002).

## Treatment of fibroids

Uterine fibroids are tumours that arise in the myometrium. They are the commonest form of pathology found in women, being present in about 30% women over the age of 35. They are composed predominantly of smooth muscle with a variable amount of connective tissue. Three subtypes are recognized, depending on their situation in relation to the uterine wall, namely submucous, subserous and intramural. Submucous fibroids are often implicated in menorrhagia, while those in other sites may be innocent bystanders. The proportion associated with objective menorrhagia is not well documented. They are commonly multiple and may result in considerable uterine enlargement. Fibroids are frequently asymptomatic, but may present with menorrhagia, pelvic pain or pressure symptoms.

Fibroids are thought to be oestrogen dependent since they do not occur prior to puberty and become smaller after the menopause. It is currently believed that oestrogen exerts an effect on fibroid growth, by the stimulation of growth factors.

Uterine fibroids are usually diagnosed clinically but they may be difficult to differentiate from ovarian masses. Ultrasound is useful in this situation, but again there may be difficulty in distinguishing between pedunculated subserous fibroids and solid ovarian tumours. If any doubt remains, patients need referral, and laparoscopy or laparotomy may be considered.

The management of women with uterine fibroids depends on size, associated symptoms, as well as her age and reproductive wishes. Small asymptomatic fibroids rarely require treatment but need to be monitored regularly, say with annual ultrasound because of concern with sarcomatous changes in fibroids, although this is very low (less than 0.2%). Women with fibroids and menorrhagia are usually treated by hysterectomy. For those wishing to conserve their fertility, myomectomy may be offered. Endoscopic techniques allow removal of subserous and intramural fibroids by laparoscopy and submucous fibroids by hysteroscopy, and thus avoid laparotomy. Local destruction by techniques such as laser or electrocoagulation are currently being evaluated.

There is considerable demand for an alternative to surgery in the management of fibroids. Prostaglandin synthetase inhibitors are probably of limited effect in reducing heavy menstrual bleeding. The 19-norsteroids danazol and gestrinone may be effective and may indeed shrink uterine volume. A therapeutic innovation is the use of GnRH analogues to induce a temporary and reversible menopausal state. These analogues produce amenorrhoea and fibroid shrinkage. Unfortunately, shrinkage is rarely complete and not sustained after cessation of therapy. Another concern is the bone mineral loss associated with a prolonged hypo-oestrogenic state, limiting the use of analogues to 6 months. GnRH analogues are especially useful prior to hysterectomy, making the operation technically easier and reducing operative blood loss. The combination of the GnRH analogue goserelin and endometrial resection as an alternative to hysterectomy for fibroids is extremely encouraging (Rees *et al.* 2001).

Uterine embolization involves interruption of the uterine blood supply. The technique involves selectively cannulating both uterine arteries and embolizing them, usually with polyvinyl alcohol particles, to the point of complete or near-total occlusion. No attempt is made to only embolize the fibroids as opposed to the remainder of the uterus. Following the procedure, pain and discharge (sometimes fragments of fibroids may be passed) are common. The most significant complication is infection and some deaths have been reported. Data are limited and protocols need to be established and randomized controlled trials undertaken. Myoma coagulation or myolysis by way of the laparoscope or hysteroscope is another addition to the armamentarium of treatments for fibroids which again needs evaluation (Goldfarb 2000).

## Dysmenorrhoea

Derived from the Greek meaning difficult monthly flow, the word dysmenorrhoea has come to mean painful menstruation. Dysmenorrhoea can be classified as either primary or secondary. In the former type, there is no pelvic pathology while the latter implies underlying pathology which leads to painful menstruation.

### Primary dysmenorrhoea

In general, primary dysmenorrhoea appears 6–12 months after the menarche when ovulatory cycles have become established. The early cycles after the menarche are usually anovular and tend to be painless. The pain usually consists of lower abdominal cramps and backache and there may be associated gastrointestinal disturbances such as diarrhoea and vomiting. Symptoms occur predominantly during the first 2 days of menstruation. Primary dysmenorrhoea tends not to be associated with excessive menstrual bleeding; it is rare for women to have both dysmenorrhoea and menorrhagia.

Primary dysmenorrhoea is associated with uterine hypercontractility characterized by excessive amplitude and frequency of contractions and a high 'resting' tone between contractions. During contractions endometrial blood flow is reduced and there seems to be a good correlation between minimal blood flow and maximal colicky pain, favouring the concept that ischaemia due to hypercontractility causes primary dysmenorrhoea.

It is now generally agreed that the myometrial hypercontractility pattern found in primary dysmenorrhoea is associated with increased prostaglandin production. More recently, elevated levels of leukotriene C4, D4, and E4 (substances allied to prostaglandins) have been found in endometrium collected from dysmenorrhoeic women. Increased vasopressin levels have also been implicated.

Although excessive levels of prostaglandins, leukotrienes, and vasopressin have been found in primary dysmenorrhoea, the primary stimulus for their production remains unknown.

## Secondary dysmenorrhoea

Secondary dysmenorrhoea is associated with pelvic pathology such as endometriosis, adenomyosis, pelvic inflammatory disease, submucous leiomyomas and endometrial polyps. The use of a non-hormonal intrauterine contraceptive device may also lead to dysmenorrhoea. Secondary dysmenorrhoea tends to appear several years after the menarche and the patient may complain of a change in the intensity and timing of her pain. The pain may last for the whole of the menstrual period and may be associated with discomfort before the onset of menstruation. The mechanism by which various pathologies cause pain is uncertain and again prostaglandins may be involved, though the evidence is less clear.

## Assessment: 10-minute consultation

The 20-year-old patient has increasingly painful periods, not improving with paracetamol, which used to work. Her partner is using condoms.

### What should you ask?
- For how long have periods been painful?
- Has there been any change?
- When does the pain occur?
- Is there pelvic pain at other times or dyspareunia?
- Is there flooding or passage of clots?
- How long do periods last and how often do they occur?
- Is there any intermenstrual bleeding or postcoital bleeding?
- Is there a history of infertility or pelvic inflammatory disease?
- What contraception is being used?
- Are cervical smears up to date?

### What should you do?
- Arrange pelvic examination if required and cervical smear if due.
- If history is suggestive of primary dysmenorrhoea, menstruation is regular with no abnormal bleeding, and examination normal with no need for hormonal contraception, prescribe either ibuprofen or mefenamic acid for 3 months and arrange follow-up appointment.

- If hormonal contraception is required, consider the combined oral contraceptive pill or depot progestogens.
- If history is suggestive of secondary dysmenorrhoea, menstruation is irregular, or there is intermenstrual/postcoital bleeding, or pelvic examination abnormal, refer.

### Frequently asked questions

- Why are my periods painful?
- What are you going to give me?
- What are the side effects?
- Do I need any tests?
- Does it mean I can't have children?

A full gynaecological history is an essential part of the investigation. The onset of dysmenorrhoea and its relation to menstruation usually differentiate between primary and secondary dysmenorrhoea. The presence of an intrauterine contraceptive device or a history of infertility should also be noted. In young girls one can usually assume a diagnosis of primary dysmenorrhoea and it is probably unnecessary to examine them. If the history is suggestive of secondary dysmenorrhoea, a bimanual pelvic and speculum examination should be performed. A particular search should be made for polyps protruding through the cervical os and for enlargement, tenderness or fixity of the uterus or adnexae.

Referral to a gynaecologist may be necessary if pathology is suspected and the investigations may include ultrasound, MRI scans, hysteroscopy and laparoscopy.

### Treatment

The clear involvement of prostaglandins in primary dysmenorrhoea has led to the use of prostaglandin synthetase inhibitors such as mefenamic acid, naproxen, ibuprofen and aspirin to treat the disorder. Meta-analysis shows that they are all effective and that ibuprofen is the preferred analgesic because of its favourable efficacy and safety profiles (Zhang *et al.* 1998). Commencing treatment before the onset of menstruation appears to have no demonstrable advantage over starting treatment when bleeding starts. This observation is compatible with the short plasma half-life of prostaglandin synthetase inhibitors. The advantage of starting treatment at the onset of menstruation is that it prevents the patient treating herself when she is unknowingly pregnant, which would only become apparent when a period is missed. Cyclo-oxygenase is the major enzyme in the prostaglandin synthetic pathway. It exists in at least two isoforms, COX-1 that is constitutive and COX-2 that is inducible. Highly selective COX-2 inhibitors have recently been introduced and one of them, rofecixib, has now been licensed for the treatment of dysmenorrhoea (Morrison *et al.* 1999).

The presence of elevated leukotriene and vasopressin levels may explain why not all women respond to prostaglandin synthetase inhibitors. The role of the various agents that affect the leukotriene pathway has not yet been fully evaluated in the treatment of primary dysmenorrhoea. Vasopressin antagonists have been examined but are not available for routine use at present. The efficacy of an orally active vasopressin receptor antagonist has recently been reported (Brouard *et al.* 2000). Transdermal glyceryl trinitrate is being evaluated (Moya *et al.* 2000). It must not be forgotten that the combined oestrogen/progestogen oral contraceptive pill is a useful agent for the treatment of primary dysmenorrhoea, especially when contraception is required. The pill is effective in 80–90% of women and probably acts by reducing the capacity of the endometrium to produce prostaglandins.

Concern remains about the 10–20% of the patients with primary dysmenorrhoea who fail to respond either to prostaglandin synthetase inhibitors or to oral contraceptives. Some of these women may really be suffering from secondary dysmenorrhoea with pelvic pathology, requiring appropriate investigation, but the concern has led to the examination of new agents such as leukotriene and vasopressin antagonists.

Effective treatment of secondary dysmenorrhoea must be based on a correct diagnosis since different pathologies require different therapies. In addition, the type of treatment offered must take into account the patient's age, her desire for conception, the severity of the symptoms and the extent of the disease.

## Amenorrhoea (absence of menstruation) and oligomenorrhoea (infrequent menstruation)

Absence of periods disturbs women just as much as other disturbances of menstruation, especially since it has implications of loss of a normal bodily function related to fertility. While some women may be concerned about loss of femininity, others will worry about an unwanted pregnancy. It seems relatively clear that women wish to menstruate regularly, not too much or too little, but not to be without altogether. There is also the connotation that amenorrhoea for 6 months or more can increase the risk of osteoporosis and bone density should be ascertained. It is prudent to start investigations if menstruation has ceased for 6 consecutive months in a woman with previously regular periods.

**Table 1.3** Main causes of amenorrhoea

---

*Hypothalamic – pituitary disorders*

Prolactin hypersecretion ± prolactin-secreting pituitary adenoma

Tumours

Weight loss – anorexia nervosa

Obesity

Psychogenic

Post-oral contraception

Isolated gonadotrophin deficiency (Kallman's syndrome)

*Ovarian, uterine, or vaginal disorders*

Polycystic ovarian disease

Ovarian failure (premature menopause)

Gonadal dysgenesis (e.g. Turner's syndrome)

Absence of uterus (e.g. testicular feminization) or vagina

Haematocolpos

*Other diseases*

Thyroid hormone deficiency or excess

Adrenal disorders (e.g. Cushing's disease, congenital adrenal hyperplasia)

Severe general disease (e.g. leukaemia or Hodgkin's disease treated with chemotherapy)

---

Oligomenorrhoea may defined as periods occurring less frequently than every 35 days. The most common cause is polycystic ovary syndrome (PCOS).

To menstruate, women require a functioning hypothalamic–pituitary–ovarian axis with a responding endometrium and genital outflow tract in the absence of endocrine or systemic disease or drug therapy, and in the presence of a normal chromosome complement. In the vast majority of women presenting in general practice, the cause will be hormonal. There has been a preoccupation in the past in distinguishing between primary and secondary amenorrhoea, but this should probably be defused since there is so much overlap between the two. Most causes of secondary amenorrhoea can also cause primary amenorrhoea if they occur before the menarche. Instead, the differential diagnoses should be based on the pathological categories (Table 1.3).

### Assessment

The initial step in the work-up of the amenorrhoeic/oligomenorhoeic patient is exclusion of the possibility of pregnancy even in a woman with primary amenorrhoea. It is important that the general practitioner should warn women that they are not necessarily infertile and are at risk of pregnancy should a sporadic ovulation occur.

## History and examination

- Age at menarche
- Development of secondary sex characteristics, pubic and axillary hair, breasts, menstrual history before amenorrhoea
- Galactorrhoea
- Recent change in body height and weight; and level of exercise
- Medication: oral contraception, chemotherapy
- Family history of genetic anomalies
- Recent emotional upsets
- Hirsutism, balding, acne as markers of androgenization; voice changes, clitoromegaly as signs of virilization
- Hot flushes and sweats and dry vagina
- Previous surgery: curettage, oophorectomy, other endocrine organs
- Symptoms of endocrine disorders: thyroid, pituitary, adrenal
- Systemic, abdominal and pelvic examination with special attention to reproductive tract and inguinal hernias, though in young girls pelvic examination is best replaced by ultrasound: acanthosis nigricans is hyperpigmented thickening of the skin folds of the axilla and neck and is a sign of profound insulin resistence and is associated with PCOS.

## Investigation

*Endocrine* tests to determine the cause of amenorrhoea involve measurement in serum in all cases of the anterior pituitary hormones FSH and LH, as well as prolactin and thyroid function tests. If FSH and LH are elevated, they need repeating. Testosterone should be measured in women with hirsutism or where testicular feminization is suspected. Oestradiol levels are usually of little value. Prolactin levels can be elevated in a number of conditions including stress (having a blood test), a recent breast examination, hypothyroidism and PCOS. A positive response to a progestogen challenge test will distinguish women with PCOS-related prolactinaemia (since they still produce oestrogen) from those with hyperprolactinaemia and polycystic ovaries on ultrasound (since they are oestrogen deficient).

The *karyotype* should be checked if there are suspicions of a chromosomal disorder such as testicular feminization and Turner's syndrome. It is important to remember that the presence of a Y chromosome requires surgical removal

**Table 1.4** Laboratory findings in major causes of amenorrhoea

|  | FSH | LH | Prolactin | Testosterone | Karyotype |
|---|---|---|---|---|---|
| Hyperprolactinaemia | Normal | Normal | High | Normal | Normal |
| Premature menopause | Very high | High | Normal | Normal | Normal |
| Polycystic ovarian disease | Normal | Slightly raised | Normal or slightly raised | Slightly raised | Normal |
| 'Hypothalamic' | Normal | Normal | Normal | Normal | Normal |
| Turner's syndrome | High | High | Normal | Normal | 45XO or mosaics |
| Testicular feminization | High | High | Normal | High | 46XY |

of the gonadal areas because the presence of testicular components carry a 25% risk of malignant tumour formation. Even gonads of XY individuals (e.g. mosaicism of XO/XY, etc.) who lack testicular tissue should have their gonads removed since there is up to a 50% chance of gonadoblastoma formation. About 30% of patients with a Y chromosome will not develop signs of virilization. Therefore this investigation should be undertaken also in women presenting with primary amenorrhoea and normal secondary sexual characteristics where gonadotrophin levels are high (Table 1.4).

If a patient is referred for specialist opinion, the following investigations may be undertaken. In cases of hyperprolactinaemia, an MRI scan is used to evaluate the pituitary fossa. Vaginal ultrasound, which may be followed by laparoscopy and examination under anaesthetic, are used to evaluate pelvic organs. The endometrial cavity can be examined by hysteroscopy when a diagnosis of Asherman's syndrome (endometrial adhesions) is suspected. Assessment of the renal tract may be instigated since abnormalities of this system are associated with developmental defects of the reproductive organs. Bone density will need assessment since bone mass is oestrogen dependent in women.

## Specific causes of amenorrhoea

### Delayed menarche

*Age of menarche*   The menarche occurs between the ages of 10 and 16 in most girls in developed countries. The first cycles tend to be anovular and there is wide variation in cycle length, and the menstruations are usually pain free and occur without warning. By 6 years after the menarche, 80% of cycles are ovulatory, and by 12 years more than 95% are ovulatory.

There has been a secular trend to earlier menarche over the past century with a decrease of about 3–4 months per decade in industrialized countries (Europe, USA, Japan). Thus the average age of menarche in 1840 was 16.5 and now averages 13. The reasons for the fall of menarcheal age are unclear but one interpretation is that it reflects improvement in health and environmental conditions. It now appears that this trend is levelling off in many countries such as Britain, Iceland, Italy, Poland and Sweden. Indeed, there appears now to be a reversal of the fall with a gradual increase in the age of menarche in Britain since the birth cohort of 1945. However, in other countries, the fall in age is still continuing.

The age of menarche is determined by a combination of factors, which include genetic influences, socioeconomic conditions, general health and well-being, nutritional status, certain types of exercise, and family size. The importance of genetic factors is illustrated by the similar age of menarche in members of an ethnic population and in mother/daughter pairs. Similarly, twin studies have shown a closer relationship in menarcheal age in identical (3 months) than in non-identical twins (12 months). Social class differences are disappearing in many countries. It is well known that delayed menarche is a feature of chronic disease.

The role of body weight and proportion of body fat has received considerable attention. It is well known that anorexia and malnutrition are associated with delayed menarche, and both conditions can induce secondary amenorrhoea. A regular menstrual cycle will not occur if the BMI is less than 19 kg/m$^2$. Fat appears to be critical to a normally functioning hypothalamic–pituitary–gonadal axis. It is estimated that at least 22% of body weight should be fat to maintain ovulatory cycles. The candidate mediator is the hormone leptin, which is secreted by fat cells which affects GnRH pulsatility. The composition of diet in childhood can also affect menarcheal age. Girls who consume more (energy-adjusted) animal protein and less vegetable protein at ages 3–5 years have an earlier menarche. Conversely, a diet high in fibre is associated with a delayed menarche.

Intense exercise such as athletics, gymnastics and ballet is associated with a delayed menarche, and it has been suggested that each year of premenarcheal training delays menarche by 5 months. However, the mechanisms involved are not fully understood, though a more linear physique may be involved. It is thought that there is a combination of biological selection and social factors.

Family size and birth order influence age of menarche. There is a tendency to later menarche in girls from larger families and there is a tendency to precocity in girls born later in the family. Again the mechanisms are unclear. The significance of early-life exposure to environmental or hormonally active chemicals is also a growing area of debate. In a follow-up of 594 children from the North Carolina Infant Feeding Study, born between 1978 and 1982, a slight (but not statistically significant) decrease in age at sexual maturation (defined using Tanner scores based on the acquisition of secondary sexual character-istics) was noted in girls exposed to higher transplacental levels of polychlor-inated biphenyls or dichlorodiphenyl dichloroethene, whilst girls that were bottle fed showed a tendency (non-significant) to mature later (Gladen *et al.* 2000). Accidental contamination of the Michigan food chain with polybrom-inated biphenyls (PBBs) led to the exposure of more than 4000 individuals in 1973. Breast-fed girls exposed to high levels of PBB *in utero* had an earlier age at menarche (mean age = 11.6 years) than breast-fed girls exposed to lower levels of PBB *in utero* (mean age = 12.2–12.6 years) or girls who were not breast-fed (mean age = 12.7 years) (Blanck *et al.* 2000). These associations clearly need further investigation.

*How and when should the general practitioner investigate* How long should a general practitioner wait before investigating the girl who has never menstruated? Since most girls will have menstruated by the age of 16, it could be considered to be the upper age of the normal menarche. However, referral is essential earlier if secondary sex characteristics have not developed, or there appear to be anatomical disorders of the genital tract or signs of a chromosome abnormality. Rarer possibilities are androgen insensitivity syndrome, previously known as testicular feminization (maturation of breasts with absent axillary and pubic hair, absent uterus with normal or short vagina; 46XY with intra-abdominal testes) or Turner's syndrome (many variants, but with typical short stature, sexual infantilism, webbing of the neck, cubitus valgus, 45XO with streak gonads). Absent development of the lower genital tract resulting in haematocolpos is another rare cause where secondary sexual development will be normal. There may be intermittent lower abdominal pain, a lower abdominal cystic swelling (confirmed on ultrasound) and a tense blue coloured membrane may be seen at the introitus. Referral is obviously necessary for incision and drainage.

If secondary sexual development is normal or appears to be progressing satisfactorily, and there is no anatomical problem, then the likely cause is hormonal, which can elucidated with an endocrine screen.

### 'Hypothalamic' amenorrhoea

This is the commonest cause of amenorrhoea seen in general practice. Hypo-thalamic problems are usually diagnosed by exclusion of structural pituitary or hypothalamic lesions and are the most common category of hypogonadotrophic amenorrhoea. They usually present as secondary amenorrhoea. The condition normally should be investigated if the woman has been for 6 months or more without periods. Biochemically, it is found that gonadotrophins are normal or low with a normal prolactin.

The clinical picture is usually associated with weight changes, vigorous exercise, stress, and cessation of the combined oral contraceptive pill, where the induced regular bleeds have masked an ongoing problem. Since weight loss and anorexia nervosa may lead to amenorrhoea, it is important for the general practitioner to enquire about recent weight changes and to check weight for height. Normal BMI is 20–25 kg/m$^2$, with amenorrhoea occurring if BMI is less than 19 kg/m$^2$. Where the problem is thought to be weight loss, it is better to achieve a return of menstruation via weight gain than drug therapy; where there is no response to weight gain, specialist referral should be considered. If weight gain is not being achieved, then the doctor must consider whether the patient has anorexia nervosa and is thus in need of psychiatric help to prevent the serious consequences of that condition.

Despite reassurance, many women find it difficult to accept amenorrhoea, which is perceived as a loss of femininity. Some may want to know that their endocrine system can be switched on, and clomiphene may occasionally be used, but it should only be used for a limited amount of time and then reserved for achieving pregnancy. However, it must be remembered that in women with idiopathic or congenital (Kallman's syndrome) hypothalamic amenorrhoea, associated with absent puberty, there is no response to clomiphene.

Rare causes of hypothalamic amenorrhoea include hypothalamic lesions such as craniopharyngiomas, sarcoidosis, tuberculosis, head injury or cranial irradiation which destroy the normal tissue.

Recent concerns are the long-term consequences of the hypo-oestrogenic state on bone density and the cardiovascular system. Women with 6 months or more of amenorrhoea should have a bone density measurement. Cyclical oestrogen/progestogen hormone replacement therapy may be used, but it must be stressed that this is not contraceptive. If contraception is needed, the combined oral contraceptive pill is a better option.

### Hyperprolactinaemia

Hyperprolactinaemia is the most common pituitary cause of amenorrhoea. Galactorrhoea is present in up to 30% of hyperprolactinaemic women but galactorrhoeic women who do not have menstrual disturbance only rarely have hyperprolactinaemia. About 5% of women present with visual field defects. High prolactin levels cause amenorrhoea by inhibiting the normal pulsatile secretion of GnRH by the hypothalamus.

There are many causes of hyperprolactinaemia, the most important that need to be diagnosed being prolactin-secreting tumours of the anterior pituitary and non-functional tumours such as craniopharyngiomas which impede the passage of dopamine to the pituitary and hence increase prolactin levels (prolactin levels 1000–3000 mU/l). Craniopharyngiomas need surgical removal. Prolactinomas less than 1 cm in diameter are referred to as microadenomas (prolactin levels 1500–4000 mU/l), and those greater than 1 cm as macroadenomas (prolactin levels 5000–8000 mU/l). The exact incidence of the clinical problem is uncertain with between 9 and 27% of pituitary glands in routine autopsy series having been found to contain adenomas. Women with hyperprolactinaemia (i.e. prolactin >1000 mU/l) should therefore have an MRI scan and visual field assessment.

It must be remembered that the commonest cause for a moderately elevated serum prolactin level is stress (even stress during a breast examination which is often done before a blood test!) and therefore it is important to take a repeat blood sample with the patient more relaxed, if that is possible. Drugs, including metaclopromide, phenothiazines, reserpine, methyldopa and cimetidine, may also cause hyperprolactinaemia and thus an accurate drug history is important.

Menstruation, ovulation, and fertility can be restored in patients with hyperprolactinaemia with drugs such as bromocriptine, cabergoline and quinagolide, which can be used for macro- as well as microadenomas. If a patient wants her fertility restored, then obviously she should be treated with bromocriptine and similar agents, which can be stopped during pregnancy. Twice-weekly cabergoline is now the agent of choice since the side effects are fewer than with bromocriptine. But there is controversy in patients with microadenomas who do not wish to become pregnant. If they are treated, they require contraception, preferably with a barrier method. Alternatively, they could be given hormone replacement therapy to counteract the hypo-oestrogenic effects on their bones and cardiovascular system; these women need specialist referral since oestrogen can cause enlargement of a prolactinoma. Approaches over the years have become more conservative, with documentation of a benign clinical course with spontaneous resolution in many patients. Surgical referral is required for women with macroadenomas, drug resistance, drug intolerance or suprasellar enlargement prior to pregnancy.

### Polycystic ovary syndrome (PCOS)

First described by two gynaecologists, Stein and Leventhal, in the early 1930s, this syndrome was originally ascribed to patients with amenorrhoea, hirsutism, obesity, and bilateral polycystic ovaries. On ultrasound the classical picture is a string of small follicles, 2–8 mm in diameter arranged like a necklace in the periphery of the ovary. It is clear, however, that any form of menstrual irregularity can occur: oligomenorrhoea, or menorrhagia with regular or irregular cycles. There is considerable heterogeneity of symptoms and signs among women with PCOS and these may change over time in any individual. PCOS is familial and various aspects of the syndrome may be differentially inherited. There is now a problem of definition. The European view is that PCOS encompasses any of the following: polycystic ovaries on ultrasound scan, signs of androgen excess, menstrual cycle disturbance and elevated androgen and/or LH levels. In the USA the syndrome is denoted by the combination of hyperandrogenization and ovulatory dysfunction in the absence of non-classical adrenal hyperplasia without necessarily a need to identify polycystic ovaries on ultrasound.

The condition involves:

◆ the presence of an excessive number of small follicles placed peripherally in the ovaries with a relative failure of follicular selection processes which should produce a dominant follicle;

◆ a continuous background of oestrogen production by the small follicles;

◆ ovarian stromal hyperplasia associated with excessive androgen production;

◆ conversion of androgens in peripheral fat to oestrone, resulting in adequate oestrogenization;

◆ insulin resistance, leading to hypersecretion in both obese and slim women with PCOS; insulin stimulates androgen secretion by the ovarian stroma;

◆ disturbed ovarian pituitary feedback, resulting in elevated secretion of LH. However, the expression of excessive androgen production depends not simply on blood levels of testosterone and androstenedione, but on the peripheral metabolism of testosterone to dihydrotestosterone in the specific androgen-sensitive end-organs (the hair follicles). This is the main difference between hirsute and non-hirsute women with PCOS.

Several studies have tried to estimate the prevalence of polycystic ovaries in normal women and found it to be about 20% on ultrasound scan, whilst up to 10% will be symptomatic. There are concerns about the long-term risks of developing type 2 diabetes and cardiovascular disease as well as endometrial hyperplasia and cancer due to unopposed oestrogen exposure. Genetic studies have shown abnormalities in both the steroidogenic pathway for androgen biosynthesis and in the regulation of expression of the insulin gene.

A recent survey of 1741 women with PCOS referred to a specialist clinic showed that 39.8% and 29.8%, respectively, had raised serum LH and/or testosterone concentrations, while symptoms of obesity, hyperandrogenization and menstrual cycle disturbance occurred in 38.4, 70.3 and 66.2% of patients, respectively (Balen *et al.* 1995). Obesity was associated with hirsutism and an elevated serum testosterone concentration and was also correlated with increased rates of infertility and cycle disturbance. The rates of infertility and cycle disturbance also increased with serum LH concentrations (>10 IU/l). A rising serum concentration of testosterone was associated with an increased risk of hirsutism, infertility and cycle disturbance.

Hypersecretion of LH is associated with menstrual disturbance, reduced conception rates and increased miscarriage rates in both natural and assisted conception cycles. If the testosterone level is >4.8 nmol/l, the patient needs to be investigated to exclude androgen-secreting tumours, Cushing's syndrome, and congenital adrenal hyperplasia.

Treatment is symptom orientated and also is determined by whether fertility is desired. The chronic anovulatory state in PCOS causes menstrual irregularity and increases the risks of endometrial hyperplasia and cancer. Cyclical progestogens can be given for 12 days each month, but this regimen is not contraceptive. Alternatively, a combined oral contraceptive pill can be used. If hirsutism is a problem, a contraceptive pill containing the antiandrogen drug cyproterone can be used; however, the role of waxing and electrolysis should not be forgotten. Laser is more expensive but should be considered if hair is dark and skin fair. Women with oligomenorrhoeic/amenorrhoeic PCOS appear to gain regular menstrual cycles as they get older, and therefore artificial methods of cycle control can be stopped from time to time to see if there has been a spontaneous resolution to the problem. In the women who wish to become pregnant, ovulation induction with clomiphene may prove effective. Gonadotrophin stimulation is the next step in treatment for women who are 'clomiphene resistant'; however, the results in women with PCOS are less successful, and there is controversy about the which is the best regimen (Nugent et al. 2000). In PCOS, women are at risk of ovarian hyperstimulation syndrome and multiple pregnancy and need close monitoring. Surgery in the form of laparoscopic laser or diathermy to the ovarian surface is now used instead of wedge resection. Its mode of action is uncertain, since unilateral diathermy can result in bilateral ovulation. This is believed to be less likely to cause the adhesions which were a problem after wedge resection.

Weight loss improves the endocrine profile, the likelihood of ovulation and a healthy pregnancy but may be difficult to achieve. Initial reports of the use of insulin-sensitizing agents (metformin) have been encouraging, particularly when associated with weight loss, but this requires more evaluation both in the short and long term. Spironolactone and finasteride are potential treatments of hirsutism; however, neither is licensed for this indication and contraceptive cover is required because of the theoretical risk of feminizing a male fetus. Spironolactone may have a place when combined oral contraceptives are contraindicated.

### Premature menopause

A menopause is considered to be premature if it occurs before the age of 45 and occurs in about 1% of women. It is characterized by high FSH and LH with normal prolactin levels. Other symptoms may be present, such as hot flushes and night sweats, as well as atrophic vaginitis. Sadly, premature ovarian failure can occur at any age, even in teenagers. Premature ovarian failure is difficult to distinguish from resistant ovary syndrome with fluctuating ovarian function and unpredictable ovulation. In the vast majority of cases no cause can be found. The causes are detailed below.

◆ *Chromosome abnormalities*, particularly of the X chromosome, have been implicated. X chromosome mosaicisms are the most common abnormality in women with premature ovarian failure. In Turner's syndrome (45XO), accelerated follicular loss causes ovarian failure. Familial premature ovarian failure has been linked with fragile X premutations. Women with Down's syndrome also have an early menopause.

◆ *Autoimmune disease.* Autoimmune endocrine disease such as hypothyroidism, Addison's and diabetes may be associated with premature ovarian failure.

◆ *FSH receptor abnormalities.* Mutations of gonadotrophin receptors have been reported.

◆ *Disruption of oestrogen synthesis.* Specific enzyme deficiencies (e.g. 17α-hydroxylase) can prevent oestradiol synthesis, leading to primary amenorrhoea and elevated gonadotrophin levels, even though developing follicles are present.

◆ *Metabolic.* Galactosaemia is associated with premature ovarian failure. It is thought that galactose and its metabolites may be toxic to the ovarian parenchyma.

◆ *Radiotherapy and chemotherapy.* Chemotherapy can cause either temporary or permanent ovarian damage, which depends on the cumulative dose received and duration of treatment, so that long-term treatment with small doses is more toxic than short-term acute therapy. These changes occur at all ages, but especially so in women aged more than 30 years. With regard to radiotherapy, ovarian damage is dose and age dependent.

◆ *Hysterectomy without oophorectomy* can cause ovarian failure either in the immediate postoperative period where in some cases it may be temporary, or at a later stage where it occurs sooner than the time of the natural menopause. This is an area of controversy and may depend on ovarian function preceding hysterectomy. The diagnosis may be difficult since not all women suffer acute symptoms, and in the absence of a uterus the pointer of amenorrhoea is absent. A case could be made for annual FSH estimation in women who have had a hysterectomy before the age of 40.

◆ *Infection.* Tuberculosis and mumps are infections that have been implicated. In most cases, normal ovarian function occurs after mumps infection.

If the woman is concerned about fertility, specialist referral is required. Treatment with cyclical oestrogen/progestogen therapy is indicated in women with premature ovarian failure, both to treat symptoms and to protect against premature heart disease and osteoporosis. The options are hormone replacement therapy or the contraceptive pill, depending on fertility goals. The combined oral contraceptive pill may be a more acceptable option in younger women. Bone density measurements are indicated in women who have 6 months' or more of amenorrhoea. There is some controversy about the dose of oestrogen required to maintain bone mass, which will need monitoring in these women. Some may need the addition of bisphosphonates, but again this is controversial. An autoantibody screen should be undertaken since premature ovarian failure can be associated with other endocrinopathies, e.g. hypothyroidism A karyotype should be checked, especially in young women and where there is a positive family history.

In the past these women were considered sterile and counselled that future pregnancy was impossible. However, in recent years it has become apparent that some may resume normal ovarian function, either spontaneously or while taking hormone replacement therapy, and may become pregnant. The picture has also changed with the use of oocyte donation in some IVF programmes. Therefore it is important for women with premature ovarian failure to realize that there is a possibility of pregnancy. Ovarian stimulation followed by cryopreservation of oocytes can be used prior to chemotherapy or radiotherapy in specialized centres. There are also prospects of cryopreservation of ovarian tissue with reimplantation after treatment. These techniques should be viewed with caution in women with fragile X premutations or Turner mosaicism, who may in the future request these techniques in adolescence. They will be best served using healthy donated oocytes.

## Scanty periods

Scanty regular menstruation needs no investigation; blood losses as low as 2 ml per month have been found in normal parous women. It may herald the menopause or, rarely, have an endocrine basis, but in general is not a worrying symptom.

## Other menstrual symptoms

### Prolonged menstruation

On average, women menstruate for 5–6 days of each cycle and anything over this may be considered prolonged. As discussed earlier, the number of days of bleeding does not relate to menstrual blood loss since most of the loss is passed in the first 3 days of menstruation whether the overall loss is light or heavy. Prolonged menstruation in itself does not require investigation, but may go along with other complaints such as menorrhagia. The main menstrual flow can be prolonged by being preceded or succeeded by spotting in association with a non-hormonal IUCD or the progestogen-only pill: reassurance is usually all that is required. Several days of spotting before a period can be a sign of an endometrial or cervical polyp or even malignancy; visualization of the cervix, a cervical smear, and pelvic examination should be carried out by the general practitioner with referral to the gynaecologist if there are suspicious findings.

### Irregular menstruation and abnormal bleeding

#### *Irregular periods*

Women often worry if their previously regular periods become irregular, but as discussed earlier, this is likely to be no more than a normal variation of hormonal changes. Irregular menstruation, both long and short cycles, is most common at the extremes of reproductive life, soon after the menarche or before the menopause. These cycles are usually anovulatory. In adolescent girls it does not need investigation and unless there are signs of obvious disease, hormonal therapy to regularize periods should be avoided. Rather, the general practitioner should reassure the girl that it is part of the normal maturation process and her periods will become regular with time. However, there are a few young girls with persistent heavy irregular periods associated with anovular cycles where the concern is the effect of sustained unopposed oestrogen exposure which may lead to endometrial hyperplasia in later life. The underlying diagnosis is usually PCOS. A useful guide as to when to refer for investigation is if the intermenstrual interval is greater than 3 months. If she requires contraception this may outweigh all other considerations and an oral contraceptive may then be used. Otherwise cyclical progestogens can be employed. In later life, nearer the menopause, irregularity of periods is extremely common. But if periods become heavy as well as irregular or there are problems such as intermenstrual or postcoital bleeding, referral to a gynaecologist is wise.

### Intermenstrual and postcoital bleeding

Investigation and management mainly depend on the age of the patient. In perimenopausal women these symptoms cannot be ignored. Speculum examination is essential to exclude a cervical lesion, malignancy, ectropion, or polyp and pelvic examination will define any obvious uterine or ovarian problems. Referral to a gynaecologist should be made in older women (over 40) unless, for example, a cervical polyp is present. This can be easily avulsed by the general practitioner using long forceps to twist off the polyp and cauterize the resulting raw area with a silver nitrate stick. It is mandatory that the polyp should be sent for histology to exclude rare malignancies. If the bleeding settles after removal of a polyp, then referral is unnecessary. In young women, midcycle bleeding is often associated with ovulation and does not require investigation. Intermenstrual and postcoital bleeding in young women is rarely associated with malignancy but again it is important that the cervix be visualized, cervical smears taken, and a bimanual pelvic examination carried out to exclude pathology (see above). If the bleeding persists over several cycles, referral should be considered.

## Postmenopausal bleeding

This always requires examination and urgent referral because of the high incidence of malignancy. Although the most common malignancy is endometrial, cancer of the cervix, vulva, or ovary may present in this way. It may, however, be due to non-malignant causes such as atrophic vaginitis or a polyp. Persistent heavy bleeding or breakthrough bleeding in women taking hormonal replacement therapy also needs investigation to exclude endometrial pathology.

## Variations in colour and smell of menstrual blood

Women may report to their doctor a change in the colour or smell of their menstrual blood which may worry them. There is no known association with pelvic pathology and these symptoms. If anything, these changes are associated with different rates of menstrual flow. Thus patients should be reassured.

# Toxic shock syndrome

The only reason for including this section here is that there is the misconception that toxic shock syndrome (TSS), an extremely rare disease, is solely associated with tampon use. In fact it was first described in children in 1978 as a multisystem disease characterized by rapid onset of fever, hypotension, hyperaemia of the mucous membranes and rash followed by desquamation and multisystem involvement. However, the descriptions of staphylococcal scarlet fever suggest that TSS was already noted in 1927. In 1980, an increase in TSS was noted in previously healthy young women with onset during menstruation. Initial studies of menstrual TSS suggested that tampon use was a risk factor for the disease, and a particular brand was implicated which was withdrawn in 1980. In the USA only half of the reported cases occur in menstruating women who use tampons. Non-menstrual cases in men, women, and children, associated with hospital-acquired infections, surgery, boils, insect bites, burns, parturition, and contraceptive barriers, have been increasingly recognized. Some women are subject to recurrences of menstrual TSS even when tampons have not been used.

The association between TSS and *Staphylococcus aureus* infection was firmly established when an exotoxin from isolates of TSS-associated *S. aureus* was isolated in 1981. The exotoxin has since been called toxic shock syndrome toxin-1 (TSST-1) and is generally considered to be the major cause of TSS. Other pathogens such as *Escherichia coli* have also been more recently implicated.

The exact role of tampons in menstrual TSS is uncertain. Initially it was thought that high absorbency of tampons such as those containing carboxymethylcellulose or polyacrylate was an important factor. Indeed, these substances are no longer used. However, the role of absorbency is now being questioned since the original studies did not distinguish the effects of absorbency from the effects of chemical composition or other tampon characteristics that are correlated with absorbency. One persistent problem in understanding the aetiology of TSS is that the vaginal environment is anaerobic but the production of TSST-1 requires the presence of oxygen. Therefore, it has been suggested that the insertion of a tampon might provide the oxygen necessary for toxin production. Another theory is that highly absorbent tampon material binds magnesium ions; in a magnesium-deficient environment, production of TSST-1 increases dramatically.

It is important to put the risk of developing TSS in perspective. It is a very rare disease probably due to the high rate of carriage of antibody against TSST-1 in the population, with no justification for women to avoid using tampons. Tampon packets now carry warnings about TSS. On the other hand, if one suspects that a woman has TSS, it is important to arrange hospital admission for appropriate antibiotic treatment since the disease has a high mortality.

# Acknowledgement

The author would like to thank Mr Adam Balen for his helpful comments and suggestions.

# Information for patients on PCOS

Leaflet: 'Polycystic ovary syndrome', Treatment Notes, Consumers' Association, April 2001. Based on information from the Drug and Therapeutics Bulletin. Website: www.verity-pcos.org.uk

# References and further reading

Balen, A., Conway, G.S., Kaltsas, G., *et al.* (1995). Polycystic ovary syndrome: the spectrum of the disorder in 1741 patients. *Human Reproduction*, **10**, 2107–11.

Blanck, H.M., Marcus, M., Tolbert, P.E., *et al.* (2000). Age at menarche and tanner stage in girls exposed in utero and postnatally to polybrominated biphenyl. *Epidemiology*, **11**, 641–7.

Brouard, R., Bossmar, T., Fournie-Lloret, D., Chassard, D. and Akerlund M. (2000). Effect of SR49059, an orally active V1a vasopressin receptor antagonist, in the prevention of dysmenorrhoea. *British Journal of Obstetrics and Gynaecology*, **107**, 614–19.

Coulter, A., Kelland, J., Long, A., *et al.* (1995). *The management of menorrhagia.* Effective Health Care Bulletin no 9. Stott Bros., Halifax.

*Drug and Therapeutics Bulletin* (2000). Which operation for menorrhagia? **38**, 77–80.

*Drug and Therapeutics Bulletin* (2001). Tackling polycystic ovary syndrome. **39**, 1–5.

Gladen, B.C., Ragan, N.B. and Rogan, W.J. (2000). Pubertal growth and development and prenatal and lactational exposure to polychlorinated biphenyls and dichlorodiphenyl dichloroethene. *Journal of Pediatrics*, **136**, 490–6.

Goldfarb, H.A. (2000). Myoma coagulation (myolysis). *Obstetric and Gynecological Clinics of North America*, **27**, 421–30.

Grant, C., Gallier, L., Fahey, T., Pearson, N. and Sarangi, J. (2000). Management of menorrhagia in primary care-impact on referral and hysterectomy: data from the Somerset Morbidity Project. *Journal of Epidemiology and Community Health*, **54**, 709–13.

Hope, S. (2000). Menorrhagia. *British Medical Journal*, **321**, 935.

Kennedy, A.D., Sculpher, M.J., Coulter, A., *et al.* (2002). Effects of decision aids for menorrhagia on treatment choices, health outcomes, and costs: a randomized controlled trial. *Journal of the American Medical Association*, **288**, 2701–8.

Kovacs, G.T. (2000). *Polycystic ovary syndrome.* Cambridge University Press, Cambridge.

Kurman, R.J., Kaminski, P.F. and Norris, H.J. (1985). The behavior of endometrial hyperplasia. A long-term study of 'untreated' hyperplasia in 170 patients. *Cancer*, **56**, 403–12.

Marshall, S.F., Hardy, R.J. and Kuh, D. (2000). Socioeconomic variation in hysterectomy up to age 52: national, population based, prospective cohort study. *British Medical Journal*, **320**, 1579.

Morrison, B.W., Daniels, S.E., Kotey, P., Cantu, N. and Seidenberg, B. (1999). Rofecoxib, a specific cyclooxygenase-2 inhibitor, in primary dysmenorrhea: a randomized controlled trial. *Obstetrics and Gynecology*, **94**, 504–8.

Moya, R.A., Moisa, C.F., Morales, F., Wynter, H. and Ali, A. (2000). Narancio transdermal glyceryl trinitrate in the management of primary dysmenorrhea. *International Journal of Gynaecology and Obstetrics*, **69**, 113–18.

Nugent, D., Vandekerckhove, P., Hughes, E., Arnot, M. and Lilford, R. (2000). Gonadotrophin therapy for ovulation induction in subfertility associated with polycystic ovary syndrome (Cochrane Review). *Cochrane Database System Review* **4**, CD000410.

O'Brien, P.M.S., Cameron, I.T. and Maclean, A.B. (eds) (2000). *Disorders of the menstrual cycle.* RCOG Press, London.

Pasquali, R., Gambineri, A., Biscotti, D., *et al.* (2000). Effect of long-term treatment with metformin added to hypocaloric diet on body composition, fat distribution, and androgen and insulin levels in abdominally obese women with and without the polycystic ovary syndrome. *Journal of Clinical Endocrinology and Metabolism*, **85**, 2767–74.

Pelage, J.P., Le Dref, O., Soyer, P., *et al.* (2000) Fibroid-related menorrhagia: treatment with superselective embolization of the uterine arteries and midterm follow-up. *Radiology*, **215**, 428–31.

Peterson, H.B., Jeng, G., Folger, S.G., Hillis, S.A., Marchbanks, P.A. and Wilcox, L.S. (2000).The risk of menstrual abnormalities after tubal sterilization. *New England Journal of Medicine*, **343**, 1681–7.

Pugeat, M. and Ducluzeau, P.H. (1999). Insulin resistance, polycystic ovary syndrome and metformin. *Drugs*, **58**(S1), 41–6; discussion 75–82.

Rees, M. (1991). Role of menstsrual loss measurement in management of excessive menstrual bleeding. *British Journal of Obstetrics and Gynaecology*, **98**, 327–8.

Rees, M.C.P. (1998a). Medical treatment of menorrhagia. In: Cameron, I.T., Fraser, I.S. and Smith, S.K. (eds), *Clinical disorders of the menstrual cycle*, pp. 155–66. Oxford University Press, Oxford.

Rees, M.C.P. (1998b) Perimenopausal contraception with levonorgestrel intrauterine levonorgestrel system. In: Johansen (ed.), *Mirena: the levonorgestrel intrauterine system*, pp. 53–66. EDB. Parthenon Press, Camforth.

Rees, M.C.P. (1998c) Menarche. In: Stanhope, R. (ed.), *Adolescent endocrinology*, pp. 39–44. Bioscientifica, Bristol.

Rees, M.C.P., Chamberlain, P. and Gillmer, M.D. (2001). Management of uterine fibroids with goserelin acetate alone or goserelin acetate plus endometrial resection. *Gynaecological Endoscopy*, **10**, 33–5.

Reid, P.C., Coker, A. and Coltart, R. (2000). Assessment of menstrual blood loss using a pictorial chart: a validation study. *British Journal of Obstetrics and Gynaecology*, **107**, 320–2.

Royal College of Obstetrics and Gynaecology (1998). *The initial management of menorrhagia. Evidence-based guidelines 1*. RCOG Press, London.

Royal College of Obstetrics and Gynaecology (1999). *The management of menorrhagia in secondary care. Evidence-based guidelines 5*. RCOG Press, London.

Sheth, S. and Sutton, C. (eds) (1999). *Menorrhagia*. Isis Medical Media Ltd, Oxford.

Turner, E., Bowie, P., McMullen, K.W. and Kellock, C. (2000). First-line management of menorrhagia: findings from a survey of general practitioners in forth valley. *British Journal of Family Planning*, **26**, 227–8.

Vollman, R.F. (1977). *The menstrual cycle*. W.B. Saunders, Philadelphia.

Zhang, W.Y., Li Wan Po, A. (1998). Efficacy of minor analgesics in primary dysmenorrhoea: a systematic review. *British Journal of Obstetrics and Gynaecology*, **105**, 780–9.

# Chapter 2

# Premenstrual syndrome
## Fiona Blake

From earliest times men have written about women's changing moods and behaviour and attributed them to their female anatomy and their menstrual cycle. In the twentieth century, Frank (1931) coined the term premenstrual tension (PMT). He perceived a link between symptoms in the latter half of the menstrual cycle and the fluctuations of the reproductive hormones. From the 1950s, Dalton has campaigned for the better recognition and treatment of such symptoms and widened the concept, calling it premenstrual syndrome (PMS). Since then, PMS has received much publicity, in both the lay and medical press. There is still much debate about the syndrome's definition, aetiology and treatment, but following considerable research and debate, there is now a better understanding of PMS and a range of ways of managing the problem. It is a complex and fascinating topic that raises many questions about the interactions between hormones and physiological changes and life events and stress. Women today are taking an active and positive role in acquiring knowledge and information about health issues and many women hear about PMS and identify similar symptoms in themselves. With information, patience, and encouragement, women can work out ways to understand and manage their symptoms and this may include seeking medical advice from their general practitioner (GP).

## Definition

Many women notice change in their emotional and physical feelings during the menstrual cycle. While for the majority such changes are acceptable, for others they are distressing. These distressing premenstrual changes are now described as 'premenstrual syndrome' rather than 'premenstrual tension', in recognition of the variable nature of the symptoms, which may not always include tension. The definition of PMS has been fraught with problems, since the type of symptoms and their severity can vary enormously both between women and between cycles for individual women. There are a number of definitions of PMS available. O'Brien (1990) gives a widely accepted example:

... a disorder of non-specific somatic, psychological or behavioural symptoms recurring in the premenstrual phase of the menstrual cycle. Symptoms must resolve completely by the end of menstruation leaving a symptom-free week. The symptoms should be of sufficient severity to produce social, family or occupational disruption. Symptoms must have occurred in at least four of the six previous menstrual cycles.

He does not specify which symptoms, because these can be so variable. More than 150 symptoms have been described, but the commonest include: low mood, irritability, anxiety, tension, clumsiness, poor memory, food craving, sleep disturbance, bloating, breast tenderness, abdominal pain, back ache, weight gain, fatigue.

Some women notice only mood changes, others only physical symptoms, but it is more common for both to be experienced together. There are no specific symptom clusters and individual women tend to report their own unique combination of symptoms. However, most of the women looking for help have a predominance of psychological symptoms because these interfere most with relationships in everyday life.

Recently, a severe premenstrual syndrome with predominantly mood symptoms has been defined in the appendix of the American Psychiatric Association's Diagnostic and Statistical Manual (DSM IV, 1994), called 'premenstrual dysphoric disorder' (PMDD). Operational criteria have been described so that research into this severe condition can be more consistent. Epidemiological data using these criteria reveal a subgroup of women with a disorder that is very like an affective disorder and which may be best treated as one. This has allowed women with the most disabling pattern of PMS symptoms to be researched specifically, with encouraging results for all sufferers. While being yet another medical label for women, this may be helpful with regard to management approaches (see later).

Distressing changes may start up to 14 days before menstruation, although it is more common for the symptoms to last for up to a week, and disappear at or shortly after the start of menstrual bleeding. Many women say that the severity varies from cycle to cycle, depending on general life events and stresses. Until the timing in relation to menstruation is established, PMS can be confused with more general problems such as anxiety or depression, and may be misdiagnosed or mistreated. Hence, the first step in diagnosis is careful and regular symptom recording to establish the nature and timing of the problems. Women should be asked to complete menstrual charts, recording their moods and other symptoms for at least two cycles. Various menstrual diaries are available (Fig 2.1), or a simple practical alternative is to customize a diary for the individual based on the predominant symptoms (Fig 2.2).

## SYMPTOM CHART

**Name:**

**Month:**

**Date:**

| Day of Menstrual Cycle | 1 | 2 | 3 | 4 | 5 | 6 | 7 | 8 | 9 | 10 | 11 | 12 | 13 | 14 | 15 | 16 | 17 | 18 | 19 | 20 | 21 | 22 | 23 | 24 | 25 | 26 | 27 | 28 | 29 | 30 | 31 | 32 | 33 | 34 | 35 | 36 | 37 | 38 | 39 | 40 | 41 | 42 | 43 | 44 | 45 | 46 | 47 | 48 |

**Symptoms**

Bleeding
Breast Tenderness
Bloated
Headache
Pelvic Pain
Backache
Irritable
Depressed
Tense
Anxious
Fatigue
Clumsy
Disorganised
Alcohol
Unattractive
Low Self Image
Weight Change

Fill in the chart daily commencing on the first day of your period, as follows:

**BLEEDING** - If you have bleeding, shade in the box ■  for spotting , mark ●

**SYMPTOMS** - Record symptoms every evening as follows:

None = leave blank
Mild = 1 (present but tolerable)
Moderate = 2 (interferes with normal activities)
Severe = 3 (incapacitating)

**Fig 2.1** Premenstrual assessment chart for clinical use. (O'Brien 1987, based on the Prism calendar).

## Daily Symptom Diary

Choose the four symptoms that trouble you most, (eg irritability, depression, tiredness), list them at the top of the columns. Score these symptoms each evening as follows:

None      =   0
Mild      =   1   (present but tolerable)
Moderate  =   2   (interferes with normal activities)
Severe    =   3   (incapacitating)

Add any relevant comments about what is happening in your life in the last column. Note bleeding with an M (for menstruation) in the "Bleeding" column

| Date | Bleeding | Symptom 1 | Symptom 2 | Symptom 3 | Symptom 4 | Comments |
|------|----------|-----------|-----------|-----------|-----------|----------|
|      |          |           |           |           |           |          |
|      |          |           |           |           |           |          |
|      |          |           |           |           |           |          |
|      |          |           |           |           |           |          |
|      |          |           |           |           |           |          |
|      |          |           |           |           |           |          |
|      |          |           |           |           |           |          |
|      |          |           |           |           |           |          |
|      |          |           |           |           |           |          |
|      |          |           |           |           |           |          |
|      |          |           |           |           |           |          |
|      |          |           |           |           |           |          |
|      |          |           |           |           |           |          |
|      |          |           |           |           |           |          |
|      |          |           |           |           |           |          |
|      |          |           |           |           |           |          |
|      |          |           |           |           |           |          |
|      |          |           |           |           |           |          |
|      |          |           |           |           |           |          |
|      |          |           |           |           |           |          |
|      |          |           |           |           |           |          |
|      |          |           |           |           |           |          |
|      |          |           |           |           |           |          |

**Fig 2.2** A daily symptom diary that can be customized for particular symptoms.

Some women complain of symptoms that seem to be related to the menstrual cycle but wax and wane at other times in the cycle, e.g. at ovulation. Some definitions allow such variations, e.g. Magos (1990):

. . . distressing physical, psychological and behavioural symptoms not caused by organic disease which regularly recur during the same phase of the menstrual cycle and which significantly regress or disappear during the remainder of the cycle.

Again it is crucial to establish the pattern by prospective daily symptom diary kept over several cycles.

## Prevalence

It is hard to evaluate how many women experience PMS since the experience of cyclical changes is so common and what makes them distressing and disabling is so subjective. Epidemiological studies indicate that between 75 and 90% of ovulating women experience cyclical changes at least some time in their lives. For many these are in no way a problem. They can indeed be a positive part of their lives and could be regarded as normal 'physiological' aspects of the menstrual cycle. Logue and Moos (1988) found that between 5 and 15% of women actually feel better in the premenstrual phase, experiencing increased well-being, energy, and activities before menstruation. About 5–10% of women have PMS that is severe and disabling, depending on sample and definition (Connelly, 2001). This leads to a significant number of consultations for PMS in the surgery. It is likely that what brings a woman to seek medical help is the effect of PMS on her life. Women seek help when symptoms interfere with personal, home, or working life and in particular with relationships with family, children, partner, friend, or colleagues.

## Effects of PMS

PMS is undoubtedly distressing for many women, not only for themselves but also for those around them. Women with small children too young to understand PMS may feel extra stress and be worried about the effect their feelings are having on their children. Cyclical mood changes, particularly if seemingly unpredictable, may be a problem in relationships with a partner, unless PMS is discussed, understood and accepted. Women whose colleagues at work are unsympathetic and dismiss suggestions or complaints on their part as 'it's that time of the month again' will obviously find PMS hard to bear. Women often worry that their performance at work may be impaired before menstruation but studies have shown that this is largely not the case (Cockerill *et al.* 1994). Many women who suffer with PMS organize their work and home life so that they avoid stressful events premenstrually. Evidence suggests, however, that women who are admitted to psychiatric hospital, attempt suicide, or commit crimes are more likely to be in the luteal phase of their cycle. This is not to say that all premenstrual women are at risk of these events, but women who are likely to require psychiatric admission or commit crimes and who experience PMS, may be more vulnerable in the premenstrual phase.

PMS may well influence women's sexuality, and there is no doubt that mood changes interact with sexual feelings. A woman who experiences severe premenstrual tiredness or breast tenderness may find this reduces her interest in sexual activities before menstruation, although sexual interest may well increase after menstruation once she feels an improvement in well-being. However, some women feel more sexually interested in the premenstrual phase. Fluctuations in sexual interest may cause worry to a woman and possible problems in relationships unless links to the menstrual cycle are understood. Problems of varying sexual interest linked to PMS may be one reason for consulting the GP.

## Who experiences PMS?

There appears to be no distinctive 'type' of woman likely to experience PMS, although in general it appears to be more common in women in their thirties and forties and in women who have children. Certain events may be linked to the onset of PMS, such as stopping the oral contraceptive, the birth of a child, or sterilization, which suggests a hormonal connection. PMS can still be experienced following hysterectomy if the ovaries remain (Bäckström *et al.* 1981). PMS seems to be common across all social classes although it seems that women who seek medical help specifically for PMS are more likely to be in social classes I and II. Therefore, the primary health care team should be alert to the possibility of PMS in women consulting for other problems, such as anxiety or depression. There also appears to be a general link between adverse life events and PMS. Women tend to experience PMS as more of a problem during times of stress, such as when there are problems at home or at work, or during examination times or when moving house.

Despite some views that PMS is a complaint of 'neurotic' women, there is no consistent relationship between women's personalities and PMS. There do, however, appear to be links between PMS and general psychological health. Women who are psychiatrically ill may experience more, and more severe, premenstrual psychological symptoms than psychologically healthy women. Women with PMS are more likely to have had a depressive illness in the past and more likely to have had postnatal depression (Halbreight 1996). Recently, interest has focused on PMS in perimenopausal women. During the time leading up to the menopause, PMS can become more severe and blur into the menopause. It is possible that some women are more vulnerable than others to hormonal fluctuations and are therefore at risk of problems with PMS, the menopause, and a mild form of postnatal depression and so require extra support at these times.

## Causes of PMS

There has been no shortage of hypotheses to explain PMS. The most plausible include abnormal tissue responses to normal levels of ovarian hormones, abnormalities of serotonin and other neurotransmitters. Endocrinological studies have not shown any convincing abnormalities, particularly none in the luteal phase (Roca *et al.* 1996). Nevertheless, medical suppression of the ovarian cycle with gonadotrophin-releasing hormone or surgical ablation by bilateral oophorectomy has been proven to eliminate PMS. There may be interactions between hormones and neurotransmitters. For example, there may be increased sensitivity to progesterone due to serotonin deficiency (Rapkin *et al.* 1997). Recent studies showing the efficacy of serotonin reuptake inhibitors have strengthened the evidence for involvement of the serotonin system (Eriksson 1999). To these can be added nutritional theories, including deficiencies of pyridoxine, essential fatty acids, hypoglycaemia and low magnesium or calcium levels. Cultural, psychological, and social theories have also been put forward (Rodin 1992).

PMS probably results from a combination of physical, psychological, and social factors interacting with life events.

## Management

PMS is a common problem which deserves sympathetic attention and appropriate management. Many women find that with support and encouragement they can work out solutions for themselves; and if problems persist, then various medical treatments can be tried. Now that many practices have well woman and family planning clinics, the 'best person' to deal with PMS may be any member of the team. It is probably helpful to have someone able and willing to deal with the complex interaction between psychological and physical symptoms, relationship and social difficulties. A purely medical approach will fail to engage the woman in examining her situation on a broad front and may encourage her to pin too much hope on pharmacological solutions for problems that may benefit from adjustments to lifestyle and stress.

Health visitors, counsellors, and nurses as well as GPs should be aware of PMS and how it may be affecting their patients. Primary care team members, because of their knowledge of an individual woman and her circumstances, are ideally placed to help her work out whether PMS is the main cause of her distress or whether other factors in her life are actually to blame.

PMS is a problem that is best dealt with by empowering the woman to do as much as she can to help herself and collaborate positively in evaluating any medical treatments prescribed.

Women coming to the surgery with PMS need time to work out what the problems and solutions are and so a number of appointments may be necessary. The initial consultation should seek to establish a therapeutic relationship, identify the woman's complaints and begin to prioritize the difficulties.

## History

Assessment starts with the history of the main troublesome symptoms, the timing in the menstrual cycle, the severity, and the impact on the woman and those around her. Ask her why she is seeking help now. There may have been a crisis, an unmanageable extra stressor, or she may have heard about a new treatment that she would like to try. She will not have the definitions of PMS to hand and so may rely on magazine articles, a friend's suggestion, or a scan of the Internet to prompt her presentation. As many as half of women who present complaining of PMS do not have cyclical symptoms after diary keeping so another label needs to be found, and guidance towards a more useful focus. Unfortunately, many women come already certain of their diagnosis and do not want to contemplate an alternative. This may be because they fear the stigma of depression or relationship difficulties and are not confident about solutions to such issues.

## Social and relationship context

Women often feel responsible for the emotional well-being of those around them. They blame themselves when things go wrong and look for internal reasons for social and relationship problems. It may be easier to blame the hormones than confront the misery of an absent partner or wayward children. Some social problems are intractable but can be borne except when further strained by premenstrual symptoms.

## Cultural norms, expectations and fears

Many women cannot deal with their own anger and are very upset about irritable outbursts, especially when directed at 'innocent victims' such as their small children. A typical example of this might be as follows: a woman is overwhelmed with guilt and depression because of an irritable outburst with partner or children. She is appalled at her behaviour and seeks an explanation that allows her to retain her image of herself as self-controlled and loving and reject the side of herself that becomes angry or demanding because it is not how women should behave, even if the anger is justified. She may describe herself as 'Jekyll and Hyde' and does not accept her different reactions as part of normality but instead feels out of control and therefore ill. The most frequent fear is that this represents 'madness' and PMS offers a hormonal explanation that avoids this conclusion. Reassurance about her sanity and the role of stress may allow exploration of psychological factors.

## Previous treatments

The patient may be very familiar with her PMS and better versed in the options for treatment than her professional adviser. She may have already tried a number of strategies and have strong views about the next step. A history of past treatments and the outcomes will enable rational and acceptable choices for the future.

## Past medical history

PMS is a chronic disorder and a history of gynaecological events, previous illnesses, psychological and other will help put PMS in the context of the woman's previous experience of health and illness.

## Daily symptom diary keeping

A clear history of PMS is useful in planning treatment but research has shown that women are rather poor at remembering the detail of fluctuating symptoms and tend to attribute negative symptoms to PMS premenstrually and to external events post-menstrually. Thus a daily symptom diary can provide further information about timing and circumstances that enables better definition and management of the situation. It may indicate a pattern of symptoms that confirms PMS, but if it does not then the woman herself will be the first to speculate on alternative explanations (Fig 2.3). The chart is also valuable in determining whether advice or treatment is helping and the woman should be encouraged to keep it for several months. Knowing in some detail how she is likely to feel at particular times of the cycle gives the woman some sense of the predictability of her symptoms and allows her to plan for the difficult times. It is very helpful to make allowances for PMS, and many women have benefited from fairly simple rearrangements to their schedules of work and other activities to reduce the stress during premenstrual days.

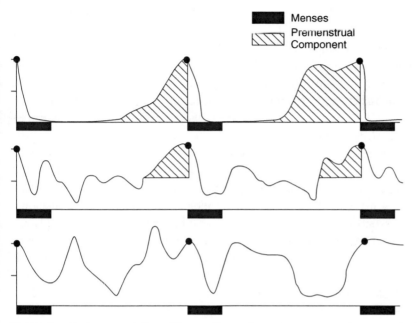

**Fig 2.3** Graphical representation of three patterns of symptoms common in premenstrual complaint: (a) 'pure' PMS; (b) premenstrual exacerbation of an underlying disorder; (c) symptoms that are non-cyclical, perhaps part of another disorder, e.g. depression. (Adapted from Sampson 1989).

## Education, understanding and support

Talking to her GP, health visitor, or practice nurse may open the door for a woman to talk to others such as her partner, family, friends, or colleagues. This means that problems are brought out into the open rather than the woman feeling isolated or 'going round the bend'. A woman can learn more about her body, about normal functions of her female self, and what might be abnormal. Talking to others can also reveal a wealth of remedies and strategies for dealing with PMS. Many women spend their time looking after others and an important part of the strategy to combat PMS is for the woman to look at *her* needs and to nurture herself.

## General health promotion and review of health status

A check on general health is useful. Health promotion is worthwhile for all and the evidence for such advice lies in the broader epidemiological studies on the value of low fat, high fibre diet, exercise and the dangers of smoking and excess alcohol. A person will probably be fitter and able to deal better with stress if eating a balanced 'healthy' diet and incorporating some form of exercise and relaxation into her lifestyle.

It is also possible that women are more sensitive to changes in blood sugar levels in the premenstrual days, resulting in feelings of weakness, fatigue, and carbohydrate cravings. Careful attention to diet can help, eating frequent small protein-rich meals, particularly if the woman tends to skip meals or eat sugary snacks. It is well worth looking at caffeine intake, since caffeine can increase levels of anxiety and irritability. Many people drink more tea and coffee than they realize and cutting down or cutting these drinks out completely can be helpful. Alcohol consumption may influence PMS. Many women drink more alcohol in response to PMS but excessive intake can make symptoms worse.

There may be links between smoking and premenstrual symptoms and cutting down or stopping smoking is part of general health advice. Exercise can help many of the physical and emotional symptoms of PMS, including tiredness, anxiety, irritability, and bloating. If breast tenderness is a problem, a well-fitting sports bra may help. Learning simple relaxation techniques or meditation can help too. Isolation and lack of control over life's demands is known to be stressful. Encouraging fun, time with friends, personal time, and regular sleep can reduce dysphoria and anxiety and give a sense of control.

One of the most distressing symptoms of PMS is aggressive irritability, which women say affects their activities and relationships. Although in our culture women are generally brought up to be more passive and nurturing than men, it is possible that PMS may bring out real anger about real problems in an otherwise easy-going woman. She and those around her may perceive this as irritability and dismiss the underlying problems, which need to be explored. The premenstrual days may not be the best time to tackle problems that are making her angry, but this is not a reason for ignoring them.

This assessment illustrates the importance of taking a holistic approach to PMS and looking at every woman's circumstances, particularly before embarking on medical treatments. It is important to remind women that good habits of life are best practised in the 'good' weeks, as it is much more difficult to start when things are already overwhelming. Books on PMS are available with sections on diet, relaxation and exercise (Sanders 1985; Duckworth 1990; Harrison 1991). There is a useful address for women's health at the end of the chapter. If no women's health group is run in the surgery, there may be a local group to which women can be referred.

## Evaluating the evidence for treatments for PMS

There are many options for the specific treatment of PMS. The evidence for effectiveness varies in both quality and quantity. Much remains unclear. Effective treatment is evidence based if there are controlled trials of a certain quality that indicate the treatment confers benefit compared with placebo or alternative treatment. In PMS a good trial should be double-blind and placebo-controlled, preferably with a crossover design. The trial should establish the presence of PMS in the subjects prior to the trial by the use of prospective daily symptom charts that have been validated for the purpose. There should be at least one cycle prior to randomization of placebo treatment to exclude women who respond to any intervention. The trial should include sufficient cycles to allow for variation in severity that naturally occurs (usually two pretreatment cycles and two or more treatment cycles). Few trials meet these criteria. Variations between samples due to diagnostic differences, sample sources, and outcome measures also add to the difficulty when comparing current information.

Nevertheless, some provisional conclusions can be offered to guide management, especially as some treatments are promoted with much fanfare and negative evidence. Other strategies using common sense are cheap and can do no harm and therefore may be tried without concern while researchers pursue further studies to consolidate the evidence.

## Non-drug treatments

### Psychological approaches

There have been various psychological approaches to the management of PMS, including counselling, psychotherapy, and hypnotherapy, although none has been evaluated in controlled trials. Group therapy or self-help groups allow women to share their experiences and approaches to PMS (Kirkby 1994). Groups for women with PMS, run in the surgery or in a local community centre, can be very valuable for women with PMS and their partners or families. Some women may be helped by a discussion about PMS as part of a series of meetings on women's health issues where they can obtain information and discuss their problems. Specific PMS groups have been run by GPs and psychologists, giving women a chance to air their feelings, try out self-help techniques such as relaxation, and discuss medical treatments.

## Cognitive behavioural therapy (CBT)

This is one of the few psychological treatments that has been evaluated in controlled trials and the evidence is mixed. Three controlled trials have found CBT better than other measures or a waiting list, but two others have found no extra benefit. Variations between the trials are greater than their similarities, so further research is required. Meanwhile, the principles of CBT are useful to promote satisfactory management of this chronic disorder. The rationale for why it may be helpful for PMS is explained below. There are no harmful effects. Such treatment is also likely to improve other areas of poor health and functioning.

CBT has been shown to be an effective treatment for many psychological problems, such as anxiety and depression, which are common components of PMS (Hawton *et al.* 1989). Cognitive therapy may be particularly suitable for PMS, being brief, time-limited, structured, and collaborative. Therapist and patient work together to help the patient work out solutions to the problems she is facing. It is a common-sense approach that is particularly acceptable to people who are wary of psychological therapy implying that the symptoms are 'all in the mind'. The focus of therapy is on the woman's psychological response to emotional and physical changes and the therapy aims to help the individual to examine patterns of negative thinking and her assumptions about the symptoms and to learn more adaptive and helpful thoughts and behaviours.

The cognitive model of PMS proposes that the woman's cognitive appraisal of the premenstrual changes, in the context of the woman's circumstances and personal assumptions, determines whether she sees the changes as normal and a manageable part of her life, or distressing. For example, interpreting physiological changes in the luteal phase in a negative way is likely to lead the individual to become more distressed and upset by the symptoms, thereby increasing the woman's overall level of distress. The symptoms may be magnified by vicious circles of negative thinking, thereby increasing the woman's anxiety, irritability, or low mood. In particular, the woman may find that physiological changes interfere with her normal coping mechanisms, leading her to predict that she is going to lose control. These thoughts lead the individual to feel tense and anxious, leading to indecision and inability to concentrate. These changes are then interpreted as further evidence that she is losing control and so on in a vicious circle (Blake 1995), as illustrated in Fig 2.4.

The rationale for cognitive therapy is that whilst psychological factors do not, in their own right, cause premenstrual distress, psychological factors influence the response to both psychological and physiological symptoms, thereby modifying the degree of distress. For many women, directly targeting the symptoms with physical treatments alone has proved unhelpful; therefore reducing the distress about the symptoms is a more useful strategy.

In a small, controlled trial of cognitive therapy for severe PMS in Oxford, the treated group had a significant relief of premenstrual symptoms compared with a waiting list group (Blake *et al.* 1998). The common-sense nature of the approach makes it a valuable addition to the range of treatments for PMS and can be modified for use in primary care.

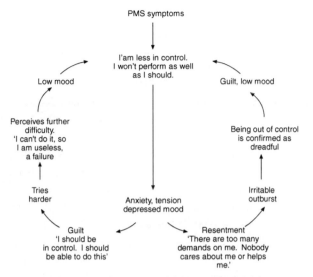

**Fig 2.4** Vicious circles of negative thinking in PMS. (Blake 1995. Reproduced with permission of the Association for Advancement of Behaviour Therapy).

## Medical treatments

There are many different medical approaches for PMS although, as for self-help remedies, there is still a scarcity of well-conducted clinical trials. One problem in evaluating the efficacy of drug treatments is that most trials conducted show a very large placebo effect, particularly in the first month of treatment: in one study (Magos *et al.* 1986), 94% of the women in the placebo group showed a significant improvement. Hence any drug trial should be placebo-controlled and ideally crossover, with each phase continuing for at least 3 months. In addition, definitions of PMS vary so widely that it is difficult to generalize from a clinic-based study to sufferers in primary care.

As far as possible, medical treatments should be used when there is a clear indication. Women should be encouraged to think of medical treatment as just one element in the management of PMS. Attention to lifestyle and relationships is still required. The development of healthy habits will enhance any medical effects, especially as drug treatments may not be sustainable or efficacious in long-term use when the disorder is chronic. Most drugs mentioned here have potentially harmful side effects. Any treatment used for PMS must be thought about in terms of its possible hazards in pregnancy and women should be warned about these, particularly with endocrine treatments.

A number of hospitals run out-patient PMS clinics and referral to a specialist clinic can be useful for severe PMS, for complex cases, or when considering one of the more specialized treatments discussed below. Menopause clinics may also see women with PMS; it is useful to check what facilities are available locally. Simply referring women to a gynaecologist may be unhelpful unless the gynaecologist has an interest in PMS and is sympathetic to the problem.

### Selective serotonin re-uptake inhibitors (SSRIs)

These drugs have had a significant impact on the treatment of depression in recent years. The symptom overlap between depression and PMS has been pointed out (Roy-Byrne *et al.* 1987) and depression itself is often exacerbated premenstrually. Serotonin may play a role in PMS, particularly the affective and mood-related symptoms (Rapkin 1992) and therefore SSRIs have been studied for their possible efficacy in this disorder. Fluoxetine has been shown in well-conducted, randomized, double-blind, placebo-controlled trials to be effective in women with both general PMS (Menkes *et al.* 1992) and PMDD (Steiner 1995; Steiner *et al.* 1995). Women who experience predominantly mood-related and affective symptoms (including tension, irritability, and depressive symptoms) to a severe degree seem to be most helped by SSRIs, but even the physical symptoms are relieved by these drugs. There has now been a systematic review (Dimmock *et al.* 2000) that finds that SSRIs give significant improvement in overall symptoms compared with placebo. This included fluoxetine, sertraline, citalopram, paroxetine, and fluvoxamine. It is likely that the SSRIs will also be suitable for women with premenstrual exacerbation of underlying depression, but there are no studies of this so far.

Recent studies of intermittent (luteal) use of SSRIs suggest that this is also effective (Steiner *et al.* 1997). In one trial using citalopram, intermittent doses were *more* effective than continuous dose or placebo (Wikander *et al.* 1998). The improvement in symptoms is immediate, unlike the delay experienced when treating depression. This suggests a different mechanism of action. In general they are well tolerated but side effects can be unpleasant and include headache, nausea, insomnia, anxiety, and sexual dysfunction.

### Other antidepressants and anxiolytics

In randomized controlled trials (RCTs), the serotonergic tricyclic antidepressants clomipramine and nortryptiline were better than placebo for PMS but have significant side effects, which cause problems with adherence. They cause dry mouth, sedation, constipation, dizziness, and blurred vision. Other new non-SSRI antidepressants are under investigation. Lithium is ineffective. Anxiolytics such as alprazolam and buspirone have some positive effects and have been favoured in the USA. RCTs are mixed, so it remains unclear what role, if any, they should have in treating PMS. In Britain, the fear of tolerance, addiction, and withdrawal problems make them unacceptable to most women and their GPs for use in the long term.

## Prostaglandin inhibitors

Prostaglandin inhibitors are used widely for dysmenorrhoea and two double-blind, controlled trials of naproxen demonstrated relief of physical premenstrual symptoms related to pain but not of mood-related symptoms. Mefenamic acid has also been shown to relieve some PMS symptoms (Moline 1993). All RCTs available show an effect compared with placebo.

## Hormone treatments

These either attempt to abolish the menstrual cycle or to moderate hormonal fluctuations. Women often arrive at the surgery saying 'it must be a hormone imbalance, doctor'. Some informed patients may ask for hormone measurements. Unless the GP feels the woman may be menopausal or suffering from some other complaint such as a thyroid disorder, hormonal measurements are inappropriate. It is important to remember that apart from oral contraception, and the possible use of the progestogen-containing IUCD (IUS) in the future as an adjunct to oestrogen therapy, endocrine therapies cannot be guaranteed to prevent pregnancy.

## The combined oral contraceptive pill (COC)

Surprisingly few trials have examined the use of COCs for PMS although many women report relief while on the COC or first experience PMS after stopping the COC. Unfortunately, only RCTs will separate out the effects of the hormones from the effects of circumstances that lead women to use or cease using COCs. Three RCTs found no benefit over placebo. One found relief for bloating and breast pain. While some women have experienced an exacerbation of premenstrual symptoms with the COC, probably as the result of progestogens, many women, in practice, are helped. In women for whom PMS is exacerbated by anticipation of periods with pain and heavy bleeding, COCs, possibly used continuously for several months, will offer relief. The COC does offer the chance to regulate the timing of the cycle and to try another hormonal milieu. Many women need this effective method of contraception anyway. Further research may elucidate which combinations are most likely to be helpful.

## Oestrogen therapy, hormone replacement therapy (HRT)

Evidence from RCTs suggests that oestrogen relieves PMS. Magos *et al.* (1986) studied oestradiol implants, which abolished ovulation. There was a significant improvement in severe symptoms. Unfortunately, implants can cause problems with tachyphylaxis, so oestradiol patches were considered. An initial RCT using high doses showed that these were more effective than placebo in relieving most PMS symptoms (Watson *et al.* 1989). More recent work showed that 100 μg patches can control symptoms (Smith *et al.* 1995).

In clinical practice it is preferable to start at conventional HRT doses and work up from there until symptoms are controlled. Cyclical progestogen must be used in women who have a uterus. Different progestogens can be tried. Currently, dydrogesterone or medroxyprogesterone acetate look like being the least likely to cause PMS-type symptoms. Progestogen should probably be given for 10 days per month, but for women who find it really hard to tolerate, some gynaecologists working in the field are giving 7 days only. It is now possible to give oestrogen systemically while protecting the endometrium with a progestogen-containing IUCD (IUS). This has the advantage of minimal systemic absorption of progestogen, thereby circumventing the PMS-like side effects. The IUS is licensed for contraception at present but it has great potential for use in PMS. Studies are in progress to evaluate oestradiol patches in conjunction with the levonorgestrel IUCD for PMS.

Side effects of oestrogen include headaches, breast tenderness, bloating, and nausea. Patches may cause skin irritation, and there is a slight increased risk of breast cancer with long-term oestrogen use in menopausal women (see Chapter 3).

### Gonadotrophin-releasing hormone agonists (GnRH agonists)

GnRH agonists have been shown to be more effective than placebo in several well-conducted trials (Hammarback and Bäckström 1988). Ovulation is abolished and a menopausal state follows. Unfortunately, the induction of low oestrogen levels makes them unsuitable for long-term use because of the symptoms of the menopause (sweats and flushes, vaginal dryness) and the risk of osteoporosis. The bone loss caused by low oestrogen has been well documented (Dodin *et al.* 1991). These adverse effects can be counteracted by 'add-back' therapy with oestrogen and progestogen HRT. So much hormonal manipulation may seem drastic but women with severe PMS find life so intolerable that they will try anything. The best use for GnRH analogues may, however, be in making a definitive diagnosis of PMS in women who are suffering severely but for whom treatment does not appear to be working. Treatment with GnRH analogues is usually initiated in a specialist clinic rather than in general practice.

### Danazol (GnRH antagonist)

The advent of oestrogen therapy has relegated danazol very much to the sidelines in PMS treatment. Danazol is an anti-gonadotrophin and in large doses (400–800 mg daily) inhibits ovulation, thus alleviating PMS by abolishing the cycle. Most women find this dose intolerable because of side effects such as weight gain, acne, bloating, and hirsutism (Watts *et al.* 1987). In RCTs it is better than placebo and two trials of intermittent treatment (luteal phase) suggest some effect, particularly for breast pain. It should be prescribed under specialist supervision.

### Progesterone and progestogens

Many women are still being prescribed progesterone for PMS because Katerina Dalton has advocated it. Her books make interesting reading and she has done much to publicize the plight of women with PMS. However, results of well-conducted trials of progesterone (usually in the form of pessaries or suppositories) have been disappointing. A systematic review of 14 RCTs using progesterone against placebo and other treatments found no improvement in overall symptoms (Wyatt *et al.* 2000). For example, a double-blind crossover study of 168 women (Freeman *et al.* 1990) showed no difference between progesterone in a dose of 400 mg or 800 mg daily from day 16 to day 28 of the cycle and placebo. Adverse effects include abdominal pain, headache, dizziness, dysmenorrhoea, and excessive bleeding.

Although dydrogesterone has also been used in PMS, results of placebo-controlled trials are conflicting. Three out of seven RCTs found improvement using dydrogesterone, four showed no effect. Some women experience PMS-like symptoms when taking progestogen as part of HRT (Magos *et al.* 1986). Thus progesterone and progestogens have little place in the treatment of PMS at present.

### Tibolone

Two small RCTs show some evidence of benefit. One trial compared tibolone with placebo and the other with a vitamin supplement. No significant adverse effects were noted.

### Bromocriptine

None of the 14 RCTs showed any effect on overall symptoms but it does relieve breast tenderness. Bromocriptine has many side effects and thus is no longer used for PMS.

## Complementary treatments

Women have sought help for PMS from various complementary or alternative practitioners including acupuncturists, homeopaths, and herbalists. There is little systematic evidence for such treatments, but many offer considerable psychotherapeutic support alongside specific techniques. Some encourage lifestyle improvements as outlined above, though perhaps with a different rationale. The placebo response is likely to be large, but until such treatments are subject to controlled trials, the extent of treatment efficacy is unknown. There are some treatments that have been researched, usually in the realm of dietary supplements, that can be evaluated in conventional ways. These include pyridoxine, magnesium and calcium, evening primrose oil, vitex agnus castus fruit and chiropractic therapy. It should be remembered that some complementary treatments have significant adverse effects and risks, especially herbal remedies. Some Chinese herbal treatments and some dietary supplements contain potent substances that are not covered by the usual legal safeguards for pharmaceuticals. Women who are trying to conceive may not be made aware of the possible teratogenic effects of these substances.

## Nutritional supplements

### Pyridoxine (vitamin B6)

Trials of vitamin B6 have been of poor quality. A systematic review (Wyatt *et al.* 1999) found no high quality RCTs and three further RCTs gave conflicting results. Wyatt noted that none of the trials met the criteria for inclusion in a systematic review, so it remains an unevaluated treatment, but the trend from the existing studies suggest that the limited evidence is positive.

Whatever the evidence, it is usually the first treatment that women try as it is freely available without prescription. High doses (>200 mg/day) should be avoided because of the risk of peripheral neuropathy.

### Oil of evening primrose

One systematic review (Budeiri *et al.* 1996) conducted some time ago found eight RCTs of oil of evening primrose for PMS. The numbers involved in the studies and size of the effect were small. Therefore, there continues to be insufficient evidence for its use for general symptoms of PMS except for premenstrual breast tenderness for which the product is licensed in the UK.

### Mineral supplements

Magnesium, manganese, and calcium have been investigated in controlled trials for their usefulness in PMS. Results have been so mixed that it is hard to draw any conclusions from them.

### Vitex agnus castus extract

This plant extract is used by herbalists for control of premenstrual symptoms. A recent RCT (Schellenberg 2000) has suggested that it is indeed effective in relieving a range of PMS symptoms. It was well tolerated.

## Chiropractic therapy

One RCT has compared chiropractic therapy with placebo therapy and found benefit. However, there was a crossover and women who had placebo first got no better with subsequent chiropractic therapy.

## Surgical treatments

### Oophorectomy and hysterectomy

For women with extremely severe PMS, perhaps particularly for those who also have menstrual problems, oophorectomy and hysterectomy with subsequent oestrogen replacement therapy will result in a cure for PMS. RCTs confirm this and show a reduction in symptoms even with hysterectomy alone, though some women continue to experience the symptoms as ovulation continues. However, women and their GPs must make an informed decision about this, as it is a major step. The risks are those of a major operation and fertility is lost. Its use is rare and GPs may be mediators between women and gynaecologists to ensure that the best decision is made for a particular woman. No evidence is available for other surgical procedures such as laparoscopic oophorectomy or endometrial ablation.

# Conclusion

Premenstrual syndrome includes a wide range of physical and emotional changes which vary in severity, duration, and effects on a woman's life. It is unlikely that there is a single or simple cause, and any consideration of the aetiology of PMS must take into account psychological, physiological, and social factors. Management of PMS is not simple, but it is certainly aided by a greater understanding and acceptance of the problem and the development of a range of approaches and remedies. Women need to devote time to experiment to find an appropriate solution, and may require help from the primary health care team to evaluate how they can help themselves and, if necessary, what medical treatments might be useful. In any individual woman it is essential to determine whether or not she has PMS, what her main problems are, and the circumstances that led her to seek medical help. The first steps are sympathetic discussion of the problems and reorganization of aspects of her life to cope with times of feeling low. Attention to general health and lifestyle is the key to dealing with PMS. Following this, a woman may try a variety of self-help approaches, but may need to call upon the primary care team further to explore the range of effective treatments, both medical and non-medical.

If a woman is not helped by any of the approaches available in primary care, even more attention must be paid to correct diagnosis and what is going on in her life more widely. Referral to a specialist PMS clinic may be indicated. Gynaecologists vary in their interest in this topic but, as research is progressing rapidly in this field, it is a great boon for the team and the woman if up-to-date expert advice and treatment are available.

# Frequently asked questions

## Do I have PMS?

It is likely that you have PMS if you have distressing and disabling symptoms that appear in the premenstrual phase of your menstrual cycle, that are relieved by the onset of menstruation and you have at least a week post-menstrually with few or no symptoms. The pattern should bother you most months, though there can be a lot of variation. No symptoms are specific. It is easy to think that randomly changing symptoms have something to do with hormones even when they do not. There are no tests for it. Instead the doctor relies on you charting your symptoms every day so that the pattern of symptoms is written down for him or her to see. It is usually clear from such a diary whether you have 'pure' PMS, PMS on top of background symptoms which are there all month, or that the symptoms vary randomly. Doctors also try to avoid making an illness out of ordinary experiences, so if it does not bother you much it will not be called PMS.

## If this isn't PMS, what is it?

You can usually give the doctor some good ideas yourself. It could be stress at home or work, difficult relationships, or too much to do. You may not be looking after yourself properly and better and more regular meals, sleep, and fun times might be needed. You may be ill and a health check will reveal the problem. It could be that you have got so run down that you are depressed and then everything becomes dreary and difficult to manage. Your doctor will try to help you think about what is wrong.

## What works for PMS?

Many things have been tried for PMS. No single treatment is 100% effective, which may explain why so many things have been tried. It seems that actively managing your lifestyle to make it as balanced and healthy as possible can be very helpful. This is not easy for many women and may be why PMS becomes an issue when women have the most demands. It also helps to talk things through and to have a positive attitude. Women report they may benefit from aerobic exercise and extra vitamin B6. Some hormone treatments are known to help, and certain antidepressants, a painkiller called mefenamic acid, and herb extracts. If these don't help, gynaecologists can also try switching off the cycle (though this is usually only temporarily) and have a few other special hormone treatments to offer. In rare severe cases the womb and ovaries are removed surgically to stop the cycle for good.

## How can I help myself?

Careful recording of the symptoms and when they occur is the first step. With this knowledge you can then begin to predict difficult situations and prepare for them better.

Here are a few ideas. It may be that you get tired premenstrually. Some early nights may allow you to cope better as the period approaches. Perhaps you generally work through lunch and do not eat until evening. This will probably lead to more stress premenstrually, so book yourself lunch more often. Perhaps you are not doing much exercise. Exercise helps PMS, so plan to walk or cycle more or go to an exercise or dance class. If you need to, think seriously about cutting down on alcohol or cigarettes. Get out and have some fun. Have time to yourself. Meet up with friends. Talking to a friend or counsellor can enable you to see that you have some choice in how you manage your life and offer you vital encouragement to help you break unhelpful habits.

## What about hormones?

Hormones ought to be what PMS is all about. Yet there are no measurements of hormones that really give the doctor a good idea of what is happening for sufferers. Changing the balance of the hormones has some effect, but not all hormone supplements are truly effective. Oestrogen patches (the same as hormone replacement therapy, HRT) help many women, but it is not clear whether the combined oral contraceptive pill does or not. For women who need the Pill anyway, a change of type of Pill can improve PMS. It is worth a try. We know from many studies that progesterone suppositories (which used to be a real favourite) are no better than a sugar pill. It is probable that the contraceptive progesterone-only pill does not work very well either.

There are other special hormone treatments but they are fairly strong with lots of side effects. These are used by gynaecologists for the desperate sufferer!

### What about diet and vitamin supplements?

Lots of diets and supplements have been suggested for PMS. A healthy mixed diet is always sensible but there is no evidence that special foods cure PMS. The research into supplements is still limited but probably vitamin B6 helps (but don't take too high a dose), evening primrose oil helps breast tenderness, and extract of agnus castus fruit relieves symptoms.

## 10-Minute consultation

A woman comes to see you complaining of premenstrual syndrome (PMS). She has had it for years. It was less of a problem before her children arrived because she could arrange her life to suit the time of the month, but it has been getting harder to manage in the last few years. This is the first time she has consulted a doctor for it, though she has spoken with friends and tried vitamins and oil of evening primrose. Now she has come because she got so cross with her 12-year-old son when he refused to leave his computer game and come for tea, that she threw his meal in the bin. It was 2 days before her period was due. Now she is mortified that she lost her temper so completely. Her 14-year-old daughter told her to see the doctor.

### What issues you should cover

- Ask about the typical premenstrual symptoms – what they are, when they wax and wane, and which are most troublesome. Was this month's upset different from the usual pattern or simply had a more distressing outcome?
- Ask about her social situation.
- Ask about recent events and stressors. Is anything making life, as well as PMS, more difficult *now*.
- What does she know about PMS?
- What has she tried so far? How long did she persist with the strategy? Did it help?
- Has she any other medical needs? Consider particularly gynaecological complaints that may make PMS worse – heavy or irregular periods, painful periods, menopausal symptoms, dyspareunia, etc. Are her contraceptive needs met?
- Ask about psychological problems – does she have general low mood, tearfulness, anxiety, sleep disturbance, appetite change, and lack of enjoyment in life indicative of depressive illness?

- Ask what does she hope to get from the consultation?
- Clarify that you agree on a working definition of PMS – not specific symptoms but any that occur regularly in the premenstrual phase of the cycle with relief at menstruation and a week post-menstrually with few or no symptoms.

## What you should do?

- Acknowledge the perceived link between the symptoms and the cycle and remind her where appropriate of the possibility that many factors contribute to PMS complaint. Remind her that there are no magic answers but that she can play her part in learning how her body and mind reacts and what strategies improve her well-being.
- Show her a symptom diary and how to complete it. Stress its importance for understanding her pattern of symptoms and testing the effectiveness of advice and treatment.
- Outline suitable lifestyle changes if indicated and be sympathetic where these have been difficult to achieve. Note whether there is a general openness or hostility to your explorations of possible self-help. This will indicate whether she is open to trying to help herself or whether she hopes that medical management will fix things.
- Mention the possible role of her social situation, stressors, and relationships, if this has not already been covered.
- Mention a few possible treatments which you would consider. If she has already tried various measures, establish which of the remainder would be top of your list.
- Physical examination is only indicated if symptoms suggest other disorders.
- Investigations only as indicated, e.g. full blood count if tiredness, prominent dizziness, or excessively heavy periods.
- Plan to review after 2 months of diary keeping.
- Offer an opportunity to see the practice nurse (or counsellor) to discuss how diary keeping is going, how she is coping and whether she has been able to utilize any self-help advice. This might occur within a month and gives another opportunity to review general health (e.g. cervical smear) and be reminded of healthy lifestyle issues.

## Options for medical treatment

Ideally, medical treatments should come *after* diary keeping, but many women will simply not manage it so the following treatments remain as therapeutic tests for such women.

- ◆ Over the counter
  - (a) vitamin B6 (50–100 mg/day)
  - (b) agnus castus fruit extract
- ◆ Prescription
  - (a) oral contraceptive pill (or a different progestogen if already on it)
  - (b) mefenamic acid (for symptomatic days)
  - (c) oestrogen patches (HRT) plus cyclical oral progestogen (dydrogesterone) unless she has had a hysterectomy. Start at 50 μg patches twice weekly and increase over 2–4 months as required
  - (d) SSRIs
    - (i) fluoxetine or citalopram 20 mg only in luteal phase
    - (ii) fluoxetine or citalopram 20 mg continuously, particularly useful when (1) there is premenstrual exacerbation of underlying depression and anxiety, (2) the symptom pattern is unclear, (3) the patient still insists that a random pattern is PMS, (4) the patient has failed to respond to intermittent doses
- ◆ Specific symptoms
  - (a) pain: naproxen or mefenamic acid
  - (b) breast tenderness: oil of evening primrose
  - (c) bloating: spironolactone
  - (d) headaches: naproxen or mefenamic acid.

## Useful address

Women's Health
52 Featherstone Street, London EC1Y 8RT
Tel: 020 7251 6580

## References

American Psychiatric Association (1994). *Diagnostic and statistical manual of mental disorders*, 4th edn. Washington, DC.
Bäckström, T., Boyle, H. and Baird, D.T. (1981). Persistence of symptoms of premenstrual tension in hysterectomised women. *British Journal of Obstetrics and Gynaecology*, **88**, 530–6.

Blake, F. (1995). Cognitive therapy for premenstrual syndrome. *Cognitive and Behavioural Practice*, **2**, 167–85.

Blake, F., Gath, D., Salkovskis, P., *et al.* (1998). Cognitive therapy for the premenstrual syndrome: a controlled trial. *Journal of Psychosomatic Research*, **45**, 307–18.

Budeiri, D.J., Li, W.P. and Dornan, J.C. (1996). Is evening primrose oil of value in the treatment of the premenstrual syndrome? *Controlled Clinical Trials* **17**, 60–8.

Cockerill, I.M., Wormington, J.A. and Nevill, A.M. (1994). Menstrual cycle effect on mood and perceptual motor performance. *Journal of Psychosomatic Research*, **38**(7), 763–71.

Connelly, M. (2001). Premenstrual syndrome: an update on definitions, diagnosis and management. *Advances in Psychiatric Treatment*, **7**, 469–77.

Dimmock, P.W., Wyatt, K.M., Jones, P.W. and O'Brien, P.M. (2000). Efficacy of selective serotonin-reuptake inhibitors in premenstrual syndrome: a systematic review. *Lancet*, **356**, 1131–6.

Dodin, S., Lemay, A., Maheux, R., *et al.* (1991). Bone mass in endometriosis patients treated with GnRH agonist implant or danazol. *Obstetrics and Gynaecology*, **77**, 410–15.

Duckworth, H. (1990). *Premenstrual syndrome: your options.* Attic Press, Dublin.

Eriksson, E. (1999). Serotonin reuptake inhibitors in the treatment of premenstrual dysphoria. *International Clinical Psychopharmacology* **14**(S2), S27–33.

Frank, R.T. (1931). The hormonal causes causes of premenstrual tension. *Archives of Neurological Psychiatry*, **26**, 1053–7.

Freeman, E., Rickel, K., Sondhemer, S.J., *et al.* (1990). Ineffectiveness of progesterone suppository treatment for premenstrual syndrome. *Journal of the American Medical Association*, **264**, 349–53.

Halbreight, U. (1996). Premenstrual syndromes. In: *Psychiatric issues in women*, pp. 667–86. Baillière Tindall, London.

Hammarback, S. and Bäckström, T. (1988). Induced anovulation as a treatment of premenstrual tension syndrome – a double-blind crossover study with LRH agonist versus placebo. *Acta Obstetrica et Gynecologica Scandinavica*, **67**, 159–63.

Harrison, M. (1991). *Self help with PMS.* Macdonald Optima, London.

Hawton, K., Salkovskis, P.M., Kirk J. and Clark, D.M. (eds) (1989). *Cognitive behaviour therapy for psychiatric problems.* Oxford University Press, Oxford.

Kirkby, R.J. (1994). Changes in premenstrual symptoms and irrational thinking following cognitive-behaviour coping skills training. *Journal of Consulting and Clinical Psychology*, **62**, 1026–32.

Logue, C.M. and Moos, R.H. (1988). Positive perimenstrual changes: towards a new perspective on the menstrual cycle. *Journal of Psychosomatic Research*, **32**, 31–40.

Magos, A.L. (1990). Advances in the treatment of the premenstrual syndrome. *British Journal of Obstetrics and Gynaecology*, **97**, 7–10.

Magos, A.L., Brincat, M. and Studd, J.W.W. (1986). Treatment of premenstrual syndrome by subcutaneous oestradiol implants and cyclical oral norethisterone: placebo controlled study. *British Medical Journal*, **292**, 1629–33.

Menkes, D.B., Taghavi, E., Mason, P., *et al.* (1992). Fluoxetine treatment of severe premenstrual syndrome. *British Medical Journal*, **305**, 346–7.

Moline, M.L. (1993). Pharmacologic strategies for managing premenstrual syndrome. *Clinical Pharmacy*, **12**, 181–96.

O'Brien, P.M.S. (1987). *Premenstrual syndrome.* Blackwell, Oxford.

O'Brien, P.M.S. (1990). The premenstrual syndrome. *British Journal of Family Planning*, **15**(S), 13–18.

Rapkin, A.J. (1992). The role of serotonin in premenstrual syndrome. *Clinics in Obstetrics and Gynaecology*, **35**, 629–36.

Rapkin, A.J., Morgan, M., Goldman, L., *et al.* (1997). Progesterone metabolite allopregnanolone in women with premenstrual syndrome. *Obstetrics and Gynaecology*, **90**, 709–14.

Roca, C.A., Schmidt, P.J., Bolch,M., *et al.* (1996). Implications of endocrine studies of premenstrual syndrome. *Psychiatric Annals*, **26**, 576–80.

Rodin, M. (1992). The social construction of premenstrual syndrome. *Social Science and Medicine*, **35**, 49–56.

Roy-Byrne, P.P., Hoban, M.C. and Rubinoiw, D.R. (1987). The relationship of menstrually-related mood disorder to psychiatric disorders. *Clinics in Obstetrics and Gynaecology*, **30**, 386–95.

Sampson, G.A. (1989). Premenstrual syndrome. *Baillières Clinical Obstetrics and Gynaecology*, **3**, 687–704.

Sanders, D. (1985). *Coping with periods*. Chambers, Edinburgh.

Schellenberg, G. R. (2001). Treatment of premenstrual syndrome with Agnus Castus fruit extract: a prospective, randomized, placebo-controlled study. *British Medical Journal*, **322**, 134–8.

Smith, R.N.J., Studd, J.W.W., Zamblera, D. and Holland, E.F.N. (1995). A randomized comparison over 6 months of 100 mg and 200 mg twice-weekly doses of transdermal oestradiol in the treatment of severe premenstrual syndrome. *British Journal of Obstetrics and Gynaecology*, **102**, 475–84.

Steiner, M. (1995). Intermittent fluoxetine dosing in the treatment of women with premenstrual dysphoria. *Psychopharmacological Bulletin*, **33**, 771–4.

Steiner, M., Steinberg, S. and Stewart, D. (1995). Fluoxetine in the management of premenstrual dysphoria. *New England Journal of Medicine*, **332**, 1529–34.

Steiner, M., Kovzekwa, M., Lamont, J. *et al.* (1997). Intermittent fluoxetine dosing in the treatment of women with premenstrual dysphoria. *New England Journal of Medicine*, **332**, 1529–34.

Watson, N.R., Studd, J.W.W., Savvas, M., *et al.* (1989). Treatment of severe premenstrual syndrome with oestradiol patches and cyclical norethisterone. *Lancet*, **2**, 730–2.

Watts, J.F., Butt, W.R. and Logan-Edwards, R. (1987). A clinical trial using danazol for the treatment of premenstrual tension. *British Journal of Obstetrics and Gynaecology*, **94**, 30–4.

Wikander, I., Sundblad, C., Andersch, B., *et al.* (1998). Citalopram in premenstrual dysphoria: is intermittent treatment during luteal phases more effective than continuous treatment throughout the cycle? *Journal of Clinical Psychopharmacology*, **18**(5), 390–8.

Wyatt, K.M., Dimmock, P.W. and O'Brien, P.M.S. (1999). Vitamin B6 therapy: a systematic review of its efficacy in the premenstrual syndrome. *British Medical Journal*, **318**, 1375–81.

Wyatt, K.M., Dimmock, P.W., Jones, P.W. and O'Brien, P.M.S. (2000). Progesterone therapy: a systematic review of its efficacy in the premenstrual syndrome. *Neuropharmacology*, **23**, S2.

Chapter 3

# The menopause and hormone replacement therapy

Elizabeth Barrett-Connor

## Introduction and definitions

Natural menopause is the permanent cessation of menstruation resulting from the loss of ovarian follicular activity. It is confirmed after 12 consecutive months of amenorrhoea for which there is no other obvious cause. The average age at natural menopause, about 51 years, has been constant for centuries. A majority of women experience natural menopause between ages 45 and 55 years. Cigarette smoking, a vegetarian diet, and simple hysterectomy are each associated with an earlier (by 1–2 years) average age at menopause. Premature menopause (last menstrual period before age 40) can follow bilateral oophorectomy, chemotherapy, or radiation (i.e. induced menopause), or be caused by premature ovarian failure.

The menopause transition (perimenopause) is usually defined as the interval before menopause when hormone levels fluctuate and fall. When the menopause transition begins depends on its definition: reduced fertility typically begins about 10 years before the last menstrual period, hormone changes are apparent about 8 years before the last menstrual period, and menstrual irregularities with or without vasomotor symptoms, disturbed sleep, and mood changes usually begin about 4 years before the last menstrual period.

Postmenopause describes the years after the menopause. Late postmenopause, defined as 10 or more years after the last menstrual period, is more important than chronological age for conditions that are clearly related to low postmenopausal oestrogen levels, such as osteoporosis.

## The perimenopause

### Hormone changes and their utility for diagnosis of menopause

During the menopause transition, the ovaries produce less and less oestradiol and progesterone, causing an increase in follicle-stimulating hormone (FSH), and a later lesser increase in luteinizing hormone (LH) levels. After the menopause, levels of circulating oestrogen (mainly oestrone, average concentration 20 pg/ml) are much lower and are derived from the peripheral aromatization of adrenal androgens, not from the ovary. The low blood levels of oestradiol (average 13 pg/ml) in postmenopausal women are not further reduced by oophorectomy.

Although the postmenopausal ovary does not produce oestrogen, it does produce testosterone. Testosterone levels are only slightly lower in postmenopausal women with intact ovaries than in premenopausal women. Testosterone levels are much lower in women who have had bilateral oophorectomy, and somewhat lower after hysterectomy with ovarian conservation.

The menopause transition can be diagnosed clinically in the majority of women based on age, menstrual pattern, and vasomotor symptoms. Oestradiol levels are not diagnostic because striking episodic increases in oestradiol occur during this period, and postmenopausal levels may not be seen until 6 months or longer after the onset of amenorrhoea. Two serum FSH levels greater than 30 IU/ml obtained at least one month apart document that ovarian function has ceased, but this test is rarely necessary unless the woman is less than 40 years of age, has hot flushes after a hysterectomy with one ovary conserved, or her oophorectomy status is unknown. Evaluation of menopause-like symptoms accompanied by menstrual irregularities or amenorrhoea in a sexually active heterosexual woman of reproductive age should include a pregnancy test.

### Symptoms

Some women sail through the menopause with no complaints; others are miserable; and most have symptoms that are somewhat bothersome. More severe symptoms follow an induced menopause. Not all symptoms that occur during the menopause transition are due to hormone changes; symptoms may in reality reflect problems with work, personal relationships, inadequate social supports, or another medical condition. The only symptoms unequivocally associated with oestrogen deficiency are those that have been consistently shown to respond better to oestrogen than to placebo in clinical trials – these are vasomotor and urogenital symptoms. Other common symptoms including mood swings, depression, and disturbed sleep are less consistently improved by oestrogen in controlled clinical trials.

Specific symptoms and their severity vary by ethnicity and culture, even within countries. For example, the Study of Women's Health Across the Nation (SWAN) in the USA found that Japanese- and Chinese-American women reported menopause symptoms less frequently than Americans of northern European ancestry, while African-American women reported more vasomotor symptoms and vaginal dryness (Gold *et al.* 2000). In another North American study, symptoms were more common in women of lower socioeconomic status, women who smoked cigarettes, women who were less physically active, and (contrary to popular opinion) in overweight women (Greendale *et al.* 1998). In a study of Australian women, hot flushes were reported by 27%, night sweats by 17%, vaginal dryness by 17%, and trouble sleeping by 17% (Dennerstein *et al.* 2000).

## Menses

During the menopause transition, ovarian follicles become less sensitive to circulating gonadotrophins, shortening the follicular phase and the menstrual cycle length. Nearly all women experience changes in menstrual cycles for 4–8 years before menopause, and any menstrual pattern is possible. Cycles become irregular and bleeding may be increased or decreased. Heavy, painful, or irregular bleeding may reflect stimulation of the endometrium by unopposed oestrogen. Sometimes women of late reproductive age miss several menstrual periods and then restart apparently normal menses.

## Vasomotor symptoms

A hot flush (also called a hot flash) is a sudden wave of heat sensation, typically spreading over the upper body and face. The aetiology of hot flushes is unknown. In the USA and UK, about 30% of still regularly cycling women as young as age 35 report hot flushes. At some point in the menopause transition, hot flushes are experienced by about 75% of women. Without oestrogen therapy, hot flushes typically become less severe but persist for several years. Some women continue to report hot flushes in old age. Severe hot flushes can cause embarrassing visible changes in skin colour and sweating. Severe night sweats require change of bedding and interfere with sleep.

## General overview of hormone replacement therapy (HRT)

Oestrogen is the treatment of choice for women who seek relief from vasomotor symptoms. At least 40 randomized controlled clinical trials have shown that

HRT reduces the severity of vasomotor symptoms, often with improvement beginning within the first week (Rymer and Morris 2000). Transdermal oestradiol, intranasal 17β-oestradiol spray, and oral oestrogen are equally effective. Standard oestrogen products and doses are shown in Table 3.1.

Women prescribed oestrogen who have an intact uterus must take a progestogen for a minimum of 12 days per month or daily in order to prevent endometrial hyperplasia and cancer. Doses shown in Table 3.1 protect the endometrium. Approximately 70% of women given oestrogen with cyclical progestogens will have predictable cyclical bleeding as long as this treatment is continued. Continuous combined oestrogen plus progestogen causes unpredictable light spotting or bleeding, which ceases in the first year of treatment in 90%. Young women may prefer cyclical regimens to avoid unpredictable bleeding, whereas older women usually prefer continuous regimens without cyclical bleeding. Women with a longer duration since menopause have less bleeding when beginning HRT. Regimens combined in one tablet or patch (Table 3.1) offer convenience and the added safety of ensuring that the progestogen is taken. A well-referenced review of HRT prescription options has been published (McNagny 1999).

**Table 3.1** Range of hormone replacement therapy for menopause symptom management

| Type | Name | Oestrogen | Progestogen | Form |
|------|------|-----------|-------------|------|
| Sequential combined therapy | Adgyn Combi | Oestradiol (2 mg) | Norethisterone (1 mg) | Tabs |
| | Climagest | Oestradiol (1 mg, 2 mg) | Norethisterone (1 mg) | Tabs |
| | Cyclo-progynova | Oestradiol (1 mg, 2 mg) | Levo/norgestrel (0.25 mg/0.5 mg) | Tabs |
| | Elleste Duet | Oestradiol (1 mg, 2 mg) | Norethisterone (1 mg) | Tabs |
| | Estracombi | Oestradiol (50 μg) | Norethisterone (0.25 mg) | Patches |
| | Estrapak | Oestradiol (50 μg) | Norethisterone (1 mg) | Patches + Tabs |
| | Evorel-Pak | Oestradiol (50 μg) | Norethisterone (1 mg) | Patches + Tabs |

**Table 3.1** (*continued*)

| Type | Name | Oestrogen | Progestogen | Form |
|------|------|-----------|-------------|------|
| | Evorel Sequi | Oestradiol (50 µg) | Norethisterone (170 µg) | Patches |
| | Femapak | Oestradiol (40 µg, 80 µg) | Dydrogesterone (10 mg) | Patches + Tabs |
| | Femoston | Oestradiol (1 mg, 2 mg) | Dydrogesterone (10 mg) | Tabs |
| | Femoston 2/20 | Oestradiol (2 mg) | Dydrogesterone (20 mg) | Tabs |
| | Nuvelle | Oestradiol (2 mg) | Levonorgestrel (75 µg) | Tabs |
| | Nuvelle TS | Oestradiol (50 µg, 80 µg) | Levonorgestrel (20 µg) | Patches |
| | Premique Cycle | Conj.oestrogens (0.625 mg) | Medroxy progesterone (10 mg) | Tabs |
| | Prempak-C | Conj. oestrogens (0.625, 1.25 mg) | Norgestrel (150 µg) | Tabs |
| | Tridestra | Oestradiol (2 mg) | Medroxy progesterone (20 mg) | Tabs |
| | Trisequens | Oestradiol (2 mg, 2 mg, 1 mg; 4 mg, 4 mg, 1 mg) | Norethisterone (1 mg) | Tabs |
| Continuous combined therapy | Climesse | Oestradiol (2 mg) | Norethisterone (0.7 mg) | Tabs |
| | Elleste Duet Conti | Oestradiol (2 mg) | Norethisterone (1 mg) | Tabs |
| | Evorel Conti | Oestradiol (50 µg) | Norethisterone (170 µg) | Patches |
| | Femoston Conti | Oestradiol (1 mg) | Dydrogesterone (5 mg) | Tabs |
| | Indivina | Oestradiol (1 mg, 2 mg) | Medroxy progesterone (2.5 mg, 5 mg) | Tabs |
| | Kliofem | Oestradiol (2 mg) | Norethisterone (1 mg) | Tabs |

**Table 3.1** (*continued*)

| Type | Name | Oestrogen | Progestogen | Form |
|------|------|-----------|-------------|------|
| | Kliovance | Oestradiol (1 mg) | Norethisterone (0.5 mg) | Tabs |
| | Nuvelle Continuous | Oestradiol (2 mg) | Norethisterone (1 mg) | Tabs |
| | Premique | Conj. oestrogens (0.625 mg) | Medroxy progesterone (5 mg) | Tabs |
| Gonado-mimetic | Livial | Tibolone (2.5 mg) | | Tabs |
| Unopposed oestrogen (if uterus is intact, progestogen *must* be used) | Adgyn Estro | Oestradiol (2 mg) | | Tabs |
| | Aerodiol | Oestradiol (150 μg) | | Spray |
| | Climaval | Oestradiol (1 mg, 2 mg) | | Tabs |
| | Dermestril | Oestradiol (25, 50, 100 μg) | | Patches |
| | Dermestril September | Oestradiol (25, 50, 75 μg) | | Patches |
| | Elleste Solo | Oestradiol (1 mg, 2 mg) | | Tabs |
| | Elleste Solo MX | Oestradiol (40, 80 μg) | | Patches |
| | Estraderm MX | Oestradiol (25, 50, 100 μg) | | Patches |
| | Estraderm TTS | Oestradiol (25, 50, 100 μg) | | Patches |
| | Evorel | Oestradiol (25, 50, 75, 100 μg) | | Patches |
| | Fematrix | Oestradiol (40 μg, 80 μg) | | Patches |
| | FemSeven | Oestradiol (50, 75, 100 μg) | | Patches |
| | Harmogen | Oestrone (0.93 mg) | | Tabs |
| | Hormonin | Oestriol oestradiol /oestrone (1 strength) | | Tabs |

**Table 3.1** (*continued*)

| Type | Name | Oestrogen | Progestogen | Form |
|---|---|---|---|---|
| | Menorest | Oestradiol (37.5, 50, 75 μg) | | Patches |
| | Menoring | Oestradiol (50 μg) | | Vaginal ring |
| | Oestrogel | Oestradiol (1.5 mg) | | Gel |
| | Premarin | Conj. oestrogens (0.625, 1.25 mg) | | Tabs |
| | Progynova | Oestradiol (1 mg, 2 mg) | | Tabs |
| | Progynova TS | Oestradiol (50, 100 μg) | | Patches |
| | Sandrena | Oestradiol (0.5 mg, 1 mg) | | Gel |
| | Zumenon | Oestradiol (1 mg, 2 mg) | | Tabs |
| Progestogens | Adgyn Medro | | Medroxy progesterone (5 mg) | Tabs |
| | Crinone | | Progesterone (4%) | Vaginal gel |
| | Duphaston HRT | | Dydrogesterone (10 mg) | Tabs |
| | Micronor HRT | | Norethisterone (1 mg) | Tabs |

A commonly used HRT in the UK and USA is conjugated equine oestrogen (0.625 mg) given alone to women who have had a hysterectomy or in combination with progesterone for at least 12 days per cycle to women with a uterus. This combined daily regimen was used in the Heart and Estrogen/Progestin Replacement Study (HERS), the largest published controlled clinical trial of HRT and symptoms, which included 2763 women aged 44–79 years. Among HERS women who reported severe hot flushes at baseline, 85% had improved after one year of hormone therapy (Prempro) compared to 48% of women on placebo (Hlatky *et al.* 2002). Nevertheless, nearly all women said their hot flushes had not completely resolved. Among women who reported trouble sleeping before treatment, a similar low proportion on HRT (37%) and placebo (33%) reported improvement after one year.

The lowest effective dose of oestrogen is presumably the safest dose (although there is no convincing evidence of a dose–response effect for cancer risk). For years the standard dose of oestrogen was 0.625 mg/day of Premarin or its equivalent, based on bone maintenance (Table 3.1). It is now clear that many women have satisfactory symptom relief, bone preservation, and less bleeding with half this dose. For example, in one trial (Utian *et al.* 2001) conducted in women who reported 8–10 hot flushes per day, daily Premarin doses of 0.625, 0.45, or 0.3 mg in combination with medroxyprogesterone acetate (MPA) (at doses of 2.5 or 1.5 mg/day) were equally effective in reducing the severity and number of hot flushes in the first year of treatment; when oestrogen was given without a progestogen, however, the 0.625 dose was more effective than the lower doses. But in another trial of norethindrone plus ethinyl oestradiol (femhrt®) in women who reported at least 10 hot flushes a week, there was a dose-related decrease in hot flush frequency and severity with the best response at the highest dose (Speroff *et al.* 2000).

Women with premature ovarian failure or induced menopause may need higher doses for symptom relief. Some, but not all, studies suggest that adding testosterone to oestrogen reduces the oestrogen dose necessary to relieve hot flushes after induced menopause (Rymer and Morris 2000). After women reach the age of natural menopause, some can be encouraged to reduce the dose gradually to the lowest level compatible with their symptoms.

Some women respond well to one dose, drug, or route of administration when another regimen is unacceptable. It is unknown whether differing responses reflect differences in therapy or differences in women. Not all women prescribed HRT feel wonderful, and a majority quit therapy within 2 years. Bleeding, breast pain, and fear of cancer are frequent reasons for non-adherence. On the other hand, women who abruptly stop hormones after years of use (for example, in response to news headlines about oestrogen's risks) often restart – in order to 'feel like their old selves' again. Oestrogen side effects and contraindications to HRT are shown in Table 3.2.

**Table 3.2** HRT side effects and contraindications

| Side effects of short-term HRT | Contraindications to HRT |
| --- | --- |
| Mastalgia | Pregnancy |
| Heavy bleeding | History of deep vein thrombosis or embolism |
| Bloating | Breast cancer* |
| Headaches | Uterine cancer* |
| Gallbladder disease | |
| Deep vein thrombosis and embolism | |

*Partial contraindication.

# Alternative treatment for vasomotor symptoms

Tibolone is a synthetic steroid that is inactive until metabolized to products with oestrogenic, progestogenic, and androgenic activity. Tibolone does not stimulate the endometrium and is therefore not prescribed with a progestogen. In a large clinical trial (Hammar *et al.* 1998), tibolone was as effective as continuous HRT (17β-oestradiol 2 mg plus norethisterone acetate 1 mg) for hot flushes, sweating, and vaginal dryness; the bleeding pattern was superior, in that almost no women had bleeding or spotting after the third month of tibolone, compared with an average of 7 months of bleeding with HRT.

Other prescription medications shown in clinical trials to relieve hot flushes include high-dose medroxyprogesterone acetate (MPA) (20 mg/day) or megestrol acetate (20 mg b.i.d.) (used for breast cancer patients), selective serotonin reuptake inhibitors including sertraline, venlafaxine (25 mg/day) and paroxetine; the antihypertensive clonidine, either oral (0.1–0.4 mg/day) or transdermal (0.1 mg/day); and veralipride 100 mg per day (used in patients treated with GnRH agonists) (Freeman 2001).

## Complementary management of vasomotor symptoms

Many women wanting to avoid oestrogen seek 'natural' relief of symptoms. Black cohosh extract is now available in teas and tablets; the most favourable clinical trial results are reported for a German quality-controlled product, Remifemin. A dose of 40 mg twice a day compares favourably with a standard dose of oestrogen for relief of menopause symptoms. Clinical trials have not shown that dong quai or evening primrose oil (gamolenic acid) is more effective than placebo for the treatment of hot flushes. Vitamin E has only a small benefit (about one fewer hot flush per day).

The infrequency of hot flushes reported by Asian women has been attributed to phyto-oestrogens in their high soya diet, but clinical trials show mixed results. For example, one study of 94 women found no significant difference in symptoms after 3 months of treatment with phyto-oestrogen-rich soya supplements compared with casein placebo (Kotsopoulous *et al.* 2000), but another study of similar size and duration found isolated soya protein reduced hot flushes by 45%, compared to a 30% reduction in women treated with casein ($P < 0.01$) (Albertazzi *et al.* 1998). Different results may relate to differences in women (not all women absorb phyto-oestrogens equally well) or differences in the products tested.

Some small lifestyle changes may be helpful, including wearing layered clothing that can be removed as necessary; reducing the intake of spicy foods, caffeine and alcohol; not smoking; and increasing physical activity.

## Quality of life, mood, and depression

Randomized placebo-controlled trials of less than two years duration have reported improved quality of life (estimated by standard quantitative tests) in oestrogen-treated women (Rymer and Morris 2000). This benefit is only clearly documented in women who have vasomotor symptoms (Skarsgard *et al.* 2000). In a recent publication from the HERS trial, women treated with Prempro who had no menopause symptoms at baseline reported less vigor and well being than women on placebo (Hlatky *et al.* 2002).

The relation of oestrogen to depressed mood during the menopause transition is controversial. A 1995 review of 14 clinical trials (Zweifel and O'Brien 1997) concluded that oestrogen therapy improved depressed mood during the menopause transition or after oophorectomy, but most of these trials included women with vasomotor symptoms and impaired sleep. Women with clinical depression do not usually improve on standard oestrogen regimens. However, very high doses of transdermal oestradiol may provide significant benefit, as suggested by small short trials (Schmidt *et al.* 2000; Soares *et al.* 2001).

Progestogens may worsen perimenopausal depressive symptoms (Halbreich 1997). Women who had premenstrual syndrome before menopause are more likely to have negative mood effects during the progestogen phase of HRT (Bjorn *et al.* 2000). A trial of progestogen withdrawal should be considered for any woman who becomes depressed after starting HRT.

St Johns Wort has been recommended as an alternative therapy for menopausal depression, based on a meta-analysis of 23 trials in 1757 women with depressive disorders (Linde *et al.* 1996); the authors concluded that St John's Wort was superior to placebo and comparable to standard antidepressant medication; Linde and Mulrow's subsequent review of 27 trials in 2291 women reported similar results (Linde and Mulrow 2002). By contrast, two other clinical trials in a total of 540 women with major depression found no benefit (Shelton *et al.* 2001; Hypericum Depression Trial Study Group 2002).

### Headaches

Women may report either increases or decreases in migraine frequency or severity with menopause or hormone therapy. Women who had few or mild headaches premenopause report worsening with HRT (Silberstein 2000). One clinical trial reported a significant increase in the frequency and duration of migraines after oral but not transdermal oestrogen and no effect of HRT on tension headaches (Nappi *et al.* 2001).

# Weight gain

Weight gain is common during the menopause transition, and has been attributed to both oestrogen deficiency and oestrogen therapy. A quantitative review (Norman *et al.* 2001) of 22 randomized controlled trials found no evidence that postmenopausal oestrogen alone or with a progestin promotes or prevents weight gain. A clinical trial has shown that weight gain during the menopause transition *can* be prevented by diet and exercise (Kuller *et al.* 2001): premenopausal women were randomly assigned to an intervention of reduced saturated fat plus increased physical activity or to assessment only; after the menopause transition, weight had decreased 0.2 lb in the intervention group and increased 5.2 lb in the control group, and waist circumference had decreased 2.9 cm compared to 0.5 cm in the control group.

# Sexuality, urogenital symptoms, and libido

## Genital complaints

After the menopause, the urogenital mucosa becomes thinner, less elastic, and less vascular. By late menopause the vagina is shortened and narrowed, with a thin, friable surface. Vulvovaginal symptoms, which do not necessarily parallel clinical findings, include dryness, pruritis, discharge, dyspareunia, and post-coital bleeding. Nevertheless, many older women report a satisfactory sex life without HRT. In the Massachusetts Women's Health Study (Avis *et al.* 2000), factors such as marital status and sexual dysfunction of partner, physical and mental health, and cigarette smoking had a greater impact on sexual functioning than menopause status.

Oral, transdermal, and intravaginal oestrogen (cream, tablet, or vaginal ring) have been shown to relieve vaginal symptoms in at least ten randomized placebo-controlled trials (Cardozo *et al.* 1998). Among HERS women treated with oral oestrogen, 61% on HRT and 47% on placebo reported improvement in genital dryness (Hulley *et al.* 1998).

Topical oestrogen appears to be more effective for vaginal dryness than oral oestrogen and may be required *in addition to systemic oestrogen* in some women. A vaginal ring containing 2 mg of oestradiol can be inserted by the patient or health-care provider once every 3 months. Oestradiol tablets (oestradiol hemihydrate – Vagifem) are inserted vaginally daily for 2 weeks and twice a week thereafter. Oestradiol or Premarin creams can be applied by plastic applicator or finger one to three times a week. The vaginal ring and tablets do not increase circulating oestrogen levels, and are considered safe for breast cancer survivors, although some oestrogen is systemically absorbed

**Table 3.3** Topical oestrogen preparations for atrophic vaginitis*

| Preparation | Administration | Comment |
|---|---|---|
| Conjugated oestrogen (0.625 mg) Premarin Vaginal Cream | 0.5–2 g/day intravaginally | Reduce to one-half initial dosage over 1–2 weeks to maintain vaginal mucosa at the lowest possible dose |
| Oestriol (0.01%) Ortho-Gynest Vaginal Cream | Initial: 1–2 applicatorsful/day for 1–2 weeks  Maintenance: 1 applicatorful 1–3 times/week | Reduce to one-half initial dosage over 1–2 weeks to maintain vaginal mucosa at the lowest possible dose |
| Oestriol (0.1%) Ovestin Vaginal Cream | Initial: 2–4 g daily for 1–2 weeks  Maintenance: 1 g 1–3 times/week | Reduce to one-half initial dosage over 1–2 weeks to maintain vaginal mucosa at the lowest possible dose |
| Oestradiol (25 μg) Vagifem | Initial: 1 tablet inserted vaginally once daily at same time each day  Maintenance: 1 tablet inserted vaginally twice weekly | |
| Oestradiol ring (75 μg)† Estring | Insert ring into upper one-third of vaginal vault | Keep in place continuously for 3 months, then remove and replace with new ring |

*Attempt to discontinue or taper medication at 3- to 6-month intervals.
†The only topical oestrogen therapy for which there is no evidence of endometrial stimulation.

(Table 3.3 lists topical oestrogen preparations). For women who wish to avoid oestrogen, vaginal dryness can be managed with vaginal moisturizers and lubricants. Replens decreases vaginal pH, as does oestrogen.

## Libido

Although adequate lubrication can improve arousal and orgasm, there is no evidence that reduced sexual desire with onset during the menopause transition is caused by oestrogen deficiency or improved by oestrogen replacement. In fact, oral oestrogen increases sex hormone binding globulin, which can then reduce bioavailable testosterone (Slater *et al.* 2001). In two clinical trials, oestrogen plus testosterone improved sexual enjoyment, desire, and arousal more than oestrogen alone (Rymer and Morris 2000). Testosterone regimens shown to improve libido produce circulating testosterone levels above the physiological range, with potential side effects of acne, facial hair, and deepening of the voice. Trials of low-dose testosterone patches are under way. Tibolone, an oestrogen substitute with androgenic effects, has been shown in clinical trials to improve vaginal dryness, libido, and sexual satisfaction.

## Urinary complaints

Urinary tract symptoms attributed to oestrogen deficiency include dysuria, frequency, nocturia, stress incontinence, urge incontinence, coital incontinence, and urinary tract infection. Of these only the frequency of *recurrent* urinary tract infection has been shown in clinical trials to be reduced by oestrogen treatment, presumably by reversing the postmenopausal decrease in vaginal flora and increase in vaginal pH caused by lack of oestrogen (Raz and Stamm 1993; Eriksen 1999). However, HRT did not prevent urinary tract infections in women without a prior history of urinary tract infections (Brown *et al.* 2001).

There is no good evidence that HRT protects against stress or urge incontinence. In the largest reported trial, women assigned to oestrogen plus a progestogen reported *increased* incontinence compared to women assigned to placebo (Grady *et al.* 2001).

# Hormone replacement therapy to prevent chronic diseases

The last 25 years was a time of great enthusiasm for the concept of oestrogen deficiency diseases, and the potential of HRT to prevent diverse conditions that are common in later life. Observational studies reported that women using

HRT had fewer fractures, less heart disease, less colon cancer, and less dementia, but other factors could explain some or all of these putative benefits
(Barrett-Connor and Grady 1998). For example, women physicians in Britain
with continued hormone use are more likely than non-hormone-using physicians to report a healthy diet and vigorous physical activity (Issacs *et al.* 1997).
Only randomized, placebo-controlled clinical trials that control for the effects
of known and unknown differences between women who chose to take or continue hormones can provide the basis of 'evidence-based medicine'. Nowhere
has the importance of clinical trials been so evident as in recent HRT trials
where results differed from expectations, as discussed below.

## Osteoporosis and fractures

### Bone loss

Osteoporosis is due to imbalance between bone formation and bone resorption, leading to loss of bone quantity and quality. Throughout life there is
constant removal and replacement of bone in myriad small bone remodelling
units on bone surfaces. Low bone mineral density (and even osteoporotic
fractures) can occur before the menopause in young women with anorexia
nervosa or extreme physical activity. In these young women, amenorrhoea is a
classical feature of malnutrition-related bone loss, which is usually reversible
with adequate nutrition.

The balance between bone formation and bone resorption is disturbed
during the menopause transition before menses cease when FSH levels are
high but oestrogen levels are relatively normal. Bone loss is often accelerated
for several years after menopause, averaging 2% per year (range <1%–5%),
after which there is a steady slow bone loss of about 0.5%/year; however,
some women show little change in bone mineral density after menopause
(Greendale *et al.* 2000). With advanced age, bone loss accelerates, reflecting
immobility, illness, poor nutrition, or secondary hyperparathyroidism due to
vitamin D deficiency.

### Peak bone mass

The age when a woman has osteoporotic bone levels depends on her peak bone
mass and the rate of bone loss after menopause. The age when peak bone mass
is achieved is uncertain, but is thought to be between 20 and 30. Peak bone
mass is determined in part by small effects of multiple genes, birth weight,
childhood growth and development, not smoking, a diet adequate in protein
and calcium, and weight-bearing physical activity. Women of African heritage
tend to have higher peak bone mass and women of Asian heritage tend to have

lower peak bone mass than Caucasian women. Women who have poor diet and sedentary habits in youth and young adulthood never attain their potential peak bone mass.

## Fracture risk

Fracture risk increases with age and is also closely related to bone density, bone connectivity, body size, and the propensity to fall. A 50-year-old white woman has a 15% lifetime risk of hip fracture, usually occurring after age 70; a 40% risk of at least one spine fracture, often by age 60; and a 15% risk of Colles fracture, typically before age 60. Wrist, spine, and hip fractures can each cause functional limitations. After a hip fracture, only one-third of women regain their prefracture level of function and independence, and one in five die within the year of fracture.

## Clinical diagnosis

### The patient with a fracture

Osteoporosis is usually unrecognized until the patient has a fracture. A prior low-trauma (non-vehicular) fracture by history or on spine x-ray is the most powerful risk factor for another fracture, increasing the risk of another fracture three- to fivefold, even when bone mineral density is not very low. A history of a non-vehicular fracture before menopause (ages 20–50) doubles the risk of a postmenopausal fracture (Wu *et al.* 2002).

Surgical treatment of the first fracture will not prevent the next fracture. When a woman has a low-trauma fracture after age 45, she should be presumed to have osteoporosis and should be considered for treatment with a bone-specific medication (Lindsay *et al.* 2001). Further evaluation is necessary only to exclude other pathology. Treatment with a bone-specific agent may also improve the outcome after hip replacement. Unfortunately, less than half of women receive medical treatment for osteoporosis after surgery for hip fracture.

### The patient without a fracture

**Medical history**   The two strongest risk factors for osteoporosis are age and low body weight. A family history of osteoporosis or hip fracture (mother, father or sibling) doubles the risk. Osteoporosis is more likely if the patient has been a cigarette smoker, consumed a diet low in dairy products, has a history of intentional or unintentional weight loss, immobilization, rheumatoid arthritis, or hyperthyroidism, or has chronically used thyroid hormone, cortisone, or anticonvulsants. (Use of sex hormones or diuretics is associated with better bone density.) Women of African descent generally have better bone density and fewer fractures, and Asian women tend to have poorer bone density but not necessarily more fractures than women of northern European origin.

*Medical examination*   Very thin women are at increased risk of low bone density and fractures. Weight loss, intentional or not, is associated with bone loss. Height and weight should be measured at each visit, and compared with previously measured or reported young adult height and weight. A height loss of more than 3 cm strongly suggests one or more vertebral fractures, which can be confirmed by lateral spine radiographs. Kyphosis with onset in late menopause (the dowager's hump) does not necessarily mean the patient has osteoporotic spine fractures and is often associated with osteoarthritis.

*x-Rays*   Because one-third of bone must be lost before osteoporosis is obvious on roentgenogram, a 'normal x-ray' does not rule out osteoporosis. Lateral spine films are useful if a vertebral fracture is suspected, but most bone pain is not due to a fracture and most spine fractures do not cause pain.

*Bone markers*   Blood and urine tests can provide information on bone turnover. They are not recommended for diagnosis but, because changes are seen much earlier, they are superior to bone density for determining response to treatment and may be available routinely in the future.

*Bone scans*   The gold standard for the diagnosis of osteoporosis is a bone density test of the hip or spine using dual energy x-ray absorptiometry (DEXA), technology with a high degree of precision. Ideally both hip and spine should be evaluated because women with osteoporosis at the spine may not show low bone density at the hip or vice versa. If only one site is scanned, the hip is the preferred site for the evaluation of older postmenopausal women because vertebral osteophytes often mask low bone density in the lumbar spine. Bone density of the lumbar spine is preferred for younger women (who do not usually have osteophytes), because bone loss progresses more rapidly and is visible earlier at the spine than the hip.

Dual energy x-ray absorptiometry of the hip or spine requires a large, expensive piece of equipment, limiting its use to specialty clinics. Low bone density at the distal wrist, forearm, or heel (which can be measured with much smaller, less expensive devices) predicts future fracture risk reasonably well (Siris *et al.* 2001). Broader use of these less expensive instruments should improve the ability to diagnose osteoporosis in general practice.

Whether and when to measure bone density is controversial. In the USA, a bone density test is recommended for all women aged 65 and older, but other countries usually require additional risk factors before recommending a bone density test. Experts recommend bone mineral density measurements for relatively young postmenopausal women who have had an early menopause or other risk factors such as family history, excessive thinness, and cigarette smoking. Bone density has also been used to motivate women to accept therapy and to monitor response to therapy. Bone density is a better motivator than monitor, because bone density changes slowly, and relates poorly to change in fracture risk. A repeat bone scan to monitor treatment should be postponed until at least 2 years have passed since therapy was initiated.

*Interpretation of bone density*    The Z-score is the number of standard deviations above or below the average bone mineral density (BMD) value for a woman of the same age. A T-score is the number of standard deviations above or below the average BMD for healthy young white women. The World Health Organization defines osteoporosis as a T-score at least 2.5 standard deviations below the mean T-score for a young adult reference sample. Every standard deviation of reduction in bone mineral density doubles the risk of fracture, that is, approximately −1 T-score or −1 Z-score. This is true whether central or peripheral bones are assessed (Siris *et al.* 2001).

Bone density is used to diagnose osteoporosis. To predict future fracture risk, bone density must be considered together with clinical risk factors, including the patient's years postmenopause, frailty, and propensity to fall. Risk factors for falls are shown in Table 3.4.

A fracture risk of 5% in the next year warrants bone-specific drug therapy. This level of risk is observed in elderly women who have had a vertebral fracture, women on high-dose corticosteroids, and in some women who have

**Table 3.4** Risk factors for falls

| Individual factors associated with falls | Environmental hazards |
|---|---|
| Limited vision | Poor lighting |
| Impaired cognition | Broken handrails |
| Balance problems | Ill-fitting or poorly soled shoes |
| Alcohol excess | Improperly fitted bathroom |
| Frailty, muscle weakness | Inadequate or poor use of assistive walking devices |
| Medications, particularly sedatives | Inconvenient storage |
| | Uneven or cluttered walking surfaces |
| | Wet or slippery floors |
| | Loose area rugs |
| | Lack of grab bars in tub, shower, near toilet |

very low BMD plus several clinical risk factors (Table 3.5 lists diseases and drugs associated with osteoporosis risk). Targeting women 65+ years of age who have multiple risk factors or who show clinical evidence of osteoporosis (height loss, fracture) makes more efficient use of limited medical resources by reducing the number needed to treat to prevent one fracture (Cauley *et al.* 2001b).

**Table 3.5** Diseases and drugs associated with risk of osteoporosis in adults

**Diseases**

| | |
|---|---|
| Acromegaly | Hyperparathyroidism |
| Adrenal atrophy and Addison's disease | Hypophosphatasia |
| Amyloidosis | Idiopathic scoliosis |
| Anoxoria nervosa | Immobilization/paralysis |
| Ankylosing spondylitis | Lymphoma and leukaemia |
| Athletic amenorrhoea | Malabsorption syndromes |
| Chronic obstructive pulmonary disease | Multiple myeloma |
| Congenital porphyria | Multiple sclerosis |
| Cushing's syndrome | Nutritional disorders |
| Diabetes mellitus (type 1) | Osteogenesis imperfecta |
| Endometriosis | Pernicious anaemia |
| Epidermolysis bullosa | Rheumatoid arthritis |
| Gastrectomy | Sarcoidosis |
| Gastric operations | Severe liver disease, especially primary biliary cirrhosis |
| Gonadal insufficiency (primary and secondary) | Thalassaemia |
| Haemochromatosis | Thyrotoxicosis |
| Haemophilia | Tumour secretion of parathyroid |
| Hyperadrenocorticism | hormone-related peptide |

**Drugs/Habits**

| | |
|---|---|
| Anticonvulsants | Heparin |
| Cigarette smoking | Lithium |
| Excessive alcohol | Methotrexate |
| Excessive thyroxine | Phenothiazines Retinol supplements |
| Glucocorticosteroids and adrenocorticotropin | Tamoxifen (premenopausal use) |
| Gonadotrophin-releasing hormone agonists | |

## Prevention and treatment of osteoporosis

Deciding whether and how to intervene involves assessment of short-term fracture risk and other non-skeletal health issues.

### Exercise

Although physical activity in youth is positively associated with peak bone mass, exercise in later life has probably only a modest effect on slowing bone loss. The benefits of resistance or weight-bearing physical activity are shown in clinical trials which include striking improvements in muscle strength and function and a reduced risk of falling (by about 25%) even in very old age.

### Calcium

Calcium intake must equal obligatory calcium loss to maintain calcium homeostasis and prevent bone loss. Without dairy products, the diet rarely provides more than 300 mg of calcium per day, less than the obligatory calcium loss from skin, urine, and stool. About 1200 mg of calcium per day is recommended for postmenopausal women without HRT. This requires increased consumption of milk products (each dairy portion contains approximately 300 mg), or other calcium-supplemented foods (such as calcium-supplemented orange juice, which is particularly useful for women with lactose intolerance), or calcium supplements. More than 20 clinical trials have shown that calcium supplements improve bone mineral density, especially in elderly women (Nordin 1997). Calcium alone is not sufficient to prevent fractures, however.

### Vitamin D

Vitamin D, primarily produced in the skin after exposure to sunlight, is necessary for optimal calcium absorption. Low Vitamin D levels are relatively common in winter, and year round in the elderly who no longer go outdoors. Physiological supplements of calciferol (400–800 mg/day) increase calcium absorption, prevent secondary hyperparathyroidism, and increase bone density at the femoral neck in the elderly (Dawson-Hughes et al. 1995; Ooms et al. 1995). Vitamin D supplementation of 600–800 IU/day is recommended for housebound women and for those 65 and older.

Evidence that vitamin D prevents fracture is mixed. Two large trials of vitamin D (plus adequate calcium) for fracture prevention in the elderly had contradictory results. One (Lips et al. 1996) found no difference in fracture rates in older Dutch men and women assigned to calciferol 400 IU/day or placebo. In England, a trial of 100 000 IU of oral vitamin D given every four months for two years reduced fracture risk by 22% (Trivedi et al. 2003).

## Oestrogen

Many controlled clinical trials have shown that postmenopausal oestrogen therapy increases bone mass moderately, whether begun at the time of the menopause or in old age. Oestrogen has several bone-sparing effects, increasing calcium absorption from the gut, reducing renal calcium loss, and directly reducing bone resorption. The greatest effects are seen at the spine. Bone density increases for the first 3 years of HRT, with no evidence of significant further gain (Greendale *et al.* 2000). Bone loss resumes when oestrogen is discontinued (Cauley *et al.* 2001b; Gallagher *et al.* 2002).

Transdermal and oral oestrogens have similar effects on bone density. Although bone augmentation is better at higher doses, a majority of healthy women maintain bone with as little as 0.3 mg of conjugated equine oestrogen or equivalent (half the previously recommended 0.625 mg/day) when oestrogen is taken with adequate calcium. Studies consistently show better bone preservation in women who take both oestrogen and calcium (Nieves *et al.* 1998). Oestrogen combined with cyclical or continuous medroxyprogesterone acetate or with cyclical progesterone does not improve bone density more than treatment with oestrogen alone (Marcus *et al.* 1999), but the addition of a more androgenic progestogen or testosterone may provide additional bone benefit.

Although oestrogen unquestionably preserves bone, until recently the strongest evidence that HRT prevents fractures was based on a systematic review of 22 trials of HRT, which found a 27% reduction in non-vertebral fracture risk (Torgerson and Bell-Syer 2001). Women in these trials did not have a diagnosis of osteoporosis based on low bone mineral density. In the large HERS trial, HRT did not reduce fracture risk in older women who had heart disease but not osteoporosis (Cauley *et al.* 2001a).

The recently reported Women's Health Initiative (WHI) is the first large trial to unequivocally show that HRT prevents fractures. In this trial, 16 608 women were assigned to placebo or conjugated equine oestrogen plus medroxyprogesterone acetate (Prempro); after 5 years HRT reduced the risk of all fractures by 24% and reduced the risk of hip fractures by 33% compared to placebo (Writing Group for the Women's Health Initiative Investigators 2002).

Unfortunately, the WHI reported an early excess of cardiovascular disease and a delayed excess of breast cancer (Fig 3.1), greatly reducing the potential use of HRT for fracture prevention because continued HRT is required for bone maintenance while HRT for 4 or more years promotes breast cancer (see below). Consensus is building that HRT (oestrogen plus a progestogen) should be used only by women with menopause symptoms and ideally for no more than 4 years after age 50. This conclusion does not necessarily apply to unopposed oestrogen. Another part of WHI is examining the

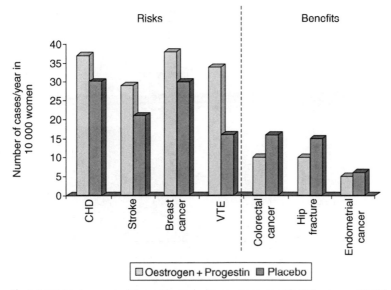

**Fig 3.1** WHI Estrogen and Progestin Trial: disease rates per 10 000 women. CHD (coronary heart disease) 1.29; stroke 1.41; breast cancer 1.26; VTE (venous thromboembolism) 2.11; colorectal cancer 0.63; hip fracture 0.66; endometrial cancer 0.83; global index 1.15.

risk–benefit ratio of unopposed oestrogen in 10 739 women; results are not yet available.

In the absence of contraindications (Table 3.2), it is usual to initiate HRT after a premature menopause, to be continued until about age 50 or 55, in order to mimic the oestrogen-replete lifespan. This treatment is reasonable, based on oestrogen's proven ability to delay postmenopausal bone loss, although not tested in clinical trials.

### Non-oestrogen medication for osteoporosis
Since 1990 the bisphosphonates, alendronate and risedronate, and raloxifene, a SERM (Selective oEstrogen Receptor Modulator) have been shown in large clinical trials to prevent spine fractures in women at high risk of fracture (women who were on average 15 years postmenopause and had low bone density or prior spine fracture). There are no head-to-head comparisons of these therapies with fracture outcomes, but each suppresses turnover and reduces fracture risk by 40–50% with overlapping 95% confidence intervals (Fig 3.2). These treatments do differ with regard to BMD increments, with greater increases for alendronate and risedronate than raloxifene. Because only small improvements in bone density are necessary to reduce fracture risk, the choice of medication should be based on considerations other than the change in bone density.

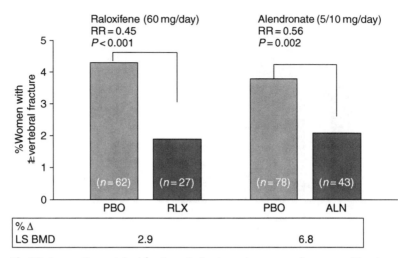

**Fig 3.2** Prospective vertebral fracture studies in postmenopausal women without prevalent fractures. ALN, alendronate; RLX, raloxifene; PBO, placebo. % ΔLS BMD versus placebo. Data for raloxifene from Ettinger, B. *et al.* (1999). *Journal of the American Medical Association*, **282**, 637–45; data for alendronate from Cummings, S.R. *et al.* (1998). *Journal of the American Medical Association*, **280**, 2077–87.

Parathyroid hormone (rhPTH) stimulates bone formation and increases bone mass more dramatically than any other medication. In a clinical trial, a 20 μg dose of rhPTH reduced the risk of new vertebral fractures by 65% over a period of less than 2 years; the number of women with new moderate or severe fractures was reduced by 90% (Neer *et al.* 2001). This drug is expensive and must be taken by daily injection, but may be life-saving for the small subset of women with severe osteoporosis who do not respond to or tolerate other treatment. Present recommendations are for one or two years of use, after which another antiresorptive medication can be initiated.

Tibolone in doses of 1.25 mg/day significantly improves BMD of both spine and hip in early postmenopausal women (Gallagher *et al.* 2001). No large clinical trial with fracture outcomes has been reported.

***Treatment choice by age*** Oestrogen or tibolone are most often prescribed to preserve bone in the early postmenopausal years. Oestrogen is effective when begun later, but the resultant bleeding and breast pain are often unacceptable for older women. Women 5–15 years postmenopause without severe osteoporosis may prefer raloxifene for its possible reduced risk of breast cancer and heart disease. Older women with osteoporotic T-scores on BMD or prior fracture(s), may prefer alendronate or risedronate for their rapid-acting bone-specific effects. Alendronate and risedronate but not raloxifene have been shown to reduce the risk of non-spine fracture by 20–25% (Black *et al.* 1996; Cummings *et al.* 1998; Harris *et al.* 1999).

There are practical reasons to focus on older women. Given a 3-year treatment that reduces fracture risk by 50%, in women aged 65 and older it would be necessary to treat 13 who have had a fracture and 63 without a prior fracture in order to prevent one new fracture. To prevent one fracture in 50-year-old women, it would be necessary to treat 50 who have had a fracture and 250 without prior fracture. In addition to the smaller number needed to treat, older women are often more willing to take and continue osteoporosis treatment because their risk of fracture is more proximate than the risk for younger women, making the risk–benefit ratio for medication more favourable. On the other hand, women who have already sustained a fracture and are treated with the strongest available bone-specific osteoporosis drug will still have a higher fracture risk than similarly treated women without prior fracture.

*Combination therapy*   For women with very advanced osteoporosis who do not respond to other therapy, rhPTH can be given in combination with antiresorptive agents such as oestrogen or a bisphosphate, with further increase in bone formation. Other than this, combined use of two osteoporosis therapies is rarely necessary, incurs greater costs, increases side effects, and only increases bone density slightly above that achieved by single-drug therapy. No clinical trials have shown an additive effect of dual therapies on fracture protection.

*Side effects*   Because all treatments have side effects, only women at high risk of fracture in the near future should be prescribed aggressive pharmacotherapy. The most serious common side effect of HRT, raloxifene, and tibolone is venous thromboembolic disease including pulmonary embolus. The risk, about two to four times that in non-users, decreases but does not disappear with continued therapy (Writing Group for the Women's Health Initiative Investigators 2002). Given the poor risk–benefit ratio for combined oestrogen plus progestogen therapy, the initiation of combined HRT for fracture prevention must be seriously questioned, particularly now that alternative treatment options are available. The risk–benefit ratio for unopposed oestrogen and fracture risk reduction is still being studied in WHI.

Raloxifene increases hot flushes, more often in younger women. In clinical trials, approximately 20% of women younger than 60 years of age and 10% of older women developed hot flushes, but symptoms were usually mild and rarely led to discontinuation of therapy. Unlike oral oestrogen, raloxifene does not increase the risk of gallbladder disease or endometrial hyperplasia.

Alendronate is most often stopped because of upper gastrointestinal symptoms, particularly in women aged 70 and older and those with active gastro-oesophageal reflux disease. Women who experience upper gastrointestinal symptoms on daily alendronate usually can tolerate 70 mg once a week, an interval that seems to allow superficial gastric erosions to heal. Trials of intermittent dosing with alendronate and risedronate have shown bone density changes equal to those achieved with daily dosing, and it is likely that most women will prefer weekly therapy.

Women who have already suffered osteoporotic fractures have a very high risk of new fractures in the future, and require a bone-specific medication such as alendronate or risedronate, each of which can reduce the risk of fracture by half within a year or two (Black *et al.* 1996). It is unknown how many years to continue bisphosphonate therapy.

*Alternative therapies*    Statin use has been reported to reduce risk of bone loss or fracture risk in some observational studies, but this was not confirmed in the largest observational study from the Women's Health Initiative (LaCroix *et al.* 2000). No clinical trial data have been reported.

Thiazide diuretics may reduce bone loss and fracture rates, as suggested by observational studies and one clinical trial (LaCroix *et al.* 2000).

Soya food (soya protein isolate at 20–25 g soya protein/day) has little or no effect on bone density, but ipriflavone, a synthetic isoflavone, reduces bone loss. No fracture trials have been reported.

Observational studies suggest vitamin C is associated with higher levels of BMD. No trials have been reported.

## Coronary heart disease

There is much confusion and conflicting evidence, mainly from observational studies, on the interaction between oestrogen and/or oestrogen and progesterone on coronary heart disease. Many lines of evidence suggest that oestrogen is cardioprotective. Multiple possible mechanisms have been observed, including improvements in LDL and HDL cholesterol, vasoreactivity, Lp(a), fibrinogen, fasting blood glucose, homocysteine, and nitric oxide. Data from more than 30 epidemiological studies showed a 30–50% reduced risk of heart disease in women using oestrogen compared to non-users. On the basis of this evidence, oestrogen has been promoted for the prevention of heart disease. Results were similar in a recent meta-analysis restricted to 18 'good quality' observational studies, but no significant reduction in coronary heart disease incidence was observed in studies that controlled for socioeconomic status (Nelson *et al.* 2002).

The first clinical trial evidence that HRT might be harmful came from a 1997 review of adverse events associated with oestrogen therapy in 22 small, short trials; this pooled analysis showed an increased cardiovascular risk in women without heart disease (Hemminki and McPherson 1997). This study was largely ignored.

In 1998, HERS, the first large clinical trial of HRT with coronary heart disease as the primary outcome, reported a 50% *increased* risk of coronary events during the first year and no overall reduction in the risk of fatal and non-fatal coronary disease or stroke after 4 years in women assigned to Premarin plus medroxyprogesterone versus placebo (Hulley *et al.* 1998). The early harm was not offset by later protection, as shown in a nearly 3-year extension of the HERS trial (Grady *et al.* 2002a). An extensive search for subgroups of women who might have been helped or harmed in HERS has not produced any convincing explanation (Furberg *et al.* 2002). Women in HERS all had heart disease at baseline and it was suggested that HRT increased the risk of cardiovascular events only in such women.

In 2002, the WHI trial of more than 27 500 healthy US women (less than 10% of whom had heart disease at baseline) also informed participants of an excess risk of cardiovascular disease (Rossouw 2001). The WHI Premarin plus MPA (Prempro) part of the trial, with 16 608 women, was stopped early based on an excess global risk largely due to a 29% increased risk of coronary heart disease, a 26% increase of invasive breast cancer, a 41% excess stroke, and a twofold greater risk of pulmonary embolism. The excess of myocardial infarction and venous clotting appeared early in the trial. The investigators calculated that there was only a 10% chance that this cardiovascular harm would reverse itself if the trial were continued longer. WHI women taking Prempro were told to stop their medication.

The Premarin-only part of the WHI trial with 10 739 women has not been stopped because the risk–benefit ratio is uncertain at this time (Writing Group for the Women's Health Initiative Investigators 2002). At this writing, WIS-DOM, a large clinical trial based in the United Kingdom, of the same hormone regimen used in WHI, has stopped recruiting new subjects.

Several other smaller trials, some using oral or transdermal oestradiol (Barrett-Connor 2002), also found no protection against coronary atherosclerosis or stroke. Thus, there is no evidence that HRT prevents cardiovascular disease, and it should not be prescribed for this reason.

## Breast cancer

In 1997 the Oxford Collaborative Group on Hormonal Factors in Breast Cancer reanalysed data from 51 of the 52 published observational studies of

HRT and breast cancer, which included more than 16 000 women, and reported that breast cancer risk increased after 5 years of hormone therapy. The 2.3% increased risk for each year of added use was the same as the increased risk for each year of delayed menopause, providing supporting evidence that oestrogen promotes breast cancer.

Subsequently, other large observational studies (each with >1000 breast cancer cases) also reported an increased risk of breast cancer in women who used HRT for more than 4 or 5 years, most notably in women taking oestrogen with a progestogen (Magnusson *et al.* 1999; Ross *et al.* 2000; Schairer *et al.* 2000).

Despite the strong epidemiological evidence and biological plausibility that oestrogen promotes breast cancer, until the WHI, no clinical trial had sufficient size and duration to test this hypothesis. The WHI found a 26% increased risk of breast cancer, first apparent after 4 years of combined treatment (Writing Group for the Women's Health Initiative Investigators 2002). The increased risk was highest in women who had used HRT before the trial. The other WHI comparison, of unopposed oestrogen versus placebo, has not been stopped, suggesting no excess in breast cancer to date.

Other clinical trial evidence that combined HRT may be more harmful than unopposed oestrogen comes from the PEPI trial, where about one-third of women taking oestrogen plus a progestin versus 15% of women taking unopposed oestrogen had increased breast density on routine mammogram (Greendale *et al.* 1999). Increased breast density is a risk factor for breast cancer in postmenopausal women (Boyd *et al.* 1995), increasing during the first year of hormone therapy, but reversible within one year of stopping it.

Indirect evidence that oestrogen increases breast cancer risk comes from studies of the selective oestrogen receptor modulators tamoxifen and raloxifene; each has been shown to reduce the risk of breast cancer in a large clinical trial (Fisher *et al.* 1998; Cummings *et al.* 1999). In an interesting sidelight to the Italian Tamoxifen Trial, overall breast cancer rates were very low except in women taking HRT: 8 of 390 women taking HRT plus placebo developed breast cancer compared to 1 of 362 women taking HRT and tamoxifen (Veronesi *et al.* 1998).

Although breast cancer is a justifiable concern, excess risk is small for an individual woman, and the risk appears to be reversible, with no excess risk 5 years after stopping oestrogen. The WHI calculated absolute excess risks per 10 000 person-years attributable to oestrogen plus progestin were eight more invasive breast cancers (Writing Group for the Women's Health Initiative Investigators 2002). In observational studies, breast cancer occurring in women taking oestrogen was usually *in situ*, node negative, oestrogen-receptor positive, and had a better prognosis than non-HRT-associated breast cancer (Natrajan *et al.* 1999). This improved prognosis may reflect more frequent mammograms with earlier diagnosis and treatment in women taking HRT, and was not reported in WHI.

## Endometrial cancer

Unopposed oestrogen causes endometrial hyperplasia, a cancer precursor. In the PEPI trial, unopposed oestrogen increased endometrial thickness assessed by transvaginal ultrasound and endometrial hyperplasia by needle biopsy by 10% per year (Writing Group for the PEPI Trial 1996). These changes were not observed in women taking oestrogen plus continuous or cyclical MPA or cyclical micronized progesterone. In another study, treatment with up to 5 years of continuous combined oestradiol (2 mg) plus norethisterone (1 mg) daily was not associated with endometrial hyperplasia; in fact, pre-existing hyperplasia reverted to normal in HRT-treated women (Wells *et al.* 2002).

Five years of unopposed oestrogen increases the endometrial cancer risk four- to five-fold; the risk for 10 years' use is increased approximately 10-fold (Grady *et al.* 1995; Beresford *et al.* 1997). A good prognosis is usual when the oestrogen-stimulated cancer causes bleeding leading to early diagnosis and treatment, but the relative risk for invasive cancer is also increased. Women who take 10–12 days of a progestogen with their oestrogen are protected from endometrial cancer; the reported exceptions may reflect non-compliance with the progestogen (Grady *et al.* 1995).

Some women who cannot tolerate a progestogen may want to take oestrogen alone. This requires a clear explanation of endometrial cancer risk and annual endometrial biopsy and/or transvaginal ultrasound. Unfortunately, a 5 mm increase in endometrial thickness by ultrasound does not always precede the development of atypical endometrial hyperplasia, a cancer precursor (Langer *et al.* 1997).

## Colon cancer

In a systematic review of 21 published observational studies of HRT and colorectal cancer, 9 reported a significant reduction in colorectal cancer, 9 reported no significant protective effect, and 3 reported a small non-significant increased risk (Hebert-Croteau 1998). WHI reported an absolute risk reduction of 6 fewer colorectal cancers per 10 000 person-years (Writing Group for the Women's Health Initiative Investigators 2002).

## Ovarian cancer

Some observational studies have reported an excess risk of ovarian cancer in women taking HRT or unopposed oestrogen (Lacey *et al.* 2002; Riman *et al.* 2002) but most have found no association. None of these studies is convincing regarding safety or harm.

## Memory loss and dementia

LeBlanc *et al.* (2001) reported a significantly reduced relative risk of dementia in women taking oestrogen but there is no clinical trial evidence that oral oestrogen slows memory loss or the progression of dementia. Only small trials in recently oophorectomized women have shown improved verbal memory (Sherwin, 1999). In HERS, approximately 1000 older intact women with heart disease completed six cognitive function tests; after 4 years, women assigned to HRT did not perform better on any test than women assigned to placebo (Grady *et al.* 2002b). The Women's Health Initiative Memory Study (WHIMS), an ancillary 4-year study of 4532 WHI women aged 65 and older, reported that more women in the estrogen plus progestogen than placebo group had a clinically significant decline in global cognitive funtion (6.7% vs. 4.5%) (Rapp *et al.* 2003) and twice as many women developed probable dementia (Shumaker *et al.* 2003). No benefit has been shown in a one-year clinical trial in which 120 women with early Alzheimer's disease were randomly assigned to placebo or unopposed Premarin (either 0.625 mg or 1.25 mg) (Mulnard *et al.* 2000); cognitive function scores on the clinical dementia rating scale were actually significantly *worse* in women assigned to oestrogen.

By contrast, raloxifene shows some promise; in a 3-year trial, older women (aged 70+) assigned to raloxifene had less decline on two of six cognitive function tests than women assigned to placebo (Yaffe *et al.* 2001).

## Venous thromboembolic disease (VTE)

There is no question that oral oestrogen increases the risk of VTE and pulmonary emboli. In observational studies of healthy women, the absolute numbers of excess VTE are about 1 in 5000 HRT users per year. In HERS women with documented heart disease, the absolute risk was much higher, about 1 per 250 users per year (even though a majority were taking aspirin and statins, medications that seem to reduce the risk of venous thromboembolism) (Grady *et al.* 2000). An increased risk of VTE persisted throughout the 4-year HERS trial, showing that not all susceptible women who will have VTE do so during the first year of treatment. In WHI, women taking oestrogen plus progestin had twofold greater rates of VTE including pulmonary emboli and deep vein thrombosis (Writing Group for the Women's Health Initiative Investigators 2002). Again, excess risk was greatest in the first year but was still apparent after 4–5 years.

Mutations in factor V Leiden or prothrombin are associated with an increased risk of VTE, but most women with VTEs do not have either genotype, and screening is not currently recommended. There are insufficient data to assume that transdermal HRT will be safer. A careful history for prior VTE should be obtained, and women with a positive history should avoid oestrogen.

## Gallbladder disease

The risk of gallbladder disease is approximately doubled by oral oestrogen. In HERS there was about one extra case per 250 HRT users per year. Observational data and laboratory studies suggest that transdermal oestrogen will have little or no effect on gallbladder disease.

## Conclusion

Despite the apparent ubiquity of oestrogen receptors in diverse human tissues, and its multiple biological effects, randomized clinical trial evidence of HRT benefit or harm is presently limited to only a few important outcomes: relief of vasomotor and genital symptoms, an increased risk of VTE that wanes a little over time, an increased risk of CHD and stroke that does not appear to be limited to the first year of treatment, an increased risk of breast cancer first apparent after 4–5 years of HRT, an increased risk of gallbladder disease, and a decreased risk of fracture and colon cancer. Overall, the benefits of the extended use of combined HRT necessary to prevent fractures and colon cancer are clearly exceeded by the risks. The risk–benefit ratio for unopposed oestrogen is not clear. Fortunately, other non-HRT medications have been shown to be effective in reducing women's risk of cardiovascular disease and fractures.

# 10-Minute consultation: osteoporosis

Mrs B is a 62-year-old Caucasian woman worried about osteoporosis after reading an advertisement in a magazine. She says she is in excellent health, has no complaints, and has never had a fracture. But her previously healthy mother died 2 years ago at age 89, within 6 months of a hip fracture.

## What would you do next?

- Obtain a menopause and HRT history (oestrogen deficiency is the commonest cause of osteoporosis).

- Obtain a diet, weight and lifestyle history to elicit risk factors for osteoporosis.

Mrs B was 48 when she had her last menstrual period and began hormone replacement therapy (HRT) on the advice of her physician. She quit HRT 2 years later after reading an article about breast cancer, and she takes no prescription medications now.

Mrs B's main exercise is walking two blocks to the shop for fresh bread and her daily pack of cigarettes. She drinks one or two glasses of wine when out with her friends. Because she dislikes milk and cheese, she has started taking 1000 mg of supplemental calcium each morning. She worries about wrinkles and skin cancer, and is thus careful to avoid sun exposure.

Mrs B's physical examination is normal. She is quite pleased that her weight, 8 stone 3 pounds, has not changed since she was 25, but she is surprised at her measured height, which at 5 feet, 5 inches is nearly 2 inches shorter than she remembers.

## Is Mrs B at high risk for osteoporosis, and why?

Mrs B has several characteristics that make osteoporosis a real possibility for her. She has lived more than 10 years with postmenopausal oestrogen levels; the short amount of time she used oestrogen would have had no sustained benefit, because estrogen must be continued to preserve bone. And she has several lifestyle risk factors.

Osteoporosis is important only because it is a risk factor for fracture. The strongest risk factor for a fracture is a previous fracture. Mrs. B's 2-inch height loss is compatible with unrecognized vertebral fractures. The next two strongest risk factors for osteoporosis are years since menopause and low body weight. Mrs. B's menopause was 2 or 3 years earlier than the average age (51 years); cigarette smoking is associated with an earlier menopause and low bone mineral density. She is also fairly thin. Low body fat and smoking are each associated with lower levels of endogenous oestrogen and with lower circulating levels of oestrogen after HRT. Limited weight-bearing exercise impairs muscle and bone strength and balance, all risk factors for a fragility fracture. She is also likely to be vitamin D deficient. Furthermore, because 1000 mg of calcium is about twice the amount the body can absorb at one time, her effective calcium supplementation is only half the amount she is taking.

On the positive side, she is in your office because she is worried about osteoporosis, which suggests that she may be receptive to bone-sparing recommendations. Also her general health is good, she has not lost weight (weight loss is a risk factor for osteoporosis), and her mother's first fracture did not occur until she was nearly 90. Although there are few data on this point, it is likely that only a family fracture occurring before age 75 or 80 is a useful predictor of increased fracture risk in another family member. Modest alcohol intake that does not replace a reasonable diet is not bad for bones, and may actually have a small positive effect on bone mineral density.

## How can you be sure the patient has osteoporosis?

Expensive tests should not be ordered unless the results will change management and patient compliance. Even without tests, this woman's concerns open the door at this and future visits to educational opportunities about positive lifestyle changes she can make and treatment options that are available.

In the absence of a confirmed previous low trauma fracture, the only way to be certain a patient has osteoporosis is to obtain a spine film and look for vertebral fractures (two-thirds of which are unrecognized without an x-ray), or to obtain a central or peripheral bone scan to determine whether her bone mineral density is at least 2.5 standard deviations below the young adult mean (i.e. a T-score of $-2.5$ or lower).

A prior fracture carries a much higher risk of subsequent fractures than an osteoporotic T-score, and in some countries documentation of a prior fracture may be required before prescription of a bone-specific agent is approved. In this case the physician chose to order spine films first, based on their very strong risk prediction, the reported height loss, and because x-rays could be obtained without waiting for a referral appointment.

## Which bone scans and when?

There is a difference of opinion about the optimal time to order a bone scan when osteoporosis is suspected but no fracture has occurred. Unless there are several risk factors, it is usually reasonable to wait until the patient is at least 5 years postmenopause, allowing some bone loss to have occurred. But a combination of such risk factors as family history, height loss, tobacco habit, and physical inactivity noted above can prompt much earlier evaluation.

The gold standard for a diagnosis of osteoporosis is dual energy x-ray absorptiometry (DEXA) of the hip. When more than one site is scanned, it is not uncommon to see considerable divergence in the results. In Mrs B, the lumbar spine T-score was $-1.5$ and total hip T-score was $-2.3$. Most clinicians would call the hip result close enough to the WHO criteria to warrant a diagnosis of osteoporosis. Although postmenopausal bone loss occurs first at the spine, it is often obscured by osteoarthritis at this site, as was the case here. Low bone density based on bone scans at peripheral sites including the forearm and heel has also been shown to predict fracture risk, and these smaller, less expensive instruments are suitable for the primary care office.

### After a diagnosis of osteoporosis, what additional work-up is necessary?

At this point in the work-up there is divergent opinion depending as much on the specialty of the physician as the characteristics of the patient. Many specialists order serum calcium, phosphate, creatinine, alkaline phosphatase, a sensitive TSH test, and vitamin D and PTH levels, and others add 24-hour urine calcium, serum protein electrophoresis (for multiple myeloma), and tests for coeliac disease to diagnose the most common of the secondary causes of osteoporosis. These tests are certainly appropriate for osteoporotic women who are young, or who have unusually severe disease, or who are otherwise ill. For the apparently well postmenopausal patient like Mrs B, these additional tests would not be ordered by most generalists unless the patient fails to respond to therapy.

### What treatment would you recommend?

Mrs B should make the following lifestyle changes:

- diet (specifically, she needs to divide the calcium into a twice-a-day regimen and add vitamin D to her diet);
- exercise (she should do more weight-bearing exercise plus resistance training); and
- smoking cessation (she should get help through a smoking-cessation programme).

In addition, the three main regimens for the treatment of osteoporosis in a patient such as Mrs B are oestrogen, raloxifene, or one of the bisphosphonates – alendronate or risedronate.

#### *Oestrogen*

HRT has been shown in multiple clinical trials to preserve bone, and the prevention of osteoporosis is a desired side effect when oestrogen is used to treat menopausal symptoms in the early postmenopausal years. However, HRT is no longer approved in the USA for the *treatment* of osteoporosis. This decision was based on the paucity of clinical trial data showing fracture prevention in women with osteoporosis. HRT does preserve bone when given to older women, but women who have been without oestrogen for more than 5 years tend to have more problems than younger women with breast pain and bleeding. In any event, Mrs B is worried about cancer and has already stopped oestrogen once, so HRT would not be a good choice for her.

### Raloxifene

This selective oestrogen receptor modulator is approved for prevention and treatment of osteoporosis, based on clinical trials showing a 40% reduced risk of spine (but not hip) fractures in women with osteoporosis with or without prior fractures. Raloxifene does not increase the risk of breast cancer (preliminary data suggest it may reduce the risk), heart disease, or stroke. The only serious side effect reported to date is venous thromboembolic disease, with rates similar to those reported with HRT. Raloxifene is not effective for the treatment of hot flushes, but instead slightly but significantly increases hot flushes. Mrs B did not have bothersome hot flashes and is worried about breast cancer, so this might be a good bone medication for her.

### Bisphosphonates

Alendronate and risedronate are oral bisphosphonates that have been shown to reduce spine fractures and hip fractures in women with osteoporosis. Although there are no head-to-head comparisons, the 40–50% spine fracture risk reduction is similar for these two bisphosphonates and also comparable to raloxifene (based on overlapping 95% confidence intervals). This is the only regimen shown to prevent hip fracture, and would also be an acceptable choice for this patient. The only common potentially serious side effect is oesophageal erosion and bleeding, so the medication should not be given to patients who report GERD or a hiatus hernia. These upper GI side effects are uncommon when the total weekly dose is given once a week instead of daily (70 mg alendronate or 35 mg risedronate).

### Follow-up

Fracture risk reduction is not concordant with the change in BMD. No repeat scan need be obtained for at least 2 or 3 years. Bone markers such as NTX or CTX can be helpful within the first few weeks of treatment, but are not used unless the patient has unusually severe osteoporosis. A new fracture does not necessarily mean treatment failure, in that the patient might have had more fractures or more severe fractures without the medication.

Further encouragement for lifestyle change, especially smoking cessation, is the most important follow-up activity for this patient.

## References

Albertazzi, P., Pansini, F., Bonaccorsi, G., Zanotti, L., Forini, E. and De Aloysio, D. (1998). The effect of dietary soy supplementation on hot flushes. *Obstetrics and Gynecology*, **91**, 6–11.

Avis, N.E., Stellato, R., Crawford, S., Johannes, C. and Longcope C. (2000). Is there an association between menopause status and sexual functioning? *Menopause*, **7**, 297–309.

Barrett-Connor, E. (2002). Looking for the pony in the HERS data. *Circulation*, **105**, 902–3.

Barrett-Connor, E. and Grady, D. (1998). Hormone replacement therapy, heart disease, and other considerations. *Annual Review of Public Health*, **19**, 55–72.

Beresford, S.A., Weiss, N.S., Voigt, L.F. and McKnight, B. (1997). Risk of endometrial cancer in relation to use of oestrogen combined with cyclic progestagen therapy in postmenopausal women. *Lancet*, **349**, 458–61.

Bjorn, I., Bixo, M., Nojd, K.S., Nyberg, S. and Backstrom, T. (2000). Negative mood changes during hormone replacement therapy: a comparison between two progestogens. *American Journal of Obstetrics and Gynecology*, **183**, 1419–26.

Black, D.M., Cummings, S.R., Karpf, D.B., *et al.* (1996). Randomised trial of effect of alendronate on risk of fracture in women with existing vertebral fractures. Fracture Intervention Trial Research Group. *Lancet*, **348**, 1535–41.

Boyd, N.F., Byng, J.W., Jong, R.A., *et al.* (1995). Quantitative classification of mammographic densities and breast cancer risk: results from the Canadian National Breast Screening Study. *Journal of the National Cancer Institute*, **87**, 670–5.

Brown, J.S., Vittinghoff, E., Kanaya, A.M., Agarwal, S.K., Hulley, S. and Foxman, B. for the Heart and Estrogen/Progestin Replacement Study Research Group (2001). Urinary tract infections in postmenopausal women: effect of hormone therapy and risk factors. *Obstetrics and Gynecology*, **98**, 1045–52.

Cardozo, L., Bachmann, G., McClish, D., Fonda, D. and Birgerson, L. (1998). Meta-analysis of estrogen therapy in the management of urogenital atrophy in postmenopausal women: second report of the Hormones and Urogenital Therapy Committee. *Obstetrics and Gynecology*, **92**, 722–7.

Cauley, J.A., Black, D.M., Barrett-Connor, E., *et al.* (2001a). Effects of hormone replacement therapy on clinical fractures and height loss: The Heart and Estrogen/Progestin Replacement Study (HERS). *American Journal of Medicine*, **110**, 442–50.

Cauley, J.A., Zmuda, J.M., Ensrud, K.E. and Bauer, D.C. (2001b). Timing of estrogen replacement therapy for optimal osteoporosis prevention. *Journal of Clinical Endocrinology and Metabolism*, **86**, 5700–5.

Collaborative Group on Hormonal Factors in Breast Cancer (1997). Breast cancer and hormone replacement therapy: collaborative reanalysis of data from 51 epidemiological studies of 52,705 women with breast cancer and 108,411 women without breast cancer. *Lancet*, **350**, 1047–59.

Cummings, S.R., Black, D.M., Thompson, D.E., *et al.* (1998). Effect of alendronate on risk of fracture in women with low bone density but without vertebral fractures: results from the Fracture Intervention Trial. *Journal of the American Medical Association*, **280**, 2077–82.

Cummings, S.R., Eckert, S., Krueger, K.A., *et al.* (1999). The effect of raloxifene on risk of breast cancer in postmenopausal women: results from the MORE randomized trial. Multiple Outcomes of Raloxifene Evaluation. *Journal of the American Medical Association*, **281**, 2189–97.

Dawson-Hughes, B., Harris, S.S., Krall, E.A., Dallal, G.E., Falconer, G. and Green, C.L. (1995). Rates of bone loss in postmenopausal women randomly assigned to one of two dosages of vitamin D. *American Journal of Clinical Nutrition*, **61**, 1140–5.

Dennerstein, L., Dudley, E.C., Hopper, J.L., Guthrie, J.R. and Burger, H.G. (2000). A prospective population-based study of menopausal symptoms. *Obstetrics and Gynecology*, **96**, 351–8.

Eriksen, B. (1999). A randomized, open, parallel-group study on the preventive effect of an estradiol-releasing vaginal ring (Estring) on recurrent urinary tract infections in postmenopausal women. *American Journal of Obstetrics and Gynecology*, **180**, 1072–9.

Fisher, B., Costanino, J.P., Wickerham, L., *et al.* (1998). Tamoxifen for prevention of breast cancer: report of the National Surgical Adjuvant Breast and Bowel Project P-1 Study. *Journal of the National Cancer Institute*, **90**, 1371–88.

Freeman, R. (2001). Hot flashes. Prescription alternatives to ERT/HRT. *Menopause Matters*, **26**, 63–4.

Furberg, C.D., Vittinghoff, E., Davidson, M., *et al.* (2002). Subgroup interactions in the Heart and Estrogen/progestin Replacement Study: lessons learned. *Circulation*, **105**, 917–22.

Gallagher, J.C., Baylink, D.J., Freeman, R. and McClung, M. (2001). Prevention of bone loss with tibolone in postmenopausal women: results of two randomized, double-blind, placebo-controlled, dose-finding studies. *Journal of Clinical Endocrinology and Metabolism*, **86**, 3618–28.

Gallagher, J.C., Rapuri, P.B., Haynatzki, G. and Detter, J.R. (2002). Effect of discontinuation of estrogen, calcitriol, and the combination of both on bone density and bone markers. *Journal of Clinical Endocrinology and Metabolism*, **87**, 4914–23.

Gold, E.B., Sternfeld, B., Kelsey, J.L., *et al.* (2000). Relation of demographic and lifestyle factors to symptoms in a multi-racial/ethnic population of women 40–55 years of age. *American Journal of Epidemiology*, **152**, 463–73.

Grady, D., Gebretsadik, T., Kerlikowske, K., Ernster, V. and Petitti, D. (1995). Hormone replacement therapy and endometrial cancer risk: a meta-analysis. *Obstetrics and Gynecology*, **85**, 304–13.

Grady, D., Wenger, N.K., Herrington, D., *et al.* (2000). Postmenopausal hormone therapy increases risk for venous thromboembolic disease. The Heart and Estrogen/progestin Replacement Study. *Annals of Internal Medicine*, **132**, 689–96.

Grady, D., Brown, J.S., Vittinghoff, E., Applegate, W., Varner, E. and Snyder, T. (2001). Postmenopausal hormones and incontinence: the Heart and Estrogen/Progestin Replacement Study. *Obstetrics and Gynecology*, **97**, 116–20.

Grady, D., Herrington, D., Bittner, V., *et al.* (2002a). Cardiovascular disease outcomes during 6.8 years of hormone therapy: Heart and Estrogen/progestin Replacement Study follow-up (HERS II). *Journal of the American Medical Association*, **288**, 49–57.

Grady, D., Yaffe, K., Kristof, M., Lin, F., Richards, C. and Barrett-Connor, E. (2002). Effect of postmenopausal hormone therapy on cognitive function: the Heart and Estrogen/progestin Replacement Study. *American Journal of Medicine*, **113**, 543–8.

Greendale, G.A., Reboussin, B.A., Hogan, P., *et al.* (1998). Symptom relief and side effects of postmenopausal hormones: results from the Postmenopausal Estrogen/Progestin Interventions Trial. *Obstetrics and Gynecology*, **92**, 982–8.

Greendale, G.A., Reboussin, B.A., Sie, A., *et al.* (1999). Effects of estrogen and estrogen-progestin on mammographic parenchymal density. Postmenopausal Estrogen/Progestin Interventions (PEPI) Investigators. *Annals of Internal Medicine*, **130**, 262–9.

Greendale, G.A., Wells, B., Marcus, R. and Barrett-Connor, E. (2000). How many women lose bone mineral density while taking hormone replacement therapy? Results from the Postmenopausal Estrogen/progestin Interventions Trial. *Archives of Internal Medicine*, **160**, 3065–71.

Halbreich, U. (1997). Role of estrogen in postmenopausal depression. *Neurology* **48**(S7), S16–19.

Hammar, M., Christau, S., Nathorst-Böös, J., Rud, T. and Garre, K. (1998). A double-blind, randomised trial comparing the effects of tibolone and continuous combined hormone replacement therapy in postmenopausal women with menopausal symptoms. *British Journal of Obstetrics and Gynaecology*, **105**, 904–11.

Harris, S., Watts, N.B., Genant, H., *et al.* (1999). Effects of risedronate treatment on vertebral and nonvertebral fractures in women with postmenopausal osteoporosis: a randomized controlled trial. Vertebral Efficacy with Risedronate Therapy (VERT) Study Group. *Journal of the American Medical Association*, **282**, 1344–52.

Hebert-Croteau, N. (1998). A meta-analysis of hormone replacement therapy and colon cancer in women. *Cancer Epidemiology Biomarkers and Prevention*, **7**, 653–9.

Hemminki, E. and McPherson, K. (1997). Impact of postmenopausal hormone therapy on cardiovascular events and cancer: pooled data from clinical trials. *British Medical Journal*, **315**, 149–53.

Hlatky, M.A., Boothroyd, D., Vittinghoff, E., Sharp, P. and Whooley, M.A. (2002). Quality-of-life and depressive symptoms in postmenopausal women after receiving hormone therapy: results from the Heart and Estrogen/progestin Replacement Study (HERS) trial. *Journal of the American Medical Association*, **287**, 591–97.

Hulley, S., Grady, D., Bush, T., *et al.* (1998). Randomized trial of estrogen plus progestin for secondary prevention of coronary heart disease in postmenopausal women. Heart and Estrogen/Progestin Replacement Study (HERS) Research Group. *Journal of the American Medical Association*, **280**, 605–13.

Hypericum Depression Trial Study Group (2002). Effect of *Hypericum perforatum* (St John's Wort) in major depressive disorder. A randomized controlled trial. *Journal of the American Medical Association*, **287**, 1807–14.

Issacs, A.J., Britton, A.R. and McPherson, K. (1997). Why do women doctors in the UK take hormone replacement therapy? *Journal of Epidemiology and Community Health*, **51**, 373–7.

Kotsopoulos, D., Dalais, F.S., Liang, Y.-L., McGrath, B.P. and Teede, H.J. (2000). The effects of soy protein containing phytoestrogens on menopausal symptoms in postmenopausal women. *Climacteric*, **3**, 161–7.

Kuller, L.H., Simkin-Silverman, L.R., Wing, R.R., Meilahn, E.N. and Ives, D.G. (2001). Women's Healthy Lifestyle Project: A randomized clinical trial: results at 54 months. *Circulation*, **103**, 32–7.

Lacey, J.V., Mink, P.J., Lubin, J.H., *et al.* (2002). Menopausal hormone replacement therapy and risk of ovarian cancer. *Journal of the American Medical Association*, **288**, 334–41.

LaCroix, A.Z., Ott, S.M., Ichikawa, L., Scholes, D. and Barlow, W.E. (2000). Low-dose hydrochlorothiazide and preservation of bone mineral density in older adults. A randomized, double-blind, placebo-controlled trial. *Annals of Internal Medicine* **133**, 516–26.

Langer, R.D., Pierce, J.J., O'Hanlan, K.A., *et al.* (1997). Transvaginal ultrasonography compared with endometrial biopsy for the detection of endometrial disease. Postmenopausal Estrogen/Progestin Interventions Trial. *New England Journal of Medicine,* **337**, 1792–8.

LeBlanc, E.S., Janowsky, J., Chan, B.K. and Nelson, H.D. (2001). Hormone replacement therapy and cognition: systematic review and meta-analysis. *Journal of the American Medical Association,* **285**, 1489–99.

Linde, K. and Mulrow, C.D. (2002). St John's Wort for depression. *Cochrane Reviews.* http://www.med.exact.com/medexact/dispatcher.jsp?country=us&section=cochrane_home&; accessed 4/8/02.

Linde, K., Ramirez, G., Mulrow, C.D., Pauls, A., Weidenhammer, W. and Melchart, D. (1996). St John's wort for depression – an overview and meta-analysis of randomised clinical trials. *British Medical Journal,* **313**, 253–8.

Lindsay, R., Silverman, S.L., Cooper, C., *et al.* (2001).Risk of new vertebral fracture in the year following a fracture. *Journal of the American Medical Association,* **285**, 320–3.

Lips, P., Graafmans, W.C., Ooms, M.E., Bezemer, P.D. and Bouter, L.M. (1996). Vitamin D supplementation and fracture incidence in elderly persons. A randomized, placebo-controlled clinical trial. *Annals of Internal Medicine,* **124**, 400–6.

McNagny, S.E. (1999). Prescribing hormone replacement therapy for menopausal symptoms. *Annals of Internal Medicine,* **131**, 605–16.

Magnusson, C., Baron, J.A., Correia, N., Bergstrom, R., Adami, H.O. and Persson, I. (1999). Breast cancer risk following long-term oestrogen- and oestrogen-progestin-replacement therapy. *International Journal of Cancer,* **81**, 339–44.

Marcus, R., Holloway, L., Wells, B., *et al.* (1999). The relationship of biochemical markers of bone turnover to bone density changes in postmenopausal women: results from the Postmenopausal Estrogen/Progestin Interventions (PEPI) trial. *Journal of Bone and Mineral Research,* **14**, 1583–95.

Mulnard, R.A., Cotman, C.W., Kawas, C., *et al.* (2000). Estrogen replacement therapy for treatment of mild to moderate Alzheimer's disease: a randomized controlled trial. Alzheimer's Disease Cooperative Study. *Journal of the American Medical Association,* **283**,1007–15.

Nappi, R.E, Cagnacci, A., Granella, F., Piccinini, F., Polatti, F. and Facchinetti, F. (2001). Course of primary headaches during hormone replacement therapy. *Maturitas,* **38**, 157–63.

Natrajan, P.K., Soumakis, K. and Gambrell, R.D. Jr (1999). Estrogen replacement therapy in women with previous breast cancer. *American Journal of Obstetrics and Gynecology,* **181**, 288–95.

Neer, R.M., Arnaud, C.D., Zanchetta, J.R., *et al.* (2001). Effect of parathyroid hormone (1–34) on fractures and bone mineral density in postmenopausal women with osteoporosis. *New England Journal of Medicine,* **344**, 1434–41.

Nelson, H.D., Humphrey, L.L., Nygren, P., Teutsch, S.M. and Allan, J.D. (2002). Postmenopausal hormone replacement therapy. Scientific review. *Journal of the American Medical Association,* **288**, 872–81.

Nieves, J.W., Komar, L., Cosman, F. and Lindsay, R. (1998). Calcium potentiates the effect of estrogen and calcitonin on bone mass: review and analysis. *American Journal of Clinical Nutrition*, **67**, 18–24.

Nordin, B.E. (1997). The calcium controversy. *Osteoporosis International* **7**(S3), S17–23.

Norman, R.J., Flight, I.H.K. and Rees, M.C.P. (2001). Oestrogen and progestogen hormone replacement therapy for peri-menopausal and post-menopausal women: weight and body fat distribution. *Cochrane Reviews*. http://www.cochranelibrary.com/CLI . . . = 724&T = (OESTROGEN+and+ PROGESTOGEN); accessed 4/26/01.

Ooms, M.E., Roos, J.C., Bezemer, P.D., van der Vijgh, W.J., Bouter, L.M. and Lips, P. (1995). Prevention of bone loss by vitamin D supplementation in elderly women: a randomized double-blind trial. *Journal of Clinical Endocrinology and Metabolism*, **80**, 1052–8.

Rapp, S.R., Espeland, M.A., Shumaker, S.A. *et al.* for the WHIMS Investigators (2003). Effect of estrogen plus progestin on global cognitive function in postmenopausal women. The Women's Health Initiative Memory Study: A randomized clinical trial. *Journal of the American Medical Association*, **289**, 2663-72.

Raz, R. and Stamm, W.E. (1993). A controlled trial of intravaginal estriol in postmenopausal women with recurrent urinary tract infections. *New England Journal of Medicine*, **329**, 753–6.

Riman, T., Dickman, P.W., Nilsson, S., *et al.* (2002). Hormone replacement therapy and the risk of invasive epithelial ovarian cancer in Swedish women. *Journal of the National Cancer Institute*, **94**, 497–504.

Ross, R.K., Paganini-Hill, A., Wan, P.C. and Pike, M.C. (2000). Effect of hormone replacement therapy on breast cancer risk: estrogen versus estrogen plus progestin. *Journal of the National Cancer Institute*, **92**, 328–32.

Rossouw, J.E. (2001). Early risk of cardiovascular events after commencing hormone replacement therapy. *Current Opinion in Lipidology*, **12**, 371–5.

Rymer, J. and Morris, E.P. (2000) Extracts from 'clinical evidence': menopausal symptoms. *British Medical Journal*, **321**, 1516–19.

Schairer, C., Lubin, J., Troisi, R., Sturgeon, S., Brinton, L. and Hoover, R. (2000). Menopausal estrogen and estrogen-progestin replacement therapy and breast cancer risk. *Journal of the American Medical Association*, **283**, 485–91.

Schmidt, P.J., Nieman, L., Danaceau, M.A., *et al.* (2000). Estrogen replacement in perimenopause-related depression: a preliminary report. *American Journal of Obstetrics and Gynecology*, **183**, 414–20.

Shelton, R.C., Keller, M.B., Gelenberg, A., *et al.* (2001). Effectiveness of St John's wort in major depression: a randomized controlled trial. *Journal of the American Medical Association*, **285**, 1978–86.

Sherwin, B.B. (1999). Can estrogen keep you smart? Evidence from clinical studies. *Journal of Psychiatry and Neuroscience*, **24**, 315–21.

Shumaker, S.A., Legault, C., Rapp, S.R. *et al.* for the WHIMS Investigators (2003). Estrogen plus progestin and the incidence of dementia and mild cognitive impairment in postmenopausal women. The Women's Health Initiative Memory Study: A randomized clinical trial. *Journal of the American Medical Association*, **289**, 2651-62.

Silberstein, S.D. (2000). Sex hormones and headache. *Revue Neurologique (Paris)*, **156**(S4), S30–41.

Siris, E.S., Miller, P.D., Barrett-Connor, E., *et al.* (2001). Identification and fracture outcomes of undiagnosed low bone mineral density in postmenopausal women.

Results from the National Osteoporosis Risk Assessment. *Journal of the American Medical Association,* **286,** 2815–22.

Skarsgard, C., Berg, G.E., Ekblad, S., Wiklund, I. and Hammar, M.L. (2000). Effects of estrogen therapy on well-being in postmenopausal women without vasomotor complaints. *Maturitas,* **36,** 123–30.

Slater, C.C., Zhang, C., Hodis, H.N., *et al.* (2001). Comparison of estrogen and androgen levels after oral estrogen replacement therapy. *Journal of Reproductive Medicine,* **46,** 1052–6.

Soares, C.N., Almeida, O.P., Joffe, H. and Cohen, L.S. (2001). Efficacy of estradiol for the treatment of depressive disorders in perimenopausal women: a double-blind, randomized, placebo-controlled trial. *Archives of General Psychiatry,* **58,** 529–34.

Speroff, L., Symons, J., Kempfert, N. and Rowan, J. (2000). The effect of varying low-dose combinations of norethindrone acetate and ethinyl estradiol (femhrt®) on the frequency and intensity of vasomotor symptoms. *Menopause,* **7,** 383–90.

Torgerson, D.J. and Bell-Syer, S.E.M. (2001). Hormone replacement therapy and prevention of nonvertebral fractures: a meta-analysis of randomized trials. *Journal of the American Medical Association,* **285,** 2891–7.

Trivedi, D.P., Doll, R. and Khaw, K.T. (2003). Effect of four monthly oral vitamin $D_3$ (cholecalciferol) supplementation on fractures and mortality in men and women living in the community: randomized double blind controlled trial. *British Medical Journal,* **326,** 1 March, 1–6; bmj.com--accessed March 20, 2003.

Utian, W.H., Shoupe, D., Bachmann, G., Pinkerton, J.V. and Pickar, J.H. (2001). Relief of vasomotor symptoms and vaginal atrophy with lower dose of conjugated equine estrogens and medroxyprogesterone acetate. *Fertility and Sterility,* **75,** 1065–79.

Veronesi, U., Maisonneuve, P., Costa, A., *et al.* (1998). Prevention of breast cancer with tamoxifen: preliminary findings from the Italian randomized trial among hysterectomised women. Italian Tamoxifen Prevention Group. *Lancet,* **352,** 93–7.

Wells, M., Sturdee, D.W., Barlow, D.H., *et al.* (2002). For the UK Continuous Combined Hormone Replacement Therapy Study Investigators. Effect on endometrium of long term treatment with continuous combined oestrogen-progestogen replacement therapy: follow-up study. *British Medical Journal,* **325,** 239–43.

Writing Group for the PEPI Trial. (1996). Effects of hormone replacement therapy on endometrial history in postmenopausal women. The Postmenopausal Estrogen/Progestin Interventions (PEPI) Trial. *Journal of the American Medical Association,* **275,** 370–5.

Writing Group for the Women's Health Initiative Investigators (2002). Risks and benefits of estrogen plus progestin in healthy postmenopausal women. Principal results from the Women's Health Initiative Randomized Controlled Trial. *Journal of the American Medical Association,* **288,** 321–33.

Wu, F., Mason, B., Horne, A., *et al.* (2002). Fractures between the ages of 20 and 50 years increase women's risk of subsequent fractures. *Archives of Internal Medicine,* **162,** 33–6.

Yaffe, K., Krueger, K., Sarkar, S., *et al.* (2001). Cognitive function in postmenopausal women treated with raloxifene. *New England Journal of Medicine,* **344,** 1207–13.

Zweifel, J.E. and O'Brien, W.H. (1997). A meta-analysis of the effect of hormone replacement therapy upon depressed mood. *Psychoneuroendocrinology,* **22,** 189–212.

# Chapter 4

# Contraception
## John Guillebaud

About 75% of women choose to consult their general practitioner (GP) for contraception, although some still prefer the anonymity and specialization of the Family Planning Association (FPA) clinic. General practitioners are potentially in the most favourable position to offer good advice, being already familiar with the patient's health and life circumstances. But some practices perpetuate the myth that contraception equates to 'the Pill' (like vacuum cleaners equate solely to 'Hoovers') and so deprive their patients of other choices, or devote too little time and skill to counselling. Research shows that not being given enough information about contraceptive methods is associated with women being dissatisfied, with not using methods correctly, and with abandoning contraception even if they do not want to get pregnant (Contraceptive Education Service 1996).

It is clear that consumer choice needs to be preserved. Although most advice is provided by the doctor, a very important contribution can and should be made by nurses. The midwife, health visitor, or other domiciliary nurse is well placed to motivate and guide those in need. Much of the routine counselling and follow-up can be fruitfully delegated to a fully family planning-trained practice nurse – with usually a gain rather than a loss in standards. Cap-fitting, pill-teaching, IUD-checking, and cervical smear-taking are all duties that can be appropriately delegated to the practice nurse, as well as the supervision of those who choose methods based on fertility awareness.

For GPs, the postgraduate training for the Diploma of the Faculty of Family Planning and Reproductive Health Care (DFFP) includes theoretical teaching and practical experience in all the methods, aside from intrauterine contraceptive techniques and the insertion and management of subdermal implants, for which there are separate courses leading to Letters of Competence.

Everyone involved in this work should also be equipped to receive the often hidden signals about related, often complex, psychological and emotional factors in any family planning consultation. Further training is available through the Institute of Psychosexual Medicine.

Each contraceptive client should be helped by the doctor or nurse to formulate her own assessment of the risks and benefits of the available methods based on up-to-date opinion and information, backing their counselling with good literature. The latest UK FPA leaflets are ideal in this respect, user-friendly (in contrast to most package inserts) yet accurate and adequately comprehensive, thereby providing strong medico-legal back-up for practitioners who may later be asked to justify their actions in the increasingly likely event of litigation. FPA leaflets may thus be regarded as an essential supplement to, but by no means as a replacement for, the counselling time by doctor and/or nurse, who must also routinely keep accurate and contemporary records. Records assume even greater importance on the not infrequent occasions when best practice requires that a licensed product has to be used in an unlicensed way (see page 220).

## Trends in contraceptive usage

The methods of contraception used by couples have changed over the years and there have been changes within the social classes. Oral contraceptive usage declines periodically in response to 'pill scares', but remains at around three million users. Sterilization rates in the UK are the highest in Europe, maybe too high in the young, and by the mid-forties close to 50% of women rely on their own or their partner's sterilization. Newer choices such as implants, improved copper IUDs, and the levonorgestrel intrauterine system (LNG-IUS) are proving slow to 'catch on' in the numbers that their many advantages would support. But further inroads into the supremacy of the pill must be expected.

## Choice of method

In choosing a method to match their circumstances and needs, most women prioritize both high contraceptive effectiveness and avoidance of adverse effects and health risks in their eventual choice (Fig 4.1). Success with the methods that are free of all systemic risk, like the condom, depends greatly upon correct and consistent use, and this is not a common commodity.

Yet condemnation of, for example, coitus interruptus, does not guarantee either adoption or successful use of a theoretically more effective method. Indeed, it may lead to non-use even of this method in 'emergency' situations. With 'so far successful' users it may instead be worth exploring with the couple the use, say, of a spermicide as an adjunct to the withdrawal method. It is safe to say that 'any method is better than none, but some are better than others'.

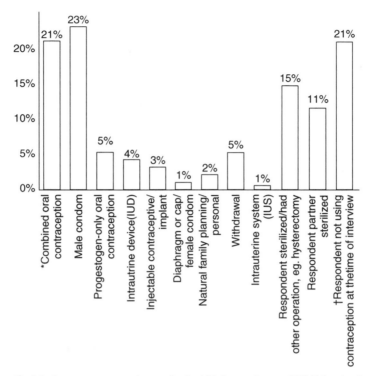

**Fig 4.1** Current contraceptive use in the UK. From a Report (2001) for the Department of Health, using the 1999 Omnibus survey of the Office for National Statistics. Percentages sum to more than 100% as respondents could give more than one answer. *Includes 3% not sure which type of pill. †Includes 15% not in current sexual relationship.

Fashions also change. During the last 20 years male barriers and the Pill have been the most widely used reversible methods. Actually, both these, like the fertility awareness methods, are less than ideal for many by virtue of having the wrong 'default state' – meaning the state of conception if there is a significant user-error (default)! Methods like injectables, implants, IUDs, and the LNG-IUS have the more appropriate default state, of continuing contraception until a defined action is taken to reverse them.

There are also important related problems that may confront the prescriber. They may be physical or psychological (i.e. physically or mentally disabling) or psychosexual. Unless they are considered in an understanding and flexible manner, the couple may have great difficulty with the use of contraception and unwanted pregnancies may then occur. With regard to the much-neglected topic of disability, there is a great quote in the book by Cooper and Guillebaud (1999) attributed to Alf Morris MP:

a society in which there is genuine respect for the handicapped; where if years cannot be added to the lives of the very sick, at least life can be added to their years.

Table 4.1 gives an updated (2002) indication of reliability ranges which can be quoted to couples. Widely varying limits are frequently quoted because the results of any study are bound to be influenced by the age, motivation, and sexual activity of the population concerned, and by the enthusiasm of the investigator and the degree and duration of follow-up achieved.

## Sexual health

Since the first edition of this book almost 20 years ago there is an urgent additional concern, to advise people of all ages who are sexually active on how they may minimize their personal risk of infection with the human immunodeficiency virus (HIV). But in the UK the other sexually transmitted infections are far more prevalent, especially *Chlamydia*, that great scourge producing tubal-factor infertility. The Government's Sexual Health Strategy (Department of Health 2001) encourages a holistic approach, with ever more 'joined-up working' between genitourinary medicine (GUM) and primary care contraception services, whether GP- or clinic-based.

In practical terms, wherever and however any sexually active person presents, surely by now in 2002 there should be no residual embarrassment about taking a good sexual history: at minimum, at every reproductive health consultation, by the screening question, 'Have you had sex with someone different in the last 3 (or 6) months?', followed by more detailed probing according to the tenor and body language of the response. The question cleverly covers both a change of partner during 'serial monogamy' and any possible brief encounter within a basically long-term relationship. The answers often show how wrong our assumptions can be: the young woman with multiple body piercings may be in a mutually monogamous relationship, while the 'pillar of society' may have frequent partner changes.

Wherever acceptable, monogamy is a behaviour pattern to be encouraged (on medical grounds, for optimal emotional as well as reproductive security). This must be supplemented, in the real world, by enthusiasm for the condom – for best results, ideally in addition to a recognized, non-barrier contraceptive (the 'double Dutch' approach).

## Eligibility criteria

WHO's classification of contraindications (Box 4.1) is an enormous help when discussing all methods, not only the combined oral contraceptive (COC). This classification will be used throughout the chapter. Unless otherwise stated,

**Table 4.1** User-failure rates for different methods of contraception per 100 woman-years (2002)

| | Range in the world literature[1] | Oxford/FPA Study[2]–all women married and aged above 25 | | |
|---|---|---|---|---|
| | | Overall (any duration) | Age 25–34 (≤2 years' use) | Age 35+ (≤2 years' use) |
| Sterilization (Lifetime risk, per 100 women) | | | | |
| Male | 0.05 | 0.02 | 0.08 | 0.08 |
| Female | 0.5 | 0.13 | 0.45 | 0.08 |
| IUS | | | | |
| Levonorgestrel-IUS | 0–0.2 | | | |
| Injectable (DMPA) | 0–1.0 | | | |
| Etonogestrel implant (Implanon™) | 0–0.07 | | | |
| Combined pills | | | | |
| 50 µg oestrogen | 0.1–3 | 0.16 | 0.25 | 0.17 |
| <50 µg oestrogen | 0.2–3 | 0.27 | 0.38 | 0.23 |
| IUD | | | | |
| T-Safe Cu 380A | 0.1–0.3 | | | |
| Multiload Cu 375 | 0.3–1.0 | | | |
| (375 designed for longevity appears more effective than 250, latter no longer recommended) | | | | |
| Nova-T 380 | 0.5–0.8 | | | |

**Table 4.1** (*continued*)

| | Range in the world literature[1] | Oxford/FPA Study[2]–all women married and aged above 25 | | |
|---|---|---|---|---|
| | | Overall (any duration) | Age 25–34 (≤2 years' use) | Age 35+ (≤2 years' use) |
| Flexi-T 300 | c. 1.5 | | | |
| Gyne Fix | 0.1–0.5 | | | |
| Progestogen-only pill (not desogestrel-containing) | 1–2 | 1.2 | 2.5 | 0.5 |
| Diaphragm | 4–8 | 1.9 | 5.5 | 2.8 |
| Condom | 2–15 | 3.6 | 6.0 | 2.9 |
| Female condom | 5–15 | | | |
| Coitus interruptus | 8–17 | 6.7 | | |
| Spermicides alone | 4–25 | 11.9 | | |
| Fertility awareness | 2–20 | 15.5 | | |
| No method, young women | 80–90 | | | |
| No method at age 40 | 40–50 | | | |
| No method at age 45 | c. 10–10 | | | |
| No method at age 50 (if still having menses) | c. 0–5 | | | |

[1] Excludes atypical studies giving particularly poor results and all extended-use studies.
[2] Vessey *et al.* (1982)

Notes: 1. Ranking of efficacy, but overlap of ranges in the first column
2. Influence of age: all the rates of the fourth column being lower than those in the third column. Lower rates still to be expected above age 45
3. Much better results obtainable in other states of relative infertility, such as lactation (see below)
4. Rates for female and male sterilization come from Peterson *et al.* (1996) and Philp *et al.* (1984). They are expected lifetime rates per 100 operations performed.
5. Desogestrel POP has a much greater efficacy than other POPs, See p.167.

either WHO's own categorization is given or (where there is disagreement or WHO has not yet pronounced) the category accords with UK and Faculty best practice.

---

**Box 4.1 WHO classification of contraindications (2001) with some amplifications by John Guillebaud (2001a)**

**WHO 1:** A condition for which there is no restriction for the use of the contraceptive method (the scheme can be applied to ALL methods, not just the hormonal ones)

◆ 'A' is for ALWAYS USABLE

(e.g. COC with history of candidiasis or amenorrhoea due to anorexia)

**WHO 2:** A condition where the advantages of the method generally outweigh the theoretical or proven risks

◆ 'B' is for BROADLY USABLE

(e.g. COC in smoker age 20, or migraine without aura)

**WHO 3:** A condition where the theoretical or proven risks usually outweigh the advantages. But respecting the patient/client's autonomy – if she accepts the risks and rejects or should not use relevant alternatives, given the alternative risks of pregnancy the method can be used – with caution/ additional care

◆ 'C' is for CAUTION/COUNSELLING, if used at all

(e.g. COC in diabetes without known tissue damage, or above age 35 with significant migraine without aura)

**WHO 4:** A condition which represents an unacceptable health risk

◆ 'D' is for DO NOT USE, at all

(e.g. migraine with focal aura, COC with personal history of VTE)

*Note:* Clinical judgement is required, always in consultation with the contraceptive user, especially:

◆ In all category WHO 3 conditions – which do mean an alternative would really be preferable to the method first requested

◆ If more than one condition applies. As a working rule, two category 2 conditions moves the situation to category 3; and if any category 3 condition applies, the addition of either a 2 or a 3 condition normally means WHO 4 (DO NOT USE)

Ref: WHO (2000)

Eligibility criteria – downloadable from www.who.int/reproductive–health.

# Hormonal contraception

## The combined oral contraceptive (COC)

The following subjects demand brief discussion:

- benefits versus risks;
- choice of users ('safer women'), considering separately the risk factors for venous and arterial thrombosis;
- choice of pills ('safer pills'), taking account of:
  - (a) what is known about their side-effect profile;
  - (b) biological variation in the pharmacology of contraceptive steroids;
  - (c) endometrial bleeding as a possible 'threshold bioassay' of their blood levels;
- supervision and follow-up, including implications of the monthly pill-free week.

### Benefits versus risks

Capable of providing virtually 100% protection from unwanted pregnancy and taken at a time unconnected with sexual activity, the Pill provides enormous reassurance by the associated regular, short, light, and usually painless withdrawal bleeding at the end of the 21-day pack. Inevitably, most of this section will be on possible risks and hazards associated with taking the Pill, but the positive aspects should not be forgotten; they are listed in Box 4.2. Although some of these findings await full confirmation, such good news is rarely mentioned while the suspected risks are widely publicized and often over-stressed.

Understanding of potential unwanted effects is based largely on the reported findings and analyses of three valuable prospective studies, two in this country, that of the RCGP and the Oxford FPA Study, which both commenced in 1968, and the American Nurses Health Study. The first compares morbidity, mortality, and pregnancy outcomes in users and non-users, whilst the second has either IUD-users or diaphragm-users as controls. The third uses data collected from more than 121 000 nurses, among whom are users of the Pill and all alternatives available in the USA, starting from 1976 to the present. The main findings have been confirmed by numerous case – control studies. Space does not allow full discussion of all the work that has been published in the 40 years during which the Pill has been available in this country. Practitioners should form their own opinion of the risks and benefits by their own reading, but the following may help to summarize present medical opinion upon which contemporary prescription of the Pill is based.

## Box 4.2 **Beneficial effects of the combined pill**

### Contraceptive

Highly effective

Highly convenient, non-intercourse related

Reversible

### Non-contraceptive

A reduction in the rate of most disorders of the menstrual cycle:

+ less heavy bleeding; therefore
+ less anaemia
+ less dysmenorrhoea
+ regular bleeding, and timing can be controlled (for example, no pill-taker need have 'periods' at weekends)
+ fewer symptoms of premenstrual tension overall
+ no ovulation pain

Less functional ovarian cysts – since abnormal ovulation prevented

Fewer extrauterine pregnancies – since normal ovulation inhibited

Less pelvic inflammatory disease (PID)

Less benign breast disease

Possible reduction in the rate of endometriosis

Fewer symptomatic fibroids

Reduced incidence of severe rheumatoid arthritis in current users

Possibly less thyroid disease (both overactive and underactive syndromes according to RCGP study)

Fewer sebaceous disorders (oestrogen-dominant COCs)

Possibly fewer duodenal ulcers – this effect is not well established and could be due to anxious women avoiding COCs

Possibly less *Trichomonas vaginitis*

Possibly less toxic shock syndrome

Beneficial effect on risk of cancer of the ovary and endometrium – see text

Possible beneficial effect on colorectal cancer risk

No toxicity if overdose is taken

Obvious beneficial social effects

Reassuringly, since the last edition, Beral *et al.* (1999) have shown from the RCGP study database that COCs have their main (small) effect on every known cause of mortality during current use and for some varying time thereafter: 10 years after use ceases, mortality in past users is indistinguishable from that in never users.

## Tumours

No medication continues to receive so much scrutiny and investigation as the Pill. For some time fears have been expressed about its possible connection with breast, cervical, and liver cancers.

### Breast cancer

The incidence of this disease is high and therefore it must inevitably be expected to develop in women whether they take COCs or not. Since the recognized risk factors include early menarche and late age of first birth, use by young women was rightly bound to receive scientific scrutiny.

The literature to date is copious, complex, confusing, and contradictory! Research is complicated by the problems related to *latency, changes in formulation, time of exposure*, and *high-risk groups*. A major cause of discrepancies may be the fact that long-term use of the COC by young women is a relatively recent and variable phenomenon between populations.

The 1996 publication by the Collaborative Group on Hormonal Factors in Breast Cancer reanalyses original data which relate to more than 53 000 women with breast cancer and more than 100 000 controls from 54 studies in 25 countries. This is 90% of the world epidemiological data. The model for the Pill-associated increased risk for breast shows disappearance of the risk in ex-users and highlights recency of use of the COC as the most important factor: with the odds ratio unaffected by age of initiation or discontinuation, use before or after first full-term pregnancy, or duration of use. The main findings are summarized in Table 4.2 and below.

COC pill-users can be reassured that:

◆ while the small increase in breast cancer risk for women on the Pill noted in previous studies is confirmed, the odds ratio of 1.24 signifies an increase of 24% only while women are taking the COC, diminishing to zero after discontinuation, over the next few years;

◆ beyond 10 years after stopping there is no detectable increase in breast cancer risk for former Pill-users;

◆ the cancers diagnosed in women *who use or have ever used* COCs are *clinically less advanced* than those who have never used the Pill, and are less likely to have spread beyond the breast;

**Table 4.2** The increased risk of developing breast cancer while taking the pill and in the 10 years after stopping (Collaborative Group on Hormonal Factors in Breast Cancer 1996)

| User status | Increased risk |
| --- | --- |
| Current user | 24% |
| 1–4 years after stopping | 16% |
| 5–9 years after stopping | 7% |
| 10 plus years an ex-user | No significant excess |

♦ this reanalysis shows that these risks are not associated with duration of use, the dose or type of hormone in the COC, and there is no synergism with other risk factors for breast cancer (e.g. family history).

However, if the background risk for the individual is larger, whether because of increased age or a family history, the applicable increase in Table 4.2 necessarily means more attributable cases than in younger women without an added risk factor. Irrespective of the use of hormonal contraception, the cumulative risk of breast cancer in young women is very small, being one in 500 in women up to age 35. Thereafter age becomes itself the most important risk factor, the cumulative risk increasing with age to one in 100 at age 45 and one in 12 by age 75. The increase in attributable cases as age of last use increases has been calculated and is shown in Table 4.3.

Most importantly, for a given age at last use the excess risk is little affected by a women's prior duration of oral contraceptive use. In this 1996 reanalysis, the risks for progestogen-only contraceptives (POP and injectable) showed a similar trend but failed to reach statistical significance, and therefore the issue is not normally raised with users in routine prescribing for oestrogen-free products.

The collaborative group concede that their findings in ever-takers of the pill, of less advanced cases being identified but more of them at a given age, could be explained wholly or in part by surveillance bias (pill-takers both during and after the years of use of the method perhaps being more 'breast aware' than non-takers). However, the present consensus interpretation is that the Pill is a weak co-factor for this cancer, but that for some reason the resulting tumours are less aggressive.

### Clinical implications
The Faculty of Family Planning has concluded that pill-users should be informed of the above data but reiterates the advice given by the Committee on Safety of Medicines (CSM) that there need be no change in prescribing practice.

**Table 4.3** Cumulative risk of breast cancer by recency of use. Showing usage in different age groups, the cumulative numbers of breast cancer cases per 10,000 women in never-users of oral contraception and the cumulative number per 10,000 women who had used oral contraception for 5 years and who were followed up for 10 years after stopping

| Pill use for 5 years, or any duration[1] | To age 20 | To age 25 | To age 30 | To age 35 | To age 40 | To age 45 |
|---|---|---|---|---|---|---|
| Breast cancers diagnosed by | Age 30 | Age 35 | Age 40 | Age 45 | Age 50 | Age 55 |
| Never-users | 4 | 16 | 44 | 100 | 160 | 230 |
| Users who stopped 10 years earlier | 4.5 | 17.5 | 49 | 110 | 180 | 260 |
| Excess number of cases of breast cancer per 10,000 women | 0.5 | 1.5 | 5 | 10 | 20 | 30 |

[1]Since the researchers state that for a given age at last use the excess risk is little affected by a woman's prior duration of oral contraceptive use

◆ The breast cancer issue should now normally be addressed, in a sensitive way, as part of routine pill counselling for all women. This discussion should be initiated opportunely, and not necessarily at the first visit if not raised by the woman, along with encouragement to report promptly any unusual changes in their breasts at any time in the future ('breast awareness'). The balancing protective effects against at least two malignancies (ovary and endometrium – see below) should also be mentioned. The known contraceptive and non-contraceptive benefits of COCs may seem so great to many (but not to all) as to compensate for almost any likely lifetime excess risk of breast cancer.

◆ In explaining the breast cancer risk model to a pill-taker, I use the fourth column of Table 4.3, dividing the numbers by 10, and ask her to visualize two concert halls each holding 1000 women. Imagine that the first is filled with 1000 pill-takers, all now aged 45, but all having used the COC for varying durations of time, then stopping when they reached age 35 (a common scenario). The (cumulative) number of cases of breast cancer would be 11 in concert hall 1. However, in hall 2, filled with never-takers of the pill also all currently aged 45, there would be 10 cases; i.e. there is only one extra case in hall 1. Moreover, if the pill acts as a co-factor (see above), it is possible that she was a woman who would have developed the disease without the pill at a later age anyway. And the remaining 989 women in hall 1 will from this time on have only the same risk of breast cancer as the women of hall 2, i.e. no ongoing added risk because it is over 10 years since their last pill. This is a very important finding, with the overall risk rising so much with age. Finally, the cancers diagnosed among the pill-takers in hall 1, already and in future, will tend to be less advanced than those in hall 2.

◆ *What about pill use by the older women?* As Table 4.3 shows, there is no change in relative risk but an increased attributable risk (3 extra cases per 1000 for 10th year ex-users now aged 55). This must be explained and may be acceptable to many with the balancing (see below) from the established protection against cancer of the ovary and endometrium. But to my mind these data about the COC combined with new choices now available should lead to more older women choosing other contraceptive options, including the new IUS (see pages 213–14).

◆ *Women with benign breast disease* (BBD) or with the family history of a *young first-degree relative with breast cancer under age 40* have a larger background risk than the generality of women, but only the same as women slightly older than their current age but free of the risk factor. The 24% increment of risk will mean more attributable cases, so that these are fairly strong *relative contraindications (WHO 3)*. If the woman chooses the COC as she is entitled to do, given its benefits, it should be a low-dose formulation, for a limited duration, with specific counselling and extra surveillance. If the woman with BBD had a breast biopsy, the histology should be obtained: if epithelial atypia (premalignant) was found, the situation for the COC changes to WHO 4.

◆ If a woman develops carcinoma of the breast, COCs should be discontinued, and women with a history of this cancer should normally avoid COCs (WHO 4).

The results of a major US study are reassuring (Marchbanks et al. 2002). 4575 women aged 35 to 64 with breast cancer were compared with matched controls. There was no pill-associated increased risk of breast cancer. This applied both to those exposed to the pill at a young age or before their first pregnancy and to the older age group overall.

## Cervical cancer

A prospective study (Vessey *et al.* 1983) showed a twofold increase of cervical neoplasia in long-term users of the Pill compared with IUD users. Studies before and since that date on cervical cancer are complicated by the problem of getting accurate information relating to different patterns of sexual activity, both for women and their partners. Some authorities maintain that the Pill is more likely to be a factor in the induction of adenocarcinoma. The prime carcinogen for the commonest (squamous) cancer is clearly sexually transmitted, and probably a virus or combination of viruses.

The COC is at least a co-factor, probably speeding transition through the pre-invasive stages (Smith *et al.* 2003). Long-term users of oral contraceptives should have regular cervical smears, but 3-yearly is still considered adequate unless there are other risk factors. The COC may continue to be prescribed in cases under treatment and/or monitoring for pre-invasive lesions (see relative contraindications WHO 2, below).

## Liver tumours

The benign *liver tumours* are rare conditions but do occur more frequently in COC users – with an extremely low incidence estimated at no more than three additional cases in 100 000 users (Tuckey 2000). The risk is believed to increase with duration of use of older high-dose products and all cases had significant liver enlargement. Rarely, long-term use of the pill may also be associated with primary liver cancer, but without evidence of summating with the increased risk associated with cirrhosis or hepatitis B infection.

### Choriocarcinoma

This was more common among women given the Pill in the presence of active trophoblastic disease (with elevated hCG) in some studies – but not in others from the USA, where chemotherapy is used form the outset in almost all cases of trophoblastic disease so that any possible adverse effect of the COC cannot manifest itself. In UK practice, with less aggressive management the COC is avoided initially, but may be used as soon as trophoblastic activity is undetectable by hCG measurement (supervised by the Reference laboratories).

### Carcinoma of the ovary and of the endometrium

These two cancers are *less* frequent in COC-users. Numerous studies have shown that, in round terms, for both cancers there is a reduction to one-half in the incidence among all users; to one-third in long-term users; and a protective effect can be detected in ex-users for up to 10–15 years. Suppression of ovulation and of normal menstruation in COC users probably explains the similarity of the findings.

### Colorectal cancer

There are suggestive data, though the case is not yet proven, that the Pill may also *protect* against this cancer (Tuckey 2000).

Other cancer links (either way) have been mooted but not confirmed, and women who are apparently cured by local surgery for neoplasia of the ovary, cervix, and for malignant melanoma may all use COCs. The 'bottom line' when counselling women is as follows: *populations using the Pill may develop different benign or malignant neoplasms from control populations, but there is no proof that the overall risk of either type of neoplasia is increased.* (It could even be reduced, though there is no proof of that either.)

## Cardiovascular disease

### Arterial diseases: acute myocardial infarction (AMI), haemorrhagic stroke (HS) and ischaemic stroke (IS)

These can be quickly dealt with, since recent epidemiology, led by the WHO (Farley *et al.* 1999), has shown that the COC was not the prime cause of most of the arterial events occurring in Pill-takers, whether within or outside research studies. The COC was blamed for the adverse outcome really caused by other factors. Principally in terms of frequency these are smoking and hypertension, plus all arterial risks do increase with age. Migraine is a specific, independent risk factor for ischaemic stroke. But all arterial diseases are exceptionally rare in healthy women, Pill-taking or not, during the reproductive years.

### Acute myocardial infarction (AMI)

The RCGP study (Croft and Hannaford 1989), the Oxford/FPA study (Vessey *et al.* 1989), the American nurses study (Stampfer *et al.* 1988) and more recently the large case-control MICA Study (Dunn *et al.* 1999) were all unable to detect any increased risk of myocardial infarction in Pill-takers (either current, or long-duration, or past) *unless they were also smokers.* In that case the odds ratio (OR) went up to 10, and there was double jeopardy, since the case-fatality rate of AMI when it occurs in smokers who *also* use the COC is also much higher (RCGP 1983).

Exceptionally, Tanis *et al.* (2001) did find a statistically increased OR 2.5, with confidence intervals (CIs) 1.5–4.1, for AMI in pill-takers, but this was focussed among users of levonorgestrel (LNG)-containing pills ('second generation', see below). The AMI risk for users of desogestrel or gestodene-containing pills was not significantly increased, odds ratio 1.3 and CIs 0.7–2.5. Yet the difference between the two groups of pills was not significant, and moreover the similar well-designed MICA study showed a trend (also not significant) for the LNG pills to be the preferable ones for AMI risk. There continues to be uncertainty on this issue.

### Haemorrhagic stroke (HS), including subarachnoid haemorrhage

Again, the WHO and other studies have failed to show any increased risk due to the COC under age 35 unless there is also a risk factor such as hypertension (OR 10) or smoking (OR 3). The risk increases with age and this effect (unlike with AMI) is magnified by current COC use, but with no effect of past or long-duration use.

### Ischaemic stroke (IS)

Here there is a detectable increase in the OR due to Pill-taking in the range of 1.5–2. Much of this risk seems to be focused within the subpopulation who suffer from migraine of varying type and severity (see below). The OR for hypertension is 3, and for smoking also 3+.

### Effect of dose/type of hormone

It is reasonable to assume, though never proven, that the modern low-oestrogen pills do minimize the arterial risks, as has been shown (at least for the comparison between less than and more than 50 µg doses) for venous thromboembolism (VTE). Whether the type of progestogen in the COC separately affects the arterial conditions above is still uncertain.

### Venous thromboembolism (VTE)

Much work both in haemostasis and in epidemiology established early on, within 10–15 years of first marketing of COCs, that ethinylestradiol (EE) could be (slightly, but significantly) prothrombotic in susceptible individuals, and the dose normally given was promptly lowered to sub-50 μg. The progestogen content was only later implicated as an independent risk factor for VTE (Committee on safety of Medicines, 1995).

There has been a range of expert views about the four main publications (references in Farley *et al.* 1999) of December 1995 and January 1996, on the combined oral contraceptive and VTE. They were highly congruent, describing a doubling of the OR for users of desogestrel/gestodene products (DSG/GSD) in comparison with the remainder (here termed non-DSG/GSD pills). Initially many authorities agreed with the pill manufacturers that the whole of the association might be explained, not by cause and effect, but by confounding, especially through:

- prescriber bias (prescribers being selectively more likely, prior to October 1995, to use DSG/GSD products for first-timers and women thought to be at risk of VTE);

- the 'attrition of susceptibles' or 'healthy-user effect' (non-DSG/GSD pills being more commonly used by longer-term users and parous women who would be less likely as a population to suffer a VTE, since those who had would no longer be using the method);

- diagnostic bias resulting from prescriber bias, in that women on DSG/GSD pills, because of a perceived higher risk, might then be more likely to be referred for accurate investigations leading to this easily-overlooked diagnosis.

The initial WHO findings about two specific pill pairs seemed to confirm confounding, and made assessment of the new data difficult, for those of us who were honest seekers after the truth at the time, given the then current very heated debate in progress between the CSM and the pill manufacturers. The rate of VTE was higher in users of Mercilon than Marvelon and in Dianette 35 users compared with Diane 50 users, despite the first of each pair containing less oestrogen. The prothrombotic effects of EE were and are accepted by all, even the pill manufacturers: but if one adds the notion that progestogens can influence this, how could the effects of a lower EE dose be greater than a higher, when the progestogen plus its dose are constant?

This finding can only be explained by confounding of some kind, and partly explains the delay in mainstream acceptance of the whole 'third-generation' story as it relates generically to marketed pills. The advent of new haemostasis data – first from Rosing and co-workers in the Netherlands and more recently from the Margaret Pyke Centre (MPC) study showing lower levels of Protein S in Marvelon than in Microgynon users – much enhanced the biological plausibility of the difference between 'generations' (Mackie *et al.* 2001). It also confirmed my view that levonorgestrel (LNG) and norethisterone (NET), not

DSG and GSD, are the '*different*' progestogens. DSG and GSD seem not to hinder EE in exerting its oestrogenicity, whereas LNG and to a lesser extent NET interact by functionally anti-oestrogenic effects, making them in combination with EE less likely to benefit acne, for example, but that disadvantage appears to be ineradicably linked (through the same fact of less oestrogenicity) with a lower risk of VTE. Hence in my view we should in future consider all formulations as functionally either less or more oestrogenic, and move towards dropping the 'generation' terminology.

In July 2001, the European Committee for Proprietary Medicinal Products independently concluded almost exactly as had the 1998 Review of the whole issue by the UK Medicines Commission, summarized in the useful 1999 Press Release quoted here:

> An increased risk of venous thrombo-embolic disease (VTE) associated with the use of oral contraceptives is well established but is smaller than that associated with pregnancy; which has been estimated at 60 cases per 100,000 pregnancies. Some epidemiological studies have reported a greater risk of VTE for women using combined oral contraceptives containing desogestrel or gestodene (the so-called third generation pills) than for women using pills containing levonorgestrel (LNG) – the so-called second generation pills' [*sic:* category also includes norethisterone (NET) pills]. The spontaneous incidence of VTE in healthy non-pregnant women (not taking any oral contraceptive) is about 5 cases per 100,000 women per year. The incidence in users of second generation pills is about 15 per 100,000 women per year of use. The incidence in users of third generation pills is about 25 cases per 100,000 women per year of use: *this excess incidence has not been satisfactorily explained by bias or confounding.* The level of all of these risks of VTE increases with age and is likely to be increased in women with other known risk factors for VTE such as obesity.
>
> Women must be fully informed of these very small risks. Provided they are, the type of pill is for the woman together with her doctor or other family planning professionals jointly to decide in the light of her individual medical history.

Table 4.4 helps to put this in perspective; VTE has a low mortality and the difference in risks between different progestogen pills is small in comparison with the risks which are taken in everyday life. Using the absolute rates given, and assuming an estimated 2% mortality for VTE, there is only around two per million difference in annual VTE mortality between DSG/GSD products and LNG/NET products. This difference equates to choosing, in a whole year, to risk one extra 2-hour drive in the country rather than sitting in one's garden. Therefore, if, for example, a woman chooses to switch from a LNG/NET to a DSG/GSD brand because she finds it preferable for her quality of life and so-called minor side effects which are important to her, such as acne, headaches, depression, weight gain, breast symptoms, or for cycle control: if she avoids using Britain's roads for 2 hours in the next year, she will maintain her level of VTE risk at that of her previous product!

**Table 4.4** Comparative risks – estimates 1996. Annual risks per million women

| Activity | Cases | Deaths |
|---|---|---|
| Having a baby, UK (all causes of death) | | 60 |
| Having a baby (venous thrombosis) | 600 | 10 |
| Using DSG/GSD Pill (venous thrombosis) | 250 | 4 |
| Using non-DSG/GSD Pill (venous thrombosis) | 150 | 2 |
| Non-user, non-pregnant (venous thrombosis) | 50–110 | 1 |
| Risk from *all causes* through COC (healthy non-smoking woman) | | 10 |
| Home accidents | | 30 |
| Playing soccer | | 40 |
| Road accidents | | 80 |
| Scuba diving | | 220 |
| Hang-gliding | | 1500 |
| Cigarette smoking (in next year, if aged 35) | | 1670 |
| Death from pregnancy/childbirth in rural Africa | | 6000–10 000 |

*Sources*: Dinman, B.D. (1980), *Journal of the American Medical Association*, **44** 1226–8
Anon (1991) *British Medical Journal*, **302**, 743
CSM (1999)
Strom, B. (1994) *Pharmacoepidemiology*, 2nd ed., pp. 57–65. Wiley, Chichester

## Prescribing guidelines (Faculty of Family Planning 2000a, b)

First and foremost, Hannaford and Webb (1996) help to put the small print into perspective, highlighting what really matters:

> Current scientific evidence suggests only two prerequisites for the safe provision of COCs: a careful personal and family medical history with particular attention to cardiovascular risk factors, and an accurate blood pressure measurement.

Blanket (untargeted) screening by any blood test is not justifiable (too many false negatives plus false positives if defined as the occurrence of disease events). Moreover breast and pelvic examinations are irrelevant to the COC *per se*.

- Multiple risk factors, or any one arterial or venous factor as shown in Tables 4.5 and 4.6, combined with age above 35 years, means that all COCs should be avoided (WHO 4).
- All marketed pills may now be considered first line. Given the tiny, not yet finally established difference in VTE mortality between the two generations, the woman's own choice of a DSG or GSD product after (well-documented) discussion must be respected: even if based on no more than the presence

**Table 4.5** Risk factors for venous thromboembolism (VTE). WHO categories in (—)

|  | Absolute contraindication (4) | Relative contraindication |
|---|---|---|
| Family history (parent or sibling under 45) | Clotting abnormality or tests not done | Clotting factors done, normal (2) |
| Overweight–high body mass index (BMI) | BMI >39 | BMI 30–39 (3) |
| Immobility | Confined to bed | Wheelchair life (3) |
| Varicose veins | Past thrombosis | Extensive VVs (2) |

*Notes*: 1. A single risk factor in relative contraindication column indicates use of non-DSG/GSD pill, if any COC used
2. NB synergism, such that more than one factor in the relative contraindication column means COC method is absolutely contraindicated
3. There is conflict in the literature on the association of smoking with venous thromboembolic disease.
4. There is an increased risk of VTE with age.

of acne, or a friend's recommendation, or the need for better cycle control, indeed her perception of any issue of quality of life. 'The informed user should be the chooser'.

◆ Young first-time users: despite what just said, a LNG or NET product should in my view remain the **usual** first choice. Reasons:

(a) they will include an unknown subgroup who are, for congenital or acquired reasons, VTE-predisposed, and the risk is therefore highest during the first ever year of use

(b) VTE is a more relevant consideration than arterial disease at this age and

(c) the pills are cheaper.

◆ Single risk factor for *venous* thrombosis : LNG or NET product preferred, if COC used at all (WHO 3 if BMI >30; but WHO 4 if >39 ).

*Women with possible hereditary thrombophilia*: if one or more young first-degree relatives (defined in Table 4.5) suffered idiopathic VTE, the index woman should, in my view, in this country, not be prescribed any COC until thrombophilia has been excluded. The main abnormalities to be sought are factor V Leiden (the genetic cause of activated protein C resistance) which is the most prevalent; and deficiencies of protein C, protein S, and antithrombin III. Any of these, if found, absolutely contraindicate all EE-containing pills (WHO 4). Even if they are not found, the woman cannot be totally reassured and the COC should remain WHO 3 for her, since by no means all the predisposing abnormalities of the complex haemostatic system causing idiopathic VTE have yet been identified. Moreover, a LNG or NET product should be used.

**Table 4.6** Risk factors for arterial cardiovascular system (CVS) disease WHO categories in (—)

| Risk factor | Absolute contraindication (4) | Relative contraindication | Remarks |
|---|---|---|---|
| Family history (FH) arterial CVS disease in parent or sibling <45 | Known atherogenic lipid profile—or tests not available | Normal blood lipid profile or first attack in relative >45 | POP usually a better choice oral method method in all relative contraindications + consider LNG-IUS (see text) |
| Cigarette smoking | ?40+ cigarettes/day | 5–40 cigarettes/day (2–3) | |
| Diabetes mellitus (DM) | Severe or diabetic complications present (e.g. retinopathy, renal damage) | Not severe/labile, and no complications; young patient with short duration of DM (3) | |
| Hypertension (↑ BP) | BP >160/95 mmHg on repeated testing | ↑ BP but ≤160/95 mmHg (3) (see text) | WHO permits up to 100 mm diastolic as WHO 3 |
| Excess weight | BMI >39 | BMI 30–39 (3) | |
| Migraine | Focal aura symptoms; severe, or ergotamine-treated | Migraine without focal aura (2); sumatriptan treatment (2) | Relates to stroke risk. Consider tricycling, if non-focal aura headaches mainly in pill-free interval |
| Increasing age | If >50 (safer alternatives=fully effective) | >35 (2) | |

Notes: 1. Synergism: if more than one relative contraindication applies, including if woman aged >35, do not use COC
2. Some of the numbers selected are arbitrary and perhaps too strict if they are the sole problem (for example, the COC might actually be allowed reluctantly for a current healthy 25-year-old admitting to two packs of cigarettes a day). They also relate to use solely for contraception. Use of COCs for medical indications often entails a different risk benefit analysis, i.e. the extra therapeutic benefits may outweigh expected extra risks

Commonly, however, the 'family history' is weak – e.g. a more distant male or female relative, and perhaps there was a good reason for the VTE occurring (it was not idiopathic). If so, screening for thrombophilia is not indicated and the situation is WHO 2, though again a LNG or NET product should be used.

*Acquired thrombophilia* The most important of these is the anti-phospholipid syndrome occurring in connective tissue disorders, notably systemic lupus erythematosus (SLE). If identified this syndrome contraindicates the COC (WHO 4).

- Single definite *arterial* risk factor, e.g. smoking, usually after a number of years of VTE-free use, which is reassuring with regard to that condition (but only moderately, because the risk steadily rises with age); and also if COC is used at all (WHO 2) by older healthy and risk-factor-free women above age 35.

Arterial diseases are not only commoner among *smoking* pill-takers (but not non-smokers, see above), the case-fatality rate of acute myocardial infarction (AMI) is also much higher (RCGP 1983), and oddly enough in one unconfirmed study highest in users of LNG-containing pills. So on that basis, added to the apparently better lipid effects of DSG and GSD products, and the evidence above from Tanis *et al.* (2001), which differs from the MICA study (Dunn *et al.* 1999) in finding that the LNG products had a statistically increased risk of AMI (above non-users of any COCs): changing to a 20 μg EE-containing DSG or GSD product may be discussed with women in this category.

The primary reason, therefore for changing to a more oestrogenic product, such as a DSG/GSD brand, is for the control of side effects occurring on a LNG/NET product.

### What about other progestogens?
### Norgestimate, the progestogen in Cilest
There remains considerable uncertainty here, through lack of epidemiological data, and the CSM's October 1995 letter did not recommend any change in prescribing practice for Cilest. Intriguingly, one of its main metabolites is levonorgestrel (22% by weight, equivalent to about 55 μg). Since, as we saw above, this is functionally an anti-oestrogenic progestogen, one might expect some counteraction of the oestrogenicity and maybe therefore the thrombogenicity of the extra 17% of ethinylestradiol (35 μg rather than 30 μg) which Cilest contains, in comparison with other monophasic low-oestrogen products. At present we cannot be certain that Cilest should not be put in the 'third-generation' category for VTE risk.

For the time being Cilest can be considered as a useful option, tending to be oestrogen dominant but with no special limitations as to its use in the new prescribing environment prevailing in the UK since October 1995.

EVRA, a dermal patch delivering a combination of EE with norelgestomin, the active metabolite of norgestimate, is shortly expected on the UK market in May 2003 (Audet *et al.* 2001). The patch delivers through the skin a daily dose equivalent to an oral tablet of Cilest, with a similar side-effect profile and contraindications, but without diurnal fluctuations or the usual oral peak dose given to the liver. Each patch is worn for 7 days, three patches to be used for 21 days, and there is at least 2 days' 'margin for error' if the user forgets to put on a new one. This aids compliance, but it will still be essential never to lengthen the patch-free (contraception-free) interval (see below).

*Cyproterone acetate (CPA) as in Dianette*  This is an anti-androgen and in Dianette a dose of 2 mg is combined with ethinylestradiol (EE) 35 μg, for the oral treatment of moderately severe acne and mild hirsutism in women. These are its indications; but it is also a reliable anovulant like other COCs, and has similar back-up mechanisms, rules for missed tablets, interactions, absolute and relative contraindications. However, animal studies unconfirmed in humans suggest a risk of feminization of male fetuses and so it is absolutely contraindicated in pregnancy and lactation.

Otherwise, practically everything in this chapter on the COC applies to Dianette. But it is definitely an oestrogen-dominant product, as shown by its desired effect in the polycystic ovary syndrome (PCOS) of permitting EE to raise Sex hormone binding globulin (SHBG). So it might potentially also allow the oestrogen to have relatively greater effects in a prothrombotic direction than a levonorgestrel product would (see above). Although there are no clear epidemiological data, my current working hypothesis is therefore to put it in the same category as a 'third-generation' desogestrel/gestodene product and follow broadly the prescribing guidelines above.

Duration of treatment with Dianette needs to be individualized. In the Summary of Product Characteristics (SPC) it is recommended to 'withdraw when resolution' (of the acne or hirsutism) 'is complete', but repeat courses may be given if the conditions recur. There is a concern that prolonged high-dose treatment with CPA can cause benign and malignant liver tumours in rats, and hepatotoxicity has been described with the much higher 50 μg-plus doses used by dermatologists and for prostate cancer therapy. There is some evidence, but no certainty, that the 2 μg dose does not increase the risk of such tumours or of cholestatic jaundice any more than all other COCs, which are (rarely) also implicated. In my experience patients develop a very strong 'brand loyalty', but I encourage them to switch (commonly to Marvelon, which is usually satisfactory as maintenance therapy) when their condition is controlled, usually after one or two years. But if they do not tolerate the alternative they may return to and continue with Dianette for much longer, assuming they accept the unlikely but possible hepatic and prothrombotic risks.

*Drospirenone, the progestogen used in Yasmin* Yasmin is a new (2002) monophasic combined oral contraceptive marketed by Schering. Each tablet contains 3.0 mg drospirenone and 30 µg of ethinylestradiol (EE). Drospirenone differs from other progestogens in COCs, it has diuretic properties due to anti-mineralocorticoid activity comparable to a 25 mg dose of spironolactone, according to the SPC. This may help to oppose the salt and fluid-retaining effects of EE and so help symptoms like bloatedness. It has also been associated in a small trial, comparing it with Microgynon 30, with a very small (statistically but not clinically significant) lowering of blood pressure – a real difference from all other products tested which slightly raise mean pressure. This potentially important effect deserves further study.

It acts as an anti-androgen, so the combination may be an alternative to Dianette for conditions like PCOS.

Drospirenone with EE is an oestrogen-dominant combination, and so cannot be expected *a priori* to have the lower risk of VTE associated with the somewhat anti-oestrogenic levonorgestrel of, for example, Microgynon. But the epidemiological data to establish this either way are not available.

NO WEIGHT GAIN? There is a published European multi-centre randomized trial (Foidart *et al.* 2000), which definitely shows statistically lower body weight changes as compared with desogestrel-containing Marvelon. However, after 12 months, the slope of the Yasmin mean weight chart increases again, in parallel with that for Marvelon-users, and by 24 months mean weight of the users has returned to baseline value. Most authorities conclude that the small (1%) decrement in weight is due only to the diuresis, so there would be a maintained slight reduction of total body water in long-term use compared with controls. The subsequent steady gain in mean weight would then be the superimposed background increase observed regularly in European populations, as the years go by.

Interestingly, Yasmin will add some new WHO 4 conditions for pills: this particular brand should not be used in patients at risk of high potassium levels (i.e. renal insufficiency, hepatic dysfunction, and adrenal insufficiency).

Yasmin is welcomed as a new choice for appropriate women, an alternative to Dianette (i.e. unlike the latter, not primarily marketed for its acne/hirsutes benefits). It is relatively costly however, and until we have more data from studies we will not know to what extent, if any, it has real advantages over other oral contraceptive, (DTB, 2002). Until then, this should be seen as a second-line product. It can be used where the following criteria apply:

- need for oestrogen/anti-androgen therapy (significant acne, PCOS);
- raised blood pressure, the level being such as to make the clinician consider a change from the current formulation of combined pill – but COC still

clinically usable – i.e. above 140/90 but below the 160/95 level, which in UK is seen as WHO 4, (with careful follow-up and transfer to another contraceptive method if no benefit is seen);

◆ during COC follow-up, as a useful oestrogen-dominant second choice for empirical control of minor side effects, especially those attributed to fluid retention.

NB: However an existing weight problem with a BMI above 30 would normally indicate a less oestrogen dominant LNG-product, see p.131 (2nd bullet).

## Absolute and relative contraindications

Each packet of pills contains an insert, whose wording can often cause anxiety to both women and prescribers! But the personal and family history may unearth a range of contraindications, which are comprehensively summarized in Boxes 4.3 (WHO 4) and 4.4 (WHO 3 and 2 conditions). These are, in reality,

---

### Box 4.3 **Absolute contraindications to combined oral contraception (Guillebaud 1999)**

There are some conditions in which all brands of the COC are absolutely contraindicated (WHO 4):

*Past or present circulatory disease*

◆ Any past proven arterial or venous thrombosis

◆ Ischaemic heart disease or angina

◆ Severe or combined risk factors for venous or arterial disease (see Tables 4.5 and 4.6)

◆ Atherogenic lipid disorders

◆ Known prothrombotic abnormality of coagulation/fibrinolysis, congenital thrombophilias with abnormal levels of individual factors; from at least 2 (preferably 4) weeks before until 2 weeks after mobilization following elective major or leg surgery; during leg immobilization or varicose vein treatment; and during short-term exposure to high altitude (above 4000 metres)

◆ Migraine with focal aura or severe >72 hours; migraine requiring ergotamine treatment

◆ Transient ischaemic attacks even without headache

◆ Past cerebral haemorrhage, which can be secondary to cerebral venous thrombosis (also to avoid hypertension if past subarachnoid bleed)

## Box 4.3 (continued)

- Most types of structural heart disease (discuss with cardiologist), including atrial septal defect (risk of paradoxical embolism), major valve defects, pulmonary hypertension, risk of significant arrhythmias, especially atrial fibrillation

### Disease of the liver

- Active liver disease (whenever liver function tests currently abnormal, including infiltration and cirrhosis); recurrent cholestatic jaundice, or history of cholestatic jaundice in pregnancy; Dubin–Johnson and Rotor syndromes

   Following (viral) hepatitis or other hepatocellular damage, COCs may be resumed 3 months after liver function tests have returned to normal.

- Liver adenoma, carcinoma
- Porphyrias – acute (see text)

### History of serious condition affected by sex steroids or related to previous COC use

- Chorea
- COC-induced hypertension
- Pemphigoid gestationis
- Haemolytic uraemic syndrome
- Stevens–Johnson syndrome (erythema multiforme), if causation by COC is diagnosed
- Trophoblastic disease but only until β-hCG levels are undetectable. (In the USA and by WHO, this is not considered a contraindication even when hCG present, partly because chemotherapy is given to almost all cases of trophoblastic disease anyway)

### Pregnancy

### Undiagnosed genital tract bleeding

### Oestrogen-dependent neoplasms

- Breast cancer (some oncologists permit COCs in selected cases after prlonged remission)
- Past breast biopsy showing premalignant epithelial atypia

**Box 4.3** (continued)

*Woman's anxiety re COC safety unrelieved by counselling*

Note that several of the above are not necessarily permanent contraindications. Moreover, over the years, many women have been unnecessarily deprived of COCs for reasons now shown to have no link, such as thrush, or positively benefited by the method, such as fully investigated amenorrhoea with hypo-oestrogenism.

## Box 4.4 Relative contraindications to COCs (WHO 3 unless otherwise stated)

The following conditions are relative contraindications, signifying that the COC method is usable in context with: the benefit–risk evaluation for that individual; the acceptability or otherwise of alternatives; and sometimes with special advice (e.g. in migraine, to report a change of symptomatology) or monitoring (e.g. more frequent blood pressure measurements). In cases with excess risk of venous thrombosis, if the pill is used at all, it should be a non-DSG/GSD variety.

- Risk factors for arterial or venous disease (Table 4.6) provided normally that only one is present, and not to a marked degree. Which formulation to choose is discussed on pp. 131–3

- Homozygous sickle-cell disease (see text)

- Long-term partial immobilization, e.g. in a wheelchair (use non-DSG/GSD pill)

- Sex steroid-dependent cancer (including after treatment for malignant melanoma)

- Oligo-/amenorrhoea (COCs may be prescribed after investigation, to supply oestrogen in a woman needing contraception or to control the symptoms of PCOS)

- Hyperprolactinaemia (relative contraindication for patients under specialist supervision, with treatment in progress)

- Very severe depression, if likely to be exacerbated by COCs (but unwanted pregnancies can be very depressing)

- Some chronic diseases (WHO 3): inflammatory bowel disease, which produces prothrombotic changes, especially in exacerbations, including

**Box 4.4** (*continued*)

Crohn's disease (one form can also be brought on by COCs); diabetes; essential hypertension, well-controlled; gallstones (WHO 2 if surgically treated in past); otosclerosis (some authorities permit supervised COC use). See also text re 'intercurrent disease'

◆ Diseases that require long-term treatment with drugs which might interact with COCs (see text)

### Weak relative contraindications (WHO 2):

◆ If a young first-degree relation has breast cancer (p. 124–5)

◆ The presence of established benign breast disease (p. 124–5)

*Note:* Gilbert's disease (isolated raised bilirubin), past history of HELLP (hypertension, elevated liver enzymes and low platelets) syndrome, and mitral valve prolapse are all WHO 1 for the COC.

---

extensions of Tables 4.5 and 4.6, but now also including contraindications which are unrelated to cardiovascular disease.

### Intercurrent diseases

It is impossible to list every known disease which might have a bearing on COC prescription and for many the data are unavailable. A working rule is to ascertain whether or not the condition might lead to *summation* with known major adverse effects of COCs, particularly with the risk of any circulatory disease. This usually means WHO 4, sometimes 3. If there is no summation, in most serious chronic conditions the patient can be reassured that COCs are not known to have any effect, good or bad; they may then be used (WHO 2), though with the most careful monitoring and alertness for the onset of new risk factors. Reliable protection from pregnancy is often particularly important when other diseases are present.

*Diabetes* The formulations with desogestrel or gestodene and only 20 μg ethinylestradiol can be valuable (but still WHO 3 in my view) for limited periods, under careful supervision and provided that there is no arteriopathy, retinopathy, neuropathy, or renal damage (or smoking), all of which mean WHO 4, and preferably if the duration of the diabetes has been less than 20 years. (WHO places diabetes, with 20 years since diagnosis, as the sole additional factor into category WHO 4.) The progestogen-only pill (POP) is acceptable and usually very reliable, but copper IUDs, the *LNG-IUS (p. 199) and Implanon (p. 173) are even better choices for most diabetics,* even if nulliparous. Sterilization is often preferred when the family is complete, but the LNG-IUS should still be offered if the woman suffers with heavy or painful periods.

*Hypertension*   Hypertension is an important risk factor for heart disease and stroke. In most women on COCs there is a slight increase in both systolic and diastolic blood pressure within the normotensive range. Approximately 1% become clinically hypertensive: the rate increases with age and duration of use and when pill-induced (UK definition being above 160 systolic over above 95 diastolic, this absolutely contraindicates the combined hormonal method in future, though not the progestogen-only methods. If women with essential hypertension and no history of exacerbation in a past pregnancy are successfully treated with antihypertensives, another method is preferable but the COC may be used under careful supervision, WHO 3 (Box 4.4).

Past severe pregnancy-induced hypertension does not predispose to hypertension during later COC use, but it is a risk factor for myocardial infarction, very markedly so if the women also smokes (Croft and Hannaford 1989). The COC is therefore best avoided (WHO 4) in such cases.

*Sickle-cell disorders*   Sickle-cell trait has no bearing on the COC (WHO 1). Both sickle-cell disease in the homozygous conditions (SS and SC genes) and the COC individually lead to an increased risk of thrombosis, possibly superimposed during the arterial stasis of a crisis. Hence, many authorities and most manufacturers have for many years included the frank sickling diseases among the absolute contraindications (WHO 4) to the COC. However, the WHO reviewing studies in West Africa and the West Indies proposes that sickle-cell disease should only be considered a weak relative contraindication (WHO 2), especially when balanced against the particularly serious risks of pregnancy. In this country, injectables , implants or the POP are normally preferred hormonal options.

## Choice of pills and users

### Initial choice of preparation

Having excluded those women with absolute contraindications (Box 4.3), and proceeding with due caution/extra monitoring in the presence of (WHO 2 and 3 type) relative contraindications (Box 4.4, along with Tables 4.5 and 4.6), the practitioner is faced with a variety of formulations (Table 4.7). Which should be chosen?

**Table 4.7** System of summarizing pills according to progestogen content ('ladders')

| Pill | | µg | µg |
|---|---|---|---|
| | | *Levonorgestrel* | *Ethinyl oestradiol* |
| Eugynon 30 (Schering) | | 250 | 30 |
| Ovranette (Wyeth) | | 150 | 30 |
| Microgynon 30 (Schering) | | 150 | 30 |
| Microgynon 30ED = Microgynon 30 + 7 inert tablets | | | |
| Trinordiol (Wyeth) (triphasic) | 6 tablets | 50 | 30 |
| Logynon (Schering) (triphasic) | 5 tablets | 75 | 40 |
| | 10 tablets | 125 | 30 |
| Logynon ED = Logynon + 7 inert tablets | | | |
| | | *Norethisterone* | *Mestranol* |
| 2. Norinyl-1 (Searle) | | 1000 | 50 |
| | | *Norethisterone* | *Ethinyl oestradiol* |
| Norimin (Pharmacia) | | 1000 | 35 |
| BiNovum (Janssen-Cilag) | | 7 × 500; 14 × 1000 | 35 |
| TriNovum (Janssen-Cilag) | | 7 × 500; 7 × 750; 7 × 1000 | 35 |
| Synphase (Pharmacia) | | 7 × 500; 9 × 1000; 5 × 500 | 35 |
| Ovysmen (Janssen-Cilag) | | 500 | 35 |
| Brevinor (Pharmacia) | | 500 | 35 |
| | | *Norethisterone acetate* | *Ethinyl oestradiol* |
| 3. Loestrin 30 (Parke-Davis) | | 1500 | 30 |
| Loestrin 20 (Parke-Davis) | | 1000 | 20 |
| | | *Desogestrel* | *Ethinyl oestradiol* |
| 4. Marvelon (Organon) | | 150 | 30 |
| Mercilon (Organon) | | 150 | 20 |
| | | *Gestodene* | *Ethinyl oestradiol* |
| 5. Femodene (Schering) | | 75 | 30 |
| Minulet (Wyeth) | | 75 | 30 |
| Femodene ED = Femodene + 7 inert tablets | | | |

**Table 4.7** (continued)

| Pill | μg | μg |
|---|---|---|
| Femodette (Schering) | 75 | 20 |
| Triadene (Schering)/ | 6 × 50; 5 × 70; | 6 × 30; 5 × 40; |
| Tri-Minulet (Wyeth) | 10 × 100 | 10 × 30 |
| | *Norgestimate* | *Ethinyl oestradiol* |
| 6. Cilest (Janssen-Cilag) | 250 | 35 |
| | *Drospirenone* | |
| 7. Yasmin (Schering) | 3000 | 30 |
| 8. Dianette (Schering) | *Cyproterone* 2mg | *Acetate* 35 |

We have already discussed how to take account of venous and arterial risks. Much has been written about matching pills to the apparent 'hormonal profiles' of individual prospective pill-takers, but the systems have no practical value. Each prescriber needs to be familiar with the composition of the available preparations. Women may react unpredictably and several types may have to be tried before a suitable one is found. Some women are never suited. This is hardly surprising. Individual variation in motivation and tolerance of minor side effects is well recognized. But there is also marked individual variation in blood levels of the exogenous hormones and in responses at the end organs, especially the endometrium (Guillebaud 1999). Thus it is a false expectation that any single pill will suit all women.

After initial selection according to the guidelines, prescribers should try to identify, if necessary, over a series of initial visits as about to be described, the lowest dose for each woman which is effective yet does not cause the annoying symptom of breakthrough bleeding (BTB). It is believed that this will minimize adverse side effects, both serious and minor.

During follow-up, the aim is to give, long term, the *lowest acceptable* amount of both hormones. To achieve this, the following important concepts need to be brought together:

- *Individual* variation in absorption and metabolism causes blood levels of all contraceptive steroids to vary tenfold, or more accurately, the area-under-the-curve varies approximately threefold (Back *et al.* 1981). There are also variable end-organ responses.

- It is hypothesized that those with the highest blood levels are likely to be the most affected metabolically, and also more at risk of both major and minor side effects from abnormal bleeding patterns.

- It is also probable that women with the lowest blood levels tend to manifest this by BTB – as do women whose blood levels are lowered by enzyme inducers.
- Absence of BTB signifies either high or adequate blood levels of the administered steroids.

How then can we avoid giving to any woman who tends to have the highest blood levels a stronger formulation than she requires? Pending the availability of direct measurements in the clinic or surgery, we can 'titrate' the dose given against the occurrence of BTB, using the endometrium as an approximate 'threshold bioassay'. The aim should be that each woman receives the least long-term metabolic impact that her uterus will allow, i.e. the lowest dose of contraceptive steroids which is just, but only just, above her own bleeding threshold. In practice this means:

- *If there is good cycle control* at the time of repeat prescription, the possibility of trying a lower-dose brand (if available) should always be considered. On the other hand;
- *If BTB occurs* and is unacceptable or persists beyond two cycles, provided that none of the important alternative explanations applies (Box 4.5), the next strongest brand up the 'ladder' in Table 4.7 should be tried. Phased pills may be particularly useful for purposes of cycle control, especially if the chief complaint is absent withdrawal bleeding. Dianette is also worth a try for this symptom.

I still prefer to avoid the excessively progestogen-dominant brand Eugynon 30, since it markedly lowers HDL cholesterol, especially in smokers, unless indicated for therapeutic reasons, e.g. in the treatment of endometriosis (see Table 4.8). But if cycle control can only be achieved by a 50 μg pill, (Norinyl-1)it for that particular woman the latter need not be considered a 'strong' brand. This 'titrating' process is not helped by the lack of provision by the manufacturers of a good range of doses, especially for the newer progestogens.

Above all, though, check first through Box 4.5, and remember especially *Chlamydia* as the alternative and likely explanation of what appears to be 'BTB'; also if any cervix bleeds readily when a smear is taken.

### Second choice if there are non-bleeding side effects

The use of contemporary pills has reduced the reporting of so-called 'minor' side effects. When symptoms do occur, it is generally bad practice to give further prescriptions such as diuretics, anti-migraine treatments, or antidepressants for weight gain, headaches, or depression, respectively. For the last

## Box 4.5 **Checklist in cases of possible 'breakthrough bleeding' (BTB) in pill-takers**

A note of caution: first eliminate other possible causes! The following checklist is modified from Sapire (1990):

◆ *Disease* – examine the cervix. It is not unknown for bleeding from an invasive cancer to be wrongly attributed to BTB. *Chlamydia* can cause a blood-stained discharge

◆ *Disorder of pregnancy* causing bleeding (e.g. recent abortion, trophoblastic tumour)

◆ *Default* – missed pill(s). Remember that the BTB may start 2 or 3 days later and be very persistent thereafter

◆ *Drugs* – especially enzyme inducers (see text), also smoking, a common cause

◆ *Diarrhoea with* **vomiting** – diarrhoea alone has to be very severe to impair absorption significantly

◆ *Disturbance of absorption* – likewise, has to be very marked to be relevant, e.g. after massive gut resection. Coeliac disease does not pose a significant absorption problem

◆ *Diet* – gut flora involved in recycling ethinylestradiol may be reduced in vegetarians. Could sometimes be a factor in BTB, but a very unlikely cause

◆ *Duration too short* – minimal BTB which is tolerable may resolve after 2–3 months' use of any new formulation. The opposite problem may sometimes apply during 'tricycling' (see text); the duration of continuous use may be too long in that individual for the endometrium to be sustained. If so, 'bicycling' of two packets in a row may be substituted

*Finally,* after the above have been excluded:

◆ *Dose* – if she is taking a monophasic, try a phasic pill; increase the oestrogen or progestogen component; try a different progestogen.

of these, pyridoxine 50–100 mg daily may be beneficial. Otherwise there are two preferred, if empirical, courses of action namely:

◆ decrease the dose of either hormone, if still possible – in the limit, oestrogen can be eliminated by a trial of the progestogen-only pill;

◆ change to any different progestogen (Table 4.7), not forgetting norgestimate, drospirenone and cyproterone acetate as options (see above).

Some more specific guidance for common side effects and conditions associated with a relative excess of either steroid may be obtained from Tables 4.8 and 4.9. Note the cautions in the important notes at the bottom of each table. And note also that modern pills have been shown NOT to cause an increase in the prevalence of candidiasis, which is common in all women.

## Supervision and long-term follow-up

Each woman needs individual teaching, backed by a good instruction leaflet (ideally the one produced by the UK FPA). Starting on day 1 (or by day 3)

**Table 4.8** Which second choice of pill? Relative oestrogen excess

| Symptoms | Conditions |
|---|---|
| Nausea | Benign breast disease |
| Dizziness | Fibroids |
| 'Premenstrual tension' and irritability | Endometriosis |
| Cyclical weight gain (fluid) | |
| 'Bloating' | |
| Vaginal discharge (no infection) | |
| Some cases of breast swelling/pain | |

Treat with progestogen – dominant COC, such as Microgynon 30, Loestrin 30, Eugynon 30 (but with caution regarding lipids, and risk of arterial disease in those with the relevant risk factors, see p. 132). Loestrin 20 is an oestrogen-deficient option: the other 20 $\mu$g products, Mercilon and Femodette, are less so, functionally.

**Table 4.9** Which second choice of pill? Relative progestogen excess

| Symptoms | Conditions |
|---|---|
| Dryness of vagina | Acne/seborrhoea |
| Some cases of | Hirsutism |
|    Sustained weight gain | |
|    Depression | |
|    Loss of libido | |
|    Breast symptoms | |

Treat with oestrogen-dominant COC, such as Ovysmen/Brevinor, or Marvelon; then Yasmin (p. 135) or Dianette, (see text, p. 134). (Caution necessary in that oestrogen-dominance may correlate with a slightly higher risk of venous thrombosis, especially if relevant risk factors present, see p. 131).

avoids the requirement to take extra precautions (see Table 4.10). However, in some cases it may be more relevant that cycle control in early cycles has been shown to be better with a day 5 than with a day 1 start. It is important to remind the woman that the packet must be completed regardless of any bleeding; also that the 7 tablet-free days are only 'safe' for intercourse if the next packet follows on time.

◆ A useful check of good pill-taking at follow-up is to ask her which day each new pack is started. It should be on a specific day of the week. If her response is 'it all depends', something is amiss!

**Table 4.10** Starting routines

|  | Start when? | Extra precautions for 7 days? |
| --- | --- | --- |
| 1. Menstruating | At or after 5th day of period | Yes |
|  | 1st day/before day 5 | No[1] |
| 2. Post-partum |  |  |
| (a) No lactation | Day 22 ideal (low risk of thrombosis by then, first ovulations reported day 28+) |  |
| (b) Lactation | Not normally recommended at all (POP or DMPA preferred) |  |
| 3. Post-induced abortion/ miscarriage | Same day or day 2 | No |
| 4. Post trophoblastic tumour | One month after no hCG detected | As 1 |
| 5. Post-higher dose COC | Instant switch 3 | No |
| 6. Post-lower or same dose COC | After usual 7-day break | No |
| 7. Post-POP | First day of period | No |
| 8. Post-POP with secondary amenorrhoea | Any day (e.g. end of packet) | No |
| 9. Other secondary amenorrhoea (pregnancy risk excluded 3) | Any day | Yes |

[1] Except in the case of Logynon ED and Femodene ED – here the starting routine entails the taking of a variable number of placebos; hence extra precautions are recommended, for 14 days in fact
[2] After *severe* pre-eclampsia or the related HELLP syndrome, delay COC use until the return of normal BP and biochemistry.
[3] This advice is because of reports of rebound ovulation occurring at the time of transfer, if the usual 7-day break is taken. Alternative: normal 7-day break plus extra contraception for first 7 days of the new packet
[4] This may mean doing negative sensitive pregnancy test after there have been at least 14 days of safe contraception or abstinence

◆ The body mass index (BMI) should be calculated at the first pill visit, and its venous/arterial implications discussed in the light of Tables 4.5 and 4.6. But ongoing weighing as a *routine* follow-up procedure is unimportant and sometimes unhelpful.

◆ Blood pressure should be recorded before starting the pill and checked after 3 months (1 month in a high-risk case), and subsequently at intervals of 6 months. After about 2 years if there is no significant change this interval can be increased to annually, but the risk of hypertension never entirely disappears. A moderate increase in blood pressure may also act as a marker for an increased risk of thrombosis, especially in the presence of any arterial risk factor.

◆ Thereafter the only items which are relevant to longer-term COC follow-up are:

(a) *blood pressure* monitoring – continuing, as just described;

(b) updating of *family history* (e.g. as she and they get older, the mother or elder sister of a young client may now have had the VTE under 45 to which they were always predisposed);

(c) management of *new risk factors, diseases,* and *relevant drugs,* i.e. updating recent past history;

(d) current *symptom monitoring,* possibly pill-related side effects – see Tables 4.8, 4.9, and related text;

(e) *headache* monitoring – the most important symptom to check.

The last of these is perhaps most often neglected – see below!

Breast awareness should be taught, and checked by nurse or doctor annually. Cervical screening should be performed regularly according to local guidelines. However, it is essential to appreciate and to explain to women that such procedures are part of well-woman care, and unrelated to safe pill management.

## Migraine

Studies have shown an increased risk (OR 1–2) of ischaemic stroke in COC users. This risk is independently increased in migraine sufferers. In Lidegaard's study from Denmark, the risk through having any kind of migraine more than once a month without the Pill was increased by a little less than threefold, compared with the background risk (MacGregor 2001). The modern COC may (further) increase the risk about twofold. And there is (as usual) further risk if the woman has other arterial risk factors like smoking.

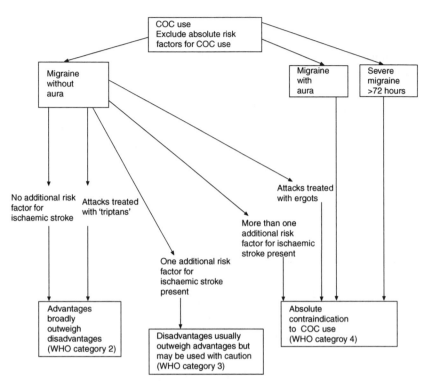

**Fig 4.2** Migraine and COC use.

Because thrombotic strokes are rare in young women (1.8 per 100 000 at age 20), the absolute (attributable) risks of having migraine, or of additionally using the COC, remain small. Using the above Danish data, there would be about 10 cases attributable to being on the COC with migraine at 20, i.e. 8 extra compared with controls without migraine or COC use. This is actually fewer than the number of venous thromboembolism cases per 100 000 attributable to either 'generation' of COCs in Table 4.4, so the situation is only WHO 2 (Fig 4.2) – but the morbidity in survivors is potentially more serious and long term. If smoking or another arterial risk factor is added, the risk goes up further (WHO 3). Moreover, the background risk at age 40–44 is at least 16 per 100 000, so all the attributable risks are 9–10 times greater, implying that women with significant migraine should cease taking the COC by that age (WHO 4).

It is also believed, though here the data are more sparse, that certain features of the headaches – i.e. migraine with aura – focus the risk of this rare catastrophe in a pill-taker. Hence the advice which follows (MacGregor and Guillebaud 1998):

## Absolute contraindications (WHO 4) to commencing or continuing the COC:

◆ Migraine with aura during which there are focal neurological symptoms (usually asymmetrical and preceding the headache itself). The significant associated symptoms during an aura *before* the headache itself are:

(a) loss of sight, or of part or whole of field of vision on one side (homonymous visual disturbance): 99% of relevant auras are visual. Teichopsia is one variety, in which a bright spot enlarges to produce a scintillating angulated line (fortification spectra) surrounding the bright area of lost vision. The latter is a bright scotoma – i.e. the lost vision is bright, not black. (*A useful tip when taking this history is to watch the hands: the woman trying to describe her visual aura will almost always wave her hand, near her head on one or other side.*)

(b) numbness, severe paraesthesia, or weakness on one side of the body (e.g. one limb, side of the mouth and tongue).

(c) disturbance of speech (nominal dysphasia).

Note the absence of photophobia or *symmetrical* blurring or 'flashing lights'; the main feature the relevant symptoms share is that they are 'focal' or interpretable as due to (transient) cerebral ischaemia. Should relevant symptoms be described, the *artificial oestrogen* of the COC should normally be stopped and thereafter avoided to minimize the risk of superimposed thrombosis causing permanent ischaemia, i.e. a thrombotic stroke.

It may be difficult to distinguish such relatively common, migraine-associated transient ischaemia from rare organic episodes – true transient ischaemic attacks or TIAs (e.g. due to paradoxical embolism which is an established risk of an atrial septal defect). Upon suspicion, these, of course, mean the same in practice, i.e. WHO 4, stop the pill immediately. But neurological investigation should also follow if an organic episode is a possibility, particularly for the following focal symptoms which are *not* typical of migraine:

(d) focal epilepsy or severe acute vertigo, ataxia, monocular blindness, aphasia, unilateral tinnitus;

(e) a severe unexplained drop attack or collapse.

TIAs are also more sudden in onset than migraine aura and last over an hour, without other migraine symptoms like nausea.

◆ Migraines which are unusually frequent/severe. 'Status migrainosus' describes attacks lasting more than 72 hours, which contraindicate the COC absolutely – *unless* they resolve after treatment for medication misuse (see below).

◆ Migraines requiring ergotamine treatment, due to its vasoconstrictor actions.

*Note*: In any of the above, any of the progestogen-only, oestrogen-free hormonal methods may be offered immediately: similar headaches may continue, but now without the potential added risk from prothrombotic haemostatic effects of the ethinylestradiol. HRT with *natural* oestrogen is also not contraindicated, if oestrogen deficiency is later suspected.

Hormonal emergency contraception may also be given by the new levonorgestrel-only method, even within an attack (MacGregor 2001).

### Relative contraindications

See Fig 4.2, which helpfully distinguishes circumstances which are WHO 2 from WHO 3. In either the COC may be used, but always with specific instruction to the woman regarding those changes in the character or severity of her symptoms which mean she should stop the method and take urgent medical advice An alternative contraceptive (e.g. the IUS) would always be preferable in the cases below if, due to the synergism highlighted in Table 4.6, there are added arterial risk factors such as heavy smoking, or diabetes or older age above 35.

- Migraine without focal aura (WHO 2). This includes migraine with photophobia, phonophobia, or any other prodromal or within-headache symptoms so long as none is localizable to the cerebral cortex or brainstem. If these or other 'ordinary' headaches occur, particularly in the pill-free interval, tricycling the COC may help (see p. 152).

- Distant past history of migraine with focal aura, i.e. a history of the last attack being more than 5 years before commencing the COC. The COC may be given a trial with the caveats above.

- The occurrence of a woman's first-ever attack of migraine of any type while on the COC. This should be stopped if she is seen during the attack, but can be later restarted with the usual forewarning about focal symptoms (and instructions if they do occur to switch to another method).

- Use of a triptan for migraine therapy in the absence of any other contraindicating factors.

### Reasons to stop the pill

Box 4.6 lists the reasons that should be understood by all well-counselled women from their first visit, for immediately discontinuing COCs and obtaining urgent further advice. They appear in lay terms in the FPA's recommended leaflet, which is one reason why, in my view, it should be given to all prospective pill-takers. Note that the first four focus on the risk of stroke in relation to migraine with focal aura and TIAs – see above.

## Importance of the pill-free week

This promotes a reassuring withdrawal bleed (WTB) – and indeed, if this does not occur in two successive cycles, it is best to exclude pregnancy. However, its importance might be greater than that, in allowing some degree of recovery

---

### Box 4.6 **COCs should be stopped immediately pending investigation and treatment if the following occur:**

- Unusual or severe and very prolonged headache
- Disturbance of speech (nominal dysphasia)
- Loss of sight, or of part of whole of field of vision on one side (homonymous visual disturbance). Teichopsia is one variety (see p. 149)
- Numbness, severe paraesthesia or weakness on one side of the body (e.g. one limb, side of the tongue); indeed, any symptom suggesting cerebral ischaemia
- Focal epilepsy or severe acute vertigo, ataxia, monocular blindness
- A severe unexplained fainting attack or collapse
- Painful swelling in the calf
- Pain in the chest, especially pleuritic pain
- Breathlessness or cough with blood-stained sputum
- Severe abdominal pain
- Immobilization, as after orthopaedic injury or major surgery (do not demand that the COC be stopped for any minor surgery such as laparoscopy) or leg surgery: stop COC and heparinize. If elective procedure and Pill stopped more than 2 weeks ahead, anticoagulation usually unnecessary

All the above could be caused by an actual or imminent thrombotic or embolic event, though other explanations may well apply. They mean that the artificial oestrogen should be stopped, but any progestogen-only method could be started immediately pending the diagnosis. Other reasons for stopping are usually less urgent.

- Acute jaundice
- Blood pressure above 160/95 on repeated measurement
- Severe skin rash (e.g. erythema multiforme)
- Detection of a new risk factor, e.g. onset of diabetes or SLE, diagnosis of a structural heart lesion such as ASD, detection of breast cancer

from systemic effects of the pill. In one study, for example, HDL-cholesterol suppression by the COCs studied was eliminated by the end of the pill-free interval (Demacker *et al.* 1982) and unpublished work from MPC shows the same regular trend for some coagulation factors. Hence it is probably wise only to cut out the gap between packets either:

♦ in the short term, upon request to avoid a bleed on special occasions. If a phasic pill is in use either the final phase of a spare pack should be used, or for longer postponement the whole pack from an equivalent monophasic pill to that final phase (e.g. Microgynon for Logynon; or Norimin if the current pill is TriNovum) OR:

♦ for specific indications such as the occurrence of regular hormone-withdrawal headaches.

The *tricycle regimen* is often used, in which three or four packets of a monophasic pill are taken in succession, followed by a pill-free gap. This leads to 10-week or 13-week cycles, only four or five WTBs per year and, in this example, only that number of headaches annually. Other important indications are given in Box 4.7 and discussed further below.

---

## Box 4.7 **Indications for the tricycle regimen (using a monophasic pill)**

♦ Headaches, including migraine without aura and other bothersome symptoms occurring regularly in the withdrawal week

♦ Unacceptably heavy or painful withdrawal bleeds

♦ Paradoxically, to help women who are concerned about absent withdrawal bleeds (this concern therefore arising less often!)

♦ Epilepsy: this benefits from relatively more sustained levels of the administered hormones (see also below for another reason related to the anti-epileptic treatment)

♦ Enzyme-inducer therapy (see text)

♦ Endometriosis – a progestogen-dominant monophasic pill may be tricycled for maintenance treatment after primary therapy (e.g. Eugynon 30, sometimes Microgynon 30)

♦ Suspicion of decreased efficacy

♦ At the woman's choice

*Note: In view of the possibility that the monthly pill-free interval is beneficial (see pp. 151–2), one of these special indications should normally apply.*

Biochemical and ultrasound data also demonstrate return of pituitary and ovarian follicular activity during the pill-free time in about one-fifth of pill-takers, in some women to a marked extent (Guillebaud 1999). Therefore, breakthrough ovulation is most likely to follow any lengthening of the pill-free (meaning contraception-free) interval. Such lengthening may result from omissions, malabsorption, and drug interaction involving pills either at the start or at the end of a packet.

Smith *et al.* (1986) showed that even if only 14 or even as few as seven pills had first been taken, no women ovulated after seven pills were subsequently missed – implying at the very least that three or four pills may be missed mid-packet with impunity! This and other work may be summarized:

- seven consecutive pills are enough to 'put the ovaries to sleep' (therefore pills 8–21 in a packet simply 'keep them asleep')

- seven pills can be omitted without ovulation, as in the regular pill-free week

- more than seven pills missed *in total* increases the conception risk.

The '*7-day rule*', as now used by the UK FPA and also the UK manufacturers, is summarized in Fig. 4.3. The part of the advice for when fewer than 7 tablets remain is critically important and can be explained:

It would be silly to let your ovaries have another break from the effect of your contraceptive, so soon after the break you made by mistake (by the pills you missed).

Fig 4.3 gives a useful flow diagram for patients: note the important footnote regarding emergency contraception. Emergency contraception is only indicated if pill omissions lead to a lengthening of the pill-free time to 9 days (or more), *or* if any combination of pills from the first seven have been omitted such as to amount effectively, in the prescriber's view, to a 9-day interval since effective pituitary/ovarian suppression. In such a case, the woman should still use condoms as well during the first 7 days of renewed pill-taking, and also be asked to return in 4 weeks to exclude conception.

Otherwise, unless very many pills are missed (arbitrarily the Faculty states four or more), the studies, including Smith *et al.* quoted above, indicate that emergency contraception would be redundant since the advice in Fig 4.3 will maintain normal or above-normal efficacy, mid-cycle and at the end of a pack.

### Vomiting of tablets (within 2 hours and not successfully replaced within 12 hours), and severe diarrhoea

Extra contraceptive precautions should start from the onset of the (maybe short) illness and continue for 7 days after it ends, with elimination of the pill-free interval as indicated by the above advice. Diarrhoea alone is not a problem, unless it is of cholera-like severity!

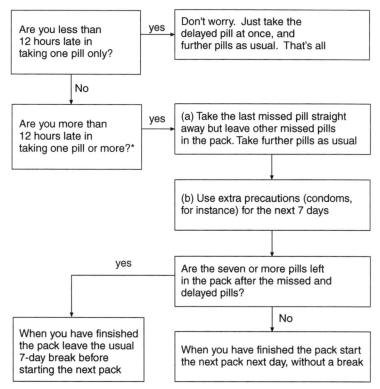

*If two or more pills missed AND if they were all from the first seven in your pack, and if you have had unprotected intercourses since the end of your last pack, talk promptly to your doctor. You may need emergency pills AS WELL AS continuing with instructions A and B above.

**Fig 4.3** Advice for missed combined oral contraceptive pills (21-day packaging).

## Women who have had a previous combined pill failure

They may claim perfect compliance or perhaps admit to omission of no more than one pill. Either way, since surveys show that most women miss tablets quite frequently but very few conceive, the ability to do so selects out those women who are likely to have low levels of hormones, or ovaries with above-average return to activity in the pill-free interval. So all women in this group should, in my view, either consider a different method or be advised to consider taking three (or four) packets in a row, the so-called *tricycle regimen*, followed by a shortened pill-free gap. Often 6 days is a good choice in these cases since it is easy to remember, with each tricycle's start day now being identical to the finish day (but contrast the more cautious 4 days recommended below, for use during potent enzyme-inducing drug treatments).

We understand that WHO will soon be issuing new guidelines for missed COCs, which will differ from those described above, though based on the same concepts. They are similar to those described in a Review some years ago, which was part-authored from MPC (Korver *et al.* 1995). Since they will not be generally authorized until new UK FPA leaflets are agreed and available for all users, for the present, the scheme summarized in Fig 4.3 should continue in use. Details are available to download (Selected Practice Recommendations) from www.WHO.int/reproductive-health.

## Drug interactions (Elliman 2000)

These may reduce the pill's efficacy, mainly in two ways. The first and by far the more important is by induction of liver enzymes, which leads to increased elimination of both oestrogen and progestogen. Alternatively, disturbance by certain antibiotics of the gut flora, which normally split oestrogen metabolites arriving in the bowel, can reduce in a very small – but unknown – minority of women the reabsorption of reactivated oestrogen. (Note: this effect on the enterohepatic cycle is not a factor in the maintenance of progestogen levels and so is irrelevant to the progestogen-only pill.) See Table 4.11 and the latest edition of the British National Formulary (BNF), Appendix 1, for the most important drugs and the clinical implications.

### Short-term use of any interacting drug/long-term use of broad spectrum antibiotic

Extra contraceptive precautions are advised for the duration of the treatment followed by the '7-day rule' as above, according to when in the pill packet the last potentially less effective pill was taken. Rifampicin is such a powerful enzyme inducer that even if it is given only for 2 days (as for instance to eliminate carriage of the meningococcus), increased elimination by the liver must be assumed for 4 weeks thereafter (Orme 1991, personal communication). Extra contraception or a stronger pill with elimination of one or more pill-free intervals (see below) should be recommended to cover that time.

With broad-spectrum antibiotics there is the useful fact that the large bowel flora responsible for recycling oestrogens are reconstituted with resistant organisms in about 2 weeks. In practice therefore, if the COC is commenced in a woman who has been taking a tetracycline long term (for acne, for example), there is no need to advise extra contraceptive precautions. There is a potential problem only in the reverse situation, when the antibiotic is first introduced to treat a long-term pill-taker. Even then, extra precautions need to be sustained only for a maximum of 3 weeks, with elimination of at most one pill-free interval.

### Long-term use of enzyme inducers (Table 4.11)

This is a WHO 3 situation and therefore an alternative method of contraception such as an intrauterine device or system, implant, or possibly depot

**Table 4.11** The more important drug interactions with COCs

| Class of drug | Approved names of important examples | Main action | Clinical implications for COC use |
|---|---|---|---|
| **Drug which may reduce COC efficacy** | | | |
| *Anticonvulsants* | Barbiturates (esp. phenobarbitone) Phenytoin, Primidone, Carbamazepine, Oxcarbazepine Topiramate | Induction of liver enzymes, increasing their ability to metabolize *both* COC steroids | WHO 3 so offer another method first. If COC preferred tricycling advised using 50 µg oestrogen COCs, increasing to max 100 µg if BTB occurs. Sodium valproate, gabapentin, lamotrigine, vigabatrin and all the benzodiazepines are anticonvulsants *without* this effect |
| *Antibiotics* | | | |
| (a) Antitubercle | Rifampicin Rifabutin | *Marked* induction of liver enzymes | Short term, see text. Long term, use of alternative contraception is preferred. e.g. Depo-Provera with 10 week injection intervals |
| (b) Antifungal | Griseofulvin | Enzyme inducer | As for anticonvulsants. Beware, griseofulvin is a teratogen. |
| (c) Other antibiotics | Penicillins, especially Ampicillin and relatives Tetracyclines | Change in bowel flora, reducing enteroheptic recirculation of ethinyloestradiol (EE) only, after hydrolysis of its conjugates | Short courses – wisest to use additional contraception during illness and follow 7-day rule. Long-term, low-dose tetracycline for acne – no apparent problem, probably because resistant organisms develop, within about 2 weeks. NB: POP is unaffected by this type of interaction |

**Table 4.11** (*continued*)

| Class of drug | Approved names of important examples | Main action | Clinical implications for COC use |
|---|---|---|---|
| *Miscellaneous* | Modafinil<br>Tacrolinus<br>Several anti-retroviral drugs St. John's word (SJW) | Induction of liver enzymes | ◆ See above, as for anti-convulsants.<br>◆ Take the advice of Consultant treating an HIV/AIDS patient, as relevant.<br>◆ CSM advises that the combination of SJW with COC should be AVOIDED |

**Drugs which may increase COC efficacy**

| | | | |
|---|---|---|---|
| | Co-trimoxazole,<br>Sulphonamides<br>Enythromycin | Inhibit EE metabolism in liver | None, if short courses given to low-dose COC user |

*Note:* Recent studies show no significant effect of mega-dose ascorbic acid in raising blood levels of ethinyloestradiol (as previously reported)

medroxyprogesterone acetate with a shortened (10-week) injection interval is preferable and should be discussed.. If rifampicin or rifabutin are prescribed long term, they are so potent that the COC should be avoided altogether. The same advice has been given by the CSM if the woman elects to continue using St John's Wort (Table 4.11), apparently (A. Breckenridge, 2000, personal communication) because the enzyme-inducing potencies of this so-called 'nature's Prozac' can vary up to 50-fold between batches as sold.

Otherwise, if the combined pill is deemed appropriate, the first choice initially is a 50–60 µg oestrogen pill combination (eg. Microgynon30 × 2 tablets) There is now only one such brands on the market, but with Norinyl-1 it is actually doubtful whether the dose is any higher than with Norimin, since there is on average only about 70% conversion of mestranol to ethinylestradiol. Probably more important than the increased dose is *also* to recommend the tricycle regimen described above (Box 4.7). This reduces the number of contraceptively 'risky' pill-free intervals (PFIs). It is particularly appropriate for epileptics since as a bonus the frequency of attacks is often reduced by the maintenance of steady hormone levels. At the Margaret Pyke Centre we recommend that the PFI is also shortened at the end of each tricycle, usually to 4 days, and in our experience of numerous referrals who have had one or more breakthrough pregnancies through enzyme induction (usually where the woman had been given no specific advice at all) this regimen nearly always succeeds in restoring COC efficacy.

If the preferred progestogen is not marketed as a 50 µg pill, an entirely logical if expensive alternative is to use combinations of tablets, e.g. Loestrin 30 + Loestrin20, or, if an oestrogen-dominant pill is preferred, one Mercilon plus one Marvelon daily. If so, very careful records are essential (following the full routine described on p. 220) since this is an unlicensed, though definitely evidence-based, use of a licensed product.

Breakthrough bleeding (BTB) may be the first clue to a drug interaction and should also be used as an indication to make appropriate alteration to the pill prescription, or to advise a change of method. If the long-term user of an enzyme inducer develops BTB, after first carefully checking against the 'D' checklist of Box 4.5, the next step is to give two or more tablets a day, if necessary to provide a combined oestrogen content of up to 100 µg (a very rare maximum), titrated against the BTB.

In this way the usual policy, which is to give the minimum dose of both hormones to finish just above the threshold for bleeding, can be followed. The woman can be reassured that she is metaphorically 'climbing a down escalator'. In other words, her increased liver metabolism means that her system is still basically receiving a low-dose regimen. She is exposed to more metabolites, but

this is not known to be harmful (and for some women the available alternatives are just not acceptable).

### Discontinuing enzyme-inducers

Enzyme induction may take numerous days to reach its peak when the drug
is introduced and it may be 4–8 weeks before the liver's level of excretory
function reverts to normal when it is withdrawn. Hence if any enzyme inducer
has been used for a month or more (or *at all* in the case of rifampicin) it is
therefore recommended (Orme 1986, personal communication) that there is
a delay of about 4 weeks before the woman returns to a standard low-dose pill
regimen. This should be increased to 8 weeks after more prolonged use of
rifampicin or barbiturates; and logically there should then also be no gap
between the higher- and the low-dose packets.

### Effects of COCs on other drugs

COC steroids are weak inhibitors of hepatic microsomal enzymes. They thus
slightly lower the clearance of, for example, tricyclic antidepressants, and
diazepam. This theoretically increases the risk of side effects – seriously only in
the case of the drug cyclosporin. Otherwise the change is very unlikely to be
noticed clinically.

As COCs tend to impair glucose tolerance, sometimes cause depression, and
raise the blood pressure, they naturally tend to oppose the action of antidia-
betic, antidepressant, and antihypertensive treatments. Similarly the prothrombotic effects of the COC tend somewhat to reduce the anticoagulant activity of
warfarin. This combination would very rarely be appropriate anyway, and in
the other examples very little, if any, upward dose adjustment is ever required
clinically.

## Congenital abnormalities and fertility

There are many conflicting reports in the world literature, not helped by small
numbers studied and confounding factors such as smoking, alcohol, and
other drugs which have not always been considered. Two per cent of all full-
term fetuses have an important malformation. The conclusions of a WHO
scientific group (1981) have not been materially challenged subsequently.
These were:

- no established evidence for any adverse effects on the fetus of oral contraceptives used prior to the conception cycle;
- with regard to oral contraceptive use after conception, the evidence for an
  increased risk of congenital malformations is unclear; but if such a risk
  exists, it must be very small.

It is always wise to warn women against taking any medication if they believe themselves to be pregnant. If the GP is asked the question: 'Should I come off the Pill for say 2 months before getting pregnant?' there is no dogmatic answer. It should certainly do no harm and most metabolic changes studied have, indeed, returned to normal well within that timescale. But there is no objective evidence that it is worth the effort. Certainly any woman finding herself pregnant almost immediately after stopping the COC should be strongly reassured.

There is no known benefit, either to fertility or health, to be gained by taking short breaks of 6 months or so every few years, as was once recommended. One-quarter of young women taking such short breaks had unwanted conceptions in one study. Moreover, a pill-taker can be reminded she has regularly given her body 'breaks' from the COC totalling 13 weeks in each year.

The first period after stopping the Pill is often delayed for some weeks. However, 'post-Pill amenorrhoea' is not a valid diagnosis and amenorrhoea for 6 months should always be investigated (Chapter 1), whether or not it occurs after stopping this method. With or without amenorrhoea, conception may be delayed by a few months on average on stopping the Pill, but there is no evidence that the Pill causes long-term irreversible infertility. Indeed, its beneficial effects (Box 4.2) protect against several causes of infertility.

## Duration of use

Though still uncertain, it remains possible that increased duration of use may adversely affect the risk of circulatory disease in some current users, though reassuringly it clearly now does not do so in ex-users (Stampfer *et al.* 1988). Recency of use, not duration, was important in the latest analysis of the world data on breast cancer (see p. 123) and regardless of duration after 10 years, all ex-users had the same subsequent mortality as never users (Beral *et al.* 1999).

Pending more information, it remains prudent to restrict total *accumulated* duration of use to a maximum of 15 years in those with definite arterial or venous risk factors. Where risk factors exist (Tables 4.5, 4.6 and Box 4.3), whether WHO 3 or WHO 2 conditions, the COC should be stopped at age 35. For healthy, risk factor-free women, which includes those free of any significant form of migraine, there is no strict upper limit. Some women may therefore choose to continue, normally using one of the 20 μg products, to age 50 – so achieving perhaps over 30 years' use – and even then switch thereafter to HRT. This is difficult to oppose when so many of the benefits (especially the protection from ovarian cancer) are clearly enhanced as duration of COC use increases. But breast cancer risk also definitely increases significantly with age, without the COC, and probably more so with it. This should be discussed with all. The availability of new choices such as the IUS must be expected in future to reduce COC use in later reproductive years.

## Summary

The combined pill provides highly acceptable contraception for many. Individuals vary, however, and best results follow from always maintaining the user's autonomy. Presentation of multiple side effects in spite of trying many different low-dose products may indicate the need for a different method, but excessive anxiety about consequences should first be suspected and possible psychosexual aspects discussed. No matter how carefully those with contraindications are excluded, a few women will experience adverse effects. Supervision is essential, monitoring above all blood pressure and headaches,

---

### Box 4.8 **Take-home messages for a new pill-taker**

- Your FPA leaflet: this is not to be read and thrown away; it is something to keep safely in a drawer somewhere, for ongoing reference
- The pill only works if you take it correctly: if you do, each new pack will always start on the same day of the week
- Even if bleeding like a 'period' occurs (breakthrough bleeding), carry on pill-taking. This, like other symptoms (e.g. nausea), will usually stop if you persevere. Ring for advice if necessary
- Lovemaking during the 7 days after any packet is only safe if you do go to the next packet
- Never start your next packet late. This is because the pill-free time is obviously a time when your ovaries are not getting the contraceptive, so might anyway be beginning to escape from its actions. (This simple explanation should always be given – it greatly improves compliance)
- What to do if any pill(s) are more than 12 hours late? (See Fig 4.3)
- Other things that may stop the pill from working include vomiting and some drugs (pp. 154–7)
- See a doctor at once if . . . (p. 151)
- You can avoid bleeding on holidays, etc., by running 2 packets together
- As a one-off manoeuvre, you can shorten one pill-free gap to make sure your withdrawal bleeds avoid weekends
- Finally: use a condom *as well* with any new partner, or whenever there might be an infection risk

and it is important that the woman feels able to report back at any time; often to the practice nurse.

The first visit for this method is by far and away the most important and should never be rushed: there is a lot of ground to cover (Box 4.8).

## Progestogen-only pill (POP)

Note: this section relates only to POPs as a category which excludes the desogestrel product cerazette, see p. 167. This is an underused and often abused method which requires maximum motivation by both patient and prescriber. Taken absolutely regularly each day within a couple of hours, without breaks, and regardless of bleeding patterns, it can provide protection from pregnancy not far short of the combined pill, especially above age 30 (for comprehensive review, see McCann and Potter 1994). The Oxford/FPA study reported a failure rate of 3.1 per 100 woman-years at age 25–29, but this improved to 1.0 at 35–39 and as low as 0.3 for women over 40 (Vessey *et al.* 1985).

Its efficacy is also enhanced during breast-feeding (but beware the young, highly fertile woman at the time of weaning).

### Mechanism of action and maintenance of efficacy

Existing databases suggest but do not prove the possibility that the failure rate is higher in heavier women, as already established for progestogen rings and a research version (not marketed) of Norplant implants. Women who weigh above 70 kg (irrespective of height, it is total body water not BMI that is thought to be relevant here) should in my view continue to be warned of this possibility (Guillebaud, 2001b). Given the amazing lack of health risk of the POP, until the conception risk is refuted by future studies, it remains practice at the Margaret Pyke Centre to offer two POPs daily, always on a 'named patient' basis (p. 220) – but *not* when conception risk is already low (e.g. through full breast-feeding or, in general, above the age 45).

Except during full lactation (when the combination regularly inhibits ovulation), there is a complex and variable interaction between the administered progestogen and the endogenous activity of the woman's ovary (Guillebaud 1999). Fertile ovulation is prevented in about 60% of cycles. In the remainder there is reliance mainly on progestogenic interference with mucus penetrability, backed by some anti-nidatory activity at the endometrium. Regularity of POP-taking is crucial to success with the method, but any regular time – without regard to the time of intercourse – appears to be satisfactory.

**Table 4.12** POPs (Progestogen-only pills)

|  |  |  |  | Number of tablets |
| --- | --- | --- | --- | --- |
| Noriday | (Searle) | 350 μg | norethisterone | 28 |
| Micronor | (Janssen-Cilag) | 350 μg | norethisterone | 28 |
| Femulen | (Searle) | 500 μg | ethynodiol diacetate | 28 |
| Neogest | (Schering) | 75 μg | dl-norgestrel | 35 |
| Norgeston | (Schering) | 30 μg | levonorgestrel | 35 |
| Cerazette | (Organon) | 75 μg | desogestrel | 28 |

(NB. 75 μg dl-norgestrel is equivalent to 37.5 μg levonorgestrel)
The choice of POP is largely empirical, though Neogest has been superseded (by the last two in table)

The starting routines are summarized in Table 4.13. Where there is interference with contraceptive activity due to missed pills, vomiting, or drug interaction, this is believed to start within as little as 3 hours. From mucus studies, contraception seems to be adequately restored if renewed pill-taking is combined with extra precautions for just 48 hours. In the UK since 1993, condom use or the equivalent has been recommended by the FPA and other bodies for 7 days, with no good evidence and based only on the POP having an anovulatory effect in over half of any population of POP users; which effect by analogy with the COC might be expected to take a week to be restored. As always with the POP, there is a paucity of good data. At the time of writing, this matter has been readdressed by WHO and the 48-hour 'rule' is being reinstated! However, this is combined with a low threshold to use emergency contraception (EC), as follows:

◆ Give EC if any tablet was taken more than 3 hours late AND the woman has had sex any time thereafter *until the 48 hours required for the mucus effect to be restored.*

Antibiotics do not interfere with the effectiveness of the POP – apart from the enzyme-inducing antibiotics rifampicin and griseofulvin. Another contraceptive method would normally be advised for all users of enzyme inducers. If nothing else is acceptable, at MPC we occasionally give two POPs per day to selected 'named patients' (p. 220) on long-term enzyme inducers, but unlike with the COC, there are no publications supporting this approach.

There is also no scientific basis on which to decide which POP to choose. The choice depends mainly on the prescriber's (and the woman's) preference, plus empirical changing to another product if side effects develop with the first one tried. Though with all POPs the dose to the infant is believed to be harmless, it appears that the least amount of administered progestogen gets into the breast milk if a levonorgestrel preparation is used.

## Indications

♦ Side effects with, or recognized contraindications to, the combined pill, in particular those believed to be oestrogen-related. Note: this includes past VTE.

♦ Older women – especially smokers above age 35.

♦ Diabetes.

♦ Obesity – but assessing the advisability in the particular case of giving two tablets daily (see above).

♦ Migraine, including varieties with focal symptoms. The woman may continue to suffer the migraines but the fear of an oestrogen-promoted thrombotic stroke is eliminated.

♦ Lactation – the combination is anovulatory. During full breast-feeding therefore – but not during or after weaning – the advice for missed pills, etc., can be based on that for the COC. At the Margaret Pyke Centre we say 12 hours overdue before (now) 48 hours of added condom use is recommended. For young women very anxious to avoid conception, the COC or an injectable/implant/IUD/IUS should be started in good time during weaning: either when breast-feeding frequency first diminishes or no later than the first bleeding episode.

♦ At the woman's choice.

## Contraindications

To the WHO 4 conditions in Box 4.9 can be added two contraindications which are 'strong relative' (i.e. WHO 3, so POP cautiously usable) and specific to the POP, namely:

♦ previous ectopic pregnancy, especially in nulliparae;

♦ past *symptomatic*, i.e. painful, functional ovarian cyst formation.

The first of these is more significant, since the POP sometimes allows ovulation with the risk of implantation in the possibly already-damaged remaining fallopian tube. An anovulant method (e.g. injectable, Cerazette, Implanon) would be preferable. The frequency of symptomatic cysts is also greater, leading to a problem in differential diagnosis among POP users with abdominal pain. Note: asymptomatic persistent follicles, which are very commonly picked up on a routine ultrasound scan, do NOT have this relevance.

## Box 4.9 **Absolute contraindications to the POP**

Absolute contraindications are few (and the last four are usually not permanent):

- Past or current *severe* arterial disease, or very high risk thereof (due to concern regarding minor lipid changes)
- Any serious side effect on the COC not certainly related solely to the oestrogen, e.g. progestogen allergy, liver adenoma
- Undiagnosed genital tract bleeding
- Actual or possible pregnancy
- Recent trophoblastic disease – until hCG is undetectable in blood as well as urine, since there is no certainty it is not the progestogen that increases the likelihood of chemotherapy being required, in some studies. In US practice this would not be seen as a contraindication (see p. 137)
- Hypersensitivity
- The woman's unrelieved anxiety about the POP method

*Relative contraindications*, which unless otherwise stated are weak (WHO 2) – so the POP is certainly broadly usable – are:

- risk factors for arterial disease, including as above under 'indications'. Atherogenic lipid disorders and the presence of more than one risk factor can be permissible, unlike with the COC;
- hypertension – either COC-related, *or* other varieties controlled on treatment. Pending more data, this use should be seen as WHO 3, in view of the preliminary WHO report (1998a), suggesting that if POP users are hypertensive the POP increases the risk (albeit non-significantly) for stroke;
- sex steroid-dependent cancer (WHO 3). Seek the agreement of the relevant hospital consultant;
- current liver disorder with persistent biochemical change (WHO 3);
- enzyme-inducer drugs (WHO 3, see above);
- chronic severe systemic diseases (see p. 219). If pregnancy is known to cause deterioration, the POP has the disadvantage of lesser efficacy than the COC. But if hormones were one day shown to aggravate the particular condition, the tiny dose in the POP should have less effect;

- past history of venous thromboembolism (see above, this is even proposed as an indication!). Because it does not significantly affect blood-clotting mechanisms, the POP may be used for such women. As confirmation: when norethisterone is taken as Primolut, no less than 45 times the daily dose in Micronor is advised – yet there is no mention in the data sheet of this past history as a contraindication. Good counselling and record-keeping are of course essential for unlicensed indications;

- acute porphyria – latent with no history of a past attack (WHO 3). Seek agreement of the metabolic consultant, and warn of possible future attack triggered by the progestogen.

## Problems and management

Negligible changes to most metabolic variables have been reported, presumably because of the low dose coupled with the counteracting effect of endogenous oestrogen still produced by the woman's incompletely suppressed ovaries. Prolonged spells of amenorrhoea occur most often in older women. Once pregnancy is excluded, the amenorrhoea must be due to anovulation so signifies very high efficacy. Unless there is evidence of hypo-oestrogenism, the method can be continued, if necessary, beyond age 50. Diagnosing the menopause in older POP users is discussed on p. 216.

Apart from the occasional complaint of breast tenderness, which is usually transient but may be recurrent and can sometimes be overcome empirically by changing from one progestogen to another, the main problem presented

**Table 4.13** Starting routines with the POP

|  | Start when? | Extra precautions? |
|---|---|---|
| Menstruating | 1st day of period | No |
|  | 2nd day or later | 7 days |
| Post-partum |  |  |
| (a) No lactation[1] | Usually day 21 | No |
| (b) Lactation[1] | Usually 21–42 days after delivery, later if LAM[2] is the initial method | No |
| Induced abortion/ miscarriage | Same day | No |
| Post-COC | Instant switch | No |
| Amenorrhoea | Any time[3] (e.g. post partum) | 7 days |

[1] Bleeding irregularities minimized by not starting immediately after delivery
[2] LAM the lactational amenorrhoea method (p. 217)
[3] Provided the prescriber is confident that there is neither sperm nor blastocyst in the upper genital tract

is that of menstrual irregularity. With advance warning, this is usually well-tolerated. It is often helpful to keep a record chart in early months, as this quickly highlights the type of problem and usually demonstrates improvement. Premenstrual symptoms are often relieved. More than half the women will have a cycle between 25 and 35 days.

Even when cycles are short, between 21 and 24 days, complaints are rare provided the bleeding is not too heavy. Two or three days of light bleeding erratically about twice a month is another common and acceptable pattern. A few women will experience prolonged and heavy bleeding and, if not relieved by changing the brand of pill, another method should be selected.

Blood pressure is regularly monitored (annually, if not raised in the first year of checks) but where previously raised during use of the combined pill, it usually reverts to normal on the POP. Indeed, if it does not do so, the woman most probably has essential hypertension.

## Cerazette – new anovulant which 'rewrites the textbooks about POPs'

This useful new product containing 75 μg desogestrel is quite different from other POPs in usually blocking ovulation. This makes it somewhat like 'Implanon by mouth' (and it may indeed be useful as a way of advance testing the acceptability of Implanon). The manufacturer, Organon UK, failed to convince the Committee on the Safety of Medicines of the acceptability of their proposed 12-hour advice for defining a missed Cerazette POP – they judged that insufficient data were presented to establish this difference from other POPs. An international study is now planned, recruiting women who are instructed to miss pills by 12, 24, 36 hours, etc., during very careful monitoring of cycles of POP use, measuring all the ultrasound and most blood markers of ovulation. Since the company does now have a licence with the existing 3-hour rule, it is now expected that they will market the product on that basis: before the definitive study supporting 12 hours can have been reported.

As with all progestogen-only methods, irregular, sometimes frequent or prolonged bleeding remains a problem, but there is a higher incidence of amenorrhoea than with existing POPs – while still apparently providing adequate, follicular phase levels of oestradiol. It may well become a first-line hormonal contraceptive for many women, given its great efficacy of better than 99.5 per 100 women years (collaborative group on desogestrel, 1998) and good margin for compliance errors, without the risks of ethinyloestradiol. Moreover, it has potentially beneficial effects on menstrual disorders, especially: dysmenorrhoea, menorrhagia, premenstrual syndrome, ovulation pain, and functional cysts. It could also be a good alternative to the COC with a past history of ectopic pregnancy.

## Injectables

There are two injectable agents available: Depo-Provera (depot medroxyprogesterone acetate or DMPA) 150 mg every 12 weeks, and Noristerat (norethisterone oenanthate) 200 mg every 8 weeks, both given by deep intramuscular injection within the first 5 days of the menstrual cycle. If given later, the FPA leaflets advise 7 days' extra precautions.

Post-partum bleeding problems are minimized if the first dose is delayed for 3–6 weeks: but much earlier use is permissible. Timing of the first dose is as for Implanon (see below).

In the UK, the only injectable currently licensed by the Committee on Safety Medicines for long-term use is Depo-Provera, and it now has additional approval as a first-line contraceptive. It has been repeatedly endorsed by the expert committees of prestigious bodies, such as the International Planned Parenthood Federation (IPPF) and WHO and, finally, in 1992, was fully approved by the US Food and Drug Administration. Its effectiveness is extremely high among reversible methods (0–1 failure per 100 woman-years), primarily because it functions by causing anovulation. *DMPA was reviewed by Bhathera (2001).*

If enzyme inducers are being taken as well long term, in the UK the injection interval has hitherto been shortened to every 10 weeks. According to the manufacturer, this practice is unnecessary, as they have data showing the clearance of DMPA is the same as hepatic blood flow, i.e. all the DMPA passing through the liver is metabolized. Therefore, the fact that liver cell enzymes have been induced and can metabolize more quickly should make no difference.

Anxiety about this method was generated by animal research of very doubtful relevance to humans. The latest WHO data imply that DMPA users have a reduced risk of cancer, with no overall increased risk of cancers of the breast, ovary, or cervix, and a fivefold reduction in the risk of carcinoma of the endometrium (relative risk 0.2). There is still the possibility of a weak co-factor effect on breast cancer similar to that suggested for COCs (see p. 121). However, this is unproven and in the WHO study the association might well have appeared because of surveillance bias in early years of use by the younger women.

The effects, whether wanted (contraceptive) or unwanted, are not reversible for the duration of the injection and this must always be explained to prospective users, backed by the approved manufacturer's leaflet. It can be stressed that most experts consider DMPA to be a safer drug than COCs, despite the adverse publicity it often receives.

After the last dose, conception is commonly delayed (median delay 9 months, which is of course only 6 months since stopping use of the method). A study in Thailand (Pardthaisong 1984) showed that within 24 months of discontinuation (i.e. from the first missed injection), 91% of DMPA users had conceived, compared with 93% of ex-IUD users, and 95% of ex-COC users. These differences were not statistically different, refuting allegations of permanent infertility caused by the drug.

## Side effects

In many users there are side effects (and in a few cases very marked). They include:

- irregular bleeding
- weight gain
- amenorrhoea.

Preliminary warning prevents anxiety about these. Menstrual abnormalities remain the greatest obstacle to any large increase in the method's popularity. Excessive bleeding may resolve if the next injection is given early (but not less than 4 weeks since the last dose). Alternatively, giving additional oestrogen may be more successful: either as ethinylestradiol 20–30 μg (usually within a pill formulation) or, if there is a past history of thrombosis or focal migraine, as natural oestrogen by any route. Either is given daily for 21 or 28 days, after which there is a withdrawal bleed. An acceptable bleeding pattern (though never perfectly regular) may follow, and if not, such courses may be repeated.

Amenorrhoea occurs in most long-term users and is usually very acceptable, with the explanation, if necessary, that 'menstruation has no excretory health benefits' and occurs in about half the long-term users. There is a concern, however, that prolonged hypo-oestrogenism through use of DMPA might lead by analogy with premature menopause to reduced bone density (supported as a risk by an overview of all published studies by Banks *et al.* 2001, but without proof of increased *fracture* risk resulting) or potentially even more importantly, to accelerated arterial disease. There is no proof that either risk is clinically significant – nor that it is not so. The 1998 WHO study of cardiovascular disease in current DMPA users was somewhat reassuring (WHO 1998a), but the numbers of very long-term users especially who started young were small. More prospective comparative data on this and on osteoporosis are urgently needed.

One thing that is clear is that low (or indeed high) oestrogen levels in users do not correlate either with measured bone density (Gbolade *et al.* 2002) or with the presence or absence of bleeding. Hence, given the present uncertainty, long-term use is of greater potential relevance to practice than amenorrhoea as such.

Every prospective user of DMPA should be informed of the association of long-term use with loss of bone mass, and lifestyle measures that are concerned with maintaining it, such as diet (milk products), exercise (enough, but without amenorrhoea), alcohol (in moderation) and cigarettes (ideally none), should be discussed (Gbolade *et al.* 2002).

## Box 4.10 **Protocol for long-term users of DMPA**

◆ After 5 years of DMPA use (or earlier only if there are possibly relevant symptoms such as hot flushes or loss of libido, and in very heavy smokers) this issue is raised.

◆ Given the absence of any proof of risk and all the advantages of the method, some women state they will wish to continue uncomplicatedly with DMPA alone, whatever the result of any test: and if so, this view of theirs is simply noted.

◆ Many other women in our experience state after discussion that now, after 5 useful years on the method, they anyway wish to make a change to another contraceptive, which will of course restore oestrogen levels – either exogenously (with the COC) or from their own ovaries. No testing is required. In the remainder, the blood oestradiol level in a sample shortly *before* the next injection is measured.

◆ If the result is above 100 pmol/l and there are no symptoms, the woman continues on DMPA as desired with the test repeated routinely in 3–5 years. If lower, a confirmatory test is arranged.

◆ Two levels under 100 pmol/l are taken as grounds for preferably a change of method as the woman now often chooses. Otherwise and more controversially, in selected well-counselled women, aware of the uncertainty whether it will be beneficial, 'add-back' natural oestrogen HRT is commenced, by any chosen route and usually continuously. Since using DMPA in this way to protect the uterus from the effects of added oestrogen is unlicensed, this must be on a 'named patient' basis.

### Comments on the above protocol

After 5 years' use, the reasons for checking for unusually low oestradiol levels (advice which differs from that of Gbolade *et al.* 2002) in the few women remaining after working through the first three bullet points in the above protocol are:

◆ oestrogen is the proximate determinant of the continuing concern about *arterial* disease

◆ oestradiol is a far cheaper test than bone density scanning.

Above age 45, DMPA users should, in my view, normally switch to another method (e.g. the POP which is after all almost 100% effective at this age) or receive additional oestrogen, unless there is good evidence that they are not oestrogen deficient.

## Indications

The main indication for an injectable is the woman's desire for a highly effective method which is independent of intercourse, when other options are contraindicated or disliked. They are welcomed by many forgetful pill-takers.

- Injectables may be used despite past thrombosis (see earlier comments for the POP), and are ideal to cover major or leg surgery. Since starting and stopping of DMPA can be overlapped with any other hormonal method, the previously used COC can be recommended 2 weeks after full mobilization, without waiting for the injection to 'run out'.
- Useful during lactation, since they have no unwanted effects on breast-milk flow and in contrast to the POP efficacy is not detectably altered by weaning.
- Injectable agents are positively beneficial in endometriosis, in sickle-cell anaemia, and in women at risk of pelvic inflammatory disease.

## Contraindications

The absolute contraindications (WHO 4) are those listed earlier (Box 4.9) for the POP. Given the uncertainty about hypo-oestrogenism discussed above, two new WHO 4 conditions would be:

- known osteoporosis already shown on a bone scan;
- long-term corticosteroid treatment.

The relative contraindications are also very similar to those for the POP, except that there needs to be more caution because the dose is larger; some studies show a reduction in HDL-cholesterol levels and there is a built-in lack of immediate reversibility. Indeed, acute porphyria is WHO 4 rather than 3 for this reason.

The presence of any single risk factor for osteoporosis can be seen as a relative contraindication, for example:

- strong family history (WHO 2);
- smoking >20 per day (WHO 2);
- amenorrhoeic athletes (WHO 3);
- anorexia nervosa/bulimia (WHO 3).

### Hypertension – either COC-related, or other varieties, when controlled by treatment

Pending more data, this use should be seen as WHO 3, in view of a study (WHO 1998a) which hints at the possibility (unconfirmed) that if DMPA users, like POP users, are hypertensive the method might increase their risk of stroke. The frequency of ectopics and ovarian cysts is reduced, unlike with the POP.

### Monitoring and management

Blood pressure (BP) is traditionally checked before each dose although, since most studies fail to show any hypertensive effect, if the first year of measurements are normal an annual check would suffice. Since (it has to be admitted) most users have a battle to avoid weight gain, the user herself usually asks to be weighed periodically.

---

### Box 4.11 **Protocol for overdue injections, i.e. patient presents beyond 12 weeks with DMPA**

- Up to 13 weeks (91 days): since the failure rate is so low at this time (every 3 calendar-months is the regular injection frequency in WHO programmes), we will give the due dose. This should abort the growth of any preovulatory follicle, like the first 7 pills do after each pill-free interval. We also advise added precautions for 7 days.

- If the next dose is late by a further 3 days (94 days): assuming intercourse has been continuing, the usual hormonal emergency contraceptive (EC) can be given plus an immediate DMPA injection.

- Up to 98 days: again, assuming regular sexual exposure, with a negative sensitive pregnancy test a copper IUD can be inserted in good faith, plus an immediate injection – unless the woman chooses to switch to the IUD as her future method.

- Beyond 98 days: EC is withheld on medico-legal grounds, since there is a remote chance of an implantation. Our usual policy is to recommend abstinence or extremely careful condom use until it is 14 days since last sex, then if a sensitive urinary pregnancy test is negative, DMPA injection can be given.

- In **ALL** these cases, added precautions for a further 7 days are advisable, plus 100% follow-up with exclusion of pregnancy about 3 weeks later. Counselling must include discussion of the (very low) potential of harm to any fetus and be fully recorded.

---

### Contraceptive implants

The implant *route* remains useful. Applying the lessons from the media and legal saga, which led to the withdrawal of Norplant since the last edition, good initial counselling is paramount, explaining the likely changes to the bleeding pattern and the possibility of 'hormonal' side effects (see below). This discussion should be backed by a good (e.g. FPA) leaflet and well-documented.

Implants contain a progestogen in a slow-release carrier. After an initial phase of several weeks giving higher blood levels, they deliver almost constant low daily levels of the hormone.

## Mechanism of action and effectiveness

Implanon™ is now (since 2000) the only marketed implant in the UK. It works primarily by ovulation inhibition, supplemented by the usual mucus and endometrial effects. It is a single 40 mm rod, just 2 mm in diameter, inserted far more simply than Norplant straight from a dedicated sterile preloaded applicator with a cleverly shaped wide-bore needle, by a simple injection/withdrawal technique. The implant contains 68 mg of etonogestrel – the new name for 3-keto-desogestrel. This is dispersed in an ethylene vinyl acetate (EVA) matrix and covered by a 0.06 mm rate-limiting EVA membrane.

- Its duration of use is for 3 years, with the unique distinction of a zero failure rate in the trials to date (2002) – though the 95% confidence interval ranges up to 7 in 10 000.
- Since in the international studies serum levels do tend to be lower in heavier women, contraceptive efficacy might be lower in the grossly obese, especially in the third year (discuss reimplanting sooner if weight above 100 kg).
- If enzyme-inducer drug treatment is necessary, additional contraceptive precautions are recommended. Condoms, the POP or oral Cerazette when available can be recommended. Use of two implants is NOT advised.

Though not difficult to insert and to remove, specific training is essential. In a comparative study, the mean insertion time was 1.1 minutes and the mean removal time 2.6 minutes. This was about four times faster for both procedures than for Norplant.

## Timing of Implanon™ insertion

- Day 1–5 of the woman's natural cycle; if day 3 or later with condom use or equivalent for the next 7 days.
- Later than day 5, this is permitted provided there has been believable abstinence up to the insertion day and additional contraception is again advised for 7 days thereafter. This is complicated in practice, so agreement at counselling to short-term use of a hormone method can be very helpful, see next bullet.
- Changing from combined pill, POP or any (other) progestogen-only method, or an IUD: Implanon™ is injected on any convenient day. This much

simplifies timing of the appointment. (Additional barrier method for 7 days would only be needed if the insertion happened to immediately follow a COC-free interval).

♦ Following first-trimester abortion: immediate insertion is best.

♦ Following delivery or second-trimester abortion: Implanon™ insertion on day 21 is recommended, and if later with additional contraception for 7 days. If still amenorrhoeic, pregnancy risk should be excluded.

♦ If breast feeding, the minimal uncertainty about the *probably* nil effects of the tiny amount of etonogestrel reaching the breast milk must be discussed (as for the POP).

## Advantages and indications

This product is suitable for women with contraindications to or problems with the COC or other common methods, who want effectiveness without the finality of sterilization.

♦ Long action with one treatment (3 years), plus very high continuation rates.

♦ Absence of the initial peak dose given orally to the liver.

♦ Blood levels are steady rather than fluctuating (as with the POP) or initially too high (as injectables). This minimizes metabolic changes.

♦ Oestrogen-free, therefore usable if past VTE.

♦ Median systolic and diastolic blood pressures were unchanged in trials for up to 4 years.

♦ Being an anovulant, special indications include past ectopic pregnancy and pain due to ovulation/functional cysts.

♦ The implant is rapidly reversible. After removal serum etonogestrel levels were undetectable within one week. Within 3 weeks, 44 out of 47 women were ovulating normally.

## Contraindications

Absolute contraindications (WHO 4) are few:

♦ Possibly progestogen-dependent tumours (liver adenoma, and in UK active trophoblastic disease)

♦ Acute porphyria

♦ Severe hepatic disease with markedly abnormal liver function

♦ Known or suspected pregnancy

♦ Undiagnosed vaginal bleeding

♦ Hypersensitivity to any component.

The manufacturer adds 'active venous thromboembolic disorder', but in my view this history (past or present) would be WHO 2. There is no evidence that Implanon™ would increase the risk.

### Relative contraindications

In my view these are as for POPs, but excluding past ectopic or ovulation pain/which are indications.

### Follow-up and management of side effects

No treatment-specific follow-up is necessary, including no BP checks. The crucial thing is an explicit 'open house' policy, to return any time to discuss her side effects, without any provider pressure to persevere if the woman really wants the implant out.

### *Altered bleeding pattern*

In the pre-marketing randomized comparative trial of Implanon™ with Norplant, the bleeding patterns were very similar, with one main difference. As expected for an anovulant method, amenorrhoea was significantly more common (20.8% versus 4.4%). The infrequent bleeding and spotting rate was 26.1%. Normal cycling was reported by 35%.

However, the combined rates for the more annoying 'frequent bleeding and spotting' and 'prolonged bleeding and spotting' totalled 18% with Implanon, almost one in five. The best treatment is short-term cyclical COC therapy, logically with 'Marvelon', or a natural oestrogen if EE contraindicated. After this the bleeding, though never completely regular, may become acceptable; if not, the oestrogen course may be repeated.

### *'Minor' side effects*

Reported in frequency order, these were: acne, headache, abdominal pain, breast pain, 'dizziness', mood changes (depression, emotional lability), libido decrease, hair loss.

In a comparative study, the mean weight increase over 2 years was 2.6% with Implanon™ and 2.9% with Norplant, but in users of an IUD the weight increase was 2.4%! Though this implies a normal increase over time, by 24 months 35% had put on more than 3 kg. As with DMPA, forewarning about weight is essential: some individuals really do put on an unacceptable amount of weight.

### *Possible hypo-oestrogenism?*

Since Implanon™ suppresses ovulation, the same questions about long-term use were asked as with DMPA. However, the initial findings on oestrogen levels and bone density in the comparative trial with IUD users have been very reassuring: there seems to be sufficient follicular activity to supply adequate oestrogen to the user.

### Local adverse effects

Discomfort at insertion and difficult removals can be minimized by good training. Infection of the site, expulsion, migration, and scarring are very infrequent. Implanon™ is very difficult to image: this greatly complicates removal after too deep insertions.

In summary, Implanon™ above all provides efficacy and convenience. If the bleeding pattern suits and hormonal side effects are minimal, it is a 'forgettable' contraceptive.


# Emergency contraception

## Choice of methods

Apart from mifepristone, still unavailable for this use, three methods are effective (Faculty of Family Planning 2000b):

- the insertion of a copper IUD, the winner for effectiveness;
- Levonelle™, the levonorgestrel-only emergency contraceptive (EC): one hormone is better than two;
- the combined oral emergency contraceptive (COEC) marketed as Schering PC4, which is now only of historical interest in the UK.


## Hormone methods

### Effectiveness

In the WHO 1998 randomized controlled trial (WHO 1998b) comparing around 1000 women given the levonorgestrel-only method and the same number given the combined hormone method *after a single exposure*, the main findings were greater efficacy and fewer side effects with the former (Table 4.14). Given that an estimated 92 of every 100 women exposed (just once) in the WHO trial would not have conceived, the true difference in efficacies of treatment within 72 hours is best stated thus: Levonelle™ prevents seven out of the eight actual conceptions that would otherwise occur and the combined method would prevent only six. A woman who relied on it every month could do a lot better, contraceptively (a cumulative failure rate of up to $13 \times 0.4$ equals around 5 per 100 woman-years), but she would be risking pregnancy more than directly risking her health.

**Table 4.14** Choice of emergency contraceptive methods

| | Copper IUD immediate insertion | Levonorgestrel 0.75 mg × 2, 12 hours apart | Combined hormone method tabs 2 × 2, 12 hours apart (historical interest only) |
|---|---|---|---|
| Normal timing after intercourse | Up to 5 days after earliest calculated day of ovulation (see text) | Up to 72 hours | Up to 72 hours |
| Overall efficacy (WHO Study: all-comers, single exposure) | About 99.9% | 99% | 97% |
| Side effects | Pain, bleeding, risk of infection | Nausea 23%<br>Vomiting 6% | Nausea 52%<br>Vomiting 19% |
| Absolute contraindications | Pregnancy | Pregnancy | Pregnancy |
| | As for copper IUDs, generally | Proven severe acute allergy to a constituent | Proven severe acute allergy to a constituent |
| | | Active acute porphyria | Active acute porphyria |
| | | Active severe liver disease | Active severe liver disease |
| | | | Current focal migraine |
| | | | Current sickle-cell crisis |

Numbers are rounded to nearest integer.

An important new finding for *both* hormone methods was that earlier treatment gave greater efficacy (Box 4.12). Every 12 hours' delay increased the failure rate by about 50%. So it is back to being best taken the 'morning after', though 'emergency pill' is still a better lay *term*, since it leaves open the fact that useful benefit can be obtained up to at least 72 hours. Moreover, it is by no means contraindicated for use even beyond that time (Box 4.12).

## Box 4.12 Failure rate of Levonelle™ when treatment is delayed, for each 24-hour period after a single exposure

Up to 24 hours: 0.4%

25–48 hours: 1.2%

49–72 hours: 2.7%

### Side effects

One of the main advantages of Levonelle™ is reduced rates of nausea and vomiting: but forewarning of this is still required, and preventive treatment is sometimes appropriate (see below).

### Contraindications

In ordinary practice there are virtually no contraindications to Levonelle™, apart from existing pregnancy, hence its suitability as an over-the-counter (OTC) product. There is no upper age limit to any of the methods if sufficient risk of conception is present.

If the woman is taking any enzyme-inducer drug, including St John's Wort, the doses with hormonal methods should be increased by 50% (one-third tablet of Levonelle™). No increase in dose is required when antibiotics are in use, aside, of course, from rifampicin/rifabutin and griseofulvin (Table 4.11).

## Copper IUD

### Effectiveness

Insertion of a copper IUD – not the LNG-IUS – in good faith before implantation, which is up to 5 days after the (earliest) possible calculated ovulation day, is extremely effective and prevents conception in almost 100% of women – even in cases of multiple exposure (Box 4.12). The judge's summing up in a 1991 Court Case (Regina vs Dhingra) gives legal support to this policy:

> I further hold ... that a pregnancy cannot come into existence until the fertilized ovum has become implanted in the womb, and that that stage is not reached until at the earliest, the 20th day of a normal 28 day cycle. . . .

### Indications and contraindications for the IUD method

There are recognized contraindications (see p. 196) and risks of pain, bleeding, or infection, as with any IUD, and this option is not first line for the nulliparous woman. She will be looking for pills but in selected cases it may be appropriate actively to suggest an IUD (Box 4.13). If so, cervical swabs are essential (for *Chlamydia trachomatis* at least, though remember this would be too soon to pick up infection at the latest intercourse) and prophylactic antibiotic cover, with contact tracing if the bacteriology is positive.

The device may always be removed following the next period, once a new long-term method is established, such as the COC or an implant, especially if there is the past history of an ectopic pregnancy. [Withholding the IUD will not lower the risk of a tubal ectopic in the current cycle (see below) but an anovulant method would often be better long term.]

Note: the LNG-IUS (Mirena™) acts by mechanisms which appear to be slower than the almost immediate effects of copper on sperm and blastocyst, and it is not recommended for this indication.

---

### Box 4.13 **Indications for emergency contraception by copper IUD**

- When the very maximum available efficacy is woman's priority
- When exposure occurred more than 72 hours earlier, up to 5 days, or in cases of multiple exposure: insertion may be up to 5 days after ovulation
- In many parous women, to be retained as their long-term method (although it may contrariwise in young nulliparae and much better to remove it just as soon as they are established on a new method such as the COC)
- Presence of absolute contraindications to a hormonal method (a very rare indication since Levonelle™)
- After vomiting of either dose within 2 hours, in a case with a particularly high pregnancy risk

### Counselling and management – a summary

◆ Careful assessment of menstrual/coital history and hence of the appropriateness of treatment is required. Earlier exposures to risk in the same cycle need particular consideration.

◆ The mode of action sometimes (not always) being post fertilization may pose an absolute contraindication to some individuals. Most modern ethicists (and this author) consider that blocking of implantation is contraception, not abortion.

◆ Medical risks should be discussed, especially:

(a) the *failure rate*. Remind the woman that the figures quoted relate to a single exposure. For the IUD method the failure rate is around 1 per 1000.

(b) *teratogenicity*. This is believed to be negligible for levonorgestrel (LNG) – although there is no proof – because before implantation the hormones will not reach the blastocyst in sufficient concentration to cause any adverse effect. Follow-up studies of women who have kept their pregnancies have so far not shown any increased risk of major abnormalities above the background 2% rate. But always warn not only that Levonelle™ may fail but also that if it does a normal baby cannot be guaranteeed.

(c) If an *ectopic pregnancy* should occur it is the result of a pre-existing damaged tube and would almost certainly have happened anyway, with or without this (pre-implantation) treatment. Actually the rate must be lowered, by the anti-fertilization effects of LNG, and by the toxic effects of the copper ion on sperm. However, a past history of ectopic pregnancy or severe pelvic infection remains a reason for forewarning re pain in the next few weeks, with either of the methods.

◆ If Levonelle™ is used, advice should be given about nausea (23%) and vomiting (6%). If an antiemetic is requested, the best seems to be domperidone (Motilium), 10 mg with each dose, although an OTC remedy might be tried.

Contraception, both in the current cycle (in case the hormonal method merely postpones ovulation) and long term should be discussed. The IUD option can cover both aspects, provided a *banded* (i.e. effective long-term) device like the T-Safe 380 A can be fitted. Less effective IUDs (Nova T 380, Flexi-T 300) may be easier to fit.

If the COC is chosen, it should normally be started as soon as the woman is sure her next period is normal, on the first or second day, without the need for additional contraception thereafter. In selected cases the COC can be started immediately, but if so, the woman must understand – with the discussion documented – that if the hormonal EC failed there would be exposure of the fetus to at least one cycle of COC (likely but not proven to be harmless).

The ground to be covered above makes clear the importance of an accurate coital and menstrual history and to promote effective arrangements for appropriate follow-up, even when the product is sold OTC.

*Vaginal examination* is NOT routinely necessary for hormonal EC and there are usually very good reasons to omit it, for example, in an anxious teenager. It should be done only if indicated on clinical grounds:

◆ at the first visit to exclude/screen for infection or to establish a baseline size and shape for the uterus (e.g. possible fibroids);

◆ at follow-up, examination is mainly indicated if there is clinical uncertainty because the next period is delayed, or in the presence of any pain.

### Special indications

These apply when the following have occurred, assuming continuing coital exposure:

◆ Missed COCs

(a) late starting of COC, by more than one day added to the 7-day pill-free interval (PFI), or

(b) any combination of pills from the first seven in the packet which in the prescriber's judgement amounts to the same thing as lengthening the PFI to more than 8 days. This is in line with the new unpublished WHO advice (2002).

After the Levonelle™ dose, the woman then returns immediately to the COC, subject to a 100% undertaking to return for follow-up 4 weeks later – and also to use additional precautions for the next 7 days. *Mid-packet* pill omissions after seven tablets have been taken never indicate emergency treatment unless at least four (WHO says 5, 2002) have been missed. Towards the *end of a packet*, so long as the woman has been properly advised, she will omit the next PFI and that makes her contraceptively safer than usual.

◆ Delay in taking a POP tablet for more than 3 hours, implying loss of mucus effect, followed by sexual exposure during the 48 hours before mucus contraception is expected to be restored. Again the POP is restarted immediately after the emergency regimen, 2 days added precautions are advised (WHO 2002), and follow-up agreed.

◆ Further exposure in the same cycle, e.g. due to failure of barrier contraception after an emergency hormonal method has been given. Additional doses of Levonelle™, for example, are acceptable if after a detailed coital history they would not be taken after implantation, from exposure earlier in the cycle. But this additional use is of course outside the terms of the licence and this should be explained and fully documented ('named patient use').

◆ Exposure more than 72 hours ago. Although Levonelle™ is licensed only up to 72 hours after the earliest act of unprotected intercourse, it may also be given later – though with uncertainty about the (diminishing) chance of success, as is clear from Box 4.12. Neither method should be used if calculations suggest that any earlier act could have led to the presence by now of an early implanted pregnancy.

◆ Overdue injections of DMPA with continuing sexual intercourse. Start the next dose from day 85–91, plus condoms to be used during the next 7 days. Later, in addition, we exclude an implanted pregnancy (so far as possible, by the coital history and a sensitive pregnancy test) and offer Levonelle™ PC4 or a copper IUD. After day 968, the next injection is best postponed until there have been 14 days of safe contraception or abstinence since whenever intercourse last occurred and a negative sensitive (25 mIU/l) pregnancy test is negative.

◆ Essential removal, or expulsion of an IUD identified, before the time of implantation, if another IUD cannot be inserted for some reason.

Research continues and alternatives methods and guidelines may supersede the above in due course.

## Intrauterine contraception

### Copper-bearing intrauterine devices (IUDs)

These have many established advantages, listed in Box 4.14. Women who are happily suited to this method love it, the rest hate it and, sadly, their views are more vigorously expressed. Women in their thirties may not request an IUD because they were told in their twenties to avoid that method. Yet for a parity 2+ 30-year-old, the devices have not changed but she has; especially if she is not yet sure that her family is complete, she is the ideal user. Currently, some doctors are complying too readily with requests for male or female sterilization which originate partly out of myths about this alternative. Too few women know that the latest copper (IUDs) are, in practice more, not less, effective that the COC (WHO 1987) and comparable with female sterilization. And then there is the IUS with its added value in medical gynaecology.

Box 4.14 **Advantages of copper IUDs**

- Safe: mortality 1:500 000
- Effective: highly (p. 000); immediately; postcoitally (not true of IUS); at pregnancy termination
- No link with coitus
- No tablets to remember
- Continuation rates high
- Reversible – even when removed for one of the recognized complications

It cannot be overemphasized that *the effectiveness and acceptability of this method depends primarily on the skill of the practitioner who inserts it.* This cannot be learnt from books: see the Faculty of Family Planning's 'apprenticeship' training scheme above. Considerable and maintained experience is an absolute essential for good technique. Among other sequelae, inadequately inserted devices are prone to be expelled or malpositioned (a cause of failure, or of 'lost threads'). Perforation of the uterus may occur, especially when it is soft (post-partum or post-abortion), or if its acutely anteverted or retroverted position is not identified and allowed for with use of atraumatic holding forceps during insertion (Table 4.15, column H).

### Effectiveness

The first-choice copper IUD for a parous woman in this country is the T-Safe Cu 380 A. It is more effective than the Nova T 380, and retains its efficacy with the passage or time – and for up to at least 10 years (initially licensed for 8).

The Multiload Cu 375 is greatly preferable to the Multiload 250 (no longer recommended) but has no established advantages over the T-Safe Cu 380 A. It does NOT have a lower expulsion rate.

### Mechanism of action

In studies, fertilized ova are almost never retrievable from the genital tract of copper IUD users, hence they must operate mainly by preventing fertilization. Their effectiveness when put in postcoitally indicates they can also act to block implantation. However, this seems to be primarily a back-up mechanism when devices are *in situ* long term.

Nevertheless, in any given cycle it might be working by blocking implantation, so there is a small risk of 'iatrogenic' conception if a device is removed after mid-cycle. Ideally, therefore, women should use another method additionally from 7 days before planned device removal or this should be postponed until

**Table 4.15** A summary of problems and complications of IUDs

| Main hazards | A Directly or indirectly threatens fertility? | B Linked with symptomatic pain? | C Linked with symptomatic bleeding? | D May present as 'lost threads'? | E Special problem in the young nullipara? | F Frequency with increasing age | G Frequency with increasing duration of use | H Can be caused by poor insertion technique? |
|---|---|---|---|---|---|---|---|---|
| 1. Intrauterine pregnancy (device *in situ*) | Miscarriage infection, see 6 | Yes | Yes | Yes | Yes | → | → | Yes, as result of 5 |
| 2. Extrauterine pregnancy | Significant mortality Loss of tubal function | Yes | Yes | No | Yes | ↑ (Little effect) | ↑ | Yes[1] |
| 3. Expulsion | Pregnancy then as 1, 6 | Yes | Yes (i.e. change of pattern) | Yes | Yes | → | → | Yes |
| 4. Perforation | Pregnancy Adhesion formation Risks of IUD removal | Yes | No | Yes | No | = | – | Yes |
| 5. Malposition | Predisposes to 1, 3, 7, 8. A cause of 'lost threads' | Yes | Yes | Yes | Yes | = | – | Yes |

Table **4.15** (*continued*)

| | Main hazards | A Directly or indirectly threatens fertility? | B Linked with symptomatic pain? | C Linked with symptomatic bleeding? | D May present as 'lost threads'? | E Special problem in the young nullipara? | F Frequency with increasing age | G Frequency with increasing duration of use | H Can be caused by poor insertion technique? |
|---|---|---|---|---|---|---|---|---|---|
| 6. Pelvic infection | Loss of tubal function | Yes | Yes | Sometimes | No | Yes | → | → | Yes[1] (See text re STDs as main cause and importance of screening pre-insertion.) |
| 7. Pain | Real underlying cause may be overlooked, see column B | – | – | Often | No | Yes | = | → | Yes as result of 5 |
| 8. Uterine bleeding | Underlying cause may be overlooked, see column C. | – | Often | – | No | No | ↑ | → | Yes, as result of 5 |

[1] If insertion introduces or exacerbates (pre-existing and undiagnosed) pelvic infection, leading to tubal damage–see text.

the next menses. If a device must be removed earlier (e.g. when treating infection) then hormonal postcoital contraception may be indicated.

### Influence of age

Copper IUDs, like all contraceptive methods, are more effective in the older woman because of declining fertility. Above age 30 there is also a reduction in rates of expulsion and of pelvic inflammatory disease (PID). The latter is not believed to be because the older uterus resists infection but because the person bearing an older uterus is in general less exposed to risk of infection (through her own lifestyle or that of her partner).

### *In situ* conception

If the woman wishes to go on to full term, the device should be removed whenever possible, having first done an ultrasound scan. This is counterintuitive: one would think this would increase the miscarriage risk. In fact, the data for all devices studied show that the miscarriage rate is at least halved by removal of the device in the first trimester. The woman should, of course, be warned that it is impossible to remove completely the IUD-associated miscarriage risk. Obviously the device should be left for removal later in theatre if the woman is going to have a termination of pregnancy. If the threads are already missing when she is seen and other causes are excluded (see below), then the pregnancy must be flagged as one of increased risk for second trimester abortion (which could be infected) and also antepartum haemorrhage and premature labour.

If the woman goes on to full term it is essential to identify the device in the products of conception, and if it is not found, to arrange a post-partum x-ray, in case the device is embedded or has perforated (see differential diagnosis in Table 4.16). There have been medico-legal cases when this was not done, leading either to sequelae from an undiagnosed perforation, or to unnecessary tests and treatments for 'infertility' when only one device was later removed for a wanted pregnancy but a much earlier embedded device remained.

There is no evidence of associated teratogenicity with conception during or immediately after use of copper devices, or indeed of cancer developing in the uterus of long-term users.

### Adverse effects of copper IUDs

These are listed briefly in Box 4.15. The first five problems in Box 4.15 share a single risk, namely of impairing future fertility. Moreover, they must be excluded as diagnoses before pain and bleeding are ascribed to the method as 'side effects'. Table 4.15 expands on this summary, which is actually a remarkably short list as compared with the COC. It also draws attention to the important interrelationships of the problems. Selection and adequate instruction of

**Table 4.16** Differential diagnosis of 'lost threads' with IUDs

| Main diagnoses<br>A. Not pregnant | Clinical clues | B. Pregnant | Clinical clues |
|---|---|---|---|
| 1. **Device in uterus**<br>Threads cut too short, or caught up around device during original insertion or avulsed at a previous removal attempt; or device itself malpositioned | (a) Periods likely to be those characteristic of IUD *in situ*<br>(b) Uterus normal size | 4. **Device *in situ* + pregnancy** | (a) Amenorrhoea<br>(b) Pregnancy test likely to be positive, with clinically enlarged uterus (sufficient to pull up thread) |
| 2. **Unrecognized expulsion** | (a) Recent periods as woman's normal pattern<br>(b) Uterus normal size | 5. **Unrecognized expulsion + pregnancy** | (a) Amenorrhoea, following one or more apparently normal periods (i.e. unmodified by IUD)<br>(b) Signs of pregnancy variably present (may be too early on first presentation) |
| 3. **Perforation of uterus** | As 2 plus (rarely) mass or actual IUD palpated on bimanual examination | 6. **Perforation of uterus + pregnancy** | As 5 plus (rarely) mass or actual IUD identified on bimanual examination |

potential users is emphasized by columns E–G of the table and the paramount importance of correct insertion is re-emphasized by column H.

---

### Box 4.15 **Adverse effects of copper IUDs**

- Intrauterine pregnancy, hence miscarriage risks
- Extrauterine pregnancy
- Expulsion – risks of pregnancy
- Perforation – risks of pregnancy/bowel and bladder adhesions
- Malposition – risks of pregnancy and frame-related pain
- Infection
- Pain
- Bleeding – increased amount; increased duration

*Note: all the first five problems have the risk of impairing **future** fertility.*

---

### IUDs with 'lost threads'

The threads are often in fact present, perhaps short or drawn up into the canal. Women should be taught how to check the strings, and if not felt, there are several other possible explanations. Looking at Table 4.15, this symptom of 'lost threads' links together numbers 1, 3, 4, and 5 in the list. As Table 4.16 shows, there are at least six causes of this condition, three with and three without pregnancy. An intra-abdominal IUD is as useless at stopping pregnancy as one that has been totally expelled. More often there is an *in situ* pregnancy (the threads having been drawn up) or the device is rotated/malpositioned. So the slogan is: 'The woman with "lost threads" is either already pregnant or at risk of becoming pregnant.' All such women therefore need to be advised to use an alternative contraceptive method until the protective presence of an IUD has been established.

### Lost strings: expulsion and perforation

*Expulsions* most commonly occur during bleeding, and soon after insertion; less than one-third are beyond the first year. Even with accurate insertion some women seem prone to expulsion, especially at reinsertion with immediately preceding removal.

For lost threads I recommend the very practical scheme in Box 4.16. Diagnosis and treatment are simultaneous in most cases, with minimum use of hospital facilities.

## Box 4.16 **Practical scheme to deal with lost IUD threads**

1. *Exclude implanted pregnancy.* Take a careful menstrual history, do a bimanual examination, and as indicated perform the most sensitive pregnancy test available. If the woman is pregnant, the management is primarily that of the pregnancy itself. In the absence of pregnancy, it is entirely appropriate (even in a GP surgery) to proceed as follows:

2. *Insert long-handled narrow forceps into the endocervical canal* – if the jaws are gently opened and shut the missing threads can be retrieved in about half of all intrauterine-located devices. If the IUD is judged still to be correctly located, no further action need be taken. But since disappearance of the threads may be a sign of malposition, it is usually advisable to remove and replace the device. If the threads are not found, the woman should be asked whether she would prefer thread retrieval (which also should quickly establish if there actually is a device *in utero*) as below or imaging first, as at step 5 below. Early recourse to imaging partly depends on her pain threshold, but is certainly much kinder than chasing a device that has actually been expelled unnoticed, or perforated.

3. *Try the use of thread-retrievers.* In the UK the most established is the Emmett Retriever, which is available presterilized and disposable, and with full instructions. Appropriate analgesia is important: as a routine mefenamic acid 500 mg should be given 20 minutes earlier, but added local anaesthesia (LA) should also be offered (see below). Most GPs will prefer to arrange hospital referral if this step fails, but if convinced after imaging by ultrasound that the device is located in the uterus, some may feel confident enough to continue – always with adequate analgesia.

4. *Next try small, blunt IUD-removal hooks* (Grafenberg pattern) or various resterilizable forceps, with short jaws (crocodile-type) or claws (e.g. the IUD-removing forceps supplied by Rocket), opening wholly in the uterine cavity. In skilled hands these metal devices will nearly always retrieve the device.

5. *Arrange appropriate imaging if not done earlier, and referral thereafter as appropriate.* An ultrasound scan may confirm correct intrauterine location within a non-pregnant uterus. This can enable the woman to continue using the same device, with periodic re-scanning; but if there is any suspicion that it is malpositioned, appropriate steps should be taken for its removal as at 4 above – preferably under local, rarely under general, anaesthesia. If the ultrasound scan shows unequivocally that the uterus is empty, and non-pregnant, an x-ray is then required to

> **Box 4.16** (*continued*)
>
> differentiate between expulsion and perforation. A uterine marker (such
> as another IUD inserted before the x-ray) may often be useful.
>
> 6. *General anaesthesia for hysteroscopy/?laparoscopy.* In a Margaret Pyke
>    Centre study, only 2.5% of 350 *in situ* intrauterine devices with missing
>    threads and no perforation required general anaesthesia for the removal;
>    this should be the norm.

### Perforation

The incidence is about one in 1000 insertions. They are often post-partum and
always insertion-related: to quote Jack Lippes: 'Devices do not perforate; for
this to occur we need a practitioner'. Both copper-carrying and LNG-releasing
devices provoke adhesions and are often found in the omentum. If imaging
confirms that perforation has occurred, removal can usually be effected by
laparoscopy, preferably by a gynaecologist with training in minimal access surgery. There should be specific advance consent to proceeding to laparotomy,
which should be a rare event. For a perforated GyneFix (see below) it is
reasonable to attempt laparoscopic removal

### Infection

This is the great fear we all have about intrauterine devices. Yet it appears
that infections have been blamed on the devices when they have really been
acquired sexually. Much of the anxiety derived from the Dalkon Shield disaster,
but this was a unique device with a polyfilament thread, increasing the risk
of transfer of potential pathogens from the lower to the upper genital tract.
Modern copper devices have a monofilament thread. They do provide no
protection against PID and the infections that occur may perhaps be more
severe through the foreign body effect; but there is increasing evidence that
they do not themselves cause PID.

The WHO study by Farley *et al.* (1992) reinforces the above view. There were
more than 23 000 insertions, worldwide. In every country but one the same
pattern emerged. There was an IUD-associated increased risk of infection for
20 days after the insertion. Significantly, the weekly infection rate 3 weeks after
insertion went back to the same weekly rate as before insertion, i.e. the norm
for that particular society. Exceptionally, in China there were no infections
diagnosed at all despite 4301 insertions.

These findings are interpreted as follows: the post-insertion infection bulge
cannot be because of bad insertion technique, restricted to the doctors outside

China. Much more probably, although the doctors in all the centres were searching for truly, mutually, monogamous women, they were only actually successful in this search in China (in the 1980s: success would be less probable now). In the other countries, PID-causing organisms (especially *Chlamydia trachomatis*) can be presumed to have been present in a proportion of the women. The process of insertion interfered with protective mechanisms and enabled the infection to spread from the lower genital tract, where it had previously resided, into the upper genital tract including the fallopian tubes. The conclusions therefore are:

◆ IUDs do not in themselves cause PID, or do so exceptionally rarely – otherwise how could all of 4300 Chinese women have escaped? Hence the IUD method is entirely appropriate (WHO 2) for appropriately screened and counselled nulliparous women (Guillebaud 2001c).

◆ The greatest risk is in the first 20 days, most probably caused by pre-existing carriage of sexually transmitted diseases (STIs).

◆ The risk thereafter, like pre-insertion, relates to the background risk of STDs (high in Africa, but apparently absent in the mainland China study population).

In practical terms this implies that for best practice:

◆ Prior to all IUD insertions or reinsertions, unless the prevalence of *Chlamydia* is known to be too low to justify it, in addition to the usual 'verbal screening' concerning sexual lifestyle/change of partner(s) all prospective IUD-users should at least be screened for *Chlamydia*.

◆ Evidence at this pre-insertion visit of cervical excitation tenderness or a purulent discharge from the cervix indicates more detailed investigation, ideally at a genitourinary medicine clinic.

◆ If *Chlamydia* is detected, IUD insertion should be postponed, maybe indefinitely. The woman should be seen ideally at a GUM clinic, for further investigation for other pathogens; she should be treated vigorously (e.g. doxycycline 100 mg twice daily for 7 days if asymptomatic and 14 days if PID diagnosed) and contact tracing arranged. If the IUD has already been inserted (emergency cases) see and examine the patient urgently when the positive report is received, and otherwise proceed as above. Consider device removal if there is any suspicion of PID, especially in nulliparae.

◆ The cervix should be very thoroughly physically cleansed before the device is inserted, following the manufacturer's instructions, with minimum trauma.

◆ Arrange a first post-insertion visit after 7 days in addition to the routine 6-week follow-up visit. This is designed to pick up any women with post-insertion infection (during the 20-day 'surge' of such infections described by Farley) and in my view is essential if there has not been preliminary screening for cervical infection. An acceptable alternative to this early visit, *provided* pre-insertion *Chlamydia* screening is routinely performed, is to:

(a) explain in detail backed by an information leaflet the relevant symptoms (of PID) and

(b) agree with the woman that she will telephone the practice nurse about a week post-insertion – ideally either way, but certainly if relevant symptoms such as fever or significant pain do occur.

As an alternative to microbiological screening, questioning about recency of partner change is of relevance but never sufficient. In a Margaret Pyke Centre study during the mid-1980s, the background rate of *Chlamydia* carriage was 2.4% in the general clinic population but *higher*, 8.2%, in the pre-IUD group who had first been sensitively questioned about their likely exposure. Given the prevalence of *Chlamydia* infection in young, sexually active women in most cities of the UK today, and the fact that we as providers can only be held culpable for attacks of PID occurring post-insertion, I consider it suboptimal to fit *or refit* IUDs or IUSs without microbiological screening (Guillebaud 2001c).

Blind prescription of broad-spectrum antibiotics to cover all insertions is second-best, not only because it precludes contact tracing. In those cases who might be benefiting, reinfection (possibly worsened by the foreign body effect) will likely occur later, from a partner who must also harbour the organism.

However, if there is any doubt about the sensitivity of the microbiology testing available, an argument can be made for doing both the screening and the antibiotic cover – e.g. with azithromycin 1 g stat.

*Management* of a clinical attack of pelvic infection, whether IUD insertion-related or later – and later means, according to the Farley WHO study, that the case must be 'coincidental' to the IUD (i.e. occurring at the same incidence as the background rate for that society) – will depend on the circumstances of the individual case. In parous women it may be possible to retain the device.

Severe cases or those where there is a diagnostic problem (especially in excluding ectopic pregnancy or pelvic appendicitis) should be referred urgently for probable laparoscopy. *Chlamydia* is the main primary causative organism, with secondary infection often by anaerobes frequently superimposed. A broad-spectrum antibiotic, preferably a tetracycline, is therefore best given together with metronidazole while laboratory reports of full GUM tests are awaited.

Two 'sins of omission' are still too often committed by hospital junior staff and the GP needs to check after the woman's discharge:

♦ Has she been counselled about the high risk of tubal occlusion should her lifestyle or lack of routine condom use in future lead to recurrences?

Westrom (1987) showed this risk would exceed 50% with just two more hospitalized attacks.

♦ Has anything been done about contact tracing?

## Actinomyces-*like organisms (ALOs)*

These are not infrequently reported in cervical smears, more commonly with increasing duration of IUD/IUS use. The user should be *seen and examined*:

♦ If there are relevant symptoms (excessive discharge, pain, dyspareunia, new intermenstrual bleeding in an established user) or signs (cervical tenderness, purulent discharge, adnexal swelling) then there should be a low threshold for hospital gynaecological referral. There the device should be removed and sent for culture, in most cases with endometrial biopsy and possibly laparoscopy to diagnose frank pelvic actinomycosis. If (very rarely) this condition is actually confirmed, appropriate antibiotic treatment may have to be for many months.

♦ Much more commonly, the finding occurs in asymptomatic women. The likelihood of frank actinomycosis occurring is believed to be lower than the pregnancy-associated morbidity from banning intrauterine contraception in such women. Accordingly, the Faculty of Family Planning protocol (Clinical and Scientific Committee 1998) recommends two possible management schemes:

(a) It is acceptable for the asymptomatic woman (especially if she is using an expensive IUS (see below) simply to be fully advised about the symptoms above with an explanatory leaflet, and monitored by symptom history *and a bimanual examination* every 6 months. There is no point in repeating the cervical smear, except at the usual screening frequency: persistence of the ALOs in the smear is likely and will not change the management in a woman completely free of relevant symptoms or signs. If at any time in future she has or develops new pelvic pain, dyspareunia, or excessive discharge, and if tenderness or an adnexal mass are noted on examination, the knowledge that ALOs are present does then indicate IUD removal plus the active gynaecological interventions above.

(b) More usually all that is required is IUD removal, with or without immediate reinsertion. Mao and Guillebaud (1984) reported the follow-up findings in three groups of women (not randomized). One group was simply monitored and the ALO finding commonly persisted, but all the women remained well. In two groups the device was removed – with or without immediate reinsertion of another copper IUD. *In both these groups follow-up smears were ALO free.*

### Ectopic pregnancy

Is this problem caused by copper IUDs? This also appears to be a myth. The main cause is previous tubal infection with one or both tubes being damaged. The non-causative association with IUDs comes about because IUDs are rather more effective at preventing pregnancy in the uterus than in the tube. Therefore the ratio of extra- to intrauterine pregnancies is higher than expected among the pregnancies. Ectopics are actually reduced in number because very few sperm get through the copper-containing uterine fluids to reach an egg, hence very few implantations can occur in a damaged tube. However, there are even fewer implantations in the uterus. Thus the denominator in the ratio is even lower than the numerator, hence allowing the *ratio* of ectopics to intrauterine pregnancies to increase when in fact both are much reduced in frequency. The risk of an ectopic in users of the T-Safe Cu 380 A and its clones is now estimated as 0.02/100 woman-years, which is at least 60 times lower than the estimated rate for sexually active Swedish women seeking pregnancy (1.2–1.6/100 woman-years).

Clinically, caution is still necessary and any IUD user with pain and a late period or irregular bleeding has an ectopic until proved otherwise. A past history *relatively* contraindicates the method (see below and WHO 3).

### Pain and bleeding

Pain may or may not be a side effect of the method which the woman accepts; but the safe slogan is 'pain ± bleeding has a serious cause until proved otherwise'. See columns B and C of Table 4.15. As well as excluding conditions like infection and an ectopic or miscarrying pregnancy, malposition of the device can cause pain as the uterus tries to squeeze the device out.

Copper devices do increase the duration of bleeding by a mean of 1–2 days, and they also increase the measured volume of bleeding by about one-third. In a population of copper IUD users, haemoglobins tend to fall, and those with the heaviest losses (above 80 ml per cycle) are prone to frank anaemia.

Bleeding problems usually settle with time. If they do not, it may be necessary to change the method of contraception, perhaps to the LNG-IUS (see below). The most successful therapies are mefenamic acid 500 mg 8-hourly and tranexamic acid 1–1.5 g 8-hourly. Unfortunately, they are not very acceptable long term and they do not seem to help the more common and often more annoying 'spotting' or intermenstrual bleeding.

### Duration of use

'Less frequent replacement would reduce the risks of pelvic inflammatory disease, uterine perforation, expulsion, and other complications that mainly occur soon after insertion . . .' (Newton and Tacchi 1990). Studies also show reduced rates of discontinuation for pregnancy, bleeding, and pain with increasing duration of use (see Table 4.15, column G). Therefore it is good news that the T-Safe Cu 380 A is fully approved for 8 years of use, and the data already support extension to at least 10 years. Moreover, any copper device which has been fitted above the age of 40 may be that woman's last device for the rest of her reproductive life (Szarewski and Guillebaud 1991).

## Which device to choose?

The T-Safe Cu 380 A appears to be the most effective copper IUD so far studied. Unlike the previous '*Slimline*' which it replaces, the device has the copper bands applied 'proud' on the plastic carrier and inset by a couple of mm from the tips of the side arms of the device. Fortunately, this rather than the *S* version was the one actually used to generate the majority of the world-wide research data, on various clones of a *T-shaped IUD with copper bands on the side arms*, the data which led to its status as the '*gold standard copper IUD*'. No copper device beats it for efficacy, against both uterine and extrauterine pregnancy, the cumulative failure rate in the two studies each of over 1000 users being only 1.4% by 5 years (Trieman *et al.* 1995).

As a consequence of this slightly different design from the previous 'Slimline' version, once loaded, the side arms of the device appear to present a rather large object to get through the cervix: yet the loaded assembly is actually quite nicely rounded and also narrower in one diameter. It usually does pass through the internal os surprisingly easily in all parous women. In nulliparae it may be but often is not necessary to dilate, up to Hegar 5.

The actual loading needs to be done either while it is still in the half-opened packet by a 'trick' which will be taught by Faculty instructing doctors; or using sterile gloves; or with the sterile plastic loading capsule supplied. *One tip:* if the capsule is used, pull back on the thread when loaded, to prevent the capsule pulling the loaded IUD out again.

All in all, this product should now be the first choice copper IUD for any likelihood of long-term use – even by nulliparae – unless there are anticipated or actual problems of fitting it.

### When to use the Nova-T 380

This would be the first choice for a nulliparous woman using it for emergency contraception and planning to have the device removed once established on a new method such as Depo-Provera.

However, in a recent randomized controlled trial (RCT) by Skjeldestad and Rauramo (2001) *Nova-T 380* was only half as effective as a banded T-380 S device (clone of the T-Safe 380 A) – failure rate by 3 years was 3.6 versus 1.7 per

100 women for the banded T ($P<0.05$). Therefore, when long-term use by a young fertile woman is actually expected, the Nova-T 380 should not therefore be chosen, unless the banded T-Safe 380 A cannot be fitted for some reason. Even then, GyneFix might be preferred on efficacy grounds.

### When to use the GyneFix?

This is a frameless device. It carries six bands of copper crimped on to a polypropylene thread bearing a knot; the latter is embedded by the special stylet-introducer in the fundal myometrium. Additional training in the insertion procedure is essential. Special indications for this product are:

◆ small uterine cavity sounding <6.5 cm

◆ distorted cavity on an ultrasound scan (if IUD usable at all)

◆ previous expulsion of any framed device

◆ previous history of needing to remove a framed device within hours or days of insertion due to excessive cramping

◆ significant spasmodic dysmenorrhoea present already pre-insertion (if Mirena IUS is not acceptable) – at least the pain cannot be added to by the presence of a frame.

The *Flexi-T-300* (Cu-Safe) is also available. Limited data from one RCT show a highish cumulative failure rate already by 2 years of 1.5 per 100 women, and a statistically higher expulsion rate, than a clone of the UK banded *T-Safe 380 A*, with which it was compared. Again therefore this is to be seen as a second-line IUD.

There do not seem to be any special advantages to any of the *Multiloads* now that the *T-Safe 380 A* is available, on the evidence: not even with respect to expulsion risk (Trieman *et al.* 1995). Moreover, if the uterus sounds to less than 6 cm the GyneFix would now be preferable to the Multiload Cu 250 Short.

All marketed IUDs in the UK are now reimbursable, on the Drug Tariff.

### Absolute (WHO 4) – but perhaps temporary – contraindications

These are the main established contraindications to Copper IUDs – but, contrast the LNG-IUS (below):

◆ suspected intrauterine or ectopic pregnancy;

◆ unexplained uterine bleeding;

◆ current or very recent active pelvic infection or pelvic tenderness, or purulent cervical discharge;

◆ recent proven STD, unless fully investigated and treated;

◆ immunosuppression (but low-dose systemic steroids acceptable).

## Absolute and permanent (WHO 4) contra-indications

- distorted uterine cavity or cavity <5.5 cm (but GyneFix usable WHO 2);
- Wilson's disease;
- known true allergy to copper;
- heart valve prosthesis, or any past history of actual attack of bacterial endocarditis.

## Relative contraindications

Copper IUD is usable with caution (WHO 2 unless otherwise stated). If intrauterine method used at all, the LNG-IUS (discussed below) is often preferable.

- Structural heart disease (bacterial endocarditis risk without history). Such women should preferably use another method (WHO 3). Otherwise the fitting should be done by an expert, with full antibiotic cover (see the recommendations of the British National Formulary). The patient would also need to be warned, more so than other IUD users, to seek prompt medical advice should she later develop pelvic pain, deep dyspareunia, or excessive discharge;
- Hip replacement or other prosthesis which could be prejudiced by blood-borne infection (antibiotic cover);
- Past history of ectopic pregnancy or other history suggesting high ectopic risk in a multipara (T-Safe Cu 380A, GyneFix or Mirena are preferred IUDs, but this is WHO 3 because even better to use an anovulant contraceptive). In young nulliparae many still consider this to be WHO 4;
- Past history of PID;
- Lifestyle risking STIs, if IUD is used advise condoms as well;
- Infection with HIV (WHO 3 – LNG-IUS definitely preferable and is WHO 1–2, given its likely reduction of transmission risk and also of infection risk with other when/if immunodeficiency develops with AIDS itself);
- Questionable fertility for any reason;
- Nulliparity/young age (if any intrauterine method chosen GyneFix or LNG-IUS may be better than framed copper IUDs);
- Severely scarred uterus (e.g. after open myomectomy);
- Severe cervical stenosis;
- Heavy periods/iron-deficiency anaemia (here LNG-IUS is WHO 1);
- Severe primary dysmenorrhoea (LNG-IUS is again indicated, WHO 1; and GyneFix also preferable to framed IUDs);

- Endometriosis – IUDs may worsen symptoms (LNG-IUS is WHO 1);
- After endometrial ablation/resection (WHO 3 – as risk the IUD may become stuck in shrunken scarred cavity, GyneFix is preferable, WHO 2, and LNG-IUS can be used electively, i.e. WHO 1 as part of menorrhagia treatment, including after submucous fibroid resection).

### Counselling (by doctor or nurse)

After considering the contraindications, there should be an unhurried discussion with the woman of the main points above, particularly regarding her infection risk, the failure rate, and the importance of reporting pain as a symptom. It must be documented that the woman gave her informed verbal consent based on her reading and understanding the current leaflet of the UK FPA or equivalent. She must be assured that in the event of relevant symptoms she will always receive prompt advice and a pelvic examination.

### Timing of insertion

It is customary to insert devices in the closing days of or just after a period. The presence of a pregnancy is thereby excluded, the procedure is easier, and any associated bleeding is accepted as part of normal loss. Recent data suggest increased risks, particularly of expulsion, if IUDs are inserted during the main flow. The normal plan is to insert between day 4 and 14, but later in selected cases.

In cases of amenorrhoea (e.g. post-partum), a very practical tip for excluding the risk of an implanted pregnancy is to use one of the most sensitive modern pregnancy tests after 14 days since the last unprotected sex, having agreed in advance that the couple will practise 'brilliantly good' birth control or abstinence.

After a recent delivery, in general practice IUDs should be inserted at 4–6 weeks, extended to 6–8 weeks after a Caesarean section. Extra care is needed to minimize the risk of perforation.

With insertion at termination of pregnancy there is no increase in complication rates if *Chlamydia* is screened for and the uterus is completely emptied. This choice is not offered often enough, especially to parous women.

### Insertion techniques

For teaching insertion techniques I strongly recommend the Faculty of Family Planning's training scheme leading to the Letter of Competence in Intrauterine Contraception Techniques. This is a one-to-one apprenticeship, supplemented by videos and preliminary practice with appropriate pelvic models, following the illustrations in each packet. Dilators Hegar 3–6 should be available:

Hegar 5 may help insertion of the gold-standard T-Safe 380 A (see above) in a nulliparous woman, but is not always needed.

Training should include more attention than in the past to the issue of analgesia; after a randomized controlled trial showed it worked, it is now routine to offer mefenamic acid 500 mg as pretreatment while in the waiting room. Parenteral cervical anaesthesia should also be taught, as well as the option of 2% lignocaine jelly inserted by quill through the external cervical os, provided enough time is allowed for it to act.

Once learned, the skills, including management of 'lost threads', must be maintained by regular practice.

## Routine follow-up

Correct location of IUDs should be confirmed 6–8 weeks after insertion. Sounding the cervical canal up to the internal os with (for example) a throat swab or Cytobrush is a valuable check for partial expulsion. Annual follow-up is then sufficient *provided* the IUD user is fully informed of the danger-signs implied in Tables 4.15 and 4.16 and has open access to return promptly to the surgery if they occur. Devices are removed as indicated for complications, for planned pregnancy, or one year after the menopause. Otherwise, Table 4.15 column G supports a flexible policy to 'leave well alone'.

# The levonorgestrel-releasing intrauterine system (LNG-IUS or 'Mirena')

This is Nova-T shaped and shown in Fig 4.4 (Andersson *et al.* 1994). It releases 20 μg/24 hours of levonorgestrel (LNG) from its polydimethylsiloxane reservoir through a rate-limiting membrane, over at least 5 years.

## Mechanisms

Its main contraceptive effects are local, by changes to the cervical mucus and uterotubal fluid which impair sperm migration (and may also somewhat inhibit 'germ' migration, see below) to the upper genital tract and by endometrial suppression. The blood levels of LNG are about one-quarter of the peak levels in users of the POP, and so ovarian function is altered less: most women continue to ovulate with or without amenorrhoea (this is primarily a local end-organ effect) and in the anovulant women sufficient oestrogen is produced from the ovary despite the amenorrhoea.

## Clinical advantages and indications

Every one of the advantages listed for the copper IUD apply to the IUS, except for the one about use as a postcoital contraceptive. It has unsurpassed efficacy,

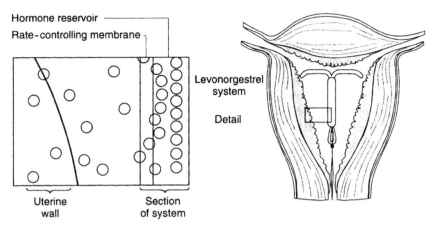

Hormone reservoir

Rate-controlling membrane

Levonorgestrel system

Detail

Uterine wall

Section of system

**Fig 4.4** The levonorgestrel intrauterine system (LNG-IUS).

around 0.1–0.2 per 100 woman-years. Return of fertility is rapid and appears to be complete. It is highly convenient, has few adverse side effects, and added gynaecological value to the menstrual cycle. It has the correct 'default state' (p. 114), unlike pills and condoms.

The above advantages are, of course, shared with the T-Safe Cu 380A S and the GyneFix, the most effective current copper IUDs. However, that is where the similarity ends, since the LNG-IUS has a range of gynaecological benefits which 'rewrite the textbooks' about IUDs. The user can expect a dramatic reduction in amount and, after the first few months (discussed below), in duration of blood loss. Dysmenorrhoea is also improved in most cases. Some of this improvement may be because it treats localized endometriosis (i.e. adenomyosis).

*This is the contraceptive method of choice for non-Pill-takers with heavy or painful menses or who are prone to iron-deficiency anaemia.*

Two unlicensed but increasingly popular uses are to provide localized progestogenic protection of the endometrium during oestrogen replacement therapy by any chosen route (with contraception as well on offer, unlike standard HRT regimens (see p. 214) or as part of the high-dose oestrogen treatment of the premenstrual syndrome. See p. 220 regarding the unlicensed use of unlicensed products.

## Menorrhagia

In an 'Effective Health Care' bulletin – *The management of menorrhagia* (Department of Health 1995), the value of this method of treating menorrhagia was acknowledged:

> Evidence from Scandinavian countries points to the effectiveness of the hormone-releasing intrauterine device as a first line of treatment of menorrhagia.

It has (since 2001) been licensed in the UK for this indication and there is no longer any concern about using the product first line for women not requiring any contraception.

## Infection

Although existing IUDs do not themselves cause pelvic inflammatory disease (PID), they fail to prevent it. There are now good data suggesting, but not proving, that this IUS really does reduce the frequency of clinical PID below the background rate, particularly in the youngest age groups who are most at risk. This and the very low ectopic rate make it possible to offer the device to some young women requesting a 'forgettable' contraceptive who would not be good candidates for conventional copper IUDs. However, the protection is not 100%, and because the superimposed foreign-body effects of an IUD or IUS may worsen an attack and bilateral monogamy is not common in most modern societies, overall the intrauterine method remains second line (WHO 2) for the young and nulliparous *woman* (and all should be specifically warned to use condoms in addition, in all relevant situations such as with a new partner).

## Ectopic pregnancy

The Progestasert and an experimental WHO device which released only 2 μg per day of levonorgestrel were both associated with an increased risk of extrauterine pregnancies. The data on file and published for the Mirena device show a definite reduction in that annual risk to about 0.06 per 100 woman-years.

## Main problems/adverse effects of the LNG-IUS (Mirena™)

- *Insertion* problems have been greatly reduced by the new (2001) inserter package.
- Like any intrauterine device, *expulsion* occurs.
- There is the usual small (approx 1 in 1000) risk of *perforation*, minimized by its 'withdrawal' technique of insertion.
- A more important problem is the high incidence in the first post-insertion months of *uterine bleeding/spotting*, which, through greatly reduced in quantity from the outset, may be very frequent or continuous and can cause considerable inconvenience. Later in the use of the method, amenorrhoea is very commonly reported. For both of these effects 'forewarned is forearmed', implying good counselling in advance of the fitting. Many women can accept the early weeks of frequent light bleeding as a worthwhile price to pay for all the other advantages, if they are well informed in advance, and coached and encouraged as appropriate while it is occurring. The prognosis that the 'dribbling' will stop is actually better than for the other progestogen-only

methods like DMPA, but the time for resolution varies between 1–6 months (rarely longer).

◆ *Amenorrhoea* should be explained and interpreted to a woman as a positive advantage of the method – not an adverse side effect, since menstruation contrary to some cultural beliefs serves no excretory functions . . . and there is no hypo-oestrogenism.

◆ *Hormonal side effects* – women should be advised that though this method is mainly local in its action, it is not exclusively so. Therefore there is a definite small incidence of steroidal side effects such as mastalgia, acne, and depression – usually but not always improving with time.

◆ *Functional ovarian cysts* are also more common, but are usually asymptomatic, and if not they should be treated as conservatively as possible as they usually resolve spontaneously.

### Main absolute contraindications (WHO 4)

◆ Sensitivity to a constituent (e.g. levonorgestrel)

◆ Suspected current intrauterine or ectopic pregnancy

◆ Unexplained uterine bleeding

◆ Current active or recurrent pelvic infection or marked pelvic tenderness, or purulent cervical discharge

◆ Recent proven STD, unless fully investigated and treated

◆ Severely distorted uterine cavity on ultrasound scan (congenital or through submucous fibroids–consider referral for resection, after which Mirena™ may be ideal, inserted under the same anaestheitic)

◆ Heart valve prosthesis, or in woman with a structural heart defect, any past history of actual attack of bacterial endocarditis or severe pelvic infection

◆ Current active arterial disease

◆ Established immunodeficiency (not low-dose systemic steroids)

◆ Recent trophoblastic disease with continuing high hCG levels (p. 000).

In addition:

◆ The IUS should not be used as a postcoital intrauterine contraceptive (a failure has been reported). Though so effective, the mechanisms of action, unlike copper, appear to take time to be established. This explains the recommended *insertion timing*, no later than the seventh day of a spontaneous cycle in a currently sexually active woman. (If there has been believable abstinence, later insertion, with condom use for the rest of the first cycle is also acceptable.)

Most of the relative contraindications listed above for copper IUDs apply but are generally no more than WHO 2; and heavy or painful periods, endometriosis, and HIV infection constitute *indications* (WHO 1).

## Insertion of the LNG-IUS

*Timing* is recommended to be in the first 7 days of the cycle. Since data for IUDs shows a higher expulsion rate when insertion was during the days of heaviest bleeding, a prostaglandin effect, this only leaves days 4–7 for most women–a veritable timing nightmare for most services.

During the initial visit, which is for counselling and the routine pre-insertion *Chlamydia* test, it is good practice to offer short-term treatment with the COC, POP, or DMPA to cover the insertion (except of course in current IUD users).

The insertion tube is wider than the Nova-T 380 (4.8 mm rather than 3.7 mm), so that, like the T-Safe 380 A, dilatation to Hegar 5 may be helpful in nulliparae. All women should be offered premedication and local anaesthesia as described above (p. 199), though the latter is rarely needed by multiparae. In the perimenopausal years a month's oestrogen pretreatment of the cervix can be invaluable.

## Conclusion

This is an excellent choice in contraception, particularly:

◆ as a safe reversible alternative to sterilization for the older woman (especially, but not exclusively, if she also needs supplementary natural oestrogen) and when there is intercurrent chronic disease;

◆ *as the* primary care alternative to hospital referral for menorrhagia and/or dysmenorrhoea – where they will likely (yet often avoidably) end up with a uterine ablation or hysterectomy.

# Barrier methods

Table 4.1 quotes efficacy rates for all these methods. 'Old fashioned' they may be, but they are once again in fashion. In spite of well-known disadvantages, they all (notably male and female condoms) provide useful protection against sexually transmitted diseases. All users of this type of method should be informed in advance about emergency contraception, in case of lack of use or failure in use.

It is also not widely enough known that vegetable and mineral oil-based lubricants, and the bases for prescribable vaginal products, can seriously damage rubber: baby oil, for example, destroys up to 95% of a condom's strength within 15 minutes. The Durex Information Service (1991) produced a useful leaflet listing common vaginal preparations, which should be regarded as unsafe to use with condoms and diaphragms (lists in Table 4.17), but they are not exhaustive. Many other everyday oils can damage rubber, as found in the bathroom or kitchen, and even suntan oils are under some suspicion.

**Table 4.17** Vaginal preparations which are safe/unsafe to use with barrier methods

| Safe | Unsafe |
|---|---|
| Aqueous enemas | *Arachis Oil Enema* |
| Aci-Jel | *Baby Oil* |
| Betadine | *Cyclogest* |
| Canesten | *Dalacin cream* |
| Clotrimazole | *E45 (and similar)* |
| Delfen Foam | *Ecostatin* |
| Double Check | *Fungilin* |
| Durex Duracreme | *Gyno-Daktarin* |
| Durex Duragel | *Gyno-Pevaryl* |
| Durex Lubricating Jelly | *Monistat* |
| Durex Senselle | *Nizoral* |
| Glycerine/glycol | *Nystan Cream* |
| Gynol II | *Petroleum Jelly* |
| KY Jelly | *OrthoDienoestrol* |
| Nystan Pessaries (not cream) | *Ortho-Gynest* |
| Ortho-Creme | *Premarin cream* |
| Ortho-Forms | *Sultrin* |
| Ortho-Gynol | *Vaseline* |
| Ovestin Cream | *Witepsol-based products* |
| Pevaryl | |
| Replens | |
| Silicones | |
| Travogyn | |

*Source*: Durex Information Service for Sexual Health (1991), updated.

## Male and female condoms

These are the only proven barrier to transmission of HIV and should be regularly used along with another contraceptive ('double Dutch'). Male condoms are everyone's second choice, second in usage to the pill under 30 and to sterilization above that age (Table 4.1). Most couples have had some experience of their use. Failure can practically always be attributed to incorrect use, mainly because of the escape of a small amount of semen either before or after the act. One GP was able to report in his study of very well-motivated couples a failure rate as low as 0.4 per 100 woman-years, but 5–15 is more representative. A clear explanation of the basics is always time well spent. At the very least mentioning how the common practice of 'putting it on just before you come' is completely unacceptable. Particularly when the COC has to be stopped after many years on medical grounds, it needs to be clearly highlighted just how 'dangerous' a drop of semen will immediately become.

Some couples are entirely satisfied with the condom. Others use it as a temporary or a back-up method. For some men and some women, however, 'spoilt' by non-intercourse-related alternatives, it is completely unacceptable, but women often do not volunteer this information about their partners. Some older men, or those who have any sexual anxiety, complain that its use may result in loss of erection. In the past, 'allergy' could also be real, to the rubber, but the arrival of polyurethane products such as Avanti™ and EZ-ON removes that excuse. For those women who dislike the smell or messiness of semen, the condom solves their problem.

EZ-ON is available mail-order (01273 230037 or sales@paladone.com), offering the first loose-fit, internally lubricated plastic male condom. It is intended to overcome the most intractable problem of the method, the undeniable interference with penile sensation during the penetrative phase of intercourse. Time will tell, whether UK men will actually vote this a truly 'user-friendly' male condom.

### Femidom

Femidom is a female condom comprising a polyurethane sac with an outer rim at the introitus and a loose inner ring, whose retaining action is similar to that of the rim of the diaphragm, though the user does not have to locate the cervix. It thus forms a well-lubricated, secondary vagina. Available over the counter along with a well-illustrated leaflet, it is considerably less likely than the male condom to rupture in use. It is also completely resistant to damage by any chemicals with which it might come into contact. Using it, the penetrative phase of intercourse can start before the man's erection is complete, and many men prefer the sensation of 'freedom' as compared with male condoms. It can be especially useful post-partum in the presence of lochia or soreness.

Reports about its acceptability are mixed, and a sense of humour (with perhaps some background music) certainly helps. But there is evidence of a group of women (with their partners) who use it regularly; sometimes alternating with the male equivalent ('his night' then 'her night'!). As the first female-controlled method, with high potential for preventing HIV transmission, it must be welcomed.

## The diaphragm and cervical caps

Many women express surprise at the simplicity of this method when first tried. Some who found it unacceptable early in their lives find it much easier later when sexual activity takes on a relatively regular pattern, perhaps with a long-term partner and anticipating childbearing in the not too distant future. Protecting the cervix from infection, neoplasia, and semen, and inserted as a routine well ahead of coitus, it can be used without spoiling spontaneity. There is little reduction in sexual sensitivity as the clitoris and introitus are not affected.

Spermicides (see below) are essential, additionally, as no mechanical barrier is complete. The jelly vehicles (gels) may provide useful lubrication for the older woman, for those in the postnatal period and others slow to lubricate as a result of sexual arousal. Although many substances are well absorbed from the vagina there is no proof of systemic harm from the use of current spermicides, chiefly using Nonoxinol 9 or its close relatives. Experience now spans over 80 years. A review by Bracken (1985) of 14 studies published to date concludes that, in particular, no association with congenital malformations or spontaneous abortion has been demonstrated. Occasionally, a sensitivity to spermicide arises but rubber allergy is rare. Direct local irritation does also occur, particularly if Nonoxinol 9 is used very frequently, as by prostitutes: this effect has recently ended the advice to use it as an adjunctive microbicide against HIV, though it does have that activity against many pathogens. In normal use, Nonoxinol 9 remains acceptable as a spermicide.

The failure rate (now quoted as 4–8 failures in the first year, even among consistent users) makes it an unsuitable choice for most young women who would not accept a pregnancy. But it does much better over the age of 35 (Table 4.1), provided it is correctly and consistently used. Correct fitting is important and can only be learnt by practical 'apprenticeship'. The complaint of discomfort implies wrong fitting. But even more important is skill in teaching placement and the vital secondary check that the cervix is covered. As for the IUD, there is no substitute for one-to-one training in this process of fitting and teaching, in which one can perhaps learn most from the older generation of skilled, family planning-trained nurses. The FPA leaflet should be provided as it includes all the (traditional if somewhat arbitrary) 'rules' of the method.

When it is apparent that a woman has great difficulty in inserting anything into her vagina, be it tampon, pessaries, or her own finger, obviously the method is not suitable. Sometimes this may be connected with some psychosexual difficulty and this may first present during the examination. Permission to discuss associated fears and anxieties may prove helpful. Simple lack of anatomical knowledge is often involved. When any barrier is rejected on account of 'messiness', this also may be due to such a problem. The offer of a less wet-feeling alternative for the spermicide, such as Delfen foam, may help.

If either partner complains that they can feel the barrier during coitus, the fitting must be urgently checked. It could be too large, or too small, or the retropubic ledge is insufficient to prevent the front slipping down the anterior vagina, or most seriously, the diaphragm may be being regularly placed in the anterior fornix. The arcing-spring diaphragm is particularly useful when this last problem is identified.

Chronic urethritis/cystitis may be exacerbated by pressure from the anterior rim and sufferers may do better with a vault or cervical cap, though spermicide-related changes to the vaginal flora may also be a factor. Diaphragms should be checked annually, post-partum, and if there is a 4 kg change in weight gain or loss. If the size remains constant, how often a new one is needed will vary. Some get misshapen, very discoloured, and worn by 1 year, and some appear pristine after 2 years.

Female barriers can be used happily and very successful by many women, but high motivation is essential. Once again a good sense of humour helps. 'Lea's shield', 'Femcap' and the Ovès cap are new plastic cervical barrier devices. The first and last have reached some markets, but at the time of writing only the latter is so far available in the UK. Better efficacy data are awaited (too little so far).

# Spermicides

Whilst invaluable as adjuncts to caps and condoms, by themselves creams, jellies, pessaries, films, and foams are usually not acceptably reliable, though there have been occasional reports of pregnancy rates under 10 per 100 woman-years. The contraceptive sponge is a useful carrier for spermicide and has reappeared since the last edition, now called Protectaid™. It is very user-friendly and inconspicuous during sex, though sadly ineffective in fertile young couples. However, along with Delfen, foam sponges are very useful for women whose natural fertility is reduced, namely:

- age over 45 with infrequent periods and perhaps suffering vasomotor symptoms plus a high FSH reading (since that alone should not be relied upon as signifying infertility); or

- above age 50 until one year after the final menstrual period, with or without HRT

- during lactation or secondary amenorrhoea.

Spermicides in any acceptable form may also be a good supplementary method for couples who consider their only contraceptive option to be the withdrawal method; or for child-spacing.

Recently, and not before time, there has been an upsurge in research interest because of the vital need worldwide, since HIV, for effective, non-irritant vaginal microbicides – which might well also (but not necessarily) be spermicides. Many candidate compounds and carrier vehicles are being screened but we still await the licensing of a product for this important indication.

The sponge and eventually a slow-release vaginal ring are likely vehicles for microbicide/virucide delivery.

## Fertility awareness: methods for natural regulation of fertility

At one time, the 'safe period method' was generally despised and only adopted by staunch Roman Catholics. Modern multiple index versions are increasingly demanded by those who prefer to use a more 'natural' method. These are more reliable, with perfect use–see the excellent review by Pyper and Knight (2001), but in Trussell's phrase they remain 'very unforgiving of imperfect use'.

The latter kind of use is common, in the real world, where the highest possible cooperation from both parties is often lacking – especially from the male whose motivation may well be suspect. (In one study the failure rate was noted to be higher when the man rather than his partner was the one in charge of interpreting the temperature charts!) To be fair to these methods, failures also commonly result from poor use of other contraceptives, such as the condom, during 'unsafe' days.

Because of variable sperm survival (averaging 3 days but achieving 7 days in rare individuals or rare cycles), maximum reliability requires many days of abstinence, especially early in the cycle. Wilcox *et al.* (2000) have shown that the 'fertile window' of a minimum of about 6 days' duration starts at a very variable time in each cycle. For maximum efficacy with any of the methods, unprotected intercourse should preferably be confined, following good evidence of ovulation, to the days after the ovum is no longer fertilizable (its average lifespan is now assessed as 17 hours).

A rise in basal temperature which has been sustained for 72 hours at least 0.2 °C above the preceding 6 days' values is the first recognized marker of the onset of the second infertile phase. This is best combined with observations of the mucus as detected at the vulva. This becomes increasingly fluid, glossy, transparent, slippery, and stretchy, like raw egg-white, under the influence of follicular oestrogen. The peak mucus day can be recognized retrospectively as the last day with such features before the abrupt change to a thick and tacky type (under the influence of progesterone). The infertile phase is defined as beginning on the evening of the fourth day after the peak mucus day, provided this is also after the third-higher morning temperature reading.

Relying only on the later of both the above signals for the onset of the post-ovulatory infertile phase for unprotected intercourse can give very acceptable failure rates of 1–3 per 100 woman-years. Accurately identifying the pre-ovulatory infertile phase is more difficult. The indicators are:

- the first sign of any mucus at all, detected either by sensation or appearance;
- calendar calculation of the shortest cycle minus 20 (or better, 21), where at least six cycle lengths are known; and the woman noted a high temperature phase in the preceding cycle to indicate that ovulation did occur in that cycle.

Whichever of these two indicators comes first indicates the requirement to abstain.

Use of both phases is only to be recommended to 'spacers', since calculations and mucus observations do not reliably predict ovulation far enough ahead to eliminate over many months or years the capricious survival of that last-surviving sperm which could cause a pregnancy. Temperature and mucus estimations are unreliable and/or give numerous 'false alarms' when some cycles are anovulatory, especially in the post-partum period and in the climacteric years. Yet lactation within certain guidelines does constitute an excellent 'natural method' – see LAM method (see Fig 4.5, p. 217).

Any who wish to use these methods deserve careful explanation and teaching. Useful instruction leaflets and further advice can be obtained from:

- The FPA, 2–12 Pentonville Road, London, N1 9FP (Tel. 020 7837 5432); www.fpa.org.uk
- The Fertility Awareness and Natural Family Planning Service, Fertility UK, 1 Blythe Mews, Blythe Road, London W14 0NW (Tel. 020 7371 1341); www.fertilityuk.org (personal teaching may be arranged)

### 'PERSONA©' – the Unipath personal contraceptive system

This innovative product, first marketed in 1996, consists of a series of disposable test sticks and a hand-held, computerized monitor. As instructed by the monitor, the test sticks are dipped in the user's early-morning urine samples and transferred to a slot in the device where the levels of both oestrone 3-glucuronide (E-3-G) and luteinizing hormone (LH) are measured by a patented immunochromatographic assay, utilizing an optical monitor. When a significant increase in the E-3-G level is detected, the fertility status is changed to 'unsafe', i.e. a red light replaces the green one on the monitor. After subsequent detection of the first significant rise of LH, the end of the fertile period is not signalled by a green light until 4 further days have elapsed. The system also stores and utilizes data on the individual's previous six menstrual cycles.

Preliminary efficacy information suggests a failure rate in consistent users of the order of 6 per 100 woman-years. This is comparable to the best previous results using fertility awareness, though higher than would be acceptable to those accustomed to the efficacy of the COC. A fertile period lasting 8 days or less was signalled to 80% of users, a definite improvement on the 10–12 days' abstinence usually demanded by the multiple index methods. For greater efficacy, it is worth suggesting to some couples that they consider using condoms very carefully in the first 'green' phase, abstinence in the 'red' phase and unprotected intercourse only in the second 'green' phase.

This approach should reduce the failure rate to about 2 per 100 woman-years, but has not been formally tested.

## Sterilization

This section is based on first-hand experience of counselling for and performing approaching 4000 vasectomies since 1970, and many hundreds of clip sterilizations, of which more than 1000 have been performed under local anaesthesia – mainly at the Elliot-Smith Clinic in Oxford.

Sterilizing procedures are still often demanded at too early an age. Yet marriages or intended long-term relationships started under age 25 now have a failure rate of more than 50%. Deferment or even avoidance of surgery is often possible by careful discussion and explanation of alternatives, particularly injectables or the modern IUDs and above all Implanon™ and the levonorgestrel-releasing intrauterine system. Older women, by contrast, are sometimes embarrassed to admit they want sex without the possibility of procreation, or at all over the age of 40–45.

## Efficacy considerations and counselling

Malpractice insurers continue to report that male and female sterilization produce far more than their share of litigation. Yet most of it would be avoidable, just by better counselling of both parties and well-documented, fully informed consent backed by a good leaflet such as that of the UK FPA (RCOG 1999). These are especially vital now the long-term efficacy of female sterilization has been called into question by Peterson *et al.* (1996). They found, in a remarkable follow-up study of 10 685 women in the US over 8–14 years, that the failure rate did not, as previously thought, stabilize after 2 years. The highest failure rate for all methods was in young women under age 30. For the only clip then available in the USA, the Hulka (not now recommended in the UK), the cumulative failure rate at 10 years approached 4%. In this country the market-leading Filshie clip is believed to have an overall failure rate–taking account of operator errors but with follow-up to, at most, 2 years–of around 0.3%, and pending more data and longer follow-up, a reasonable current estimate to give at counselling is a lifetime risk of 0.5%, or 5 failures per 1000 procedures (RCOG 1999). The ectopic risk should also be specifically mentioned.

For vasectomy, a much lower rate of one case in 2000–7000 was quoted for late failures in our own Oxford study (Philp *et al.*1984), but it is important to recognize that these followed two azoospermic semen analyses.

It must be understood by the couple that it is their responsibility to avoid conception up to the date of the procedure; the COC may be continued since it does not pose an excess risk of thrombosis at laparoscopy.

## Potential reversibility

In a series published by Winston (1980) reporting on 103 women who requested reversal between 1975–76:

- 87% were under the age of 30;
- 63% had been sterilized after delivery;
- no fewer than 75% had been unhappily married;

hence the vital importance of assessment of any disharmony or pressurizing that may be going on, in the relationship, potentially a big advantage of the counselling clinician in primary care. In my view, it is difficult to justify referral without having had the opportunity to assess the body language of the couple (by seeing them together).

Reported success of *reversal* procedures (male or female) depends enormously on patient selection especially:

- how much damage was done at the initial procedure (clips preferred);

- the age of the woman (now, less than 35 preferred);
- for vasectomy (procedure less than 10 years earlier preferred).

In the favourable cases using microsurgery, as a rule of thumb, 75–80% tubal patency is common but with achievement of healthy full-term children in only around 50%. The operations demand skill, are difficult to get, and are often expensive. It is still wise, therefore, to proceed with sterilization only when both partners can accept its permanence.

### Possible long-term side effects

The psychological sequelae of female sterilization have been looked at. Earlier studies showed considerably higher rates of psychiatric morbidity, psycho-sexual dysfunction, and regret than a prospective study (Cooper *et al.* 1982) in which women were interviewed 4 weeks prior to elective sterilization and followed up at 18 months. In this latter study, considerable regret was felt by 2% at 6 months and by 4% at 18 months, and postoperative psychiatric disturbance and dissatisfaction were largely associated with preoperative psychiatric disturbance. The poorer results in other studies may be, in part, related to sterilization in association with a termination or immediately post-partum. Regret or loss of libido are more likely if the decision is made at such a time of crisis or stress.

In a number of studies of varying designs, no difference in *menstrual pattern or volume* lost has been shown between women who have been sterilized and controls (RCOG 1999). Heavier periods may certainly be observed, but this is equally likely after vasectomy, often just because they have stopped the COC with its much lighter withdrawal bleeds. But counselling MUST include specific questioning about heaviness or pain from their own 'true' periods: this information is vital in order to promote what might be a far more appropriate decision, namely to try the LNG-IUS.

A possible benefit shown in three studies, that tubal sterilization reduces the risk of ovarian cancer, is difficult to explain but may be real (Wilson 1996).

*None* of the long-term systemic adverse effects of vasectomy for which there appeared to be some evidence has been established: notably hormone deficiency, circulatory or immune disorders, carcinoma of the testis or even the prostate (Bernal-Delgado *et al.* 1998).

### Decision-making

Many individuals who find it 'impossible' to accept continuing use of reversible contraceptive methods may just need updating about the hugely greater effectiveness and some added advantages of modern options (above all, the Mirena™ IUS, but also the T-Safe 380 A IUD and Implanon™). For others, however, an irreversible step is just what they want, and once this decision is reached, then the most appropriate procedure needs to be identified after discussion.

### Comparison of methods: the right operation, for the right person, at the right time

*Vasectomy* is very simple and safe medically, a chance for men to 'take their turn' and in primary care it should surely now have precedence in discussions, especially as it is so much more effective. Concern about some loss of potency or manliness is practically universal, so a piece of history can be very reassuring. In the early twentieth century, through the teachings of an Austrian professor named Steinach, vasectomy had a vogue as a kind of 'surgical Viagra'. It was not so, but the procedure could hardly have acquired that reputation if it did the opposite!

But men choosing vasectomy should be specifically warned:

♦ in the short term about occasionally large haematomas and

♦ longer term, about chronic *testicular pain*: a much higher incidence of the latter has been reported from America (probably from populations subject to selection bias) but our rate in Oxford is about 1%. It is almost always treated successfully by excision of the tender nodule at the operation site, often reported as a sperm granuloma.

*Tubal occlusion* remains a more invasive procedure with risk of intra-abdominal injury, even when performed, as it now can readily be, under local anaesthesia with excellent control of pain. General anaesthetics carry their own very small risk. Tubal occlusion confers immediate sterility, whilst it may be several months before the semen is clear of sperm after vasectomy. More importantly, especially once she passes the age of 40, the woman is unlikely to wish for restoration of her fertility, even with any future new partner and, unlike a man, she loses that option after her menopause. Following vasectomy, however, after death of the wife or marriage breakdown, the man (even if past 50) nearly always finds a new and younger partner, and she makes him then more likely to regret his sterility. This difference from the female operation needs to be faced by older couples during counselling.

# The over 35-year-old woman

It is primarily the (EE-containing) COC which is contraindicated above this age, in all women with a definite risk factor for circulatory disease, the most common of which, of course, is smoking. Significant migraine even without aura is WHO 3 when combined with age above 35 but becomes WHO 4 with any hint of hypertension, smoking or obesity.

If they want a pill, smokers above age 35 are usually switched to a progestogen-only brand. However, an IUS with its added (gynaecological) value might be better still, and is also increasingly being chosen by non-smokers. It is ideal not only if the periods are heavy or painful, but also if later there are symptoms of oestrogen deficiency, when as well as giving the reassurance of contraception it will protect the uterus from hyperplasia during oestrogen replacement (evidence-based, though in the UK an unlicensed use; p. 220).

For others, there is now agreement that any copper IUD fitted after the fortieth birthday may be left *in situ* until the menopause. Implanon™ is another option, but DMPA is now less often recommended because of the doubts about hypo-oestrogenism (see above).

In selected entirely healthy, slim, ideally migraine-free non-smokers, from age 35 to 50, the many therapeutic/preventive benefits outweigh, in my view, the small though definite increasing risks with age (mainly of venous or arterial thrombosis but also of breast cancer) of continuing to offer a modern 20 μg pill such as Mercilon or Femodette, if the woman has previously (as most have) used the COC for years without suffering a venous thrombosis. But as this is a WHO 3 situation, documentation of the discussion must be meticulous, and she should always be informed about the new and medically even safer alternatives above, such as the IUS. She may then elect to switch despite not being forced to do so by an incontrovertible risk factor.

In this older group, close supervision is vital, especially of women with blood pressure and headache history.

Perimenopausally, older women are not easily convinced that episodes of amenorrhoea along with less frequent intercourse mean that conception is actually much less likely to occur – and therefore that simpler methods like the contraceptive foam or sponge have acceptable efficacy, above age 45, and especially above 50 with or without HRT. The condom, cap, and diaphragm can also then be extremely reliable, though usually acceptable only if already in use since a younger age.

## When to stop contraception

Despite much research, there is no simple answer to the question: 'When can I stop contraception?' Long spells of amenorrhoea in women under 45 may indicate a premature menopause, but they may be due to other spontaneously reversible or treatable causes requiring investigation (Chapter 1). Even above that age, prolonged amenorrhoea does not rule out the chance of a later ovulation, though the risk is less if there are definite vasomotor symptoms. We now know that FSH measurements alone are most misleading – they only mean reduced feedback of ovarian hormones on the pituitary at that time; the ovaries may well still have potentially fertile ova to release. So most authorities would still advise women only to discontinue all contraception after the occurrence of complete amenorrhoea for 2 years if under age 50 (reducing to 12 months above 50).

If the combined pill is now usable in selected cases until the menopause, how may final ovarian failure be diagnosed? The 'standard' teaching above is impossible to follow with increasing use by this age of cyclical HRT, and, for healthy non-smokers, of 20 μg COCs (since the withdrawal bleeds will indefinitely mask the true menopause). The former is not safely contraceptive, and the increasing risks of the latter become unacceptable above age 50 when adequate and completely risk-free alternatives exist. A possible protocol follows.

## COC users

Measure FSH at the end of the pill-free week. If it is normal she still needs contraception but as the COC is an 'overkill' (see above), an alternative, commonly the POP (monitored thereafter as below), should be offered. If the FSH is high, above the 'menopausal' level specified by the laboratory, there are preliminary data that such a woman has begun – as a consequence of ovarian failure – to rely totally on the COC for her oestrogen. Therefore when it is stopped for just 7 days the FSH climbs rapidly. She may even report 'hot flushes' at the end of each pill-free week, the situation being comparable to sudden loss of ovarian oestrogen by oophorectomy. If she now switches to a simple barrier contraceptive (or just the Protectaid sponge or Delfen foam, which are adequate at this age) for about 6 weeks, and records into the future any subsequent bleeds, a second high FSH result without spontaneous bleeds after stopping the COC is suggestive of final ovarian failure above age 50 – particularly if she reports 'hot flushes'. After advice that the risk of later ovulation can even so not be completely excluded, the woman may then elect to discontinue all contraception, whether or not choosing to start HRT. Ultra-caution otherwise dictates some form of contraception such as the POP (or simple barrier/spermicide) for 12 more months.

## Cyclical HRT-users (using separate contraception)

Measure FSH, logically at the end of the oestrogen-only phase. A level above 25 IU/l, raised despite the HRT feedback on the pituitary, is suggestive of ovarian failure – but this should preferably be confirmed, exactly as for the COC above, after stopping exogenous hormones for 6 weeks. If, however, the woman has a normal FSH result and/or ever later menstruates while off either COC or HRT, she should assume some residual fertility and (continue to) use a simple contraceptive for the standard year, again whether or not she decides to take HRT.

### POP users

If prolonged amenorrhoea occurs as a new phenomenon along with vaso-motor symptoms suggestive of the menopause, the woman may have her FSH measured while still taking the method. If it is low, she still needs the POP, and a strength of this method is that she may continue into her late fifties. If it is high, the presence and persistence of vasomotor symptoms and a repeat high FSH value 6 weeks after stopping the treatment mean that her chances of a further fertile ovulation are extremely low, and possibly nil. With all the caveats above, she may therefore discontinue contraception (Guillebaud 1999).

Another option in selected POP-users with amenorrhoea, high FSHs, and definite vasomotor symptoms is to switch to any marketed HRT product along with continuous daily POP-taking – an unlicensed but in practice popular combination (see named-patient use), which is very likely to be con-traceptive. Once marketed, the anovulant Cerazette would be a reassuring POP for this purpose especially in sub-50 year olds. Younger women and any who want more complete reassurance may, if preferred, continue using a simple method, as usual until one year after the last non-hormonally-induced bleed.

### The Mirena IUS

Having been fitted earlier, usually to control menstrual symptoms, this is a superb way to short-circuit all these uncertainties and, in the Swedish Gynaecologist Viveca Odlind's phrase, to 'surf through the menopause'. The bottom line is that we still do not have – and badly need – a simple test of complete and final ovarian failure at the menopause.

## The woman who has just been pregnant

### If not breast-feeding

Ovulation may occur as early as 10 days after abortion and by about day 28 after delivery. Early contraception is therefore important. In women who do not breast-feed, the COC should be started no earlier than day 21 (Table 4.10) in order to minimize any extra risk of venous thrombosis. Moreover, if there has been severe pre-eclampsia or the HELLP (Hyper-tension, Elevated Liver enzymes and Low Platelets) syndrome, the COC should be not be commenced until after blood pressure and biochemical normality have both been restored. Thereafter, this past history is only WHO 1 for COC use.

## If breast-feeding

Studies have shown that ovulation is delayed among women who fully or nearly fully breast-feed their babies – with considerable individual variation related to the frequency and duration of breast-feeding episodes and the timing of introduction of food other than breast milk. In 1988 at a consensus conference in Bellagio, Italy, guidelines were produced leading to a method of family planning known as the lactational amenorrhoea method

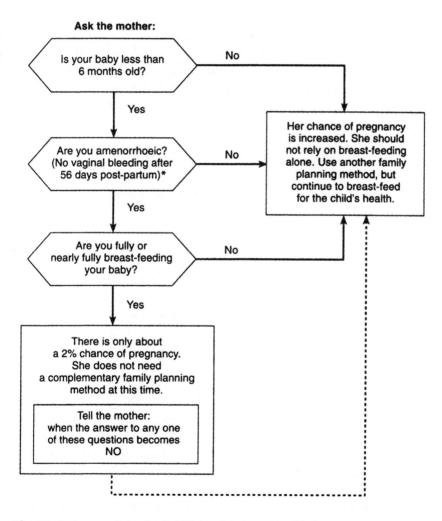

*Spotting that occurs during the first 56 days is not considered to be menses.

**Fig 4.5** LAM – use of the lactational amenorrhoea method during the first 6 post-partum months.

or LAM (Labbok *et al.* 1994). LAM is an algorithm, as shown in Fig 4.5, allowing a woman to determine when she can rely on her pattern of infant-feeding and menstruation or should add an additional method of contraception.

In the UK, despite efforts to encourage breast-feeding, only around 50% of new mothers breast-feed their babies beyond a few days, and two-fifths of them give supplementary bottle-feeds by 6 weeks. Successful breast-feeders who freely choose the lactational amenorrhoea method and accept its limitations are the only reasonable candidates for it.

The COC should be avoided as it may inhibit lactation and does enter the milk in small quantities. The POP is preferable, usually started, like the COC, on day 21. This does not interfere significantly with lactation and although traces may enter the milk, the quantity with Microval or Norgeston would be so small that it has been equated to a baby getting the equivalent of one pill in 2 years. Strangely, the natural childbirth movement nevertheless advises against its use.

Unwanted pregnancies are not uncommon when lactating POP users have not been warned that their margin for error in POP-taking will diminish at weaning. If efficacy is at a premium, they should switch to the COC (or DMPA) when their infant first takes solid food, or no later than the first bleed.

The injectable, DMPA, aside from slightly higher milk levels (which seem to be harmless to the infant) may be a preferable progestogen-only method for women who might be short-term breast-feeders and unreliable POP-takers, but want high efficacy right through weaning and thereafter. It does no detectable harm to the quality and may even improve the quantity of the breast milk. Implanon is another option despite the caution of the SPC.

The IUD or IUS is easily inserted at 4–6 weeks post-partum or 6–8 weeks after a Caesarean section, but the uterus is still soft and great care is necessary. Earlier insertion is more likely to lead to expulsion.

Condoms (especially the female condom) are useful until other methods are established. Caps and diaphragms may be refitted at 5–6 weeks and this is necessary even after Caesarean section. Aside from the LAM above, natural regulation of fertility is very difficult – the mucus signs give 'false alarms' and force prolonged abstinence on the couple if they are to obtain acceptable efficacy before normal cycling resumes.

Sterilization procedures performed at abortion or in the post-partum period carry extra operative, failure rate, and emotional risks. Surgery in both sexes is usually, and preferably, delayed for a few months.

# The very young

Although early cycles after the menarche are often anovulatory, very early conceptions do happen: and surveys show that around half of the total female population under 16 years of age have had intercourse.

A modern, low-oestrogen combined pill usually proves the most suitable method, initially. As far as we know, once periods are established it poses no special problems in teenagers, as compared with women in their twenties. However, like the condom, the COC has the wrong 'default state'. With the difficulties so many young people have in their compliance, we badly need more methods modelled on a utopian future method, reversible vaccination against pregnancy! Those already available are not perfect for teens, namely injectables, implants, IUDs, and the IUS, but according to the Government's Teenage Pregnancy Unit, set up in 2001, they should be more often offered, especially at/after a termination of pregnancy or when the COC has proved unsatisfactory for the individual.

Since teenagers generally are now at greatest risk of all sexually transmitted agents, including HIV, it is essential to promote use of the condom in addition, often, to the selected main contraceptive ('double Dutch').

Any GP faced with an under-16-year-old needs first, opportunely and non-patronizingly, to raise the medical and emotional advantages of delaying intercourse until later. The Fraser guidelines based on the Gillick case (1986) need to be taken into account. Although involvement of at least one parent is vastly preferable and we are legally obliged to discuss this, the memorandum describes circumstances in which it is good practice to proceed to prescribe the Pill without it. At all times the young person must be assured 100% of confidentiality: this usually is real enough, but the ambience of the consultation must make it also *seem* real to her; if not, this can be the greatest single deterrent to obtaining contraception.

Dedicated sessions with the right 'feel' for young people are the ideal, the model being those run by the Brook Advisory Centres. Some general practices have combined in a locality to develop highly successful drop-in centres, for the young of both sexes.

# Women with intercurrent disease

Historically, this has mainly been a problem where the condition such as diabetes, hypertension, or sickle-cell disease poses a contraindication (WHO 3 or 4) to the COC: see the discussion of 'summation'. Such women usually require maximum possible protection from pregnancy, which often has its own additional disease-related risks. The added risks of a contraceptive like the COC may sometimes be acceptable because of the reduced risk through pregnancy in comparison with medically safer, less effective reversible alternatives. Female sterilization is a possibility, but not always relevant. Likewise, the woman's healthy partner's kind offer to have a vasectomy may not necessarily be rightly accepted – e.g. if her expectation of life is very short. Clearly, each couple has to be considered individually and discussion with the consultant in charge is often mandatory, especially in cancer cases or conditions with a highly unpredictable prognosis like multiple sclerosis.

My own lecture with this title has become much shorter since May 1995, the month that the LNG-IUS first arrived on the UK market. Chiefly because of its efficacy and the virtual absence of life-endangering adverse effects, it is surprising how often this answers incoming queries about difficult contraceptive problems! But Implanon™ and the other progestogen-only methods or the T-Safe Cu 380 A are usually also good options.

## The issue of unlicensed indications (for licensed products)

Several times in this chapter unlicensed uses have been proposed. In the UK, if doctors wish to use this or any other medicinal product for an unlicensed indication, they may do so legally on their personal professional responsibility. 'Named patient prescribing' is an established process (Mann 1991) in which the doctor should ensure that he/she:

- is adopting a practice that is evidence-based and would be *endorsed by a responsible body of professional opinion* and that all practices regarding the product are acceptable to those responsible for the doctor's professional indemnity;
- has *explained to the patient* that this is an *unlicensed* prescription and provides a dedicated written handout, as appropriate;
- has explained clearly the perceived risks and benefits, so that *informed consent can be obtained and recorded* (this does not require the patient's signature);
- *keeps a record* of the patient's details and the prescription.

These arrangements should be familiar; many of us regularly use other products for indications which are not yet licensed.

# The future

Why is it that in spite of the availability of a full, comprehensive, and usually completely free contraceptive service in the UK, the requests for termination of unwanted pregnancies continue? Some women find it difficult to get contraceptive advice, and others seem unable to use any method successfully. Despite all the medico-legal obstacles, new pills, intrauterine devices and systems, injectables, implants, skin patches, new vaginal barriers, rings, condoms, and sterilization clips are known to be in the pipeline; plus shortly thereafter the long-awaited injectable/implant for *men* based on a long-acting testosterone ester, probably in combination with a progestogen. More choice has to help. However, regardless of research developments, practitioners and practice nurses in this important field of reproductive health will always need sensitivity to understand, and allow for in their counselling, the innumerable factors which affect the acceptability of contraceptive methods. There needs to be more perception by the very young of the ease of conception and by the older woman of the persistence of fertility. As a team, whether in general practice or in local clinics, we have a responsibility to make it easy for our patients to ask for advice and then to have the skill to help them use their own choice, happily and effectively.

# 10-Minute consultation

The patient is 24 and has been having sex with her present boyfriend for the last 9 months. Up until now they were using condoms but she needed emergency contraception whilst on holiday because the condom came off. She is now wondering about whether to go on the pill in case this happens again.

## What issues you should cover

- Explore the reasons for the condom failure. Teach condom techniques if necessary and stress their use against sexually transmitted infections as well as pregnancy prevention.
- Make sure she knows she can use emergency contraception again whether she continues to use condoms or the pill.
- Go over the pros and cons of taking the pill. Find out about her medical and family history to make sure there are no contraindications to her taking the pill, giving health promotion advice as appropriate.
- Explain how to take the pill, emphasizing what to do if she misses or forgets a pill and give an information leaflet.

## What you should do

◆ Discuss what she knows about the pill. Explain that the combined pill works by stopping an egg from being produced.

◆ Explain the advantages of the pill which include: 99% effective against getting pregnant if used correctly, easy to use and does not interfere with sex, gives regular and usually lighter periods (ask about periods), may reduce premenstrual syndrome (check whether PMS is a problem), protects against ovarian and endometrial cancer (check family history of these cancers).

◆ Explain the disadvantages of the pill which include lack of protection against STIs so need to use condoms.

◆ Discuss minor/nuisance side effects: headaches (check about headaches and migraines) nausea early on, mood changes (check for depression), weight (check BMI), breast tenderness, breakthrough bleeding, decreased libido. Explain it is usually possible to find a pill that suits, and that many of these minor problems do settle in the first few months of use.

◆ Discuss serious side effects: heart attacks, strokes, hypertension (check blood pressure), blood clots. Find out about family history of any of these and decide if suitable to take the pill. Explain increased risk of venous thrombosis from 5/100 000 women to 15/100 000 women in those taking 'second-generation' pills and 25/100 000 women taking the 'third-generation' pill. Emphasize the risk of smoking and the pill on heart attacks and strokes (take a smoking history).

◆ Discuss cancer risks with an increased risk of breast cancer of 1/1000 if used up to age 35. Check family history of breast cancer. There is a very small increased risk of cervical cancer on the pill but using condoms is probably protective. Remind her to have regular cervical smears from the age of 20.

## If the patient decides to go on the pill

◆ Show her a pack of pills and explain when to take them.

◆ Find out where she is in her cycle and demonstrate how to start the pill on the first day of her period. Remind her that each month she will start the new pack on the same day of the week. Demonstrate this on the pack itself and check she understands.

◆ Warn her she may get some bleeding on tablet-taking days in the first one or two cycles, also some nausea initially. Both symptoms are likely to improve if she perseveres but she can ring the Practice Nurse for advice.

◆ Go over what to do if she misses a pill, takes antibiotics or has an episode of gastroenteritis, vomiting, or severe diarrhoea. Stress that contraception is not lost if she takes a missed pill within 12 hours of her normal pill-taking time. If she forgets to take a pill for more than 12 hours, she should continue to take the pills as usual but use condoms as well for the next 7 days.

◆ Emphasize that it is more risky to miss pills at the beginning and the end of packs – describe how the pill suppresses the ovaries and stops ovulation, and how the ovaries start to 'wake up' and get ready for ovulation during the pill-free days. If this time is extended, then ovulation is more likely to occur. If she is more than 12 hours late taking a pill in the last week of the pack, she should run two packs together and use condoms for 7 days.

◆ Use the FPA leaflet, 'The combined pill', as a written reminder, pointing out the advice about missed pills, and recommend that she keeps it somewhere safe for future reference.

◆ Check whether she has any questions.

◆ Prescribe 3 months' supply of the pill and give her some condoms. Start with a second-generation progestogen (have a low threshold to try any other preparation subsequently for symptom control).

◆ Arrange to see her in 3 months before she runs out of pills. Tell her to make contact earlier if she has any worries.

◆ Make appropriate claim for family planning fee.

## Further reading for patients

Clubb, E., and Knight, J. (1996). Fertility, 3rd edn. David & Charles, London. New edition expected 2002.
Guillebaud, J. (1997). *The Pill*, 5th edn. Oxford University Press, Oxford.
Rosenberg ,M. and Long, S. (1992). Oral contraceptives and cycle control: A critical review of the literature. *Advances in Contraception*, **8**, 35–45.
Szarewski, A. and Guillebaud, J. (2000) *Contraception – a user's handbook*, 3rd edn. Oxford University Press, Oxford.
Useful patient leaflets concerning all methods and instructions in other languages can be obtained from the FPA, 2–12 Pentonville Rd, London N1 9FP.

## Useful websites

◆ Training courses on offer + useful search engine for medical FAQs; www.margaretpyke.org

◆ The FPA, 2–12 Pentonville Road, London, N1 9FP; www.fpa.org.uk

◆ WHO for Eligibility Criteria (p. 118) and new Practice Recommendations (p. 115 and p. 163) www.who.int/reproductive–health

◆ International Planned Parenthood Federation for excellent on-line Directory of Hormonal Contraception + names of equivalent pill brands used in every country; www.ippf.org.uk

◆ To inform teenagers accurately on all health subjects (Anorexia to Zits!); www.teenagehealthfreak.com.

◆ The Fertility Awareness and Natural Family Planning Service, Fertility UK, 1 Blythe Mews, Blythe Road, London W14 0NW; www.fertilityuk.org

## References and further reading

Andersson, K., Odlind, V. and Rybo, G. (1994). Levonorgestrel-releasing and copper releasing (Nova-T) IUDs during five years of use: a randomised comparative trial. *Contraception*, **49**, 56–72.

Audet, M.-C., Moreau, M., Calton, W., *et al.* (2001). Evaluation of contraceptive efficacy and cycle control of a transdermal contraceptive patch vs an oral contraceptive: a randomized controlled trial. *Journal of the American Medical Association*, **285**, 2347–54.

Back, D. J., Breckenridge, A. M., Crawford, F. F., MacIver, M., Orme, M.L'E. and Rowe, P. H. (1981). Interindividual variation and drug interactions with hormonal steroid contraceptives. *Drugs*, **21**, 46–61.

Banks, E., Berrington, A. and Casabonne, D. (2001). Overview of the relationship between use of pregestogen-only contraceptives and bonemineral density. *British Journal of obstetrics and gynaecology*, **108**, 1214–21.

Beral, V., Hermon, C., Kay, C. *et al.* (1999). Mortality associated with oral contraceptive use: 25 year follow up of cohort of 46 000 women from RCGP OC study. *British Medical Journal* **318**, 96–100.

Bernal-Delgado, E., Latour-Perez, J., Pradas-Arnal, F. and Gomez-Lopez, L.I. (1998). The association between vasectomy and prostate cancer: a systematic review of the literature. *Fertility and Sterility*, **70**, 191–200.

Bhathena, R.K. (2001). The long-acting progestogen-only contraceptive injections. *British Journal of Obstetrics and Gynaecology*, **108**, 3–8.

Bracken, M.B. (1985). Spermicidal contraceptives and poor reproductive outcomes: the epidemiological evidence against an association. *American Journal of Obstetrics and Gynecology*, **151**, 552–6.

Clinical and Scientific Committee, Faculty of Family Planning and Reproductive Health Care (1998). Recommendations for clinical practice: actinomyces-like organisms and intrauterine contraceptives. *British Journal of Family Planning*, **23**, 137–8.

Collaborative Group on Hormonal Factors in Breast Cancer (1996). Breast cancer and hormonal contraceptives. *Lancet*, **347**, 1713–27.

Collaborative group on desogestrel (1998). A double-blind study comparing the contraceptive efficacy, acceptability and safety of two progestogen-only pills containing desogestrel 75 μg/day or levonorgestrel 30 μg/day. *European Journal of Contraception and Reproductive Health Care*, **3**,169–78.

Committee on Safety of Medicines (1995). *Combined oral contraceptives and thromboembolism.* [Letter]. CSM, London.

Contraceptive Education Service (1996). *Contraceptive choices.* Family Planning Association, London.

Cooper, E. and Guillebaud, J. (1999). Author Note in Preface. *Sexuality and disability: a guide for every day practice.* Radcliffe Medical Press, Abingdon.

Cooper, P., Gath, D., Rose, N., *et al.* (1982). Psychological sequelae to elective sterilization: a prospective study. *British Medical Journal,* **284**, 461–4.

Croft, P. and Hannaford, P.C. (1989). Risk factors for acute myocardial infarction in women: evidence from the Royal College of General Practitoners' oral contraception study. *British Medical Journal,* **298**, 165–8.

Demacker, P.M., Schade, R.W., Stalenhoef, A.F., *et al.* (1982). Influence of contraceptive pill and menstrual cycle on serum lipids and high-density lipoprotein cholesterol concentrations. *British Medical Journal,* **284**, 1213–15.

Department of Health (2001). *The national strategy for sexual health and HIV.* DoH, London.

Drife, J. (2001). The third generation pill controversy ('continued'). *British Medical Journal,* **323**, 119–20.

DTB (2001). Etonogestrel implant (Implanon) for contraception. *Drug and Therapeutics Bulletin,* **39**, 57.

DTB (2002). Is Yasmin a 'truly different pill'? *Drug and Therapeutics Bulletin,* **40**, 57–9.

Dunn, N., Thorogood, M., Faragher, B. *et al.* (1999). Oral contraceptives and myocardial infarction: the results of the MICA case-control study. *British Medical Journal* **319**, 795–6.

Durex Information Service for Sexual Health (1991). *Warning: oil-based lubricants and ointments can damage condoms and diaphragms.* LRC Leaflet, 1–4.

Effective health care bulletin (1995). *The management of menorrhagia.* Bulletin 9. University of Leeds, Leeds.

Elliman, A. (2000). Interactions with hormonal contraception (FACT review). *Journal of Family Planning and Reproductive Health Care,* **26**, 109–11.

Faculty of Family Planning and Reproductive Health Care (2000a). First prescription of combined oral contraception: recommendations for clinical practice. *British Journal of Family Planning,* **27**, 27–38.

Faculty of Family Planning and Reproductive Health Care (2000b). Emergency contraception: recommendations for clinical practice. *British Journal of Family Planning,* **26**, 93–6.

Farley, T.M., Rosenberg, M.J., Rowe, P., *et al.* (1992). Intrauterine devices and pelvic inflammatory disease: an international perspective. *Lancet,* **339**, 785–8.

Farley, T.M., Meirik, O. and Collins, J. (1999). Cardiovascular disease and combined oral contraceptives: reviewing the evidence and balancing the risks. *Human Reproduction Update,* **5**, 721–35.

Foidart, J.-M., Wuttke, W,, Buow, G.M., *et al.* (2000). A comparative investigation of contraceptive reliability, cycle control and tolerance of two monophasic oral contraceptives containing either drospirenone or desogestrel. *European Journal of Contraception and Reproductive Health Care,* **5**, 124–34.

Gbolade *et al.* (2002). Depo-Provera and bone density (Fact review). *Journal of Family Planning and Reproductive Health Care*, **28**, 7–12.

Guillebaud, J. (1995). Advising women on which pill to take. *British Medical Journal*, **311**, 1111–12.

Guillebaud, J. (1999). *Contraception – your questions answered*, 3rd edn. Churchill Livingstone, Edinburgh.

Guillebaud, J. (2001a). Medical eligibility criteria for contraceptive use. *Lancet*, **357**, 1378–9.

Guillebaud, J. (2001b). Progestogen-only pills (POPs) and body weight. *Journal of Family Planning and Reproductive Health Care*, **27**, 239.

Guillebaud, J. (2001c). Intrauterine devices and infertility. *Lancet*, **358**, 1460.

Hannaford, P. and Webb, A. (1996). Evidence-guided prescribing of combined oral contraceptives: consensus statement. *Contraception*, **54**, 125–9.

Korver, T., Goorissen, E. and Guillebaud, J. (1995). The combined oral contraceptive pill: what advice should we give when pills are missed? *British Journal of Obstetrics and Gynaecology*, **102**, 601–7.

Labbok, M.H., Perez, A., Valdez, V., *et al.* (1994). The lactational amenorrhoea method (LAM): a postpartum introductory family planning method with policy and program implications. *Advances in Contraception*, **10**, 93–109.

McCann, M.F. and Potter, L.S. (1994). Progestin-only oral contraception: a comprehensive review. *Contraception*, **50**(1), S9–195.

MacGregor, E.A. (2001). Hormonal contraception and migraine (FACT review). *Journal of Family Planning and Reproductive Health Care*, **27**, 49–52.

MacGregor, E.A. and Guillebaud, J. (1998). Combined oral contraceptives, migraine and ischaemic stroke. *British Journal of Family Planning*, **24**, 55–60.

Mackie, I.J., Piejsa, K., Fers, S.-A. *et al.* (2001). Protein S levels are lower in women receiving desogestrel-containing combined oral contraceptives (COCs) than in women receiving levonorgestrel-containing COCs at steady state and on cross-over. *British Journal of Haematology*, **113**, 898–904.

Mann, R. (1991). Unlicensed medicines and the use of drugs in unlicensed indications. In: Goldberg, A. and Dodd-Smith, I. (eds), *Pharmaceutical medicine and the law*, pp.103–10. Royal College of Physicians, London.

Mao, K. and Guillebaud, J. (1984). Influence of removal of intrauterine contraceptive devices on colonization of the cervix by actinomyces-like organisms. *Contraception*, **30**, 535–45.

Marchbanks, P., McDonald, J., Wilson, H., *et al.* (2002) Oral contraceptives and the risk of breast cancer. *New England Journal of Medicine*, **46**, 2025–32

Newton, J.R. and Tacchi, D. (1990). Long-term use of copper intrauterine devices. *Lancet*, **336**, 182.

O'Brien P. (1999). Study confirms tendency towards lower risk of myocardial infarction with second generation oral contraceptives in UK. *British Medical Journal*, **319**, 1199.

Pardthaisong, T. (1984). Return of fertility after use of the injectable contraceptive, Depo-Provera: updated analysis. *Journal of Biosocial Science*, **16**, 23–34.

Peterson, H.B., Zhisen, X., Hughes, J.M., *et al.* (1996). The risk of pregnancy after tubal sterilization: findings from the US Collaborative Review of Sterilization. *American Journal of Obstetrics and Gynecology*, **174**, 1161–70.

Philp, T., Guillebaud, J. and Budd, D. (1984). Late failure of vasectomy after two documented analyses showing azoospermic semen. *British Medical Journal,* **289**, 77–9.

Pyper, C.M. and Knight, J. (2001). Fertility awareness methods of family planning: the physiological background, methodology and effectiveness of fertility awareness methods (FACT Review). *Journal of Family Planning and Reproductive Health Care,* **27**, 103–10.

RCGP (1983). Incidence of arterial disease among oral contraceptive users. *Journal of the Royal College of General Practitioners,* **33**, 75–8.

RCOG (Royal College of Obstetricians and Gynaecologists) (1999). *Male and female sterilisation* (Evidence-based Clinical Guidelines No. 4). RCOG, London.

Sapire, K.E. (1990). *Contraception and sexuality in health and disease.* McGraw-Hill, London.

Skjeldestad, F. and Rauramo, I. (2001). An open randomised trial of two copper IUDs, Nova T380 versus Gyne T 380 Slimline: 3 year results. Abstract 38 presented at 29th British Congress of Obstetrics & Gynaecology, Birmingham, July 2001.

Smith, S.K., Kirkman, R.J., Arce, B.B., *et al.* (1986) The effect of deliberate omission of Trinordiol® or Microgynon® on the hypothalamo-pituitary-ovarian axis. *Contraception,* **34**, 513–22.

Smith, J., Green, J., Berrington de Gonzalez, A., Appleby, P., Peto, J., Plummer, M., Franceschi, S. and Beral, V. (2003). Cervical cancer and use of hormonal contraceptives: a systematic review. *Lancet,* **361**, 1159–67.

Stampfer, M.J., Willett, W.C., Colditz, G.A., *et al.* (1988). A prospective study of past use of oral contraceptive agents and risk of cardiovascular diseases. *New England Journal of Medicine,* **319**, 1313–17.

Szarewski, A. and Guillebaud, J. (1991). Regular review: contraception, current state of the art. *British Medical Journal,* **302**, 1224–6.

Tanis, B.C., van den Bosch, M.A., Kemmeren, J.M., *et al.* (2001). Oral contraceptives and the risk of myocardial infarction. *New England Journal of Medicine,* **345**, 1787–93.

Trieman, K., Liskin, L., Kols, A., and Rinehart, W. (1995). IUDs–An Update. *Population Reports,* series B, no. 6. Johns Hopkins School of Public Health, Population Information Program, Baltimore.

Tuckey, J. (2000). Combined oral contraception and cancer (FACT review). *Journal of Family Planning and Reproductive Health Care,* **26**, 237–40.

Vessey, M. P., Lawless, M. and Yeates, D. (1982). Efficacy of different contraceptive methods. *Lancet,* **1**, 841–2.

Vessey, M. P., Lawless, M., McPherson, K. and Yeates, D. (1983). Neoplasia of the cervix uteri and contraception: a possible adverse effect of the Pill. *Lancet,* **ii**, 930–4.

Vessey, M. P., Lawless, M., Yeates, D. and McPherson, K. (1985). Progestogen-only oral contraception. Findings in a large prospective study with special reference to effectiveness. *British Journal of Family Planing,* **10**, 117–21.

Vessey, M. P., Villard-Mackintosh L., McPherson K. and Yeates D. (1989). Mortality among oral contraceptive users: 20 year follow-up of women in a cohort study. *British Medical Journal,* **299**, 1487–91.

Westrom, L. (1987). Pelvic inflammatory disease: bacteriology and sequelae. *Contraception*, **36**, 111–28.

WHO (1998a). Cardiovascular risk factors and use of oral and injectable progestogen-only contraceptives and combined injectable contraceptives. *Contraception*, **57**, 315–24.

WHO (1998b). Randomised controlled trial of levonorgestrel versus the Yuzpe regimen of combined oral contraceptives for emergency contraception. *Lancet*, **352**, 428–33.

WHO (2001). Medical eligibility criteria for contraceptive use, 2nd edn. WHO/RHR/00.02, Geneva.

WHO Scientific Group (1981). *The effect of female sex hormones on fetal development and infant health*. Technical report series, 657. WHO, Geneva.

WHO Scientific Group (1987). *Mechanism of action, safety and efficacy of intrauterine devices*. Technical Reports Series, 753. WHO, Geneva.

Wilcox, A.J., Dunson, D. and Baird, D.D (2000). The timing of the 'fertile window' in the menstrual cycle: day specific estimates from a prospective study. *British Medical Journal*, **321**, 1259–62.

Wilson, E. W. (1996). Sterilization. In: Glasier, A. (ed.), *Baillière's Clinical Obstetrics and Gynaecology: contraception*, pp.103–19. Baillière Tindall, London.

Winston, R.M.L. (1980). Reversal of tubal sterilization. *Clinical Obstetrics and Gynaecology*, **23**, 1261–8.

# Reference books

Drife, J.O. and Baird, D.T. (eds) (1993). *British medical bulletin: Contraception*. British Council, London.

Guillebaud, J. (2000). *Contraception today: a pocket book for general practitioners*, 4th edn. Martin Dunitz, London.

Hannaford, P.C. and Webb, A.M. (eds) (1996). *Evidence-guided prescribing of the pill*. Parthenon, Carnforth.

Kubba, A., Sanfilippo, J. and Hampton, N. (eds) (1999). *Contraception and office gynaecology: choices in reproductive healthcare*. Saunders, London.

# Chapter 5

# Unwanted pregnancy and abortion

## Lis Davidson and Joanne Reeve

Most general practitioners (GPs) will be familiar with the clinical scenario of a woman who is unhappy about her pregnancy. For some this will arouse uncomfortable feelings. The doctor may feel uneasy at being asked to provide a service – referral for abortion – rather than being asked to exercise the classical medical skills of diagnosis and treatment. In addition, the doctor's attitude to abortion may make it difficult to respond to the woman's needs.

In this chapter we hope to show that there are 'diagnostic skills' that can be usefully learnt to help women through this difficult decision-making time; to give them the maximum choice in the 'treatment' that is most appropriate for them. We offer here a liberal view of the abortion laws of England, Scotland and Wales that is ethically based in a belief that the woman's view is of primary importance, and that every child should be 'wanted'. Interpreting the statistics produces many questions, many related to what service is being provided in any given area, and what are the various social and economic drivers behind the figures.

## Terminology

Although a large proportion of this chapter will be taken up discussing abortion, for a GP this actually represents a small part of the health needs of the woman sat in his/her surgery. A request for an induced abortion (also known as a termination of pregnancy) is often the result of a complex set of circumstances for any woman and is not simply the result of 'failed' family planning or 'irresponsible behaviour'. In countries such as the Netherlands where there is a good family planning service, the abortion rate is one of the lowest in the world (6 per 1000 women in 1994). However, termination of pregnancy (TOP) is still recognized to be a necessary part of fertility control (Berer 2000).

Contraception and abortion are only two elements to consider in addressing the wider sexual health needs of women. Dahlgren and Whitehead's model of health recognizes the importance of social, community, socioeconomic, and cultural factors in influencing health and thus health needs (Dahlgren and Whitehead 1991). Decisions about unwanted pregnancies will not be influenced by biomedical concerns alone. The term 'unwanted' as used in this chapter is also not without its problems. 'Unwanted' pregnancies are not necessarily those that are unplanned, but circumstances may change. A survey of women seeking a termination of pregnancy in Liverpool in 1993 found 32% of woman described their pregnancy as unplanned, but wanted. However, the women felt they were unable to continue the pregnancy for a variety of reasons. This points to the ambiguity that many women feel in relation to decisions they make about pregnancy, especially when it involves the decision to ask for an abortion.

## Abortion legislation

It is sometimes easy to forget that TOP has only been legal again in England and Wales for around 30 years. In the eighteenth century, abortion was legal as long as it was performed before the woman felt the fetus move (the point at which it was believed the soul entered the fetus). However, the 1861 Offences against the Person Act criminalized all abortion, even for medical reasons, with punishment of up to life imprisonment for the woman and the abortionist. The 1861 Act has never been repealed, but there are now permitted exceptions that protect a woman and her doctor from prosecution in certain circumstances.

The Infant Life Preservation Act 1929 amended the law in England and Wales so that abortion was permissible if carried out in good faith in order to save the mother's life. However, it stated that it was always illegal to 'destroy the life of a child capable of being born alive' – assumed to be from 28 weeks' gestation.

An important test of the interpretation of the law came in 1938 with the Bourne Judgement. Dr Alex Bourne performed an abortion on a 14-year-old girl who had been gang raped. In his defence he stated his belief that the abortion was necessary to save the life of the mother. The judge in the case found him not guilty and opened the way for more a liberal interpretation of the circumstances in which the law would allow abortion to 'preserve a woman's life'. However, there was still reluctance by many to risk testing the limits of the law. A review of the legislation was needed, but did not come until the 1960s.

The Abortion Act 1967, which came into effect on 27 April 1968, stated conditions under which an abortion could be undertaken legally. Abortions must be done by registered practitioners in either a National Health Service hospital, or a Department of Health approved clinic. For an abortion to be legal, two doctors must agree in good faith that the woman meets one or more of the criteria listed in Table 5.1. In addition, the abortion must be notified to the Chief Medical Officer of England, Scotland or Wales within a defined time period. In an emergency, abortion can be legally certified by the operating practitioner alone, as immediately necessary to save the life of the pregnant woman (F) or to prevent grave or permanent injury to the physical or mental health of the pregnant woman (G).

When considering the risk to the woman, a doctor may take account of the woman's actual or foreseeable circumstances, and may include all factors that can influence 'health' as discussed in Dahlgren and Whitehead's model (1991). A woman's social circumstances can thus be taken into account in assessing the risks to her health of continuing the pregnancy, but this doesn't constitute abortion 'for social reasons' (Royal College of Obstetricians and Gynaecologists 2000).

The majority of terminations today are performed under the grounds stated in C (Table 5.2): there is little variation from year to year.

Section 37 of the Human Fertilisation and Embryology Act 1990 made changes to the universal time limit of 28 weeks set in the Infant Life Preservation Act 1929. A time limit of 24 weeks was set for grounds C and D, whilst grounds A, B, and E are now without limit. This 1990 Act also confirmed that it was legal for a doctor to terminate the life of one or more fetuses in a woman with a multiple pregnancy in order to leave greater chances for the other(s) to live.

**Table 5.1** Statutory grounds for termination of pregnancy

| | |
|---|---|
| A | The continuance of the pregnancy should involve risk to the life of the woman greater than if the pregnancy were terminated |
| B | The termination is necessary to prevent grave permanent injury to the physical or mental health of the pregnant woman |
| C | The continuance of the pregnancy would involve risk, greater than if the pregnancy were terminated, of injury to the physical or mental health of the pregnant woman |
| D | The continuance of the pregnancy would involve risk, greater than if the pregnancy were terminated, of injury to the physical or mental health of any existing child (ren) of the family of the pregnant woman |
| E | There is a substantial risk that if the child were born it would suffer from such physical or mental abnormalities as to be seriously handicapped |

**Table 5.2** Percentage of abortions carried out on English residents according to the statutory grounds in 1996–98

|  | 1996 | 1997 | 1998 |
| --- | --- | --- | --- |
| Number (thousands) | 160.6 | 162.8 | 169.6 |
| Statutory grounds (percentage) |  |  |  |
| A (alone or with B, C or D) | 0.1 | 0.1 | 0.1 |
| B (alone or with C or D) | 1.5 | 1.2 | 1.2 |
| C (alone) | 90.2 | 91.1 | 91.4 |
| D (alone or with C) | 7.1 | 6.5 | 6.4 |
| E (alone or with A, B, C or D) | 1.2 | 1.1 | 1.1 |
| F or G | 0 | 0 | 0 |

*Source*: Office for National Statistics.

Doctors involved in abortion care are bound by the same *Duties of a Doctor* as laid down by the General Medical Council (GMC) as they are for all other aspects of clinical practice (Royal College of Obstetricians and Gynaecologists 2000). However, under the conscientious objection clause of the 1967 Abortion Act, a doctor can legally refuse to participate in an abortion on the grounds of conscience unless the woman's life is at risk. A House of Lords' ruling in the case of a doctor's secretary who refused to type a referral letter for an abortion (Janaway v Salford Health Authority 1988) looked at the definition of the word 'participate'. They concluded the clause was only intended to be applied to participation in administering treatment. The judge stated that: 'The regulations do not appear to contemplate the signing of the certificate would form part of the treatment for the termination of pregnancy.' Thus it would appear that GPs cannot claim exemption under the law from giving advice or performing the preparatory steps to arrange an abortion if the request meets the legal requirements. The British Medical Association (BMA) advise that doctors with a conscientious objection make their views known to the patient and enable the patient to see another doctor without delay if that is their wish. Doctors may explain their views to the patient if invited to do so (British Medical Association 1999).

In its advice to doctors, the BMA make a distinction between legal and ethical obligations. They argue that some things, which arguably fall outside the legal scope of the conscience clause, such as completion of the form for abortion, are an integral part of the abortion procedure. Completion of the form for abortion thus falls morally within the scope of the conscientious objection clause. The full document 'The law and ethics of abortion' provides a more detailed discussion (British Medical Association 1999).

## Abortion laws outside England and Wales

In Scotland, the 1861 and 1929 Acts do not apply. Abortion was a common law offence prior to 1967, though in practice no prosecutions occurred for therapeutic abortions done without secrecy by a gynaecologist. The 1967 Abortion Act does apply and has clarified the position such that more doctors have been willing to provide a TOP service. There are legal differences but the practical implications are as for England and Wales.

The 1967 Abortion Act does not apply in Northern Ireland. The law here is based on the Offences Against the Person Act 1861, which makes it an offence to 'procure a miscarriage . . . unlawfully'. Interpreting the term 'unlawfully' must be done using the 1945 Criminal Justice Act (Northern Ireland), under which the 1929 Infant Life Preservation Act was applied to Northern Ireland, with the precedent set by the Bourne judgement. Abortions do take place in Northern Ireland and are lawful in some circumstances with a number of examples of case law providing some clarification. Generally, the risk to the mother must be great. This has implications for many women who travel to other countries to obtain an abortion.

In the rest of Europe the picture is variable. In France abortion is legal up to 10 weeks' gestation. Italy legalized abortion up to 12 weeks in 1978 (backed by a referendum in 1981). In Germany abortion is legal but the laws are complex and require numerous tests. In Spain, the cut-off is 22 weeks whilst in the Netherlands it is 24 weeks as in the UK. With relaxation of border controls within Western Europe, abortion has now become a European rather than a national issue. Women may now travel to other countries, thus circumventing their own countries' laws.

## Interpreting the 1967 Abortion Act (amended 1990)

The 1967 Abortion Act requires two doctors to decide whether a woman has grounds for abortion. However, doctors vary enormously in their interpretation of the Act and this has been a cause of much controversy. We offer here a liberal view as a basis for discussion.

From Table 5.2 it can be seen that most abortions are performed using grounds C and D, which require the doctor to make a clinical decision concerning the risk to the physical or mental health of continuing the pregnancy compared to having the pregnancy terminated. If the woman has children already, how will their physical or mental health be affected if the pregnancy continues? What risks will be entailed for *her* if she continues this pregnancy? Here it is important to consider the psychological implications to the woman of having to continue with a pregnancy that is unwanted. How will her circumstances, both 'actual' and 'reasonably foreseeable', be affected if she were to continue with the pregnancy?

Having assessed the risks of continuing the pregnancy, these must be compared to the risks of having an abortion. This will depend, above all, on the stage at which the abortion is performed. Survey work during the initial years of the 1967 Act found that nine out of ten women who request an abortion consult their GP by 9 weeks of pregnancy (Cartwright and Lucas 1974). A more recent review of abortion globally notes: 'In countries where safe abortions are the norm, more than 90 per cent of women have abortions in the first trimester of pregnancy' (Berer 2000). Thus nearly all women who request an abortion will be within the first trimester. As discussed later, the physical and psychological risks of an abortion performed during the first trimester are very small. Taking into account the risk entailed in having a general anaesthetic, one can say that, for any woman in good health, the risk to her mental and physical health of an abortion during the first trimester is less than the risk of continuing with an unwanted pregnancy. Thus it might be argued that most women requesting an abortion would have grounds under the law. This argument has not been ventilated in court but as Kennedy comments, 'there is no logical answer to it' (Kennedy and Grubb 1989).

However, a few women do not consult their doctor until the second trimester. As pregnancy advances, the psychological risks of abortion do not increase but by 10–18 weeks, the physical risks probably outweigh those of continuing the pregnancy (see 'Risks of termination', below). This will vary from unit to unit.

Later in pregnancy, the decision is more difficult. Very few women request an abortion after 20 weeks and there are usually specific reasons for the delay. The commonest reason is fetal abnormality that is detected by amniocentesis or late scan.

Alternatively, women present late because of denial. These often very young and/or vulnerable women need particularly sensitive care.

Competency to consent is discussed in both the BMA and the Royal College of Obstetricians and Gynaecologists (RCOG) documents. The test of competency (attributed to Mr Justice Thorpe) requires a person to be able to: first, take in and retain treatment information; second, to believe it, and third, to weigh the information, balancing risks and need.

For young women under the age of 16, 'Gillick competency' is the informal term for what should more properly be termed the 'Fraser criteria', Fraser being the judge involved in the case of Gillick *v* West Norfolk and Wisbech Health

Authority (1985). These are that a clinician providing contraceptive advice or treatment to an under-16-year-old without parental consent should be satisfied that the young person:

- will understand the advice and the moral, social and emotional implications;
- cannot be persuaded to tell their parents or allow the clinician to tell them that they are seeking contraceptive advice;
- is having, or is likely to have unprotected sex whether they receive advice or not;
- is likely to suffer physical or mental ill health unless they receive the advice or treatment; and that
- it is in the young person's best interest to give advice or treatment without parental consent.

The main exception to this guidance is if the young woman is a ward of court, where the courts would need to give their approval.

Particular difficulties arise in circumstances where child abuse, incest or abuse of vulnerable women is suspected, and is discussed in the RCOG guidelines. The duty of the doctor is to protect the child or vulnerable woman and 'secure the best possible outcome' for them.

The decision to terminate a pregnancy lies with the woman and her doctors. Legally the father of the child or spouse has no right to demand or refuse a TOP.

## Statistics

Induced abortion, like unintended pregnancy, occurs in almost all societies. In some countries, abortion statistics are limited both in terms of availability and reliability. In countries such as the UK, an abortion is only legal if it is notified to the authorities. Abortion statistics are thus both accurate and reliable. Interpreting the data is still difficult, however, with abortion rates not necessarily serving as a valid indication of women's need. The laws of the land, the availability of abortion services, the importance of religious views on abortion, the public perception of abortion, and the social impact of keeping a child all influence abortion rates, and are largely socially constructed. Not all unwanted pregnancies will be terminated; not all terminations are unwanted. Interpreting abortion statistics, and in particular making comparisons between social groups, is thus difficult. In a worldwide review of women who obtained TOP, it was clear that within all demographic and socioeconomic subgroups, some women will obtain an abortion when faced with an intended pregnancy (Bankole *et al.* 1999).

## International statistics

Regional differences exist for abortion rates in different age groups. The abortion rate among adolescents is lowest in many Asian countries, in contrast to other regions where the rate of abortion (per 1000 women) is higher for the adolescent age group than for woman in their twenties. There are certainly problems with the reliability of the data. However, the data may be explained by higher levels of sexual activity (and thus unintended pregnancy) amongst young women outside Asia, in combination with a greater motivation to terminate a pregnancy, possibly because they wish to complete their education or continue working (Bankole *et al.* 1999).

Higher abortion rates are seen amongst older women in Asian and Eastern European countries, which may reflect low levels of use of modern contraceptives (Bankole *et al.* 1999). In the former Soviet republics and Eastern Europe, women relied on abortion to limit their family size since contraception, including sterilization, was not readily available (Bankole *et al.* 1999).

Attempts to identify a correlation between the strictness of the law on abortion and abortion rate fail to identify a link. This probably reflects the multifactorial nature of the reasons for abortion – legal constraints being just one of many. Both pregnancy and abortion are thus influenced by social, cultural, and legal factors.

## England and Wales and Scotland

Abortion is now one of the commonest gynaecological procedures in Great Britain. Around 180 000 terminations per year are performed in England and Wales. After the implementation of the Abortion Act in 1968, the number of legal abortions rose rapidly until 1974 when the number fell for the first time (Fig 5.1). The fall may have been at least partly as a result of the introduction of a free contraceptive service. After the 'pill scare' of 1995, the predicted rise in requests for abortions was seen. There is some evidence that this rise was due to change in contraceptive practices (Furedi 1995). However, the rise seems to be continuing.

Interpreting the changing rate of abortion is difficult (Table 5.3). Rates are generally quoted per 1000 women within a defined age range, so changing demography cannot explain the observed trends. However, there is no clear way to measure the relative fertility of the woman in this age group. Birth and conception rates are often used as proxy measures but will be influenced by factors other than fertility alone. An influx of women from countries with tighter abortion laws may account for some of the observed increase, although figures do theoretically distinguish between women living locally and from elsewhere.

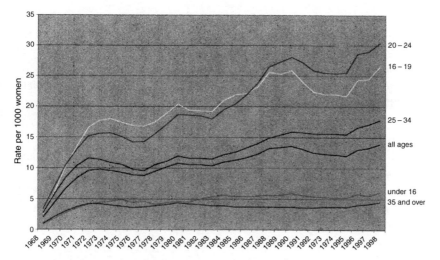

**Fig 5.1** Age-specific abortion rate, residents of England and Wales, 1968–98.
*Source*: Office for National Statistics).

**Table 5.3** Abortion numbers and rates for women in England, Scotland and Wales between 1968 and 1998

| | Abortions in England and Wales (resident women) | | Abortions in Scotland[1] | |
|---|---|---|---|---|
| | **Number** | **Rate[2]** | **Number** | **Rate[3]** |
| 1968 | 22 332 | 1.97 | 1 544 | 1.5 |
| 1969 | 49 829 | 4.38 | 3 556 | 3.5 |
| 1974 | 109 445 | 9.63 | 7 568 | 7.4 |
| 1979 | 120 611 | 10.17 | 7 784 | 7.3 |
| 1984 | 136 388 | 11.0 | 9 155 | 8.2 |
| 1989 | 170 463 | 13.36 | 10 209 | 9.1 |
| 1994 | 156 539 | 12.18 | 11 392 | 10.3 |
| 1997 | 177 871 | 13.92 | 12 109 | 11.1 |
| 1998 | 173 701 | 13.57 | 12 424 | 11.4 |

[1] Figures do not include Scottish women having abortions in England (around 1000 women a year in 1979, but dropped to 322 in 1997).
[2] Abortion rate per 1000 resident women aged 14–49.
[3] Abortion rate per 1000 resident women aged 15–44.

*Sources*: Office for National Statistics; Notifications to the Chief Medical Officer for Scotland of abortions performed under the 1967 Abortion Act.

Two service-related factors that influence abortion rates are availability and accessibility of abortion services, together with quality and efficacy of family planning services. A high abortion rate, as seen for example in Liverpool, could reflect a well-run service easily accessible to women, although there is no evidence that ease of access increases demand (Lowy *et al.* 1998). Alternatively, it could reflect a failure in the 'preventative' services, such as a problem with the family planning services in the area.

There is considerable regional variation in NHS provision of TOP services (Tables 5.4 and 5.5). In 1998, whilst more than 98% of abortions in Scotland took place in NHS hospitals, in England and Wales this figure was only 51%. A further 22% were NHS funded within the private sector – a total NHS provision of 73% (Royal College of Obstetricians and Gynaecologists 2000). The 1979 Royal Commission on the NHS recommended that 75% of abortions should be NHS funded, although this was intended as a short-term target to be raised with time as services were developed. The high Scottish provision probably reflects the relative lack of private sector provision and may therefore mask an unmet need. Certainly the provision of abortion services has traditionally been variable and dependent on the relative priorities of individual gynaecology units around the country. The recent publication of Guidelines from the RCOG should improve recognition of the need for an equitable and quality service (Royal College of Obstetricians and Gynaecologists 2000).

**Table 5.4** Regional variation in NHS provision of abortion (1999)*

|  | NHS | NHS agency | Total NHS | Non-NHS |
|---|---|---|---|---|
| England and Wales | 48.9 | 24.9 | **73.8** | 26.2 |
| England | 48.6 | 24.7 | **73.3** | 26.7 |
| Northern & Yorkshire | 77.4 | 7.2 | **84.6** | 15.4 |
| Trent | 77.5 | 9.6 | **87.1** | 12.9 |
| West Midlands | 18.9 | 53.7 | **72.6** | 27.4 |
| North West | 53.1 | 19.9 | **73.0** | 27.0 |
| Eastern | 66.8 | 11.0 | **77.8** | 22.2 |
| London | 35.7 | 29.0 | **64.8** | 35.2 |
| South East | 33.8 | 35.8 | **69.6** | 30.4 |
| South West | 69.4 | 10.6 | **80.0** | 20.0 |

Percentage of total abortions provided in NHS unit (NHS), funded by NHS but other unit (NHS agency), or private/charitable sector (Non-NHS).

*Source*: Office for National Statistics.

**Table 5.5** NHS provision of abortion in England and Wales 1969–99

| Year | Total abortions on resident women | % of total In NHS hospitals | % of total as agency (for NHS) | % of total paid for by NHS |
|---|---|---|---|---|
| 1969 | 44 829 | 67 | – | 67 |
| 1974 | 109 445 | 51 | – | 51 |
| 1979 | 119 028 | 46 | – | 46 |
| 1984 | 136 388 | 47.5 | 3.6 | 51 |
| 1989 | 170 463 | 41 | 5 | 46 |
| 1994 | 156 539 | 54.5 | 12.5 | 67 |
| 1998 | 187 402 | 50.8 | 22.0 | 72.8 |
| 1999 | 183 250 | 48.9 | 24.9 | 73.8 |

*Source*: Office for National Statistics.

**Table 5.6** Abortions (women aged 11–49 resident in England and Wales) percentage by gestational age

| Gestation | 1986 | 1994 | 1996 | 1998 |
|---|---|---|---|---|
| Under 9 weeks | 33.9 | 40.8 | 40.3 | 41.5 |
| 9–12 | 53.4 | 48.1 | 48.4 | 47.5 |
| 13–19 | 11.3 | 9.8 | 10.0 | 9.6 |
| 20 and over | 1.4 | 1.2 | 1.3 | 1.3 |

*Source*: Office for National Stastistics.

One of the key factors affecting gestational age at which abortion takes place is organization and accessibility of services. There is a slight trend towards earlier abortions (Table 5.6), but the evidence suggests this needs to improve further in the interests of women's health (Royal College of Obstetricians and Gynaecologists 2000).

## Repeat terminations

Thirty per cent of abortions were on women who are recorded as having had a previous termination. The data for one year is broken down by age in Table 5.7. As would be expected, older women are more likely to be undergoing a repeat termination.

The high proportion of repeat terminations indicates an unmet need. A study from Newcastle of 143 women showed a higher rate of contraceptive use

**Table 5.7** Showing numbers and rates of abortions and repeat abortions in England and Wales in 2000

| Age | Total number of abortions | Total number of abortions in women with history of previous abortion | % of abortions which are repeats | Rate of abortion (first time or repeat) per 1000 women | Rate of abortion in women with history of previous abortion per 1000 women |
|---|---|---|---|---|---|
| Total – all ages | 175 542 | 53 229 | 30.3 | 13.18 | – |
| <15 | 1 048 | 34 | 3.2 | 1.6 | – |
| 15 | 2 700 | 76 | 2.8 | 8.37 | 0.24 |
| 16–19 | 33 218 | 4 342 | 13.1 | 26.65 | 3.48 |
| 20–24 | 47 099 | 13 502 | 28.7 | 30.88 | 8.85 |
| 25–29 | 37 852 | 14 418 | 38.1 | 21.15 | 8.06 |
| 30–34 | 28 735 | 11 496 | 40 | 14.04 | 5.62 |
| 35–39 | 18 589 | 7 144 | 38.4 | 8.86 | 3.41 |
| 40–44 | 5 794 | 2 065 | 35.6 | 3.18 | 1.13 |
| 45+ | 459 | 144 | 31.4 | 0.27 | – |
| Not stated | 48 | 8 | 16.7 | – | – |

Rates calculated using 2000 mid-year population estimates. (–) indicates not calculated. Source: Office for National Statistics.

(with less reliance on condoms) in women having a repeat TOP compared with those presenting for the first time (Garg *et al.* 2001). However, many of these women were not using the method chosen at discharge following the first abortion. The authors suggest the need for improved contraceptive counselling and follow-up of women. Larger longitudinal studies are needed to identify causal factors and hence effective interventions.

# Methods of termination

Traditionally methods used in performing abortions have been divided into those used in the first trimester and those used later in pregnancy. The distinction is becoming less clear and it is perhaps more helpful to look at medical versus surgical techniques. The choice between them may reflect local service provision and patient choice as much as gestational age.

## Medical termination

Mifepristone was licensed as an abortifacient in France in 1988. It is currently used to induce abortion in combination with a prostaglandin in France, Sweden, China, the USA and the United Kingdom (UK) (Grimes 1997). Progesterone plays a key role in maintaining pregnancy. Mifepristone is an anti-progesterone and blocks receptor binding sites in the uterus. In addition, it promotes increased production of prostaglandins, increased sensitivity of the uterus to prostaglandins, and increased myometrial contractility. It is currently licensed in the UK to abort fetuses up to 63 days' gestation, and from 13 to 20 weeks' gestation [British National Formulary (BNF)]. As discussed later, it is increasingly being used outside those time limits. The licensed regimen uses an oral dose of 600 mg mifepristone followed 36–48 hours later by a 1 mg vaginal dose of gemeprost (a prostaglandin). However, trials have shown a dose of just 200 mg of mifepristone is equally effective, whilst the cheaper prostaglandin misoprostol is as effective as gemeprost up to 7 weeks' gestation (Royal College of Obstetricians and Gynaecologists 2000). The EC Pharmaceutical Directive 65/65/EEC specifically allows doctors to use licensed medicines for indications, or in doses/routes of administration, outside the recommendations of the licence. Details of different published regimens are given in Guidelines from the Royal College of Obstetricians and Gynaecologists (2000).

Success rates for medical terminations reported in the literature depend on the definition of success. A recent series looked at 2000 women in the UK with pregnancies of less than 63 days' gestation. It demonstrated a successful outcome (defined as no need for any further intervention) in 97.5% of women.

**Table 5.8** Percentage of women having successful abortion with no further surgical intervention required (Newhall and Winikoff 2000)

| Gestational age | % aborting successfully |
|---|---|
| 49 days | 92–96 |
| 50–56 days | 83–93 |
| 57–63 days | 86–77 |

There was an ongoing pregnancy rate of just 0.6% (Family Planning Association 1999).

An American study reported that 2–5% of women aborted with mifepristone alone. For mifepristone and a prostaglandin in combination, success was dependent on gestational age (Table 5.8). 'Success' was defined as 'no surgical intervention required' and thus included not only drug failures, but also incomplete abortion, excessive bleeding, etc. The authors stated that the different success rates may in part reflect different thresholds for doctors to intervene surgically (Newhall and Winikoff 2000).

Medical termination is not suitable for everyone (Grimes 1997; Wood 2000). Contraindications to medical termination are:

◆ being outside the appropriate gestational range;

◆ women over 35 (have been excluded from European trials);

◆ spontaneous abortion in progress;

◆ suspected ectopic pregnancy;

◆ severe asthma;

◆ cardiovascular disease;

◆ heavy smoker;

◆ a history of haemorrhagic disorder or anticoagulation;

◆ adrenal failure;

◆ long-term steroid therapy.

The advantages of medical techniques include a possible lower risk of infection requiring antibiotics in one study, and the avoidance of a physically and psychologically invasive procedure (Grimes 1997). High satisfaction levels are reported. American women who had undergone both types of abortion found the medical method more satisfactory even when the medical method had failed (Family Planning Association 1999). One American study also looked at the opinions of 77 members of staff providing the service in a unit that had just started providing medical terminations on a trial basis. Two-thirds of female and one half of male staff said they would choose the medical method. Staff reported increased satisfaction with providing a new service that offers choice and empowers women. Although there was an impact on clinic routine with the process taking longer, patients waiting around, and a greater demand on bathrooms, staff noticed a positive impact on patients. A longer time with the women gave a greater scope for education, whilst patients were noted to swap telephone numbers and provide mutual support (Ellertson *et al.* 1999). Legal as well as cultural differences exist between the USA and the UK, making direct comparisons difficult, but there seems to be some anecdotal evidence of similar findings in the UK setting.

Complications of medical abortion include drug failure. The advice in one review is that women with ongoing pregnancy in these circumstances should have suction curettage as soon as possible. However, it has been reported that some women chose to continue their pregnancy and a small number of live normal infants have been born after exposure to mifepristone early in pregnancy (Grimes 1997). Other problems associated with medical abortions include nausea and vomiting (reportedly less with vaginal rather than oral administration of the prostaglandin; Grimes 1997); pain and cramps; the increased uncertainty of the procedure with the lack of immediate confirmation of success; and an increased number of visits required to clinic (Family Planning Association 1999).

## Future developments

Some evidence is emerging of efficacy of medical termination in the 9–13 week gestation, traditionally the period in the UK at which only surgical techniques are used (Ashok *et al.* 1998). Some units report success rates of greater than 90%. There may be many factors for both the woman requesting a termination and for service providers that may make the slightly lower success rate at this gestation acceptable when balanced against the benefits of the technique.

As over-the-counter emergency contraception is introduced, what is the possibility for an equivalent service for medical abortions? An American study looked at the ability of women to use medical abortion without medical supervision. The study describes seven steps a woman would need to undertake for a medical abortion without medical supervision. These include recognizing that she is pregnant, correctly identifying the gestational age, adhering to the protocol, managing adverse reactions and seeking medical care where appropriate, and recognizing a complete abortion. Indirect evidence is presented by the authors that women are able to complete all of these tasks successfully. Differences in the abortion laws here would make it impossible to repeat this study in the UK at this time. However, there are implications for how we run medical abortion clinics, with evidence that women are able to cope with less supervision than currently undertaken (Ellertson *et al.* 1997).

In July 2002, the Department of Health announced proposals to increase access to medical terminations by offering the service within some family planning centres. The stated aim is to address unacceptable waiting times for abortion services. Since the law will remain unchanged, it is argued that the proposals will improve speed of access to services, but not increase overall abortion rates (BBC News 2002).

## Surgical termination

Menstrual aspiration was a variation of suction aspiration used prior to the development of early pregnancy testing. Performed 10–18 days after a missed period, it was used in the UK prior to the 1967 Abortion Act to alleviate 'extreme anxiety' due to delayed menstruation with no physical sign of pregnancy. Proponents of population control recommended it as a technique to circumvent abortion laws in countries where they were strict (Goldthorp 1977).

With a change in legislation and earlier pregnancy testing, the technique is no longer used. The current surgical technique employed depends on the gestational age. Under 7 weeks, the risk of missing the gestational sac increases and conventional suction termination is not considered appropriate. However, Creinin and Edwards report a personal series of 2399 early surgical abortions undertaken according to a rigorous protocol developed in Texas. They report a complete abortion rate of more than 99% (Royal College of Obstetricians and Gynaecologists 2000).

Conventional suction termination is an appropriate method of termination between 7 and 15 weeks. Guidelines from the Royal College of Obstetricians and Gynaecologists (2000) state that it is the only technique for which the evidence base is adequate to recommend its use at gestations of 9–12 weeks. However, the evidence for the efficacy of medical terminations at this gestation is increasing (Ashok *et al.* 1998). Suction termination can be done under local or general anaesthesia, and as a day patient in most cases. There is some evidence that local anaesthesia is safer than general anaesthesia (Royal College of Obstetricians and Gynaecologists 2000). Dilatation of the cervix (e.g. with mifepristone or a prostaglandin) prior to the procedure should be considered in all cases, and should be routine for all women under 18 years or at a gestation of over 10 weeks in order to reduce the risk of cervical damage or uterine perforation.

Dilatation and evacuation, preceded by cervical preparation, is safe and effective for mid-trimester abortions when undertaken by specialist practitioners (Royal College of Obstetricians and Gynaecologists 2000). It is the standard method for gestations above 15 weeks in the non-NHS abortion service in

England but is generally not favoured by gynaecologists working in the NHS. It can be unpleasant for staff and is time consuming to teach.

Complications specific to surgical techniques include problems related to anaesthesia. Damage to the external cervical os at the time of surgical abortion is seen in less than 1% of cases. The incidence is lower when abortions are performed early in pregnancy and when performed by experienced clinicians (Royal College of Obstetricians and Gynaecologists 2000). Uterine perforation as a complication of surgical techniques is rare (incidence of 1–4 per 1000 abortions). Again the risk is lower for abortions done at an earlier gestation and by experienced clinicians (Royal College of Obstetricians and Gynaecologists 2000).

### Future developments

Just as developments with medical termination offer the scope to de-medicalize the abortion procedure and give women back some control, so are there developments in the surgical field. The introduction of 'walk-in, walk-out' surgical TOP units offering '10-minute abortions' using suction aspiration under local anaesthetic has been supported by some as offering women choice. Women are reported to feel much more in control whilst the unit feels it moves away from the unnecessary clinical trappings and over-medicalization of the procedure. Opponents feel the quick service 'trivializes abortion' (Nursing Times 1998; Boorer and Murty 2001).

## Risks of termination

The absolute risk of complications following abortion is low. The RCOG Guidelines quote a recent cohort study, which found an immediate complication rate of 0.7% in a study of more than 80 000 cases (Royal College of Obstetricians and Gynaecologists 2000). Other studies have shown that increased gestational age is associated with a higher complication rate. The risk of major complication doubles when termination is carried out at 15 compared with 8 weeks' gestation (Glasier and Thong 1991). Haemorrhage and infection are possible complications of any abortion procedure. Haemorrhage complicates around 1.5 in 1000 abortions overall. The rate is lower for early abortions (1.2/1000 at <13 weeks; 8.5 < 1000 at >20 weeks). Genital tract infections of varying degrees of severity occur in 10% of cases. The risk is reduced when prophylactic antibiotics are given or when lower genital tract infection is excluded by screening (Royal College of Obstetricians and Gynaecologists 2000).

There is no evidence of an association between induced abortion and subsequent infertility or preterm delivery (Royal College of Obstetricians and

Gynaecologists 2000). Only a small minority of women experience any long-term adverse psychological sequelae after abortion. Whilst early distress is common, it is usually a continuation of symptoms present before the abortion. By contrast, mothers and their children have been documented to suffer negative effects when abortion has been denied (Royal College of Obstetricians and Gynaecologists 2000). One study followed up women for 2 years and demonstrated no difference in physical complications for women having surgical or medical terminations. However, whether the woman had a choice in the method of abortion was a significant determinant in psychological outcomes (Howie *et al.* 1997). This is another factor to consider when balancing the risks and benefits of various abortion methods.

## Service issues

Several studies have shown the benefits of a dedicated abortion service distinct from the general gynaecological out-patient service. This results in increased provision of abortions on the NHS, reduced waiting times, and a fall in the average gestational age at which abortions are performed (Glasier and Thong 1991; Hughes *et al.* 1996; Lowy *et al.* 1998). One study in Lincolnshire described the effects of setting up a dedicated abortion service. Despite fears to the contrary, the total number of abortions in the area remained the same, thus better access to a service does not necessarily 'encourage' abortion requests (Lowy *et al.* 1998).

There have been some attempts to look at the relative cost of medical and surgical terminations. A report in 1996 compared the use of suction curettage versus medical termination with mifepristone and prostaglandin in the UK setting (Hughes *et al.* 1996). The costs considered in the analysis were staffing (including time), consumables, and 'hotel costs'. They drew on a previous study that had shown that a nurse spends a mean of 75 minutes with a medically treated patient and a mean of 38 minutes with a surgical patient. The cost of TOP per patient was estimated as:

◆ for medical TOP, £346 (£333–361; 95% CI);

◆ for surgical TOP, £397 (£383–411; 95% CI).

Medical termination was thus statistically significantly cheaper than surgical TOP ($P < 0.001$). A more detailed breakdown showed that whilst staff and consumable costs were higher for medical management, this was more than counteracted by the cost of running an operating theatre. The analysis assumes (perhaps unrealistically) that the theatre costs can be released by using a medical service and it is not necessary to run both services. The study looked only at costs to the NHS and did not include any estimation of the cost–benefit ratio for patients (Hogue 1986).

A French group reported relative costs that showed the opposite (Newhall and Winikoff 2000):

- surgical TOP with local anaesthesia, £89;
- surgical TOP with general anaesthesia, £119;
- medical TOP (mifepristone/misoprostol), £129.

Cost–benefit analysis is still a relatively new discipline with ongoing debate about how to include a value for costs and benefits to patients. A decision between providing medical or surgical terminations on the grounds of cost is thus not possible from the evidence. Difficulties with employing anaesthetists to cover a TOP list, for example, may therefore be a more important question to address.

The National Strategy for Sexual Health and HIV was published by the Department of Health in 2001. It aims to improve sexual health and well-being, improve sexual health services, and address inequalities in sexual health. The document highlights the unacceptable variation in abortion services in the UK. It sets a target that, by 2005, women who meet the legal requirements should be able to have an abortion within 3 weeks of their first appointment with the referring doctor.

Ultimately, abortion services need to be viewed as one part of such a wider sexual health strategy. Current services often reflect workforce availability, local priorities, and other resource issues rather than women's needs. It may be that development of a sexual health team with multidisciplinary practitioners able to offer skills in genitourinary medicine, family planning, TOP, and health promotion and screening will go some way towards providing a needs-led service.

# 10-Minute consultation: an unwanted pregnancy

## The patient

A patient has come to see you because her period is late, she thinks she may be pregnant or has already done a test and knows she is. The pregnancy is not planned and she doesn't think she wants/is able to be a mother right now. She may or may not have been using contraception; if she was, it has clearly failed. Her fault? Your fault? Probably no one's fault. Emotions are likely to be high on her part, you as the doctor, need to be aware of your own, so that the woman can be helped impartially. If your personal values lead you to a refusal to sign the blue form (certificate A in Scotland) then you have a duty not to impose these values on your patient and to refer her to a colleague who does not hold such values.

## What issues should you cover

◆ Confirm the pregnancy. Radioimmunoassay tests detecting β-hCG in urine within 3 weeks of conception are now available as home tests and for use in GP surgeries. Most will confirm pregnancy within a few days of a missed period when used on an early-morning specimen (EMSU). To make best use of early abortion services, GPs need to offer the radioimmunoassay tests in their surgery. If the result is negative, a repeat test (on an EMSU) should be organized for a week later.

◆ Make no assumptions about what the women wants to do, but explore with her the options she has so far considered and the reasons behind these. Fill her in, as appropriate, with those she has not considered. Help her to explore the implications of the various options. For some women this can be done within the space of 10–20 minutes; for many it will need more time, either another appointment or referral to counselling.

◆ Give the woman the facts about the local termination service, the options available and the processes involved.

◆ Discuss with her, her risk of sexually transmitted infections. Explain the prevalence of *Chlamydia* and the damage it can cause if not diagnosed and treated prior to a TOP. If her sexual history suggests that she may be at some risk, encourage her to be tested. The gold standard is to refer to local GUM services for a full screening examination. An endocervical swab taken in general practice and transferred quickly is the next step down. However, if the woman is unwilling to avail herself of this, then urine sent for immunoassay testing may be a reasonable compromise. A positive result then triggers referral on, or at the very least treatment for her and her partner.

◆ Was contraception used? If yes, is there anything to be learned from why it failed? If no, does the woman have any plans for the future? This is not the moment to go into great depth about contraception, but it needs to be raised and an agreed plan made about how to follow it up.

## What should you do

◆ A pelvic examination to check gestation? This will invariably be done at the abortion unit. For a woman who is sure of her last menstrual period (LMP), the need to clarify gestation needs to be balanced against what might be considered as an excess of intimate examination. Discussing the need for examination, thus gaining consent for a joint decision, is the obvious solution.

- Refer to the appropriate service, enclosing a signed blue form if referring for termination. If the woman is undecided, it is usually wise to refer for TOP, and put in place other services such as a further appointment with yourself or a counsellor in the intervening time before the appointment with the TOP service. Give her permission to cancel the appointment for a termination, but be aware that not referring can be construed as a judgement on your part that she should not have a termination. If she does cancel, explain the need to return for referral to antenatal services.

- Arrange follow-up: in the case of termination, usually 2–6 weeks after the TOP, both to check it has been successful, and that contraception, if required, has been successfully established; in the case of a decision to continue pregnancy, then for antenatal purposes.

## Box 5.1 **Aims of counselling**

Counsellors working in primary care are a useful resource for some women, or there may be counselling services attached to local family planning services, Brook clinics or the TOP services. Some women are keen to have the opportunity to talk in depth, others are less keen, some because they already have good support networks, but others are wary through ignorance or previous bad experiences. This last group will need more effort to engage them with the concept, but are often the women who have the greatest need. The aims of such counselling (non-judgemental and non-directional) are threefold:

- to enable the woman to reach an informed decision that she will not regret;
- to lessen the emotional disturbance whatever decision is reached;
- to lessen the risk of a further unwanted pregnancy.

It may occasionally achieve far more. The crisis situation may be an important moment for a woman to understand herself and her behaviour better: her use of contraception, her attitudes to her own sexuality and any difficulties she has in intimate relationships will be at the forefront of her mind. If an increased awareness of these issues can lead her to a belief that she can exert greater control over her own life, then an unwanted pregnancy can be a trigger which leads to positive change. Too often, pregnancy counselling is seen as a barrier that a woman must pass through before she can have an abortion. To see counselling in this way is to diminish its purpose and its worth.

## Frequently asked questions

### Will I be able to have another baby?

Behind this question lies a huge anxiety for many women that having a termination will lead to later infertility. There is no evidence that women whose first pregnancy is terminated have any increased risk of subsequent infertility *unless* their abortion is complicated by pelvic infection (Hogue 1986). This question then is a useful lead-in to an exploration of sexual risk-taking, specifically in relation to risk of infection, and of particular concern, the possibility of *Chlamydia*.

### You mean I don't have to have an operation?

Many women (and some doctors) are still unaware of the relatively new medical termination techniques. Because of this, it's always important to inform women who are within the time frame of this method. There is good evidence that the acceptability of either method of TOP is greatest in women who are allowed an active choice in which method they prefer. Some women have a dread of general anaesthesia and feel going through a 'miscarriage' is somehow more natural. Others would prefer to 'just be put to sleep' and have a horror of the idea of consciously passing the fetus. Helping the women work out which group she belongs to will help her feel more in control of the decision-making process. There is one big proviso to this: both options must be available locally. If they are not, then pressure needs to be put on both the providers and commissioners of health care to provide an ideal service as recommended by the Royal College of Obstetrics and Gynaecology guidelines.

### Why can't it be done sooner?

This is a question that will be commoner in some parts of the country than others. Provision of termination is not equitable across the nation, and whilst many services are up to the Royal College's guidelines, there are still some that are wanting, with unacceptable delays that decrease the options open to women.

There may be another reason for this question: service provision may be more than adequate, but the woman particularly impatient. This sort of impatience may signal an unease with her decision, a need to 'get it over with as soon as possible' in the hope she can then forget it. It may be that services that do not give women any time to reflect on their decision can produce emotional morbidity as a result of a poorly considered decision. This consideration might be usefully reflected to the over-impatient patient.

### You're not going to tell my mother/partner are you?

Issues of confidentiality are often high on the agenda for women considering a termination. For some women this is simply a reflection of both society and their own ambivalent attitude towards abortion: a necessary evil that happens to others, not oneself.

For others it is related to either a perceived or very real fear that a partner or a parent will be hurt/angry/rejecting/violent and may even prevent them going through with their choice of solution to the unplanned pregnancy. These fears need to be explored; sometimes they dissipate when aired, or at least the woman can see her way to having a conversation with the person she initially felt unwilling to involve – but not always.

Adult women need to be reassured that their confidentiality is paramount, there is no obligation for doctors to inform partners, rather the obligation is to maintain confidentiality under all circumstances.

Young women under the age of 16 are in a particular predicament. The legality of performing a termination without parental consent is discussed earlier. Consent is advisable, and in practice few gynaecologists will perform an abortion on an under-16-year-old without such consent. Conversely, a termination should never be carried out against the wishes of a young woman who is competent to consent, whatever her parents may want.

## Questions a GP may want to ask

### Why is this pregnancy not wanted?

Not asking this question can lead to incorrect assumptions. There may be practical difficulties that the woman cannot see her way to resolving. Or she may have unrealistic fears: about fetal abnormality or about pain in labour. She may be seeking reassurance about these worries so that she can continue the pregnancy.

### Have you talked about this with anyone else?

Some women will already have discussed their situation with their partner, friends and/or family. Others may do so after discussion with you, and a few may ask for help. For example, the young woman who wants to tell her parents but just does not know how, may ask the doctor to broach it with them. Other women will remain unable to talk to anyone and they need extra support in following through whatever they decide to do.

*If you have talked with anyone, what was their reaction? What did they suggest you do?*

The point of this type of question is to ascertain whether she is being pressurized into a decision by others. We are all influenced by those close to us, but ultimately the woman needs to feel she has made her own decision.

### When you first thought you were pregnant, what did you feel about being pregnant?

Here one is concerned with the woman's view of this pregnancy. She may reveal a degree of ambivalence about being pregnant and may need help in understanding the issues behind this ambivalence. This should avoid the dangers that whatever decision she makes, she may subsequently feel that it was wrong.

### What's the worst aspect of the situation you're in?

This is a useful question to focus the woman on what is troubling her most. It also helps the doctor/nurse/counsellor remain woman-centred in responding to her particular situation.

### Before you were pregnant, what did you think about abortion?

If she finds herself having to make a decision that does not fit in with her previous and probably present values, she may need extra help in coming to terms with her decision. For example, a woman may have strong views against abortion, even believing it to be tantamount to murder, and yet she may still request an abortion because of circumstances she finds herself in. Internal conflict of this nature is likely to produce psychological problems; identification is the first step to any help that can be offered.

### Is this a one-off crisis, or just the latest in a life full of difficulties, either emotionally, practically or, most commonly, both?

If the latter, then follow-up and ongoing support from the primary care team and/or social services may well be needed to prevent or minimize further crises occurring.

### How did this pregnancy happen?

Was this the result of contraceptive failure, risk-taking ambivalence, or possibly even a desire to be pregnant? Her motives may not always be clear to the woman herself. If she can be helped to understand them, she is less likely to make the same 'mistake' again.

## Leaflets

An excellent leaflet aimed at young people is available from the Family Planning Association. Telephone 0207 837 5432.

The following three leaflets, at the end of this chapter, are reproduced with the kind permission of the Department of Gynaecology, The Women's Centre, John Radcliffe Hospital, Oxford.

## Useful websites

- www.bpas.org.uk – general information, and advice regarding British Pregnancy Advisory Services
- www.fpa.org.uk – general advice including who to turn to for abortion and contraception services
- www.mariestopes.org.uk – general information and advice regarding their services
- www.nhsdirect.nhs.uk – NHS Direct – gives addresses of support organizations and has evaluated information leaflets including links to electronic versions

## References

Ashok, P.W., Flett, G.M. and Templeton, A. (1998). Termination of pregnancy at 9–13 weeks amenorrhoea with mifepristone and misoprostol. *Lancet*, **352**, 542–3.

Bankole, A., Singh, S. and Haas, T. (1999). Characteristics of women who obtain induced abortion: a worldwide review. *International Family Planing Perspectives*, **25** (2), 68–77.

BBC news. Abortion access to be made easier, 7 July 2002. Available at www.news.bbc.co.uk/hi/health/2107700.stm.

Berer, M. (2000). Making abortions safe: a matter of good public health policy and practice. *Bulletin of the World Health Organisation*, **78**, 580–5.

Boorer, C. and Murty, J. (2001). Experiences of termination of pregnancy in a stand-alone clinic situation. *Journal of Family Planning and Reproductive Health Care*, **27** (2), 97–8.

British Medical Association (revised December 1999). The law and ethics of abortion. *BMA views*.

Cartwright, A. and Lucas, S. (1974). Survey of abortion patients for the Committee on the working of the Abortion Act. *Lane Report*, Vol III. HMSO, London.

Dahlgren, G. and Whitehead, M. (1991). *Policies and strategies to promote social equity in health*. Institute of Future Studies, Stockholm.

Department of Health (2001) *The national strategy for sexual health and HIV*. Department of Health, London.

Ellertson, C., Elub, B. and Winikoff, B. (1997). Can women use medical abortion without supervision? *Reproductive Health Matters*, **9**, 149–61.

Ellertson, C., Simonds, W., Winikoff, B., Springer, K. and Bagchi, D. (1999). Providing mifepristone-misoprostol medical abortion: the view from the clinic. *Journal of the American Medical Women's Association*, **54**, 91–6.

Family Planning Association (1999). *Medical abortion-meeting women's needs*. FPA, London.

Furedi, A. (1999). The public health implications of the 1995 'pill scare'. *Human Reproduction Update*, **5**, 621–6.

Garg, M., Singh, M. and Mansour, D. (2001). Peri-abortion contraceptive care: can we reduce the incidence of repeat abortions? *Journal of Family Planning and Reproductive Health Care*, **27**, 77–80.

General Medical Council, (1998). *Maintaining good medical practice*. General Medical Council, London.

Glasier, A. and Thong, J.K. (1991). The establishment of a centralised referral service leads to earlier abortion. *Health Bulletin*, **49**, 254–9.

Goldthorp, W.O. (1977). Ten-minute abortions. *British Medical Journal*, **2**, 562–4.

Grimes DA. (1997). Medical abortion in early pregnancy: a review of the evidence. *Obstetrics and Gynecology*, **89**, 790–6.

Hogue, C.J. (1986). Impact of abortion on subsequent fecundity. *Clinical Obstetrics and Gynaecology*, **13**, 95–103.

Howie, F.L., Henshaw, R.C., Naji, S.A. and Russell, I.T. (1997). Medical abortion or vacuum aspiration? Two year follow-up of a patient preference trial. *British Journal of Obstetrics and Gynaecology*, **104**, 829–33.

Hughes, J., Ryan, M., Hinshaw, K., Henshaw, R., Rispin, R. and Templeton, A. (1996). The costs of treating miscarriage: a comparison of medical and surgical management. *British Journal of Obstetrics and Gynaecology*, **103**, 1217–21.

Kennedy, I. and Grubb, A. (1989). *Medical law: text and materials*. Butterworth, London.

Lowy, A., Ojo, R., Stegeman, A. and Vellacott, I. (1998). Meeting women's needs for a flexible abortion service: retrospective study of a specialist day-care unit. *Journal of Public Health Medicine*, **20**, 449–54.

Newhall, E. and Winikoff, B. (2000). Abortion with mifepristone and misoprostol: Regimens, efficacy, acceptability and future directions. *American Journal of Obstetrics and Gynecology*, **183**, 44–53.

Nursing Times (1998). 'Lunch-break' abortion service seeks to expand. *Nursing Times*, **94** (25), 16.

Royal College of Obstetricians and Gynaecologists (2000). *Guidelines on induced abortion*. RCOG, London.

Wood, A.J.J. (2000). Medical termination of pregnancy. *New England Journal of Medicine*, **342**, 946–56.

# Information leaflet on early medically induced abortion

It is now possible to have termination of an early pregnancy without an operation rather than surgery with an operation. The treatment involves:

1. Hospital assessment, examination and counselling as appropriate. Completion of legal form and blood test. A blood test is taken for blood group and blood count.
2. Taking an RU-486 tablet at the hospital.
3. Being given a vaginal prostaglandin tablets in hospital 2 days later.
4. Having a final check up 1–2 weeks later with your GP or Family Planning Clinic.

## How the abortion pill (RU-486) works

You can take RU-486, also known as mifepristone or Mifegyne, up to 63 days or 9 weeks after the start of your last period. It's essential to know you are definitely pregnant: so you need to have a pregnancy test, and sometimes an ultrasound scan is necessary. RU-486 works by blocking the action of the hormone that makes the lining of the uterus or womb hold on to the fertilized egg.

The prostaglandin pessary relaxes the cervix and makes the uterus contract: this is like a normal miscarriage.

## The treatment

The RU-486 tablet is taken in the hospital; this is the first part of the treatment. You must not take the tablet unless you are completely sure about having a termination. An appointment will be made for you to return to hospital 2 days after taking the tablet. The 2 days between visits can be spent in the normal way – at home or work. During this time you may experience increased nausea, start to bleed vaginally or have period-like pains. There is a small chance that the miscarriage will occur. If you do have vaginal bleeding you should use sanitary pads and not tampons.

At the second visit, prostaglandin tablets are placed into your vagina. This causes contractions, which are usually felt as strong period-like pains. You can have painkillers if you need them. Since painkillers may take some time to be fully effective, it is best to take them early on. Bleeding will also begin and you may feel sick and have diarrhoea during this time. Most women miscarry within 4–6 hours of the tablets being given. When you miscarry you will notice largish clots of blood and tissue coming from the vagina, like a very heavy period.

It is not necessary to go to bed or lie down; you may feel more comfortable walking about. It is best to bring something with you to do and to wear comfortable clothes. You are very welcome to bring someone to stay with you while you are at the hospital. You will need to bring sanitary towels (not tampons) and toiletries. You can go home providing that someone can take you and that there is someone to stay with you at night. A small number of women do not miscarry in hospital but do so after they have gone home.

About 5 in 100 women treated in this way need to have a minor operation (D&C or scrape) under general anaesthetic to stop continuing bleeding due to some pieces of tissue left behind in the womb. One woman in 100 will not miscarry. If you do not miscarry, you are strongly advised to have a surgical termination since the treatment you have received may have caused harm to your pregnancy.

### Medicines

Some medicines can interfere with the treatment and should not be taken after you have taken the RU-486 tablets. These include painkillers such as aspirin or ibuprofen. Please tell the doctor about any medicines you take.

### Smoking/drinking

You should not smoke or drink alcohol for at least 4 days after taking the RU-486 tablets.

### What happens afterwards

You may bleed for up to 2 weeks, and some women will have a slight blood loss until their next period starts. Do not have sexual intercourse until the bleeding has stopped. Do remember to use an effective form of contraception before you resume sexual relations – ask your GP or Family Planning Clinic.

You will need to be seen at your GP's surgery, Family Planning Clinic or the hospital 1–2 weeks later to check that everything is back to normal and these arrangements will be discussed with you. It is very unlikely that your future fertility will be damaged. Almost all women who have had a termination will be able to become pregnant again if they want to. But it is not possible to guarantee future pregnancy after termination as with any other pregnancy. Very rarely a woman does not have a successful pregnancy and this may be due to a complication of the termination.

You may feel low for a short time after the termination but as your body returns to normal this should settle. Look after yourself and give yourself time to recover. If you do feel upset, it often helps to talk to someone about it. Doctors and nurses at your general practice or Family Planning Clinic and the Counsellor at the hospital are there to help you if you need them.

# Information leaflet on prostaglandin termination of pregnancy

Prostaglandin termination of pregnancy is carried out by making the womb contract like a mini-labour to expel the pregnancy tissue and is undertaken after 12 weeks of pregnancy.

The termination is only undertaken <u>after</u> you have attended a hospital clinic for assessment and examination by a doctor, completion of a legal form and counselling if required. The termination will probably involve:

1. Taking a tablet called RU-486 2 days before the termination itself is performed to prepare your womb for the termination. Once the RU-486 has been taken, the process of termination has started.

2. Being given prostaglandin either by pessaries or tablets into your vagina or by injection into your uterus to make it contract. If you have been given RU-486, the prostaglandins are given 2 days later.

3. A hormone drip of oxytocin may be given into a vein in the back of your hand or arm to help the uterus contract.

4. Having a final check-up one or two weeks later with your GP or at a Family Planning Clinic.

The method that will be used for you will be decided and discussed by the doctors and nurses seeing you at the hospital.

## Admission to hospital

1. If you normally take tablets or medicines or use inhalers, these should be taken as usual. Bring them with you.

2. If you are under 16 years of age you should bring a parent or legal guardian to sign a consent form for the procedure.

## What happens during your stay in hospital

After you have been admitted you will be checked by a midwife and a doctor. The prostaglandins will be given either by tablets or pessaries put into your vagina or by an injection into your uterus. The tablets or pessaries need inserting on two or more occasions in most patients. The oxytocin drip is given through a fine needle into a vein in the back of your hand. The effect is to make the uterus contract and induce a mini-labour like a miscarriage. The procedure may take up to 24 hours or more. You can have painkillers as you need them and they are usually given by injection, which may make you feel drowsy.

Bleeding will also begin and you may develop a temperature or have some shivering during this time. When you miscarry you will notice large clots of blood and tissue with the fetus and placenta (afterbirth) coming away.

You may be given an injection of ergometrine to help deliver the placenta. The placenta may not always come away completely and you may need a general anaesthetic to have it removed. Women whose blood group is rhesus negative are advised to have an injection of anti-D. It is best to bring something with you to do, such as something to read. You are very welcome to bring someone to stay with you during the day while you are at the hospital.

You will need to bring sanitary towels (not tampons), things for an overnight stay and toiletries. You may be able to go later the same day or you may need to stay in hospital only one night, but occasionally two or more nights are necessary.

## What happens afterwards

You may bleed for up to 2 weeks and some women will have a slight blood loss until their next period starts. This is quite normal, but if you have a lot of bleeding or lasting pain or a temperature, you must see your doctor at once. After the termination you should use sanitary towels instead of tampons until your next period, which should occur during the next 6 weeks.

Do not have sexual intercourse until the bleeding has stopped. Do remember to use an effective form of contraceptive before you resume sexual relations – ask your GP or Family Planning Clinic for advice.

You will need to be seen at your GP's surgery or Family Planning Clinic a few weeks later to check that everything is back to normal and these arrangements will be discussed with you.

It is very unlikely that your future fertility will be damaged. Almost all women who have had a termination will be able to become pregnant again if they want to. But it is not possible to guarantee future pregnancy after termination as with any other pregnancy. Very rarely a woman does not have a successful pregnancy and this may be due to a complication of the termination.

You may feel low for a short time after the termination but as your body returns to normal this should settle. Look after yourself and give yourself time to recover. If you do feel upset, it often helps to talk to someone about it. Doctors and nurses at your general practice surgery or Family Planning Clinic and the hospital Counsellor are there to help you if you need them.

# Information leaflet on early surgical termination of pregnancy

Surgical termination of pregnancy is carried out by suction under general anaesthetic and is undertaken up to 12 weeks of pregnancy. The operation is usually performed as a day case and does not involve any kind of cutting.

The procedure involves:

1. Medical assessment and examination by a doctor, completion of a legal form and counselling as appropriate at an out-patient clinic. A blood test is taken for blood count and blood group.

2. Admission to the day services unit a few days later: you will *not* be admitted the same day.

3. A short operation under general anaesthetic.

4. Having a final check-up 1–2 weeks later with your GP or at a Family Planning Clinic.

## Admission to the Day Services Unit

The following conditions must be fulfilled, otherwise it will not be possible to carry out the operation.

1. No food or drink must be taken after midnight the night before your operation.

2. If you normally take tablets or medicines or use inhalers, these should be taken as usual, with only a sip of water. Bring them with you.

3. If you are under 16 years of age you should bring a parent or legal guardian to sign a consent form for the procedure.

4. You need to be collected by a responsible adult to take you home by car or taxi during the afternoon and to look after you overnight.

Some women need to be admitted for one or two nights because of a pre-existing medical condition or if problems occur. This would be arranged at the out-patient appointment.

## What happens during the operation

After you have been admitted when all the checks have been done, it is sometimes necessary to have a small prostaglandin pessary (it is smaller than a tampon) put into the vagina. It helps to soften the cervix, which is the opening into the uterus or womb, and reduces the amount of bleeding that occurs. You may experience some cramp-like pains after the pessary is inserted. If you have any doubts about going ahead with the abortion you should tell the nurse looking after you before the pessary is inserted.

The general anaesthetic is usually injected through a fine needle into a vein in the back of your hand or arm. As soon as you are asleep, the pregnancy tissue is removed by suction and D&C (dilatation and curettage). The whole procedure takes only a few minutes.

Very rarely the wall of the womb can be damaged (perforation). In most cases no further action will be necessary and the perforation will heal up on its own, but in exceptional circumstances further surgery may be required.

## What happens afterwards

When the anaesthetic has worn off you may have some slight pain but this should soon disappear. Women whose blood group is rhesus negative are advised to have an injection of anti-D. You should be able to leave hospital within 3–6 hours after the operation.

You may bleed for up to 2 weeks and some women will have a slight blood loss until their next period starts. This is quite normal, but if you have a lot of bleeding, profuse or offensive discharge, lasting pain, or a temperature, you must see your doctor as soon as possible. The staff on the Gynaecology Ward can also advise you. These symptoms might suggest that you have an infection that will need treating or that you may need to have a D&C. After the abortion you should use sanitary towels instead of tampons until your next regular period.

Do not have sexual intercourse until the bleeding has stopped. Do remember to use an effective form of contraceptive before you resume sexual relations – ask your GP or Family Planning Clinic for advice.

You will need to be seen at your GP's surgery or Family Planning Clinic a few weeks later to check that everything is back to normal and these arrangements will be discussed with you. Very rarely the pregnancy may still continue: if your pregnancy symptoms still persist or you have no period within 6 weeks of the abortion you will need to see a doctor to check this out.

It is very unlikely that your future fertility is damaged. Almost all women who have had a termination will be able to become pregnant again if they want to. But it is not possible to guarantee future pregnancy after termination as with any other pregnancy. Very rarely a woman does not have a successful pregnancy and this may be due to a complication of the termination.

You may feel low for a short time after the termination but as your body returns to normal this should settle. Look after yourself and give yourself time to recover. If you do feel upset, it often helps to talk to someone about it. Doctors and nurses at your general practice surgery or Family Planning Clinic and the hospital Counsellor are there to help you if you need them.

# Chapter 6

# Infertility and early pregnancy loss
## Gillian M Lockwood

## The 'epidemic of infertility'

To paraphrase Tolstoy, 'all fertile couples resemble one another, but all infertile couples are unhappy in their own way'. Since about one in six couples seeks specialist help because of difficulty or delay in conceiving a first or subsequent child, the problem of infertility will continue to play a significant and increasing role in the general practitioner (GP)'s consultation load.

There are several reasons for this apparent 'epidemic of infertility'. The human species is relatively inefficient at reproducing itself and Nature offers a fairly narrow window in a woman's life in which she is reasonably fecund. Current demographic trends towards delayed child-bearing due to career or financial pressures, in conjunction with a high rate of divorce, which results in many women seeking to conceive in a new partnership and at an older age, contribute to this picture. In the United Kingdom (UK), 12% of live births are to women aged 35 years or older and *first* live births to women 35 or older now account for 7% of all births. Also, the option of adoption, especially adoption of a baby, is no longer available except to a tiny minority of childless couples. This situation is due in part to the wide availability of effective contraception and the provision of legal termination for unwanted pregnancy. Social acceptance of and financial provision for unsupported single mothers is another factor here. The media attention given to the conspicuous success of 'state-of-the-art' fertility treatments has also encouraged many couples, who in former years would quietly have tolerated their childlessness or claimed it was voluntary, to request access to investigation and treatment.

## The prime role of counselling in infertility care

Fundamental to the treatment of infertility, whether or not 'high-tech' solutions eventually need to be adopted, is the role played by counselling of the infertile couple.

It may appear, during the course of investigations, that one or other partner is primarily 'responsible' for their problem of infertility. However, it is vital that the couple's state of childlessness is seen as a shared problem, and the attribution of sole responsibility should be avoided in all but the most overt cases, a position supported by recognition of the fact that in at least one-third of all cases of infertility, there are multifactorial causes predisposing to a fertility problem.

Considered overall, and given ready access to available techniques and resources, it is likely that modern fertility practice can achieve successful pregnancies for about two-thirds of all couples referred where the woman is under 40 years of age. But the appropriate audit of success lies with how the eventually unsuccessful third are treated. If counselling helps the irrevocably childless to accept their state, but makes them aware that their sorrow and disappointment are sympathized with and appreciated – if it makes them feel that all possible avenues of assistance have at least been recognized, even if not explored – then something of great value has been achieved.

## Psychological morbidity of infertility

GPs are uniquely placed to recognize the powerful personal drives that operate in the field of infertility and it is vital that they should not allow themselves to become judgemental when viewing requests for fertility assistance from apparently unpromising or undeserving candidates. In no other field of medicine is the GP so obviously acting as a gatekeeper to facilitate or deny access to medical care. Fertility patients are particularly sensitive to any implication that they are in some sense responsible for their childlessness; they are often suffering anyway from feelings of guilt or remorse, and treating this morbidity with appropriate counselling and sympathy is often just as important as is the ability to diagnose and treat their fertility problem.

## Patient autonomy and infertility

Patients seeking help with a fertility problem are quite unusual in that the treatment they seek is elective, optional, and voluntary. They are not ill by any usual definition of illness (although their infertility may have an underlying pathological cause) and yet a medical solution to their 'problem' is likely to have a greater impact on their lives than almost any other medical intervention. Fertility patients need a high level of information about options for investigation and treatment and are often extremely well informed about their diagnosis and about the therapies that could help them. Fertility patients also differ from normal patients in that their expectations about any course of treatment are likely to be unrealistically high. Achieving successful pregnancy is an 'all-or-none' event and so failure in any given cycle of treatment [which even with a very successful treatment like *in vitro* fertilization (IVF) occurs in at least 75% of cycles] results in devastating disappointment. It is simply not possible to have infertility 'symptoms' improved by anything other than a baby, unlike the case of a less than totally successful operation which may nevertheless provide palliation or improved quality of life.

The provision of fertility services within the National Health Service (NHS) varies enormously from region to region, reflecting a widely held belief that fertility treatment is a low priority and scarce resources should be preferentially directed at life-saving and pain-relieving interventions. Although the NHS Plan clearly sets the abolition of regional inequalities (the 'post-code lottery') as a priority, the shortage of NHS treatment available has led inevitably to the proliferation of private provision of fertility care. The relatively recent development of the new reproductive technologies such as *in vitro* fertilization and embryo transfer (IVF-ET) have accelerated this trend, and nowadays the vast majority of units offering such treatments are private clinics where patients are fee-paying consumers rather than NHS recipients of medical services. More than 70% of IVF cycles in the UK are purchased by couples themselves and, where NHS provision is made, there may be strict eligibility criteria applied, long waiting lists may develop or certain types of treatment (such as treatment using donor gametes) may be excluded.

This trend has rightly focused attention on the need for audit of fertility care provision in both the private and public sectors. Drugs for IVF and similar therapies may be prescribed by GPs, but they are expensive (typically £400–600 per treatment cycle) and many practices which do prescribe may set limits to the number of cycles provided. GPs involved in counselling and referring patients must therefore be ever conscious of the need to strike a balance between offering hope to childless couples on the one hand and, on the other, not raising unrealistic expectations in the minds of a potentially vulnerable group.

## Normal fertility

The graphs in Figs 6.1–6.4 show the basic parameters of fertility within which ultimately all fertility treatment including 'high-tech' treatments must operate.

The implications of these data are that the vast majority (90%) of fertile couples where the female partner is aged under 35 will conceive within a year of starting to try. Most other fertile couples will conceive during the following

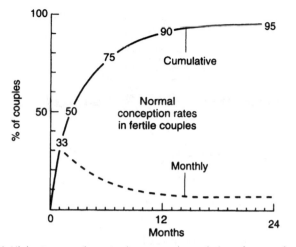

**Fig 6.1** Highest conception rates in a normal population of proven fertility.

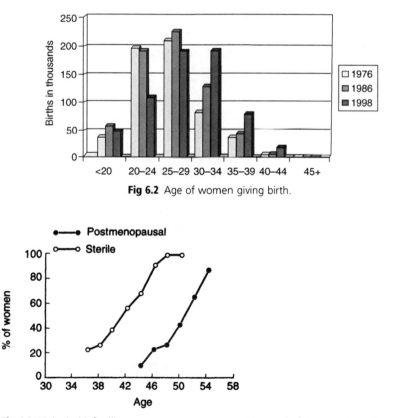

**Fig 6.2** Age of women giving birth.

**Fig 6.3** Biological infertility commences, on average, 10 years before menopause in British women.

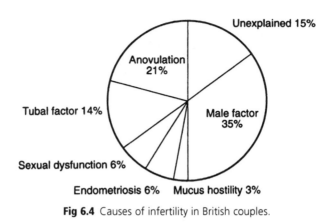

**Fig 6.4** Causes of infertility in British couples.

12 months. Referral for specialist investigation and treatment may therefore be reasonably delayed for many couples until they have been trying for 18 months or so. However, this 'wait and try' approach should not be adopted if failure to conceive is causing psychological stress and anxiety, if the infertility is primary for the couple and the female partner is in her mid-thirties or older or if there are features in the medical histories of either partner (see below) which are suggestive of underlying reproductive pathology.

## Causes of infertility

As the pie chart in Fig 6.4 shows, male factor infertility, failure to ovulate effectively, and tubal disease are by far the commonest causes of infertility in British couples. Absolute infertility is relatively rare but subfertility is common and, when two or more factors are present (such as amenorrhoea in the woman and oligospermia in the man), then the chance of a spontaneous conception occurring becomes very low indeed.

These major categories may be subdivided (Table 6.1), although, with few exceptions, making a specific diagnosis may not be particularly beneficial therapeutically. An increasingly common explanation (as opposed to diagnosis) is advanced female age i.e. ≥38 years.

## The investigation of infertility in general practice

The Royal College of Obstetricians and Gynaecologists (RCOG 1998) have recently published guidelines for the investigation and management of the infertile couple at primary, secondary, and tertiary level. The guidelines were

**Table 6.1** Major causes of infertility

| Fertility factor | Causes |
| --- | --- |
| Anovulation | Polycystic ovary syndrome (PCOS) |
| | Hyperprolactinaemia |
| | Hypogonodotrophic hypogonadism |
| | Premature ovarian failure |
| | Hypopituitarism |
| | Weight-related amenorrhoea |
| | Exercise-related amenorrhoea |
| Tubal factor | Infection (*Chlamydia*, PID, appendicitis) |
| | Endometriosis |
| | Surgical (laparotomy, tubal sterilization) |
| Sexual dysfunction | Physical (IDDM, MS, β-blockers) |
| | Psychological (loss of libido, anxiety, stress) |
| Mucus hostility | Anti-sperm antibodies |
| | Increased mucus viscosity |
| Male factor | Obstructive azoospermia |
| | Severe sperm dysfunction |
| | Primary testicular failure |
| | Congenital abnormality (cryptorchidism) |
| | Post-chemo/radiotherapy |
| | Endocrine disturbance |
| | Anti-sperm antibodies |

constructed to allow the clinician to assess the strength of the guideline by detailing both the level of the evidence and the grade of the recommendations. Fig 6.5 summarizes the RCOG guidelines for the investigation and management of the infertile couple in primary care and further information can be downloaded from the RCOG website (www.rcog.org.uk).

The problem of infertility can frequently be managed in general practice and, with appropriate investigation, advice, and treatment, many couples will achieve a successful pregnancy without recourse to the specialist fertility clinic. General practice is the ideal setting for lifestyle advice about obesity, smoking, and alcohol consumption and for preconception advice about folic acid supplements and diet.

In general practice, the couple's medical records are readily available, often dating back to birth, with a wealth of valuable family medical history that may

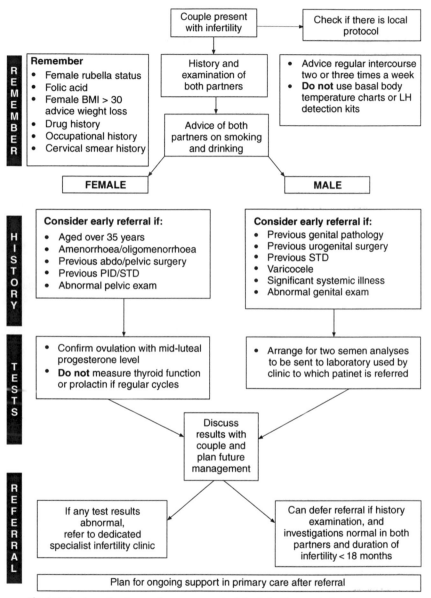

**Fig 6.5** The investigation and management of the infertile couple in primary care.

be highly relevant. These records will contain details of previous operations and diseases, in addition to psychological factors. Psychological support is one area where the GP has a great deal to contribute, not least because fertility problems can cause severe stress in a marriage, and it is often difficult for partners to support one another.

During history-taking and routine investigation, factors related to one partner's medical or reproductive history may emerge which are not known by the other partner. For example, eliciting a history of previous undisclosed paternity, termination of pregnancy, sexually transmitted disease (STD), or even sterilization may involve a breach of confidence between couples. Early on in the course of infertility consultations, it is therefore vital that an opportunity is made for the partners to be seen separately; and where significant features emerge, patients should be asked if their partners are aware of these facts. In order to provide optimal care, both partners should be encouraged to register with the same GP so that any such issues may be resolved.

## The initial consultation

It is frequently the female partner who first raises the issue of delay in conceiving with the GP, although the fertility problem may be disguised as concerns over menstrual irregularity or pelvic pain. Ideally, both partners should be present!

It is important to provide both a proposed plan of investigation and to give an outline of the diagnostic procedures that are to be undertaken. A full medical history is then taken including:

- age of both partners
- duration of infertility
- previous fertility and pregnancy outcome
- coital frequency, difficulties, and timing in relation to the 'fertile period'
- medical disorders such as diabetes, thyroid problems, hypertension, anaemia
- previous history of inflammatory disease of the reproductive tract
- surgical history of the female-abdominal, pelvic or cervical surgery
- surgical history of the male – groin or genital surgery
- drug history for both partners
- previous contraceptive use.

## Investigations in primary care

### Assessment of the menstrual cycle and confirmation of ovulation

It may be assumed that women with regular menstrual cycles in the range 23–35 days ovulate normally most months. Ovulation occurs approximately 14 days prior to the next menstruation and therefore women with particularly

short or long cycles need to be aware of their 'fertile period' Serum progesterone will be elevated to at least 30 nmol/l in the mid-luteal phase (day 21 of
a 28-day cycle) if ovulation has occurred, but timing of this test is crucial and
it is only required if the infertility is long-standing in the presence of regular
cycles, or if ovulatory therapy is being undertaken. Basal body temperature
charting to identify the tiny rise in temperature that occurs following ovulation, and the use of LH urine testing kits to identify the pre-ovulatory surge in
LH are generally both to be discouraged as they are a source of considerable
stress and are prone to mistake. Most couples may be reassured that they
will maximize their chances of conception by having intercourse every 2–3 days
from cycle day 8 to day 20.

Identifying the 'fertile period' may be readily taught in general practice and
the mucus changes associated with the ovulatory phase are recognized by most
women (Fig 6.6). There is little evidence to support the widely held belief that
a prolonged period of abstinence will 'strengthen' poor sperm and since it is

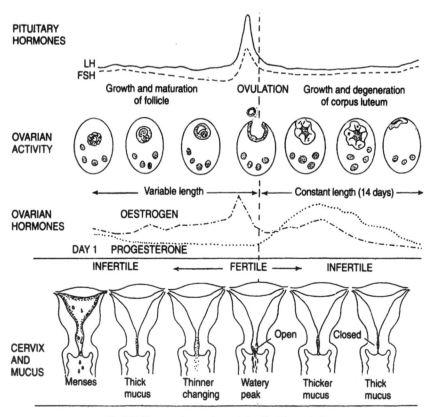

**Fig 6.6** The ovarian cycle and the 'fertile period'.

the progressive motility rather than the absolute concentration of the sperm that is crucial to its fertility, increasing the frequency of intercourse is likely to prove more helpful to couples with male factor infertility.

Even where the menstrual cycle is regular and normal, endocrine investigations should include serum follicle stimulating hormone (FSH), luteinizing hormone (LH), prolactin (PRL), testosterone, and an assessment of oestrogen status. These hormone assessments may be made from one blood sample taken in the early follicular (days 2–5) phase of the cycle. The main purpose of measuring FSH levels is to exclude primary or secondary ovarian failure, in which case the FSH level will be significantly raised (>15 IU). If the LH:FSH ratio is >3 and especially if the testosterone is elevated, the diagnosis may be one of polycystic ovary syndrome (PCOS) and these endocrine abnormalities are most likely to occur in women with oligomenorrhoea (cycle length >42 days), amenorrhoea (absence of periods >6 months), acne, hirsutism, and obesity (Balen *et al.* 1995).

The presence of galactorrhoea may suggest hyperprolactinaemia, which is an important cause of secondary amenorrhoea. The interpretation of serum prolactin levels which may be marginally raised (>800 IU/l) is difficult as PRL is a stress hormone and is often elevated by a physical examination, but in fertility patients with hyperprolactinaemia, thyroid function should be assessed as hypothyroidism is associated with this condition. Where PRL is consistently elevated (>1000 IU/l), CT or MRI scanning of the pituitary fossa should be requested to exclude a pituitary tumour. If the serum PRL is mildly elevated, but the menstrual cycle is regular and ovulatory, there is no need for treatment.

Where a woman complaining of infertility presents with secondary amenorrhoea, a progestogen challenge test will rapidly establish her oestrogen status. The test is based on the principle that an oestrogen-primed endometrium will be shed on progestogen withdrawal. A pregnancy test should be performed first, and if negative, the patient takes 10 mg oral medroxyprogesterone daily for 7 days. The majority of patients with ovulatory dysfunction and PCOS will experience withdrawal bleeding at the end of the course of progestogen and they may then proceed to ovulation induction with oral anti-oestrogens such as clomiphene citrate (see later). A negative progestogen challenge test is suggestive of severe hypothalamic–pituitary dysfunction and this group merit early referral to a specialist unit.

## Assessment of the pelvis

Tubal damage and pelvic adhesions are usually due to infection. STDs including *Chlamydia*, ascending endometritis following childbirth, miscarriage or abortion, complications of intrauterine contraceptive devices (IUCDs), etc., can all cause tubal damage. Infection often causes irreversible functional damage to the ciliated tubal lining epithelium and surgical restoration of patency may not be associated with a return of proper tubal function and increase the risk of tubal ectopic implantation. Appendicectomy and other abdominal surgery can also compromise tubal function and this was frequently the case when powdered gloves were favoured by general surgeons.

Pelvic examination will alert the GP to unexpected tenderness, immobility of the pelvic organs, or swelling in the adnexae. Formal assessment of tubal patency by hysterosalpingogram (HSG), contrast ultrasonography (HyCoSy), or laparoscopy normally requires referral, but some GPs may have access to HSG and this out-patient procedure is a useful screen for low-risk patients.

*Chlamydia* serology is a useful screening test of past 'silent' infection, indicating likely tubal damage and requiring early laparoscopy. Chlamydial antibodies are quite common in the general population and it is only when raised (immunofluorescence test or IFT titre >1/512 ) that there is a strong probability of finding otherwise unexpected tubal or pelvic inflammatory damage and adhesions. If a recent infection is suspected, both partners should be treated with a course of doxycycline and erythromycin or ciprofloxacin (see Chapter 9).

Laparoscopy remains the 'gold standard' for the investigation of tubal patency because it offers the opportunity for treatment of a range of pelvic pathologies. Tubal patency is checked by passing methylene blue dye through the cervix, and observing its passage through the fallopian tubes. Laparoscopic examination, which is usually a day-case procedure under general anaesthetic, is ideally combined with diagnostic hysteroscopy to exclude intrauterine pathology such as fibroids, septae, adhesions, and polyps. These pathologies have an uncertain impact upon fertility and they are found frequently in the fertile population; however, in the infertile population they are thought to warrant treatment.

The diagnosis of endometriosis (see Chapter 11), the presence of persisting endometrial tissue at sites other than within the uterine cavity, is frequently made during infertility investigations, although there is much debate about the relevance of this finding. Clearly significant endometriosis, which has caused structural damage to the fallopian tubes and ovaries, can lead to infertility, but it is less clear how milder forms of endometriosis contribute to the problem. Epidemiological studies have shown an increased prevalence of endometriosis in infertile women, but these studies do not indicate whether endometriosis predisposes to infertility or vice versa (Mahmood and Templeton 1990). There is no evidence to date that proves that medical treatment is beneficial in women with mild endometriosis in terms of improving their fertility outcome. Thus, many specialists now regard fertility patients with minimal or mild endometriosis as their only diagnostic finding with unexplained infertility (Thomas and Cooke 1987). However, the Endocan study, a multicentre, randomized, controlled trial (RCT) conducted in Canada on more than 300 patients with infertility and minimal/mild endometriosis, did show a significantly higher pregnancy rate in patients who had their endometrial implants ablated with electrocautery (Marcoux *et al.* 1997).

## Investigation of the male in general practice

In a third of infertile couples there is an identifiable defect either in the production or functional competence of sperm and there is evidence of a decline in sperm quality over recent decades (Skakkeback and Keiding 1994). Investigation of the male partner of a couple complaining of infertility in general practice should aim to exclude the relatively few, but sometimes reversible, disorders that may affect sperm and also identify rare but serious associated conditions such as testicular tumours. The history should include past STDs, mumps orchitis, history of scrotal, inguinal, prostatic, or bladder neck surgery, or testicular injury. Cryptorchidism (undescended testes) is the most common congenital abnormality associated with male subfertility. Early orchidopexy (before 3 years of age) is recommended, but even with early surgery there may be severe problems with spermatogenesis. The importance of maintaining the testicles at a temperature below body heat by wearing cool, loose-fitting underwear may be stressed, especially to men who drive long distances each year – long-distance lorry drivers have notoriously poor sperm parameters. Enquiry should be made about exposure to toxic agents such as radiation, cytotoxic drugs, chemicals, or drugs affecting spermatogenesis. Excessive smoking and alcohol consumption are well recognized as reducing sperm quality. Physical examination should include assessment of secondary sexual characteristics, an estimation of testicular size and consistency, a search for varicocele and assessment of the epididymes and vasa.

Semen analysis is the most important test for the diagnosis of male infertility, and the GP should stress the importance of it being produced into a sterile container after the correct period of abstinence (3–4 days), transported to the laboratory at the correct temperature (a jacket pocket is ideal), within an hour of production.

Table 6.2 shows the criteria for a normal (fertile) semen sample as defined by the World Health Organization (WHO).

A district general hospital (DGH) bacteriology laboratory will normally report volume, count, motility, and morphology. More detailed analysis,

**Table 6.2** WHO criteria for a normal sperm count

| | |
|---|---|
| Volume | 2 ml or more |
| pH | 7.2–8.0 |
| Count | 20 × 10$^6$/ml or more |
| | [Abnormal = azoospermia (no sperm) or oligospermia (reduced numbers)] |
| Motility | 50% or more with forward progression, or 25% or more with rapid progression (within) 60 minutes of ejaculation) (Abnormal = asthenozoospermia) |
| Morphology | 30% or more normal forms (Abnormal = teratozoospermia) (14% using Kruger strict criteria) |
| MAR test | Fewer than 10% of sperm with adherent particles |
| Immunoblot test | Fewer than 20% of sperm with adherent particles |

including computer assisted sperm analysis (CASA), which will provide measurements of straight line and curvilinear velocity, linearity, and lateral head displacement, can be performed by a specialist andrology service. The sperm penetration test (SpermSelect) and sperm preparation through a PERCOLL column can give valuable information about the fertility potential of the sperm, but would only normally be indicated if the initial semen analysis was abnormal. Given the great variability over quite short periods of time of serial analyses, it is vital that no great significance is attached to an isolated low count. Sperm function can only be properly tested in the context of appropriately receptive media such as pre-ovulatory cervical mucus and artificial culture fluids as used in the 'swim-up' test (see below).

In the event of low or absent (azoospermia) sperm counts, endocrine assessment should include FSH, LH, PRL, and testosterone. If FSH levels are elevated, this suggests end-organ failure. Male patients who present with azoospermia, normal sized testes, and a normal gonadotrophin profile should be referred for a urological opinion, vasogram, and testicular biopsy, since some of these patients may have a surgically correctable obstruction or sperm obtained directly from the testis by fine-needle or open biopsy may be cryopreserved and used in an ICSI-IVF treatment cycle (see later).

Where sperm parameters are exceptionally poor with low count, low progressive motility, and a high proportion of abnormal forms, then many specialists would advocate karyotyping and cystic fibrosis (CF) screening the male partner as the incidence of carrier status CF or structural chromosome defects are quite high.

## Antisperm antibodies

The MAR (mixed antiglobulin reaction) test may be performed as a routine part of standard seminal analysis, to screen for antibodies in seminal plasma. It should be requested if the sperm count reports significant 'clumping' or if the proportion of poorly progressive or non-motile sperm is high (asthenozoospermia). This finding is far more significant than a low count (<20 million per ml = oligospermia). Specific assays to detect IgA, IgG, and IgM and their binding sites are available in specialist centres, but a positive result is only likely to be significant if sperm penetration of mucus is affected.

## Sperm–mucus interaction

Sperm–mucus interaction can be tested *in vivo* (by the postcoital test, PCT) or *in vitro*. The postcoital test is ideally performed one or two days prior to ovulation (day 12 in a 28-day cycle) as this is the time that the mucus is well oestrogenized. The patient is instructed to have intercourse the night prior to attending for the test. A sample of cervical mucus is obtained from the cervical os and inspected under the microscope for the presence of motile sperm. A postcoital test is considered normal if the mucus demonstrates good Spinnbarkeit or stretchability, normal ferning pattern, and at least 5 sperm per high power field.

It is clear that the PCT is a particularly demanding investigation for patients and doctors alike! Many couples with a long-standing fertility problem find the stress of having to have intercourse at a particular time very difficult and for the female partner, to then attend for an intimate medical investigation without even being allowed to bathe first, can be quite unacceptable. From the technical point of view, if the test is done at the wrong point in the cycle, then the results are uninterpretable. Although the postcoital test has become an integral part of fertility investigations, and may readily and more conveniently be performed in the GP surgery, nevertheless a review of the literature suggests that as an assessment of sperm function, this test is rather inadequate as it has a poor correlation with pregnancy (Covaz *et al.* 1978).

# Fertility treatment: a 'ladder of assistance'

Contemporary fertility treatment is best regarded as a 'ladder of assistance', in which the lowest rungs are perhaps the most important, not least because they offer significant opportunities for early and successful intervention. The ladder shown in Table 6.3 illustrates the hierarchy of therapies available to

**Table 6.3** The ladder of assistance

| Indication | Therapy | |
|---|---|---|
| Premature ovarian failure (POF) | 'Extraordinary procedures' | ovum donation |
| Menopause | | |
| Uterine anomaly or absence | | Surrogacy |
| Very severe male factor | Micromanipulation IVF | MESA, TESA* |
| | | + ICSI* |
| | Donor insemination (DI) | |
| Blocked Fallopian tubes | | |
| Cervical hostility | Extracorporeal fertilization | IVF-ET* |
| Endometriosis | | |
| Idiopathic infertility | | |
| Oligo/asthenozoospermia | Extracorporeal gamete enhancement | GIFT, ZIFT* |
| Anti-sperm antibodies | IUI* | |
| Cervical stenosis | | |
| Anovulation | Superovulation | antioestrogens (clomiphene) |
| Oligo-ovulation | Ovulation induction | gonadotrophins |
| PCOS | | |
| | Secondary investigation | laparoscopy |
| | | hysteroscopy |
| | | HSG, PCT |
| | Primary investigation | day 21 progesterone |
| | | hormone profile |
| | | semen analysis |
| | Counselling and general health advice | |

*MESA, microepipdydimal sperm aspiration; TESA, testicular sperm aspiration; ICSI, intracytoplasmic sperm injection; IVF-ET, *in vitro* fertilization and embryo transfer; GIFT, gamete intrafallopian transfer; ZIFT, zygote intrafallopian transfer; IUI, intrauterine insemination

the infertile couple, although it must be recognized that treatment has to be guided both by the clinical findings on examination and investigation, and by the couple's own wishes.

The graph in Fig 6.7 shows the cumulative conception rates resulting from conventional management of couples with a single cause of infertility, compared with conception rates for the normally fertile. It is clear that the

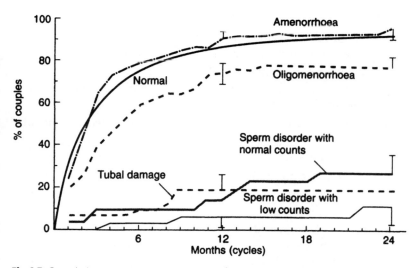

**Fig 6.7** Cumulative conception rates resulting from conventional management of couples with a single cause of infertility.

ovulatory disorders and idiopathic or unexplained infertility have the best chance of responding to relatively simple procedures such as ovulation induction and intrauterine insemination (IUI). However, great progress has been made in IVF in the last 10 years, particularly since the introduction of techniques such as intracytoplasmic sperm injection (ICSI), and now even patients with irremediably blocked fallopian tubes or where there is very severe sperm dysfunction can be offered a chance of pregnancy that is as good as normal in each cycle of treatment.

## Treatment options for infertility

### Anovulation and PCOS in general practice

Patients with irregular periods and persistent anovulation may be started on ovulation induction therapy prior to referral to a specialist unit. Clomiphene citrate is the most commonly used anti-oestrogen and it works by increasing endogenous FSH production. The treatment is successful in patients who are adequately oestrogenized (have a positive progestogen challenge test) but is less successful in hypo-oestrogenic states. Approximately 75% of anovular patients respond to clomiphene with ovulation as monitored by luteal phase progesterone elevation and the onset of regular menses, but only half of these will conceive on clomiphene alone.

The starting dose is usually 50 mg daily for 5 days, beginning on the second day of a spontaneous or induced bleed. If anovulation persists, the dose may be doubled, but at doses higher than this the deleterious effect of the anti-oestrogen on the cervical mucus becomes significant. The side effects of clomiphene therapy include multiple gestation (a sixfold increase in twin pregnancies), vasomotor symptoms such as nausea and hot flushes, weight gain, and, occasionally, visual disturbance, which is an indication for stopping treatment at once.

Recently, anxieties have been raised about an association between clomiphene and ovarian cancer (Rossing *et al.* 1994) and current guidelines restrict the prescription of clomiphene to a maximum of 6–12 cycles. Clomiphene has been quite widely used empirically in cases of unexplained infertility. There are no good studies showing a benefit over placebo for this indication and it should therefore be discouraged.

Gonadotrophin therapy, with daily injections of FSH, is indicated for women with PCOS who have been treated with clomiphene and have repeatedly failed to ovulate, show persistent hypersecretion of LH (>10 IU/l) or have a negative postcoital test due to the effect of anti-oestrogens on cervical mucus. Gonadotrophin therapy carries a significant risk of ovarian hyperstimulation syndrome (OHSS) and multiple pregnancies and in order to minimize these risks, treatment should only be undertaken at specialist units with appropriate monitoring. Monitoring should include ultrasound scanning of the developing follicles and regular assessment of oestradiol levels. Fig 6.8 shows the cumulative conception rates for 103 women with PCOS who did not ovulate with clomiphene (Balen *et al.* 1994).

Laparoscopic ovarian diathermy (LOD) has replaced wedge resection for clomiphene-resistant women with PCOS (Armar and Lachelin 1993). It is performed as a day-case procedure and is particularly useful where a laparoscopic assessment of the pelvis is also required and when the patient is not able to attend clinic for the frequent visits required for adequate monitoring of gonadotrophin therapy.

## Weight-related amenorrhoea

Anorexia nervosa accounts for 15–35% of patients with amenorrhoea, and for these women it is essential to encourage weight gain as the main therapy, since embarking upon a pregnancy when seriously underweight greatly increases the risk of intrauterine growth retardation (IUGR). A body mass index (BMI) of at least 20 kg/m$^2$ should be the goal of amenorrhoeic women who wish to conceive. Where amenorrhoea persists, even after a normal BMI has been regained following excessive weight loss, then ovulation may be induced using the GnRH pump or by injections of HMG (human menopausal gonadotrophin containing FSH and LH).

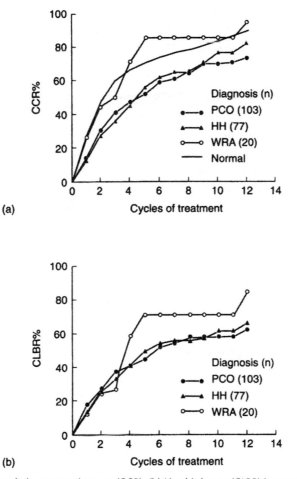

**Fig 6.8** (a) Cumulative conception rate (CCR). (b) Live-birth rate (CLBR) in women with PCOS who did not ovulate with anti-oestrogen therapy (PCO, polycystic ovaries; HH, hypogonadotrophic hypogonadism; WRA, weight-related amenorrhoea).

## Premature ovarian failure

The usual definition of premature ovarian failure (POF) is raised gonadotrophin levels with cessation of periods before the age of 40. The commonest cause is autoimmune failure, whilst infection, previous surgery, chemotherapy, and radiotherapy are also common causes. There appears to be a strong genetic predisposition to early menopause and so daughters and younger sisters of women who have had early-onset ovarian failure should be appropriately counselled. Ovarian failure before puberty, causing primary amenorrhoea, is usually due to a chromosomal abnormality (70%) or a childhood malignancy that required chemotherapy or radiotherapy. Pregnancy is possible by oocyte donation with *in vitro* fertilization and embryo transfer (see later). Women with ovarian failure should take combined hormone replacement therapy (HRT) to prevent the cardiovascular and osteoporotic consequences of oestrogen deficiency.

### Superovulation and intrauterine insemination (IUI)

Where the diagnosis is one of mild male factor (at least 5 million motile sperm are available for insemination), cervical mucus hostility, unexplained infertility or anti-sperm antibodies, then IUI may offer a fair (approximately 10–15% pregnancy rate per cycle) chance of conceiving with a relatively low-cost and low-stress technique. Since fertilization takes place within the fallopian tube, at least one of the female partner's tubes must be healthy. The treatment usually involves gentle ovulation induction with gonadotrophins to encourage the development of two to three follicles which are monitored by transvaginal ultrasonography. Ovulation is triggered with an injection of human chorionic gonadotrophin (hCG) and a sperm sample, produced on the morning of ovulation, is prepared and inserted through the cervix into the uterine cavity via a soft plastic catheter.

## Assisted conception and IVF

The treatment of infertility by assisted conception is one of the most progressive areas of modern medicine. Since the birth of Louise Brown, the world's first test-tube baby, in 1978, there have been enormous advances both in the success rates for assisted conception techniques and in the range of fertility disorders that they can treat. The original indication for IVF was tubal blockage, but it is now used for a wide range of disorders (Table 6.4).

## The technique of IVF

The IVF procedure involves removing one or more eggs from the ovary, fertilizing them in the laboratory with sperm from the male partner, and transferring some of the resulting embryos to the womb for implantation and pregnancy. Table 6.5 shows the steps in an IVF treatment cycle.

### Embryo cryopreservation

Freezing surplus embryos created in an IVF cycle increases the overall pregnancy per stimulated cycle started by 15–20%. Unfortunately, not all 'spare' embryos are suitable for freezing, as poorer quality ones do not withstand the freeze/thaw process. Where the concept of freezing is ethically acceptable to the couple, it should be encouraged, as if the fresh cycle is unsuccessful, the use of

**Table 6.4** Indications for IVF

| | |
|---|---|
| Tubal damage | Minor degrees of tubal damage may be amenable to tubal surgery such as laparoscopic adhesiolysis or salpingostomy |
| Unexplained infertility | Greater than 3 years' duration with no apparent cause identified |
| Endometriosis | Moderate and severe disease responds well to IVF although mild disease should be treated initially as 'unexplained' |
| Anovulation | Failure to conceive after 6–12 cycles of successful ovulation induction suggests an additional cause for the continuing infertility |
| Male factor | Moderate degrees of oligo/astheno/teratozoospermia will produce normal fertilization rates of oocytes *in vitro*. Men with extremely low numbers of functional sperm or obstructive azoospermia will require microassisted fertilization (MAF) techniques such as ICSI |
| Egg donation | POF, gonadal dysgenesis, iatrogenic, carriers of genetic disease, recurrent miscarriage, failed IVF |
| Failed donor sperm insemination (DI) | |

frozen embryos permits a second chance without further stimulation and oocyte recovery being required, and if the fresh cycle was successful, then the embryo quality (which often deteriorates markedly with age) will be frozen at the point that success was achieved. All the evidence available suggests that cryopreservation of embryos is safe for the future child. The frozen embryos must be thawed and transferred at an appropriate stage in the woman's cycle when the endometrium is receptive to implantation and this can be achieved in either a monitored 'natural' cycle or by creating an artificial cycle using GnRH agonists and HRT.

## Egg donation

Many women have fertility problems that can only be overcome by the use of donated eggs as part of an IVF programme (Abdalla.*et al.* 1989); however, there is a scarcity of egg donors since the treatment requires that the donor (who may be an altruistic volunteer or a friend or relative of a fertility patient who needs donor eggs) undergoes IVF treatment herself. More recently, 'egg share' schemes have developed whereby an infertile donor is prepared to donate half her oocytes from an IVF cycle to a recipient who pays the cost of both their treatments. The donor undergoes conventional IVF treatment up to the point of oocyte collection and in the meantime, the recipient's cycle is coordinated with HRT (for non-functioning ovaries) or GnRH agonist and

**Table 6.5** The technique of IVF

| | |
|---|---|
| Downregulation | Drug treatment with a GnRH agonist [daily injections (buserelin) or nasal spray (nafarelin) for 2–3 weeks] to desensitize the pituitary and suppress endogenous FSH and LH secretion. The agonist may be commenced at the start of the cycle (day 2) or in the mid-luteal phase (day 21) |
| Ovarian stimulation | Daily injections of gonadotrophin (FSH: Gonal F or Puregon) or FSH & LH (HMG: Menopur or Merional) are given to encourage the recruitment of multiple follicles |
| Monitoring of treatment | By transvaginal ultrasound to measure the growth of the follicles and by serial assay of oestradiol to individualize dosages and minimize the risk of ovarian hyperstimulation syndrome (OHSS, see later) |
| Ovulatory triggering | The average time for achieving a satisfactory follicular response is about 10 days. When approximately 3 follicles have reached a diameter of 16–18 mm, an ovulatory dose of human chorionic gonadotrophin, hCG, is given (the late-night injection) to complete the maturation of the oocytes within the follicles |
| Oocyte retrieval | This was originally carried out at laparoscopy under general anaesthetic, but now, in the majority of cases, it is carried out under ultrasound guidance using a needle passed through the vaginal vault. Intravenous sedo-analgesia is employed (customarily an opiate with a benzodiazepine). Oocyte retrieval is performed 35–36 hours after the ovulatory trigger |
| Sperm preparation | The male partner produces a semen specimen and this is prepared either by swim-up into a culture medium or passage through a PERCOLL gradient and centrifugation |
| Insemination and embryo culture | Insemination is performed 4–6 hours after the oocytes have been retrieved, depending on their maturity. The oocytes are cultured in individual petri dishes and approximately 200 000–400 000 motile sperm are added to each dish. Overnight incubation results in a fertilization rate of 65–75% for normal sperm and eggs |
| Embryo transfer | A maximum of 3 embryos are transferred to the womb 48–56 hours after collection at the 4 cell stage. 'Embryo transfer' is performed with a fine, soft plastic catheter passed through the cervix into the uterine cavity |
| Luteal support | Progesterone is given in the form of i.m. injections (Gestone) or vaginal pessaries (Cyclogest) to overcome the luteolytic effect of the GnRH agonist during the luteal phase of the cycle. Additional oestradiol is not necessary and, if implantation takes place, embryonic hCG will rescue the corpus luteum |

**Table 6.5** (continued)

| | |
|---|---|
| Pregnancy test | Relatively few women will bleed sooner than 13 days after embryo transfer (ET). Inviting patients to attend for a formal pregnancy test therefore ensures that early pregnancy monitoring can be instituted for all those with a positive test, and it is a good opportunity to discuss future plans with those couples whose cycle has not worked |

HRT (for functioning ovaries). The oocytes collected from the donor are then fertilized with sperm from the recipient's partner and the embryos are transferred as normal. If the recipient conceives, then HRT needs to be continued until luteo-placental shift has occurred (7–8 weeks).

## Surrogacy

Patients who have no uterus or in whom pregnancy is medically contraindicated can be assisted to have their own genetic offspring through surrogacy. The 'commissioning couple', who must be married, undergo conventional IVF up to the point of embryo transfer when their embryos are transferred to the host surrogate whose cycle has been synchronized to that of the 'genetic' mother. Under English law, the birth mother is the legal mother irrespective of the genetic origins of the child, but a 'fast track' adoption process is available to allow the commissioning couple to become the legal parents. Careful counselling of the 'commissioning couple' and the host surrogate (and her partner) are essential and the couples must seek legal guidance in drawing up appropriate agreements that cover issues such as care of the surrogate's existing children if she becomes ill during the surrogate pregnancy. No money (except allowable expenses) must change hands and the surrogate remains free to change her mind until the parental order process is completed.

## Microassisted fertilization (MAF) and IVF

Where there is a history of failed fertilization or very low fertilization rates with conventional IVF, then MAF techniques such as intracytoplasmic sperm injection (ICSI) may be employed. In ICSI, a single sperm is injected directly into the cytoplasm of the oocyte (Fig 6.9). With this technique, fertilization rates of 60–70% may be expected and the clinical pregnancy rates per cycle started are comparable with those of good conventional IVF (Fig 6.10).

## Other treatments for Male Factor Infertility

Where the male partner is azoospermic and no sperm can be obtained by either microepididymal sperm aspiration (MESA), percutaneous epididymal

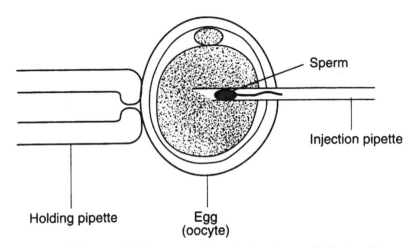

**Fig 6.9** ICSI technique. Individual sperm are injected via a microneedle 12 times thinner than a human hair, directly into the centre of the oocyte. The oocyte is stabilized by a holding pipette.

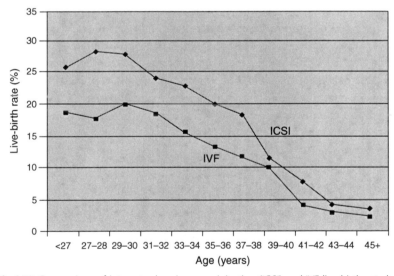

**Fig 6.10** Comparison of intracytoplasmic sperm injection (ICSI) and IVF live-birth rate by female age (using own eggs).

sperm aspiration (PESA) or testicular sperm aspiration (TESA) for use in IVF with ICSI, then artificial insemination using donor sperm (AID) may be offered.

Where the female partner has normal fertility, the cumulative conception rate in accurately timed AID cycles is close to that for normally fertile couples, and those who are not successful can proceed to IVF using donor sperm.

Donor insemination requires careful consideration and all couples should be offered counselling to discuss the legal and ethical implications of AID as covered by the Human Fertilization and Embryology Authority (HFEA). Any child conceived as a result of AID is the *legal* offspring of the social father and may be granted access to certain information (but not the identity) of the donor. It is proposed that donor anonymity may be ended, but this would not be enacted retrospectively.

## Success rates for IVF

The most important statistic for couples considering IVF is the chance that an individual couple has of having a baby following one completed cycle of treatment, the so-called 'take-home baby' rate. Table 6.6 gives the data provided by the Human Fertilization and Embryology Authority (HFEA), which licenses and inspects all units providing assisted conception treatments.

These data are average figures and many units, particularly large centres associated with research facilities, report much higher success rates (live-birth rates of 20–25% per cycle started). The HFEA now publishes annual 'league tables' giving the success rates for each unit in a standardized format; however, not all units offer all types of treatments and many centres have upper age limits or other conditions for acceptance onto a programme. The success of IVF should not be measured by one treatment cycle alone. The cumulative conception rates give a better impression of the extent to which IVF compares favourably with spontaneous conception in the natural menstrual cycle (Fig 6.7).

## Complications associated with IVF treatment

The side effects of the GnRH agonist treatment include headaches, hot-flushes, mood swings, and nasal irritation with the nasal spray. Approximately 15% of

**Table 6.6** IVF success rates by woman's age (all UK centres) – using own eggs

| Age | Treatment cycles | Clinical pregnancy rates, % per treatment | Live-birth rates, % per treatment |
|---|---|---|---|
| Under 25 | 178 | 16.9 | 9.6 |
| 25–29 | 2416 | 22.1 | 16.5 |
| 30–34 | 6806 | 19.0 | 14.6 |
| 35–39 | 6039 | 15.2 | 11.4 |
| 40–44 | 2065 | 8.2 | 4.5 |
| 45+ | 174 | 3.4 | 1.7 |

patients will develop functional follicular cysts whilst taking the agonist, especially if they had prior ovulatory dysfunction. These cysts normally disappear if the GnRH agonist administration is continued or they may be aspirated under ultrasound guidance.

Bleeding following oocyte retrieval is usually slight and the rate of infection is very low (<1%).

A new development in IVF treatment is the use of GnRH antagonists (Cetrorelix or Ganirelix), which prevents premature spontaneous ovulation during the stimulation phase of the IVF cycle and avoids the necessity of the prolonged 'downregulation' phase required with GnRH agonists.

## Ovarian hyperstimulaton syndrome (OHSS)

Mild hyperstimulation is a feature of all IVF cycles but severe OHSS occurs in 1–2% of cases and is a medical emergency requiring admission to hospital. Severe OHSS is characterized by the following features in descending order of frequency:

- gross ovarian enlargement
- ascites
- haemoconcentration
- electrolyte disorders
- pleural effusion
- clotting disorders
- pericardial effusion.

These symptoms are prolonged if conception occurs and therefore women who appear to be at risk of developing significant OHSS prior to oocyte retrieval should either have their treatment cycle cancelled, or have all their embryos frozen so no embryo transfer (ET) is performed until the symptoms have resolved.

## High-order multiple pregnancy

The transfer of three embryos at ET maximizes the pregnancy rate, but gives a high (approximately 30%) multiple pregnancy rate. The vast majority are twins (approximately 25%), but there are many sets of triplets. Since premature delivery is the most important cause of increased perinatal mortality (70 per 1000 live births), many of these tragedies will be amongst IVF triplets. In 1992, the perinatal mortality rate (PNMR) in the UK for children conceived after assisted conception was 27.4 per 1000 births compared to a general population figure of 8 per 1000. This is largely attributable to the increased PNMR associated with multiple pregnancies.

Multiple pregnancies have significant consequences that can be assessed at several levels: risks to the mother and her babies, and costs to the community resulting from the distortion these pregnancies produce in the provision of obstetric and neonatal care. There are also less tangible but nevertheless significant risks associated with even successful multiple pregnancies. 'Instant' families, produced by the arrival of triplets, are subject to great psychological, emotional, and financial stress (Botting *et al.* 1990).

Replacing only two embryos significantly reduces the risk of high-order multiple births while having little impact on overall pregnancy rates and it is the current recommendation of the HFEA that all women aged under 40 undergoing IVF should have a maximum of two embryos replaced.

## Gamete intrafallopian transfer (GIFT)

GIFT differs from IVF in that the eggs collected from the stimulated ovaries are transferred to the fallopian tubes, together with a small sample of prepared sperm, immediately after collection. Egg collection and transfer of a maximum of three eggs are carried out laparoscopically under general anaesthetic, so unlike IVF, fertilization takes place in its natural environment in the fallopian tube. GIFT, like IVF, has proved a very successful assisted conception technique and because no laboratory fertilization or embryo culture is required, GIFT can be performed in non-specialist units. However, the requirement for general anaesthesia can make GIFT more expensive than IVF (which generally has a better success rate), and its use is restricted to women with totally healthy fallopian tubes and where the sperm has previous proven fertilizing ability.

## Zygote intrafallopian transfer (ZIFT)

ZIFT is a combination of IVF and GIFT in which stimulation and egg retrieval are carried out as for IVF with fertilization occurring *in vitro* in the laboratory, but the resulting zygotes are replaced into the fallopian tubes at laparoscopy before cell division to the 4–6 cell pre-embryo stage has occurred. ZIFT is reserved for situations in which it is important to establish that fertilization has taken place, and where cervical transfer of the embryos is difficult.

## Miscarriage after IVF

Most women having IVF think of themselves as 'being pregnant' from the moment of the embryo transfer (ET) and the period that comes 2 weeks later, signifying that the cycle has not worked, can be a devastating disappointment, however well counselled the couple were about their chances of success. Even when the pregnancy test is positive, the incidence of 'biochemical' pregnancy or early pregnancy failure (missed abortion) is higher than in the fertile population (>20% and >40% in women older than 40 years). The transfer of more than one embryo can add confusion as an ongoing pregnancy can exist in spite of very heavy bleeding (from a second implantation site) and ectopic and heterotopic pregnancies occur, especially where there was pre-existing tubal damage.

### Outcome of children born following fertility treatment

The perinatal mortality and morbidity rates following treatments such as stimulated IUI and IVF are increased and, although this is primarily due to the increased incidence of multiple pregnancies, there remains a higher risk in singletons conceived after IVF compared to spontaneously conceived singletons. It is probable that maternal age, lower parity, and cause of infertility are the major reasons and it is reassuring that there is no significant increase in the incidence of congenital or chromosomal abnormalities in children conceived by IVF.

# Spontaneous and recurrent miscarriage

Reference has already been made to the relative subfertility of the human species. In fact it seems that only about half of all successfully fertilized eggs ever result in a live birth. The weak link in the chain occurs at the stage of implantation as is shown by IVF, where two or three apparently normal embryos are transferred to an appropriately prepared uterus and yet only 30–40% of women undergoing embryo transfer will get a positive pregnancy test, let alone a baby.

## Spontaneous miscarriage

In spontaneous conceptions, following a missed period and positive pregnancy test, approximately 15–20% will end in the early weeks with a heavier than average bleed (although some women may not be aware of the pregnancy having ended as they may have no bleeding and still 'feel pregnant' – a 'missed abortion'). If these miscarriages are very early, the woman may not even realize that she was pregnant and just report a delayed and heavier than usual period. Causes causes of spontaneous miscarriage are shown in Table 6.7.

Early pregnancy losses are, technically, abortions, but the association of this word with deliberate termination of pregnancy is so strong that clinicians should always use the term miscarriage, however early the pregnancy loss occurred. Women with PCOS and a raised LH level in the follicular phase (>10 IU) have

**Table 6.7** Causes of spontaneous miscarriage

| | |
|---|---|
| Chromosomal abnormalities | Approx. 50% of first-trimester abortions are chromosomally abnormal |
| Placental abnormalities | Ischaemia and retroplacental haemorrhage |
| Infection | *Listeria*, *Campylobacter*, *Brucella*, cytomegalovirus, rubella and herpes simplex |
| Uterine | Congenital anomalies such as bicornuate uterus, septae, diethylstilboestrol (DES) |
| Endocrine | PCOS, diabetes |
| Immunological | SLE, anti-phospholipid antibodies |
| Cervical incompetence | Cone biopsy, repeated mid-trimester terminations |

a higher incidence of first-trimester pregnancy loss. The frequency of PCOS in recurrent aborters is 82% compared with 23% in normal pregnancies. Trials have so far failed to demonstrate that lowering the periconceptual LH level in these women improves their pregnancy outcome.

Whenever tissue from early pregnancy failures is available for cytogenetic analysis, as is the case where the woman is admitted for an evacuation of retained products of conception (ERPOC) because of prolonged bleeding, incomplete abortion, or 'missed abortion', the chromosomal structure of the conceptus is often very abnormal. It is obviously helpful to the couple to be able to tell them that the pregnancy was doomed from the outset and also that there is no reason to believe that it is more likely than average to occur in subsequent pregnancies.

## Recurrent miscarriage

Recurrent miscarriage is defined as three consecutive miscarriages. By chance alone, one in 25 women will suffer two early miscarriages in a row and one in 125 will suffer three.

However, if subfertility has been an associated feature, with long delays between failed conceptions, or if there is a family history of miscarriage, it is reasonable to arrange a recurrent miscarriage screen. Most tertiary referral centres have a recurrent miscarriage clinic often associated with their fertility or high-risk pregnancy clinics and patients should be referred after three miscarriages or sooner if there is an associated fertility problem.

Numerous treatments for recurrent miscarriage have been tried, including passive immunization with paternal white blood cells (WBCs), suppression of LH with GnRH analogues, high-dose progesterone, prednisolone, and IVF. None of these therapies has proved more successful than close monitoring with frequent hospital visits at a dedicated clinic. Low-dose aspirin and heparin combined has been shown to help in recurrent pregnancy loss due to anti-phospholipid antibodies.

## Management of bleeding in early pregnancy

The management of threatened abortion (bleeding, minimal pain, closed cervix) is rest followed by an ultrasound scan after 6 weeks' gestation to confirm viability. No treatment has been shown to be effective, but the risk of abortion following a positive ultrasound scan (a beating fetal heart seen *in utero*) is a reassuring 5%.

Inevitable abortion (heavy bleeding, pain, open cervix) and incomplete abortion (bleeding with products of conception seen on ultrasound) have historically been treated surgically with curettage; however, the evidence from a prospective study of expectant management (Nielsen and Hahlin 1995) suggests that in the vast majority of cases surgical intervention is unnecessary and spontaneous resolution within a few days may be expected.

Missed abortion (failure of embryonic growth in spite of placental function) may be associated with a brown discharge and reduced or minimal pregnancy symptoms. Pelvic examination will suggest a uterus smaller than expected and ultrasound will reveal an empty gestational sac. Although spontaneous resolution will occur in the majority of cases within 2 weeks, evacuation of retained products of conception (ERPOC) is often advised because many women, but especially fertility patients, find this state of 'obstetric limbo' upsetting.

Ectopic pregnancy *must* be excluded in any woman presenting with pain and abnormal vaginal bleeding. Predisposing factors include previous ectopic pregnancy, congenital anomalies of the reproductive tract, previous tubal surgery, previous pelvic inflammatory disease (PID), progestogen contraceptives, and IVF and GIFT. A positive pregnancy test and an ultrasound showing an empty uterus with free fluid with or without an adnexal mass is 93% predictive of an ectopic. Although some ectopics may resolve spontaneously with a 'tubal abortion', and a conservative approach with daily serum hCG assessments may be followed if the initial hCG was <1000 IU/l, conventional management involves laparoscopy followed by laparoscopic or open surgery to remove the ectopic from the tube (by 'milking' or by linear salpingostomy) or, if the bleeding is extensive or the tube is badly damaged, salpingectomy will be performed. Direct injection of the ectopic pregnancy by hyperosmolar glucose, prostaglandin F2α, and methotrexate or intramuscular methotrexate have all been used with varying success and are unhelpful in large ectopics where there is a risk of residual trophoblastic tissue.

Rhesus isoimmunization following the sensitization of a rhesus-negative women by fetal red cells positive for the rhesus antigen can occur after even very early pregnancy loss. All women who have bleeding in pregnancy beyond 6 weeks' gestation should have serum examined for rhesus antigen and rhesus-negative women should receive anti-D γ-globulin within 3 days.

## Life after miscarriage

The advice often meted out to 'wait a few months for the cycle to settle' before trying again after a miscarriage is profoundly misguided. It was presumably felt that any uncertainty about the exact date of a last menstrual period would complicate the obstetric management of a subsequent pregnancy. But ultrasound can give a very precise dating of the pregnancy and there seems to be some good evidence for a 'rebound' enhancement of fertility in the months immediately following an early pregnancy loss. Fertility patients inevitably find the disappointment of a miscarriage much harder to bear and this psychological stress is compounded if they are discouraged from trying for another pregnancy.

## Ethical issues in assisted conception

The very rapid developments in reproductive medicine and science made during the last two decades have resulted in a fierce debate between practitioners, who wish to utilize the new reproductive technologies for the benefit of childless couples and others in society who are concerned that the existence of such techniques will lead inevitably to their application in ways that are unacceptable to the wider public.

Recent controversies have involved the fate of frozen embryos whose genetic 'parents' could not be traced by the clinics where they were being stored, the use of 'selective reduction' to reduce the number of fetuses in ongoing multiple pregnancies and the use in treatment and research of donated ovarian tissue from cadavers and aborted fetuses. The new technique of PGD (pre-implantation genetic diagnosis) allows the chromosome structure of IVF-generated embryos to be identified before embryo transfer and has raised the spectre of 'designer babies'.

Since 1st August 1991, all IVF and donor insemination (DI) centres have been licensed and regulated by the Human Fertilization and Embryology Authority (HFEA). The Authority was established by the Human Fertilization and Embryology Act 1990, which attempted to legislate for concerns about the creation and use of human embryos outside the body, and about the storage and use of genetic material for the treatment of others. Other aspects of the legislation were aimed at the concern for, and protection of, the interests of the patient, egg or sperm donor, and the child or children that may be born as a result of treatment, including the possible need for the child to have some knowledge of his or her genetic origins.

The legislation requires centres offering treatments such as IVF to take into account 'the welfare of any child who may be born as a result of the treatment (including the need of that child for a father), and of any other child who may be affected by the birth'. This may mean that the patient's GP will be asked to offer an opinion as to whether or not the couple should be treated. The HFEA does not preclude any particular category of patient from receiving treatment nor does it set an age limit on who should be treated, but it gives guidance on factors to be considered:

+ the commitment of the woman and her partner to having and bringing up children;
+ their ages and medical histories;
+ any risk of harm to any child who may be born, including the risk of inherited disorders;
+ the effect of a new baby on any existing child in the family.

It may be considered that, as the five-sixths of the population who do not require medical help to conceive, also do not have to convince anybody of their suitability to become parents, it is an unwarrantable intrusion to impose these conditions on treatment centres and hence on their patients. However, centres are generally considered to allow a fair and unprejudiced assessment of patients and it is more often the financial restrictions that, with few regional exceptions, limit access to assisted conception to those who can afford to purchase treatment in the private sector which are seen as a greater source of inequity.

## Coming to terms with childlessness

The very conspicuous success of many of the new reproductive technologies in treating what was, until recently, incurable infertility has made it particularly difficult for many couples to accept that *they* are not going to succeed. Some couples doggedly pursue treatments feeling that they cannot move beyond their infertility until they have 'tried everything' and with the rapid development of new treatments, the decision to end treatment altogether may become almost impossible to take.

Valuable work can be done in this context by specialist infertility counsellors, and the HFEA Code of Practice (1991), which applies to all fertility units offering IVF or treatments using donated gametes, specifies that three distinct types of counselling (implications counselling, support counselling, and therapeutic counselling), should be available for all fertility patients if they want it. It is difficult, however, not to empathize with the young woman whose third cycle of IVF had just failed who cried in anguish: 'I don't want counselling, I just want a baby!'

The following organizations provide useful information and support for people with fertility problems:

◆ ISSUE (the national fertility association)

Unit 9
509 Aldridge Road
Great Barr
Birmingham, B44 8NA

◆ CHILD

Charter House
43 St Leonards Road
Bexhill-on-Sea
East Sussex, TN40 1JA

◆ The Miscarriage Association

PO Box 24
Ossett
West Yorkshire, WF5 9XG

◆ British Agencies for Adoption and Fostering (BAAF)

Skyline House
200 Union Street
London, SE1 0LX

# Frequently asked questions

## I had two terminations when I was a teenager and now I can't seem to get pregnant. Will I ever be able to have a baby?

Surgical termination of first trimester pregnancy carries only a small risk (5%) of cervical damage, infection, perforation of the uterus or retention of products. If there were no serious complications, such as pelvic infection, it is unlikely that future fertility would be affected. Medical termination using mifepristone (suitable up to 9 weeks' gestation) is probably even safer since only 5% will need a surgical intervention following administration of prostaglandins.

**My partner was married before and has had a vasectomy. We want to have a baby together and I don't want to use donor sperm. What are the options?**

Reversal of vasectomy is successful in about 50% of cases as long as the original operation was uncomplicated and was performed less than 10 years before. Sperm quality may be depressed by anti-sperm antibodies and fertility treatments such as intrauterine insemination (IUI) may be required. The alternative is surgical sperm retrieval (PESA or TESA) in which sperm are obtained directly from the testis and used in an ICSI-IVF cycle.

**I was on the pill for 15 years, but came off it 18 months ago to try for a baby. My periods are very erratic now and I've noticed I've put on a lot of weight and my skin has become very greasy and spotty.**

The combined oral contraceptive pill both masks and suppresses the worst features of polycystic ovary syndrome (PCOS: oligomenorrhoea, obesity, and hyperandrogenism). The patient must be encouraged to reduce her weight to a BMI of no more than 25 with a low-fat diet and exercise and then clomiphene citrate can be prescribed to induce regular ovulation.

**I've been using LH dipsticks to identify the 'fertile period' but I never get a clear colour change and I start spotting before my next period is due.**

This sounds like an ovulatory problem with inadequate luteal phase progesterone levels. A course of clomiphene should improve the situation by boosting endogenous FSH and increasing luteal progesterone levels. If the premenstrual spotting persists when adequate progesterone levels are achieved (>30 nmol/l on cycle day 21), refer for hysteroscopy.

## 10-Minute consultation: infertility

### The patient

A 37-year-old woman comes into your surgery concerned about a delay in conceiving. She has been married for 12 years and has a stressful job as an accountant. She stopped the oral contraceptive pill 18 months ago, intending to start a family.

### What issues you should cover

- Are her periods regular? A regular cycle (23–35 days) implies normal ovulation.

- Is she aware of 'the fertile phase' (cycle days 8–20) and is intercourse occurring regularly and frequently during this time (every 2–3 days)?
- Has she had any pelvic infections or pelvic surgery? (tubal problems due to infections such as *Chlamydia*, peritonitis, endometriosis, etc., account for 25% of infertility)
- Are there any relevant features from her family history? Did her mother have problems with infertility, miscarriage, early menopause?
- Is she well (weight gain and loss, exercise, stress, and depression can all affect fertility)?
- Is there sexual dysfunction (loss of libido, anxiety, stress, performance impotence)?
- Irrespective of the cause of the infertility (male factor, tubal factor, dysovulation, 'unexplained'), modern assisted conception techniques are very effective (65 +% cumulative conception rate after three cycles of *in vitro* fertilization – embryo transfer for women under 40 years). But treatments are stressful, invasive, and expensive. Few Primary Care Trusts fund treatments such as IVF, and those that do often impose strict eligibility criteria and have long waiting lists.
- The GP should be aware that if fertility treatment fails, couples may need considerable support and counselling. Information about alternatives such as fostering and adoption should be available early, not just as a last resort.

## What you should do

- Check the rubella and cervical smear status of the woman and advise on folic acid supplementation.
- Ask about her current menstrual cycle and ensure she is having regular sexual intercourse during the fertile phase.
- Ask about previous reproductive history, past medical history, current medication, and family history.
- Stress that fertility investigations and treatment are a joint enterprise and that both partners need to be involved. It may be appropriate to arrange for the couple to meet the practice nurse to discuss health promotion such as smoking cessation, reducing alcohol intake, weight and stress management.
- Perform a pelvic examination, either during initial consultation or subsequently, to identify unexpected tenderness, immobility of the pelvic organs or swelling of the adnexae.
- Arrange fertility blood screen, including LH and FSH taken during days 1–3 of the cycle and a mid-luteal phase progesterone (day 21 in a 28-day cycle;

adjust the day of the blood test so that it falls approximately 7 days before the next period is due).

♦ Arrange follow-up appointment with patient and her partner. Semen analysis will need to be done. A freshly masturbated specimen after 2–3 days of abstinence should be delivered to the laboratory within 1 hour. If this sample is abnormal, arrange a repeat.

♦ Consider early referral for specialist advice if history or examination is abnormal in either partner, or if the woman is over 35 and the period of apparent infertility is more than 2 years.

# References

Abdalla, H.I., Baber, R.J., Kirkland, A., Leonard, T. and Studd, J.W. (1989). Pregnancy in women with premature ovarian failure using tubal and intrauterine transfer of cryopreserved zygotes. *British Journal of Obstetrics and Gynaecology*, **96**, 1071–5.

Armar, N.A. and Lachelin, G.C.L. (1993). Laparoscopic ovarian diathermy: an effective treatment for anti-oestrogen resistant anovulatory infertility in women with polycystic ovaries. *British Journal of Obstetrics and Gynaecology*, **100**, 161–4.

Balen, A.H., Braat, D.D., West, C., Patel, A. and Jacobs, H.S. (1994). Cumulative conception and live birth rates after the treatment of anovulatory infertility. *Human Reproduction*, **9**, 1563–70.

Balen, A.H., Conway, G.S., Kaltsas, G., *et al.* (1995). Polycystic ovary syndrome: the spectrum of the disorder in 1741 patients. *Human Reproduction*, **10**, 2107–11.

Botting, B.J., Macfarland, A.J. and Price, F.V. (1990). *Three, four and more. A study of triplet and higher order births*. HMSO, London.

Kovacs, G.T., Newman, G.B. and Henson, G.L. (1978). The post-coital test – what is normal? *British Medical Journal*, **1**, 818.

Mahmood, T.A. and Templeton, A. (1990). Pathophysiology of mild endometriosis: review of literature. *Human Reproduction*, **5**, 765–84.

Marcoux, S., Maheux, R. and Berube, S. (1997). Laparoscopic surgery in infertile women with minimal and mild endometriosis. *New England Journal of Medicine*, **97**, 212–22.

Nielsen, S and Hahlin, M. (1995). Expectant management of first-trimester spontaneous abortion. *Lancet*, **345**, 84–5.

Rossing, M.A., Daling, J.R., Weiss, N.S., Moore, D.E. and Self, S.G. (1994). Ovarian tumours in a cohort of infertile women. *New England Journal of Medicine*, **331**, 771–6.

Royal College of Obstetrics and Gynaecology (1998). *The Initial investigation and management of the infertile couple*. RCOG Press, London.

Skakkeback, N.E. and Keiding, N. (1994). Changes in semen and the testis. *British Medical Journal*, **309**, 1316–17.

Thomas, E.J. and Cooke, I. (1987). Successful treatment of asymptomatic endometriosis: does it benefit infertile women? *British Medical Journal of Clinical Research*, **294**, 1117–9.

Chapter 7

# Cystitis
## Sally Hope and Ian Bowler

When I makes tea I makes tea, as old mother Grogan said. And when I makes water I makes water . . . Begob, ma'am, says Mrs. Cahill, God send you don't make them in the one pot. (*James Joyce, Ulysses, 1922*)

Cystitis is an extremely common problem in women. Estimates vary but it is thought that between 10 and 20% of women are affected by a lower urinary tract infection (UTI) at some point during their lifetime. In the United Kingdom 1–3% of all consultations in general practice are for UTI. There are 5.2 million consultations per year in the USA for UTIs in women, with a billion dollar cost implication.

## Definitions

### Cystitis

Cystitis is an inflammation of the lining of the bladder. It can be produced by an infection from bacteria, viruses, or fungi. Inflammation of the trigone area can also be produced by certain chemicals. In a bacterial infection, the organisms elicit an inflammatory response in the bladder which can be identified by the excretion of polymorphonuclear leucocytes in the urine (Nicolle 1990).

### Bacteriuria

The presence of bacteria in the urine is abnormal, as bladder urine is sterile.

### Significant bacteriuria

To differentiate an infection from contamination, an arbitrary cut-off point has been uniformly recognized. This was adopted after the work of Kass in the 1950s. He quantitatively assessed the predictive value of colony-forming bacteria in urine. From his work it was established that $10^5$ colony-forming units (c.f.u.) bacteria per ml of voided urine is a highly specific threshold for true bacteriuria, but it has a low sensitivity. Recently, Stamm has argued that the threshold should be reduced to $10^2$ c.f.u. for coliforms as a sensitive indicator for infection in symptomatic women, men and children (Johnson 1991). Laboratories usually report in the range of $10^4$ to $>10^5$ c.f.u./ml. The thresholds used have different meanings in different populations, and are a compromise between sensitivity and specificity.

## Asymptomatic bacteriuria

Some women have been found to have significant bacteriuria without any symptoms. This is defined as asymptomatic bacteriuria. This is a benign condition in the elderly, but is a predictor for the development of pyelonephritis in pregnancy. It is important that pregnant women are screened for asymptomatic bacteriuria at 16 weeks by sending a urine for culture; dipstick testing for leucocyte esterase and nitrites are not adequately sensitive.

There is often vaginal contamination of a urine specimen, giving misleading results (see MSUs). Contaminated specimens usually grow a mixture of skin and faecal organisms, whereas in true bacteriuria there is usually a pure growth of a single organism. In fact, Goodfriend argues that it is virtually impossible to obtain a clean voided urine from an elderly obese female.

## Uncomplicated UTIs

An uncomplicated UTI is an infection of the bladder only, in an otherwise fit and well woman with no abnormality of her urinary tract, and no other major predisposing factors (Table 7.1).

## Complicated UTIs

Patients who have functional, anatomical, or metabolic abnormalities are defined as having complicated UTIs (Stamm and Hooton 1993). All infections of the kidneys (upper urinary tract), or any infection of any part of the urinary tract in children, pregnancy, or men should also be regarded as a complicated infection.

## Relapse or reinfection?

Recurrence of bacteriuria with a different organism from the original one is defined as a reinfection. This implies acquisition of a new pathogen. This is in distinction to the recurrence of bacteriuria with the original isolate, which is termed a relapse and implies persistence of the bacteria in the urinary tract.

A true chronic UTI is the persistence of the same organisms in the urinary tract for months or years. Reinfection is a much more common clinical entity than relapse.

## The urethral syndrome

In about 50% of all cases of women who present with acute dysuria and frequency, the urine culture is less than $10^5$ (Johnson 1991), and so is reported as 'sterile'. This is the definition of the 'urethral syndrome', also known descriptively as the frequency and dysuria syndrome. It is a topic fraught with controversy over aetiology, diagnosis, and treatment. Stamm *et al.* (1980) feels that most of the women with symptoms have a true bacterial cystitis, and should be treated accordingly. Maskell *et al.* (1979) feels that there are fastidious bacteria infecting these women, whereas O'Dowd (1995) feels that this group have more in common with irritable bowel sufferers.

Some women may have a *Chlamydia* infection (Oakeshott and Hay 1995), especially in a young, sexually active female using non-barrier contraception who has recently changed sexual partner. In the context of a 'sterile' pyuria, *Chlamydia*, gonococcal urethritis, and tuberculosis of the urinary tract should be considered.

## Presentation of cystitis

Women often present in an agony of acute dysuria, frequency, and urgency. They may have been up all night, needing to void urine every half hour to an hour. They may also have haematuria, which they may find alarming. Suprapubic pain occurs in 10% of cases.

Women with these symptoms may either have acute cystitis, acute urethritis, or acute vaginitis. The history makes the diagnosis in 90% of cases. If the woman is asked to describe the site of the pain, in acute cystitis the inflammation of the trigone area causes 'inside' dysuria (Komaroff and Friedland 1980), whereas with acute urethritis or vaginitis the dysuria feels more on the 'outside'.

If the woman presents with flank pain, low back pain, abdominal pain, fevers, rigors, sweating, headache, nausea and vomiting, malaise, or prostration, an overt upper urinary tract infection is probable. This may need in-patient hospital intravenous antibiotic treatment if she has complicating factors (Table 7.1), or is unable to take antibiotics by mouth.

The problem with 'lower urinary tract infections' is that about one-third of characteristic cases of acute cystitis also have an unrecognized infection of the upper urinary tract (Johnson and Stamm 1989).

**Table 7.1** Risk factors of occult upper urinary tract infection

| |
|---|
| *Physiological* |
| Pregnancy |
| Diabetes mellitus |
| *Anatomical* |
| Urinary tract abnormality |
| Urinary stone |
| Indwelling catheter |
| Recent instrumentation |
| *Past medical history* |
| Previous recurrent UTI, previous UTI as a child, previous pyelonephritis, symptoms present for more than 7 days before presentation, any immunosuppressive condition |
| *Urogenital ageing in the postmenopausal woman* |

## Investigations

### Leucocyte esterase and nitrite dip sticks

It is not helpful, nor cost-effective, to send routine MSUs prior to therapy on healthy, non-pregnant women presenting with acute cystitis. It is reasonable, however, to test the urine with a leucocyte esterase and nitrite dipstick (Hiscoke *et al.* 1990). This has a sensitivity of 75–95% predicting culture-proven infection (Stamm and Hooton 1993). Antibiotics should then be prescribed to those patients who have a positive result for either test. MSUs should only be sent from women with complicated UTI (Table 7.1), screening for asymptomatic bacteriuria of pregnancy, or those women who have failed to respond to first-line therapy.

### Mid-stream sample of urine (MSU)

For many years nurses have spent much time and energy collecting mid-stream urine specimens from patients. In hospital they have used the modified nursing procedure from the Royal Marsden, which requires cleansing of the external genitalia and urethral meatus with three sterile wipes before the patient is required to void the urine into a sterile bowl. The patient is asked to micturate and the mid-stream part of the urine flow is sampled. This reduces the risk of contamination by normal flora in the distal urethra, which are washed away by the initial urinary stream. In non-ambulatory patients who do not have perineal cleaning, the urine specimens are heavily contaminated with mixed faecal and skin flora. However, no difference was found between using a sterile MSU pack and non-sterile wipes in a group of women over the age of 65 (Jones 1992).

In young ambulatory patients, a study using either sterile bowls or non-sterile paper cups as a receiver for the MSU was carried out. There was no difference in the contamination rate using an easy-to-handle, cheap paper cup (White 1992).

Evaluating bacterial contamination from urine sampling techniques, it has been found in a prospective study that holding the labia apart is actually the most significant action when trying to obtain a 'clean' MSU sample. This decreased bacterial contamination from 31.1 to 13% ($P < 0.01$) in healthy young women (Baeheim *et al.* 1992). This is not surprising since the urine leaves the female urethra orifice in a broad stream, splashing on the labia, hosing down vaginal squamous cells, hairs, and bacteria into the receptacle for catching the urine. A full, clean-catch, MSU technique is difficult and time consuming to understand and perform. The simple procedure of asking the patient to hold her labia apart whilst catching the urine in a paper cup significantly decreases contaminated specimens.

Having gone to all the trouble of obtaining a reasonably reliable MSU, the urine inevitably then spends 8 hours on a hot treatment room shelf awaiting collection! This ruins the specimen by bacterial overgrowth. Ideally, the specimen needs to go to the laboratory within 2 hours. In general practice this is rarely possible, and so the urine sample should be refrigerated until transported to the laboratory.

## What follow-up is required of women with UTIs?

No follow-up and no post-urine cultures are required for a simple acute uncomplicated cystitis in a well woman. If she remains symptomatic by the third day of treatment, an MSU should be sent for culture and sensitivity. Any woman with a complex UTI, or during pregnancy, should be closely followed. Two weeks after finishing treatment for a proven complex UTI, an MSU should be sent for follow-up culture.

In the small percentage of women who have recurrent UTIs (>2 UTIs in 6 months or >3 in a year), there is concern that these women may have a stone or an obstructive uropathy as an underlying aetiology. However, on ultrasound, intravenous pyelography, or cystoscopy, fewer than 5% have a demonstrable abnormality (Hooton and Stamm 1991).

For women on continuous prophylaxis, it is essential to send an MSU if they become symptomatic, as this implies a reinfection with a resistant organism. It is imperative to know the culture and sensitivity to make the correct antimicrobial decision.

## Causes of bacterial cystitis

In 1894, Escherich cultured 'bacillus coli' in the urine of children with UTIs and described pyelitis as the disease of childhood. He gave his name to the bacteria, which caused 85% of acute UTIs. *Escherichia coli* (*E. coli*), are facultative anaerobes from the bowel flora. They ascend via the short urethra. Women who have proven *E. coli* urinary tract infections can be shown to have colonization of the vaginal introitus with *E. coli* bacteria of the same serotype. A small percentage of community-acquired infections are from other Gram-negative bacteria: *Klebsiella* and *Proteus*. *Staphylococcus saprophyticus* is the most important of the Gram-positive pathogens (Fig 7.1). Fungi and viruses are rare causes of acute cystitis in the community, but these play a more important part in hospital-acquired infections, or in people who are immunosuppressed (Measley and Levison 1991). Genital herpes may be a cause of frequency, dysuria, and even acute retention.

Bacteria can gain access to the bladder by three possible routes: ascending the very short female urethra, or by lymphatic or haematogenous spread. The overwhelming number of bacterial infections are due to local ascending infection. Infection is determined by the size of the inoculum, the host resistance or defence factors, and the virulence of the pathogen. For example, if the host defences are compromised, only a small inoculum of bacteria is required to produce an infection. In the normal woman with no abnormalities of anatomy or function, a large inoculum of virulent bacteria is required to produce a symptomatic urinary infection. Indeed, the frequent flushing of the bladder by urine is thought to defend a woman from frequent small inocula of bacteria that never proceed to actual infection. The urine itself inhibits bacteria due to its high osmolarity, high urea concentrations and low pH. Tamm–Horsfall proteins competitively inhibit the attachment of *E. coli* to the mucosal surface of the bladder and aggregate bacteria in the urine.

Much research has gone into the virulence factors that might change *E. coli* from a harmless commensal in the bowel flora to a virulent uropathogen (Sobel 1991). In order to facilitate the ascent of bacteria from vaginal introitus and the periurethral skin into the urethra and bladder, the *E. coli* needs to stick to the uroepithelial cells. There are various bacterial surface structures called adhesins and complimentary components, the host receptors, which allow binding to the epithelial surface. In normal women the bacteria have to be virulent in order to cause an infection, whereas if there is a gross underlying structural abnormality, the patient falls prey to a variety of normal bowel flora. The bacterial adhesins take the form of fimbriae; these are peptide subunits that can probe the epithelial surface for receptors. These adhesins act as virulence factors. At a cellular level expression of pili, or *fimbriae*, is much commoner in isolates from patients with cystitis. Type I fimbriae are present in all *E. coli*, and are believed to promote initial colonization. There is little difference between virulence of *E. coli* in women with recurrent or sporadic UTIs, but it seems to be the receptor repertoire for organisms on host urogenital cells that influences susceptibility. Women with recurrent infection have longer durations of vaginal colonization with uropathogenic *E. coli*, and threefold more *E. coli* adhering to the vagina, and voided uroepithelial cells (Stapleton 1999).

There are genetically determined differences in urogenital cell-receptor availability and binding characteristics, which may influence a woman's susceptibility to recurrent UTIs. Women with recurrent UTIs are three to four times more likely to be non-secretors of ABH blood-group antigens, than controls. The secretor gene encodes one of many glycosyltransferases that determine the carbohydrate composition of cell-surface glycoproteins and glycosphingolipids. Some of these serve as binding sites for uropathogenic *E. coli*. In the vaginal epithelium of non-secretors, there are two extended-chain glycosphingolipids that bind uropathogenic *E. coli* more avidly than do other glycosphingolipids (Stapleton 1999). Research is now looking at developing soluble carbohydrate inhibitors to prevent adhesion of pathogenic bacteria to the vaginal mucosa.

Certain features of the host response to bacterial attachment have also been examined. The uroepithelium produces interleukin 6 and 8 in response to a UTI. In women with acute cystitis the systemic immune response is very weak, and local antibody responses are short lived. Urogenital tissues contain antimicrobial peptides, but their role in UTIs is unknown. Much greater understanding of the host immune response is needed before a vaccine is possible. However, a group are looking at a vaccine based on *E. coli* type I fimbrial components.

The normal microbial ecology of the vagina has also caused interest. Factors that disrupt the normal flora, promote the uropathogen predominance that promotes recurrent UTIs. The most important factors are recent use of β-lactam antimicrobials, the more alkaline postmenopausal state (before treatment with exogenous oestrogen), or spermicides for contraception.

Normal vaginal bacterial commensals, lactobacilli, interfere with *E. coli* adherence to uroepithelial cells and probably have a protective effect in normal women. Lactobacillus suppositories, designed to promote the normal state of vaginal flora, are being investigated. There is a thin mucopolysaccharide coating of the transitional epithelial cells of the bladder mucosa, which also inhibits *E. coli* fimbrial attachment. It has also been suggested that antibiotic prophylaxis may work at subtherapeutic doses because the antibiotics inhibit fimbrial production, thus reducing the virulence of *E. coli*, allowing the normal host defence mechanisms of phagocytosis and mechanical flushing to prevent the bacteria colonizing the bladder.

## Treatment

Not all women presenting with the symptoms of acute dysuria and frequency have cystitis. It is reasonable to offer antibiotics to those women who have a positive leucocyte esterase and/or nitrite dipstick test (Hiscoke *et al.* 1990). There has been one recent RCT of nitrofurantoin versus placebo for treating uncomplicated UTIs in adult women (Christiaens *et al.* 2002). It showed that 77% of the group treated with nitrofurantoin showed a symptomatic improvement in 3 days, whereas there was spontaneous improvement in 54% of the placebo group. One of the placebo group developed pyelonephritis, none of the treated group did. The withdrawal rates in the two groups for 'side effects' was 9–10%. This study would not be allowed now (Leibovici 2002), as no written information or signed informed consent was required by Ghent University Hospital ethics committee. However, it is reassuring for GPs to read that we have been right to treat uncomplicated UTIs with antibiotics!

### Cranberry juice

There has been a great recent interest in cranberry juice. Some women have been taking this as an 'alternative therapy' for years, believing it to sterilize the urine. Recent work (Ofek *et al.* 1991) has shown that components in the juice may prevent UTI by inhibiting fimbrial adherence of pathogenic *E. coli*. Uropathogenic *E. coli* adhere to mucosal lining of the urinary bladder with adhesins designated MS and MR on their fimbriae. Plant juices from cranberry, blueberry, or bearberry (*Vaccinium ericaceae*) contained a high molecular weight inhibitor of MR. Attempts to isolate the active agent from cranberry and blueberry juices are being made. Women may prefer this natural remedy, which has fewer side effects, to taking courses of antibiotics. There is also evidence (Avon *et al.* 1994) that continuous prophylactic cranberry juice, as little as 30 ml twice daily, may reduce the rate of UTIs (see continuous treatment section).

## Self-help groups

Angela Kilmartin set up the 'U and I' clubs in the 1970s to help fellow sufferers gain support, knowledge, and understanding. She also wrote *Understanding cystitis* and *Cystitis: a complete self-help guide.* Although the national self-help group is no longer in existence, there are still local groups. There are also a number of free information leaflets, which give basic information about the causes of cystitis and preventive measures, which should be available in surgery waiting rooms.

## Which antibiotics work?

As a general practitioner, the primary aim is to choose the most effective antibiotic. Other considerations are: side effects, safety in potentially pregnant women, and cost. The prevalence of resistance to antibiotics in bacteria changes with time and geographical area: practitioners need to be aware of local patterns of sensitivity (Fig 7.1 and 7.2).

From the data published (Kahlmeter 2000) from 240 centres in 17 countries (the UK was one of those participating, but the USA was not), urine samples from women with uncomplicated UTIs were analysed for urinary pathogen and sensitivity. *E. coli* accounted for 80% of uropathogens in all 17 countries. The rates of resistance among *E. coli* were 30% to ampicillin and

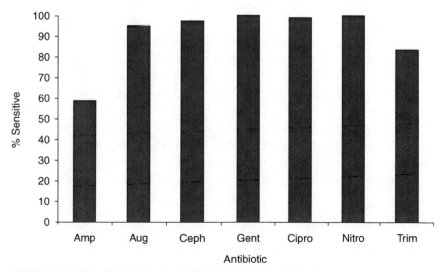

**Fig 7.1** Sensitivities of *E. coli* in urine (UK 1999). Amp, ampicillin; Aug, co-amoxiclav; Ceph, cephalosporin; Gent, gentamicin; Cipro, ciprofloxacin; Nitro, nitrofurantoin; Tri, trimethoprim.

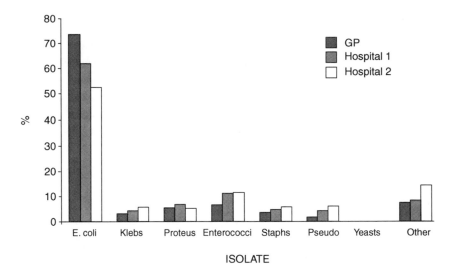

**Fig 7.2** Distribution of urinary isolates (Oxford 1999/2000). Klebs, *Klebsiella*; Staphs, *Staphylococcus saprophyticus*; Pseudo, *Pseudomonas*. [Bowler, I. (2000) *Urinary tract infections acquired in the Oxfordshire Community*. The Public Health Laboratory, John Radcliffe Hospital 01/12/1999–30/11/2000].

sulphamethoxazole, 15% to trimethoprim, 6% to nalidixic acid, 3% to ciprofloxacin, and >2% resistant to amoxicillin-clavulanic acid, mecillinam, cefadroxil, nitrofurantoin and fosfomycin. There is cause for concern that there is a rapid increase in quinolone resistance among community-acquired *E. coli* in Portugal (36%) and Spain (20%). From US data (Saint and Lipsky 1999), looking at changes in the prevalence of resistance from 1992 to 1996, there was a 20% prevalence of resistance to ampicillin, cephalothin, and sulphamethoxazole in the *E. coli* isolates. Resistance to trimethoprim changed from 9% in 1992 to 18% in 1996. Professor Stamm concludes with the ominous statement that in the USA 'trimethoprim may not be an acceptable choice for empirical first-line therapy for much longer'. By contrast, resistance to nitrofurantoin and ciprofloxacin did not change (0–2%). It is important to maintain a dialogue with your local medical microbiologist to develop local protocols for the empirical treatment, taking into account changes in local resistance patterns.

## Specific antibiotics

### Trimethoprim

Trimethoprim is still the antibiotic of choice, but may not be for much longer (Saint and Lipsky 1999) (see above). It is cheap and effective. It is just as effective as co-trimoxazole but has fewer side effects. In the UK, 78% of community-acquired *E. coli* infections will be sensitive to it. This does not mean, however, that 22% of patients will not be sensitive, when treated empirically because resistance detected in the laboratory is not always reflected in clinical failure. It should also be remembered that population-based data generated from urine specimens sent to laboratories should be interpreted with extreme caution since many simple UTIs are treated successfully without recourse to an MSU. Those specimens analysed by laboratories may represent a more complicated patient group, with a higher incidence of resistant flora. Data on antibiotic resistance patterns should be generated from populations appropriate to the patient being treated.

## Nitrofurantoin

This is returning to popularity as a first-line treatment for UTIs as 88% of community-acquired UTIs are sensitive to it. It is also useful for long-term prophylaxis. A further advantage is that it can be safely given to pregnant women, although it may cause neonatal haemolysis if used at term. It does not induce bacterial resistance in the bowel. The major problem with nitrofurantoin is compliance, since it can cause nausea and vomiting (which of course is worse in pregnancy). Nitrofurantoin should not be used for pyelonephritis. This is because it does not achieve cidal levels in the blood or kidney substance. It should only be used to treat lower UTIs. It is an excellent agent for prophylaxis, like trimethoprim.

## Cephalosporins

Most community-acquired infections are still sensitive to the cephalosporins. However, they are more expensive than trimethoprim and also disrupt the major gut flora more, thus giving potentially more side effects to the woman (vaginal thrush, etc). Cephalosporins are the empirical drug treatment of choice in pregnancy and whilst breast-feeding, because of the excellent safety profile.

## Ampicillin/amoxicillin

Unfortunately, because 40% of *E. coli* are now resistant to these drugs, they are no longer recommended for treatment of acute UTI unless the bacterial sensitivities are known. Amoxicillin is safe in pregnancy, and whilst breast-feeding.

## Co-amoxiclav

The addition of the β-lactamase inhibitor clavulanic acid to amoxicillin has improved its effectiveness against *E. coli*. At present, bacteriologists prefer this drug to be left as a second-line agent when the sensitivities are known, or in complicated UTIs. There is no evidence of teratogenicity, but manufacturers advise avoiding co-amoxiclav in pregnancy unless essential.

### The quinolones

These new agents can be used, as a second-line treatment, if trimethoprim has failed or in complicated UTIs. Unfortunately, no quinolone can be used in pregnancy (arthropathy in animal studies). 4-Quinolones should be used with caution in patients with epilepsy or a history of fits, in hepatic or renal impairment, diabetics, and patients taking theophylline or non-steroidal anti-inflammatary drugs (see BNF). The cost for a course of a 4-quinolone is approximately ten times that for trimethoprim.

## Special situations

### Pregnancy

Pregnant women have a higher prevalence of asymptomatic bacteriuria. In the non-pregnant woman, asymptomatic bacteriuria appears to be intermittent and self-limiting, but 4–7% will have bacteriuria throughout pregnancy. It is thought that pregnant women are more prone to asymptomatic bacteriuria because the higher urinary pH allows more rapid colonization by *E. coli*. The progestogen effect on smooth muscle allows relaxation of the urethral meatus, giving both easier ascent of uropathogens into the bladder, and more frequent reflux to the kidneys, causing a higher percentage of complicated upper UTI (Medicine's Resource Centre Bulletin 1995; Johnson 1991). For women with asymptomatic bacteriuria in pregnancy, there is a significant risk that they will experience a symptomatic UTI, with obstetric complications of possible premature labour, small-for-dates babies, and an increased perinatal mortality.

Routine screening of pregnant women for asymptomatic bacteriuria is advised in the 16th week of pregnancy, with an MSU (see above). If asymptomatic bacteriuria is found in these women, treatment should be given to prevent acute pyelonephritis. Pregnant women with asymptomatic bacteriuria should receive at least 7 days' treatment with an antibiotic. Most pregnant women are heavily indoctrinated not to take any drugs during pregnancy. The general practitioner must explain to the woman why she needs to be treated for an asymptomatic condition in the pregnancy, or compliance may be low, with disastrous results. Nitrofurantoin (except at term), amoxicillin and the older cephalosporins are thought to be relatively safe in pregnancy and are commonly used as first-line agents, depending on the sensitivity of the uropathogen and the allergies of the patient. Various antibiotics are not recommended in pregnancy (the quinolones, co-amoxiclav) as the potential risk to the fetus is thought to be more harmful than the potential benefit to the woman. Tetracycline should be avoided in pregnancy as they colour the fetal teeth and bones. Trimethoprim has a theoretical teratogenic risk as it is a folate antagonist, and should be avoided in the first trimester.

If there are problems with bacterial sensitivities of UTI in pregnant women, specialist advice from the local medical microbiologist should be sought. A pregnant woman with the signs of an acute pyelonephritis should be referred for hospital admission as she will probably require intravenous antibiotics.

## Diabetes mellitus

Asymptomatic bacteriuria is 40 times more common in the diabetic woman than the non-diabetic (Measley and Levison 1991). Fungal UTIs are also slightly more common as the glycosuria encourages fungal and bacterial growth. The high urinary glucose also impairs leucocyte phagocytosis. There may be an autonomic neuropathy in long-term diabetics which impairs bladder emptying, predisposing to recurrent infections. Up to 50% of diabetics have upper renal tract involvement. Long-term prophylaxis may be required in this group if there are proven underlying anatomical abnormalities, including significant residual urine due to a neurogenic bladder. Certainly diabetics should be treated immediately if there is a symptomatic infection, and some would argue for routine screening and treatment of asymptomatic patients in this subgroup (Zhanel *et al.* 1990).

## Urinary tract calculi

Stones in the urinary tract irritate the mucosa, which promotes bacterial adherence and colonization. The stone itself also acts as a focus for bacterial persistence. UTIs, in the presence of calculi, are more often caused by *Proteus mirabilis*, and other unusual organisms such as *Ureaplasma urealyticum*, *Klebsiella pneumoniae*, and *Pseudomonas aeruginosa*. The flora may give the clue to reveal an occult urinary tract calculus, particularly if *Proteus* is present. It is impossible to cure a UTI with antibiotics whilst there is a stone present. Bacteria are released from secluded sites deep in the stone, so relapse is inevitable. Treatment requires a urological referral to disrupt the stone by ultrasound, or surgical removal.

## Urogenital ageing

There is a rapid rise in the prevalence of UTIs in postmenopausal women. Women over the age of 60 have an incidence of 15% UTIs per year. In the postmenopausal woman, lactobacilli disappear from the vaginal introitus and the pH of the vagina rises. This favours colonization by *E. coli*. Entry of uropathogens into the urethral meatus may be facilitated by a urethral caruncle, and bladder and uterine prolapse cause a stagnant pool of residual urine after voiding. The vaginal and urethral mucosa is atrophic and more vulnerable to colonization with *E. coli*.

In a double-blind, placebo-controlled trial of intervaginal oestriol cream in postmenopausal women, episodes of bacteriuria were measured (Raz and Stamm 1993). Over an 8-month period, there was a considerable reduction in the frequency of asymptomatic episodes in the women using oestriol cream (nightly for 2 weeks and then twice weekly for 8 months). Of the 50 women in the treated oestriol group, there were 12 episodes of bacteriuria; the 43 in the placebo group had 111 episodes of bacteriuria ($P < 0.005$). Some women withdrew from the treatment group because of pruritis and burning from the oestriol cream. The mean vaginal pH fell from 5.5 to 3.6 in the treated group, and the re-oestrogenized women became recolonized with lactobacilli. Lactobacilli produces lactic acid, which lowers the pH of the vagina and discourages growth of uropathogens. If the vaginal pH is less than 4.5, *E. coli* do not colonize the mucosa. It has also been found in *in vitro* experiments, that fragments of lactobacilli cell wall actually prevent attachment of *E. coli* to epithelial cells. At present it is not known whether this is by stearic hindrance or specific blocking of potential attachment sites.

Although urogenital ageing has been an entity for as long as there have been women that have survived to the postmenopausal period, this is a renewed area of interest at present due to the sudden profusion of local oestrogen treatments (oestrogen pessaries, creams, and rings). There is also full systemic hormone replacement therapy (HRT) without the necessity for monthly withdrawal bleeds, a factor that had previously discouraged many postmenopausal women from continuing on medication (Hope and Rees 1995). The use of HRT in postmenopausal women who do have recurrent UTIs should be considered, and the pros and cons discussed with the patient.

There are data to suggest that if we routinely gave elderly women daily cranberry juice, there would be a significant reduction in bacteriuria and pyuria, with fewer symptomatic UTIs. In one study (Avon *et al.* 1994), 153 elderly women (mean age 78.5 years) enrolled in a double-blind trial of drinking 300 ml fruit juice with vitamin C, with or without cranberry content. Their voided urine study samples were collected at monthly intervals. Bacteriuria ($>10^5$/ml) with pyuria was 42% less after 2 months of cranberry juice, in the cranberry juice group than in the controls. Also over a 6-month period there were 16 symptomatic UTIs in the control group, and 8 in the treated group. The pH of treatment group urine was 6.0, with the mean pH of the control group of 5.5: so this is not an acidification effect.

## Urinary catheters

This is really a very complex topic, and most studies have looked at acutely ill people in the hospital setting, rather than the few, very disabled people that have urinary catheters for chronic problems in the primary care setting. Some helpful conclusions can be drawn from US data (Saint and Lipsky 1999): 25% of hospital patients have a urinary catheter sometime during their stay; 5% of those catheterized will acquire a bacteriuria per day. Thus, after 1 month nearly all will be bacteriuric. The case-fatality rate from UTI-related bacteraemia is 13%; only intravascular catheters lead to more cases of bacteraemia. Lack of proper hand-washing by health-care professionals was largely responsible for cluster outbreaks in the hospital setting, but most nosocomial UTIs reflect endemic acquisition.

### Main recommendations (Saint and Lipsy 1999)

- Avoid using a urinary catheter whenever possible. When used, remove as soon as possible. Inserting a catheter for the convenience of the nursing or medical staff is rarely appropriate.

- Always insert the catheter aseptically, use a closed drainage system, and properly maintain the catheter.

- Consider prophylactic systemic antibiotics only during short-term catheterizations (3–14 days) of patients at high risk for complications of catheter-associated bacteriuria. Most experts do not recommend routine prophylaxis for catheterized patients because of cost, potential adverse reactions, and encouraging antibiotic resistance.

- Consider using a silver alloy catheter in patients at high risk of complications, where catheter placement is relatively short term (<2 weeks).

- Suprapubic catheters may be desirable in patients needing long-term catheterization.

- A condom catheter may be sensible for incontinent men who will not manipulate the device.

- There is no good evidence that bladder irrigation, antibacterial instillation in the drainage bag, rigorous meatal cleaning, and use of meatal lubricants or creams prevent bacteriuria. They should not be used.

## Recurrent simple UTIs in the premenopausal woman

This group of women can have their lives made miserable by recurrent infection. Twenty per cent of women with UTIs have more than two UTIs in 6 months, or three or more UTIs in 12 months. For a woman with persistent recurring infections, an ultrasound of the urinary tract to exclude a stone or an obstructive uropathy may be reasonable, and a referral for cystoscopy if she has persistent haematuria. However, a cause is rarely found. Excretory urography and cystoscopy in women with recurrent urinary tract infections demonstrates anatomical abnormalities in less than 5%, with extremely few correctable lesions (Stamm and Hooton 1993). There are three management strategies for women with recurrent UTIs: postcoital prophylaxis, intermittent self-treatment, and continuous prophylaxis.

### Postcoital prophylaxis

*Next time I'm coming back as a man, he doesn't get cystitis every time we have sex.*

This is effective in women who have a very clear temporal relationship of up to 12 hours between an episode of cystitis and sexual intercourse. Retrospective and prospective studies have shown that sexual intercourse has a mechanical effect in introducing uropathogens into the bladder. Sexually active women have a greater risk ($\times 40$) of infection than non-sexually active women. Some diaphragm users have a higher rate than women using other methods of contraception. There is debate whether this is due to a mechanical effect of the diaphragm in the vagina altering the angle of the bladder neck (from urodynamic studies), or due to the change of vaginal pH from the spermicidal cream or jelly. If the woman gets recurrent postcoital dysuria and uses a diaphragm, it is certainly worth considering either checking the diaphragm for its size and fitting, changing the spermicide, or discussing the use of another form of contraception.

A residual pool of urine in the bladder may act as a reservoir for infection. The woman may be advised to empty the bladder before and after intercourse. Early post-intercourse micturition has a proven protective effect (Hooton and Stamm 1991).

In women who do develop postcoital dysuria a single dose of trimethoprim can prevent an attack if taken immediately prior or post-intercourse. The issue of antibiotics interacting with oral contraceptive drugs must be considered in this group. In a recent paper (Melekos *et al.* 1997) in 135 sexually active premenopausal women were offered either a post-intercourse dose of ciprofloxacin, or daily ciprofloxacin 125 mg. In the study, sexual intercourse rates averaged a mean of 2.52 times per week. During the year, 94% of the post coital group and 95% of the daily group remained symptom free, and had a significant drop ($\times 15$ lower) in measured introital colonization of enteric organisms. The rate of discontinuation due to adverse drug reactions was 5.3% in the continuous group and 1.3% in the postcoital group. The postcoital group consumed 33% less drug. There was a higher rate of thrush in the continuous group (3.9%), there was none in the postcoital group. It is surprising that no one in the postcoital group had thrush all year. A very important point from this trial, which has been consistently shown in other trials, was a mean relapse time after stopping antibiotics of 6–7 months for both groups (they were followed for a year). Recolonization of the vaginal introitus with pathogenic *E. coli* seems to take time after a year's treatment with antibiotics.

## Intermittent self-treatment

Most women do not like taking drugs continuously. They may only get three attacks of cystitis a year and resent having to take daily medication for this unlikely event. From their symptoms, 92% of women can correctly self-diagnose a UTI (Stamm and Hooton 1993). This is because acute cystitis usually presents with the same symptoms each time. When giving women antibiotics to start treatment on their own, they should be told that if the symptoms have not completely resolved within 48 hours they should seek medical attention. Women prefer this method as they feel more in control of their body and their medication.

## Continuous prophylaxis

A low-dose nightly antibiotic, or even twice weekly, can reduce the recurrence of urinary tract infections by 95%. If the woman relapses on prophylaxis the uropathogen is inevitably a reinfection with a different organism that is resistant to the antibiotic being used. Urinary cultures must be made to identify the uropathogen and define its sensitivity to antimicrobial agents. It seems reasonable to plan a year of treatment, and then 6 months off.

Brumfitt and Hamilton-Miller (1998) looked at 219 females aged 9–89 with recurrent UTIs, and gave them a year's prophylaxis with nitrofurantoin. They chose three different regimens: 50 mg microcrystalline nitrofurantoin twice a day, 100 mg macrocrystalline nitrofurantoin once a day, or 50 mg macrodantin daily at bedtime. In all groups there was a 5.4-fold decrease in symptomatic episodes. Women with proven abnormalities of their urinary tract responded just as well as those without a structural abnormality. In 16%, prophylaxis was not helpful, for no clear reason as they still had nitrofurantoin-sensitive UTIs: in their paper they do not mention how they tested compliance with treatment. The macrodantin group had the lowest dropout rate for adverse reactions, which were mainly nausea. Clinical improvement in all groups was maintained for 6 months after the end of prophylaxis, which was also found from the Melekos group (see post-intercourse). The conclusion was that macrocrystalline nitrofurantoin 50 mg at bedtime is an effective, safe, and appropriate choice for long-term (12 months), prophylaxis for UTIs.

## Questions doctors might raise

### When should cystitis be treated?

General practitioners are in an extremely difficult position because women with cystitis require immediate treatment. However, half of all non-pregnant women with the symptoms of urgency, dysuria, and frequency will have no detectable bacterial infection (but see: What is significant bacteriuria?). In about 50% of cases with a proven bacteriuria, symptoms may resolve through natural host defences without drug treatment in 3 days. It could, therefore, be argued that no woman should be treated for a lower urinary tract infection until they have had 3 days of symptoms. However, this is putting a large number of women potentially at risk from ascending infection, and the misery of 3 days of illness. Many women try to avoid taking antibiotics for recurrent UTIs since they know from bitter experience that the eradication of pathogenic bacteria from their urinary tract has an effect on their commensal flora of bowel and vagina (Medicine's Resource Centre Bulletin 1995). The broad-spectrum penicillins in particular destroy the commensal flora, including the lactobacilli, so facilitating the colonization of the urethral introitus with resistant Gram-negative organisms, and also allowing *Candida albicans* to gain dominance in the vagina. Many women know that they get thrush after antibiotics, but still 75% of women do not realize the link. Trimethoprim and nitrofurantoin do not usually select resistant bowel organisms and leave the urethral flora undisturbed, protecting the patient against Gram-negative colonization (Maskell 1992).

It would seem reasonable to treat only those symptomatic women who are dipstick positive for leucocytes and/or nitrites. It is also reassuring to know that the weight of evidence favours the conclusion that although UTIs can produce severe impairment of renal function, this is rare in the absence of major predisposing factors such as obstruction, stones, reflux, abnormalities of the voiding mechanisms, pregnancy, or diabetes mellitus (Kunin 1990).

### What is significant bacteriuria?

The whole topic of UTIs is fraught with problems of definition. The work by H.E. Kass defining significant bacteriuria as $>10^5$ colony-forming units (c.f.u.) per ml of voided urine was based on two groups of women, with asymptomatic bacteriuria and acute pyelonephritis. This has been widely generalized to all patient populations with UTIs but has never been evaluated for cystitis. The only reliable urine specimen is obtained by bladder aspiration or sterile catheterization; but these are invasive, uncomfortable, and not feasible in general practice. Voided urine is easy to collect, but inevitably contaminated with periurethral flora.

A general practitioner needs a test that reliably distinguishes true bladder bacteriuria from contaminated specimens. On the Kass definition of $10^5$ c.f.u./ml, many women with the symptoms of dysuria and frequency are told 'there's nothing wrong'. Stamm and Hooton (1993) argue that a new significant bacteriuria threshold should be agreed of $>10^2$ uropathogens per ml for symptomatic patients. This proves to be far more sensitive for *E. coli* (0.95), and only slightly less specific (0.85). This threshold of $10^2$ c.f.u. coliforms is a very sensitive indicator of infections since if these women are followed they will invariably reach a count of $10^5$ over the succeeding days (Johnson 1991). At present, laboratories have not taken up this revised $>10^2$ c.f.u. suggestion: in the UK laboratories report in the range of $10^5$ to $>10^5$ c.f.u./ml.

## Should I screen women for asymptomatic bacteriuria?

The first problem is what is true asymptomatic bacteriuria, and what is contamination. Of true asymptomatic bacteriuria, 30% will become symptomatic in time and the women will then seek treatment. However, most women with true asymptomatic bacteriuria appear to experience it as a transient phenomenon. Women therefore get intermittent asymptomatic bacteriuria, which can resolve without treatment (Zhanel *et al.* 1990). Since women with asymptomatic bacteriuria either present sooner or later with an acute urinary tract infection, or self-cure, there seems at present no good argument for routine screening of the whole sexually active population of women. However, there are a few subgroups that should be considered: antenatal women, women with known abnormalities of their urinary tract, and diabetics.

## When should an MSU be sent?

Given that voided urine in the general practice setting is almost inevitably contaminated (Jones 1992; White 1992; Baeheim *et al.* 1992), is there any point in sending one at all? The other major problem with sending urine for culture and sensitivity is one has to make an immediate therapeutic decision when seeing the patient about treatment, and the results from the laboratory will come back 3 days later when 80–90% of the patients seen and treated should be completely better.

In a survey of Danish GPs, microbiologists, and urologists, 48% of GPs, but only 24% of microbiologists said they would routinely send a urine sample for culture on a previously fit 30-year-old woman (Olesen and Oestergaard 1995). In Oxfordshire, the implementation of guidelines on the use of the laboratory for urine culture, has led to better patient management and more efficient use of the laboratory (Bowler *et al.* 1998).

## What length antibiotic course?

The literature is full of studies varying from single-dose antibiotics to a full 6-week course for acute UTIs (Stamm *et al.* 1987; Johnson and Stamm 1989; Bailey 1990; Nicolle 1990; Johnson 1991; Medicine's Resource Centre Bulletin 1995). The advocates of a single-dose therapy argue that this is the treatment of choice for uncomplicated UTIs in general practice since a single dose ensures compliance and cures simple cystitis. There will be an immediate relapse in the 30% who have an occult upper UTI. This can be looked on as a useful clinical guide to those patients who need further investigation, intensive treatment, and supervision. Other workers in the field are concerned that the single-dose regimen is less effective; further validation with large, controlled trials are still needed.

The 3-day course is now in vogue. It has the advantage of fewer side effects over the previously favoured 7–14-day treatment schedules, and a lower relapse rate than a single dose. However, some bacteriologists argue that although a 3-day course of trimethoprim is effective, if nitrofurantoin is used 5–7 days is better.

If an upper renal tract infection is suspected, there is evidence that a 14-day course of antibiotics is as effective as a 6-week course with fewer side effects (concomitant thrush, drug reactions such as rashes and diarrhoea, and patient compliance). There is also less likelihood of reinfection with resistant organisms.

In all uncomplicated non-pregnant female patients with lower UTIs, a 3-day course of trimethoprim or nitrofurantoin seems reasonable (Measley and Levison 1991). There is still controversy as to whether complicated UTIs (including those of pregnant women) should be treated with a 7-, 10- or 14-day course.

## Does the urethral syndrome need treatment?

There seems little doubt that the 'urethral syndrome' has several possible causes, and should be reclassified by the various aetiologies. Since 55% of patients with acute dysuria and frequency do not have 'significant bacteriuria', how should they be treated? Many women with acute symptoms are told by the receptionist that there is 'nothing wrong' when they telephone for their MSU result. This leaves the patient confused and angry.

As previously discussed, some women do have counts of $10^2$, which should be considered as 'significant' (Stamm *et al.* 1980). However, this level of bacteria would be reported as 'no growth' by a laboratory using the Kass criteria. Stamm is a strong advocate that many of these women actually have a bacterial infection, despite a 'negative' culture. He argues that women with less than $10^5$ c.f.u./ml should not be ignored if they have symptoms. Often they have low counts because they are early in the infection, and can be shown to achieve counts of $10^5$ over the following few days. Other reasons for a low bacterial count are a rapid urine flow because the women is drinking so much, a low urine pH <5 decreases the ability of *E. coli* to multiply, and possible bacteriostatic agents in the urine from over-the-counter preparations, or cranberry juice. Stamm claims that 95% of dysuric women with proven pyuria have treatable infections.

*Chlamydia trachomatis* is certainly an underdiagnosed cause of urethritis in sexually active women with pyuria (Oakeshott and Hay 1995). The prevalence of *Chlamydia* infection varies between 2 and 12% in general practice populations. Women under the age of 25 with a recent change of sexual partner, who do not use barrier contraception, are the major 'at-risk' group. They may also present with a mucopurulent vaginal discharge. On examination the cervix is friable and there is sterile pyuria. The difficulty of detecting *Chlamydia* in general practice is one that needs to be addressed, as many of these women go undiagnosed and untreated, and their contacts untraced. If cervical abnormalities are detected, such patients should be investigated for *Chlamydia* according to locally agreed protocols. The long-term sequelae of possible pelvic inflammatory disease and ectopic pregnancy must be avoided. The actual risk to an individual from one episode of *Chlamydia* has not yet been quantified.

There is still a group of women who have dysuria and pyuria who do not have *Chlamydia* or more than $10^2$ uropathogenic *E. coli*. Rosamund Maskell advocates that these women have fastidious micro-organisms that need to be grown in carbon-dioxide-dependent cultures. There is still controversy about these 'fastidious' bacteria, and her work has not been supported by other researchers in the field (Maskell *et al.* 1979; Brumfitt and Hamilton-Miller 1990).

O'Dowd (1995), feels that the syndrome has much more in common with the irritable bowel syndrome than it does with urinary tract infection. They may coexist within the same patient and he feels that these women may receive unnecessary courses of antibiotics without giving support and understanding to the psychological aspects that may be causing somatization in women who have no clear infective aetiology for their urethral symptoms.

As there has really been no satisfactory explanation for this group of women with symptoms but no isolated causative agent, this group have naturally given up on conventional medicine and turned to self-help. Women have tried changing their diet to a ketogenic one on the understanding that this might change the local environment and pH of the urethra. Women also try excluding caffeine (tea, coffee, and cola drinks), which excites the detrusor muscle of the bladder. They may try making their urine alkaline, or acid, since the optimal pH for *E. coli* is pH 6–7. If the pH is changed, some women find symptomatic relief.

However, there remains an unhappy, untreated, symptomatic group of women who have the diagnosis of urethral syndrome with (at present) no underlying aetiological factor. This group needs to be studied further.

### Should the woman be advised to drink a large quantity?

One of the few things everyone seems to know about cystitis is that the sufferer should increase their fluid intake. The normal range of urine osmolarity is 300–1200 mosmol/l; if urine becomes very dilute (<200 mosmol/l) growth of bacteria is reduced. A diuresis also helps bladder emptying, theoretically allowing the pathogenic *E. coli* to be flushed out of the system (although this ignores the *E. coli*'s ability to attach on to the bladder wall epithelium).

Women also drink substances to change the pH of their urine, to create a less favourable environment for the pathogenic *E. coli*, which further confuses the picture. However, some people argue that an excessive diuresis may actually enhance vesicouretheral reflux and in some cases actually facilitate bacteria reaching the kidneys. It also dilutes antibacterial substances in the urine, which may decrease their therapeutic efficacy. There is no prospective trial on the beneficial or detrimental use of drinking fluids in women with uncomplicated urinary tract infections. This is distinct from the beneficial effects of drinking cranberry juice, which has been found to inhibit pathogenic *E. coli* fimbrial adherence.

# 10-Minute consultation: cystitis

Consultations with a woman for a UTI can sometimes be the quickest and easiest, or the most complex; involving all the issues of that woman's lifestyle, diet, contraception, sexual activity, and stresses with relationships (Johnson and Stamm 1989; Medicine's Resource Centre Bulletin 1995).

- Take a history. Is there frequency, and burning dysuria? Is the pain inside (a trigonitis) or outside (a vaginitis)? Is there haematuria? (If just painless haematuria this should be investigated with cystoscopy.) Does the pain radiate up to the flank (complicated or upper UTI)? Is the patient having rigors? (Do they need to be admitted: immunosuppressed, diabetes out of control, pregnant).

- Test urine for leucocytes and nitrites. If positive for either, treat. If negative, think again. Examine patient if, from history, could be a *Chlamydia* urethritis, or candidiasis, etc.

- Is she pregnant, or trying to be? Ask about LMP. Prescribe appropriately, and discuss issues of safety of antibiotics in pregnancy to reach concordance.

- What contraception is she using? This may be related to the UTI. Some spermicides predispose to UTIs. Does she get UTIs after sex? Consider discussing postcoital prophylaxis. Will your antibiotic prescription make her oral contraceptive pill less effective?
- Is she having recurrent UTIs? Why? Has she been previously investigated?
- Treat a simple UTI in a non-pregnant woman with trimethoprim 200 mg twice daily for 3 days, or nitrofurantoin 100 mg twice a day for 3 days.
- Give her a urine bottle and ask her to bring in a clean-catch specimen (mid-stream with one hand holding bottle, other hand holding labia apart) in 3 days if no better.
- Advise on reasonable fluid intake; some women don't drink during the day in their offices either because of officious bosses or the disgusting state of the lavatories (this seems a real problem with school children at present). Discuss the useful prophylactic effect of small amounts of cranberry juice (30 ml twice a day).
- Agree follow-up consultation if appropriate.

# References

Avon, J., Monane, M., Gurwitz, J., *et al.* (1994). Reduction of bacteriuria and pyuria after ingestion of cranberry juice. *Journal of the American Medical Association*, **271**, 751–4.

Baeheim, A., Asbjorn, D. and Hunskaar, S. (1992). Evaluation of urine sampling technique: bacterial contamination of samples from women students. *British Journal of General Practice*, **42**, 241–3.

Bailey, R.R. (1990). Review of published studies on single dose therapy of urinary tract infections. *Infection*, **18**(S2), 553–5.

Bowler, I. (2000). Urinary tract infections acquired in the Oxfordshire community – (unpublished data). The Public Health Laboratory, John Radcliffe Hospital, Oxford.

Bowler, I., Atkins, B. and Batchelor, B. (1998). Impact on guidelines for the diagnosis of UTI. *British Journal of General Practice*, **48**, 1790.

Brumfitt,W. and Hamilton-Miller, J.M.T. (1998). Efficacy and safety profile of long-term nitrofurantoin in urinary infections: 18 years experience. *Journal of Antimicrobial Chemotherapy*, **42**, 363–71.

Brumfitt, W. and Hamilton-Miller, J.M.T. (1990). Urinary Infections in the 1990s: the state of the art. *Infection* **18**(S2), 534–9.

Christiaens, T.C.M., De Meyere, M., Verschraegen, G., *et al.* (2002). Randomised controlled trial of nitrofurantoin versus placebo in the treatment of uncomplicated urinary tract infection in adult women. *British Journal of General Practice*, **52**, 729–34.

Gupta, K., Scholes, D. and Stamm,W. (1999). Increasing prevalence of antimicrobial resistance among uropathogens causing acute uncomplicated cystitis in women. *Journal of the American Medical Association*, **281**, 736–8.

Hiscoke, C., Yoxall, H., Greig, D. and Lightfoot, N.F. (1990). Validation of a method for the rapid diagnosis of urinary tract infection suitable for a general practice. *British Journal of General Practice*, **40**, 403–5.

Hooton, T.M. and Stamm,W.E. (1991). Management of acute uncomplicated urinary tract infections in adults. *Medical Clinics of North America*, **75**(2), 339–57.

Hummers-Pradier, E. and Kochen, M.M. (2002). Urinary tract infections in adult general practice patients. *British Journal of General Practice*, **52**, 752–61.

Johnson, C. (1991). Definitions, classification, and clinical presentation of urinary tract infections. *Medical Clinics of North America*, **75**, 241–52.

Johnson, R.J. and Stamm,W.E. (1989). Urinary tract infections in women. Diagnoses and Treatment. *Annals of Internal Medicine*, **111**, 906–17.

Jones, E. (1992). In search of a fine specimen. *Nursing Times*, **88**(6), 62–3.

Kahlmeter, G. (2000). The ECOSENS project: a prospective, multinational, multicentre epidemiological survey of the prevalence and antimicrobial susceptibility of urinary tract pathogens-interim report. *Journal of Antimicrobial Chemotherapy*, **46**(S1), 15–22.

Komaroff, A.L. and Friedland, G. (1980). The dysuria-pyuria syndrome. *New England Journal of Medicine*, **303**, 452–3.

Kunin, C.M. (1990). Natural history of lower urinary tract infections. *Infection*, **18**(S2), 44–9.

Leibovici, L. (2002). Antibiotic treatment for cystitis. *British Journal of General Practice*, **52**, 708–10.

Maskell, R. (1992). Antibacterial agents and urinary tract infection: a paradox. *British Journal of General Practice*, **42**, 138–9.

Maskell, R., Pead, L. and Allen, J. (1979). The puzzle of the 'urethral syndrome': a possible answer? *Lancet*, **1**, 1058–9.

Measley, R.E. and Levison M.E. (1991). Host defence mechanisms in the pathogenesis of urinary tract infections. *Medical Clinics of North America*, **75**(2), 275–86.

Medicines Resource Centre Bulletin 6 (1995). *Urinary tract infection*, No. 8, August 1995.

Melekos, M.D., Asbach, H.W., Gerharz, E., *et al.* (1997). Post-intercourse versus daily ciprofloxacin prophylaxis for recurrent urinary tract infections in premenopausal women. *Journal of Urology*, **157**, 935–9.

Nicolle, L.E. (1990). The optimal management of lower urinary tract infections. *Infection*, **18**(S50), 50–2.

Oakeshott, P. and Hay, P. (1995). General practice update. *Chlamydia* infection in women. *British Journal of General Practice*, **45**, 615–20.

O'Dowd, T. (1995). In: McPherson, A. (ed.), *Women's problems in general practice*, pp. 288–9. Oxford University Press, Oxford.

Ofek, I., Goldhar, J., Zafriri, D., Lis, H., Adar, R. and Sharon, N. (1991). Anti-*Escherichia coli* adhesin activity of cranberry and blueberry juices. *New England Journal of Medicine*, **324**, 1599.

Olesen, F. and Oestergaard, I. (1995). Patients with urinary tract infection: proposed management strategies of general practitioners, microbiologists and urologists. *British Journal of General Practice*, **45**, 611–13.

Raz, R. and Stamm, W.E. (1993). A controlled trial of intravaginal estriol in post-menopausal women with recurrent UTIs. *New England Journal of Medicine*, **329**, 753–6.

Saint, S. and Lipsky, S.A. (1999). Preventing catheter-related bacteriuria. Should we? Can we? How? *Archives of Internal Medicine*, **159**, 800–8.

Sobel, J.D. (1991). Bacterial etiologic agents in the pathogenesis of urinary tract infection. *Medical Clinics of North America*, **75**(2), 253–73.

Stamm, W.E. and Hooton, M. (1993). Management of urinary tract infections in adults. *New England Journal of Medicine*, **329**, 1328–34.

Stamm, W.E., Wagner, K.F., Amsel, R., *et al.* (1980). Causes of the acute urethral syndrome in women. *New England Journal of Medicine*, **303**, 409–15.

Stamm, W.E., McKevitt, M. and Counts, G.W. (1987). Acute renal tract infection in women: treatment with trimethoprim-sulphamethoxazole or ampicillin for two or six weeks. *Annals of Internal Medicine*, **106**, 341–5.

Stapleton, A. (1999). Prevention of recurrent urinary-tract infections in women. *Lancet*, **353**, 7–8.

White, S. (1992). Choosing the right container. *Nursing Times*, **88**(6), 64.

Zhanel, G.G., Harding, G.K. and Guay, D.R. (1990). Asymptomatic bacteriuria. Which patients should be treated? *Arch Intern Medicine*, **150**, 1389–96.

Chapter 8

# Management of urinary incontinence in women

Ranee Thakar, Stuart Stanton and Judy Kane

## Definition and prevalence

Urinary incontinence is defined by the International Continence Society as an involuntary loss of urine that is objectively demonstrable and a social and hygiene problem (Abrams *et al.* 1988). It not only causes considerable personal suffering for the individual affected but is also of immense economic importance to the Health Service costing the nation approximately 424 million pounds per annum (The Continence Foundation, 2000). Women do not report urinary incontinence due to shame, embarrassment and ignorance regarding treatment options. Norton *et al.* (1988) found more than 25% of women with urinary incontinence delayed seeking help for 5 or more years, half of these due to embarrassment, despite significant impact on their lives.

In a survey of 10 226 adults aged over 40 (constituting a 70% response from those approached) the Medical Research Council team in Leicester have reported a 20.2% prevalence of incontinence in women (Perry *et al.* 2000). The average Primary Care Group (PCG) (population 102 700) will have more than 5600 people with urinary and more than 900 with faecal incontinence [Royal College of Physicians (RCP) 1995], with a highly conservative estimate to an average PCG being £737 000 per annum (The Continence Foundation 2000). Table 8.1 summarizes the prevalence from a variety of studies (RCP 1995). Overall, it is likely that about 3 million are regularly incontinent in the UK, a prevalence of around 40 per 1000 men and women (Norton 1996). The prevalence increases with age and is far higher among people in residential and nursing care (RCP 1995).

## Classification

Incontinence may be broadly divided into urethral sphincter incompetence (genuine stress incontinence) and the overactive bladder (detrusor instability)

**Table 8.1** Prevalence of urinary incontinence

| Women living at home | Men and women living in the Institution |
| --- | --- |
| 15–44 years: 5–7% | Residential homes: 25% |
| 45–64 years: 8–15% | Nursing home: 40% |
| 65+ years: 10–20% | Hospital – long-stay care: 50–70% |

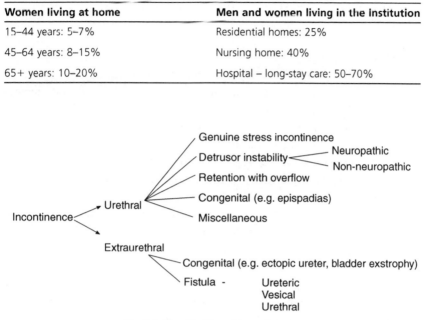

**Fig 8.1** Classification of incontinence.

Fig 8.1 shows the classification of causes. Bladder symptoms often do not correlate with the underlying diagnosis. Thus stress incontinence may occur with bladder overactivity.

# Assessment

## History

Women do not necessarily volunteer information about incontinence, but GPs must take the opportunities that exist, for example at the new patient check, to address the issue specifically. In addition, a routine inquiry about incontinence should be part of every well-woman check, be it for a cervical smear, hormone replacement therapy (HRT), or for contraceptive advice. Ante- and postnatal consultations are also valuable occasions to ask about continence.

## Constitutional

White race, obesity, and advanced age are judged by most to be risk factors for developing incontinence. White women have a shorter urethra, lower bladder neck and poorer pelvic floor muscles compared with black women, which may account for the higher incidence of incontinence in the former (Lara and Nacey 1994).

## General medical

All major system pathologies need to be ascertained to exclude conditions that would require a different approach to management. To take neurological examples first, multiple sclerosis can affect bladder function: indeed, urinary retention with overflow incontinence is sometimes the presenting symptom. Both MS and stroke also cause disabilities that can make it difficult for a patient with urge incontinence to get to a toilet in time. Similarly, a peripheral neuropathy secondary to diabetes mellitus, and Parkinsonism can be causes of incontinence. Anxiety states and dementia need to be excluded.

Chronic cough, secondary to smoking, chronic obstructive pulmonary disease (COPD), and other respiratory conditions, is a major provoker of stress incontinence. No opportunity should be missed to give smoking cessation advice, as patients are more likely to give up when there is a clear secondary gain.

Constipation, through straining, causes an increase in intra-abdominal pressure and stress incontinence. Faecal impaction makes urinary infection more likely. Faecal incontinence is associated with urinary incontinence in up to 64% of elderly nursing home patients (Ouslander *et al.* 1982). As this provides further embarrassment for the patient, it is important not to miss this part of the history, since treatment will need to be targeted at both forms of incontinence to improve quality of life.

Of the endocrine diseases that lead to frequency of micturition, diabetes is the most common, yet the occasional patient finds their way to a gynaecological out-patient department without a urine dipstick analysis having been done first. Hypothyroidism, hyperparathyroidism, and hypokalaemia can also cause urinary symptoms so need excluding.

## General pelvic

Obstetric history is required in detail to assess potential previous damage to the pelvic floor, including number of births, mode of delivery, and birth weights. Nulliparous women, compared to their parous counterparts, have less urinary incontinence. High birth weight is associated with more severe pelvic floor denervation and pudendal nerve damage (Snooks *et al.* 1984). Stress incontinence is not only more common in pregnancy, but also in the post-natal period and subsequent pregnancies (Chaliha *et al.* 1999).

Menstrual history may also provide important information. Stress incontinence is more common in the week preceding a period and menorrhagia may indicate the presence of a large fibroid.

Previous abdominal and pelvic surgery, such as hysterectomy and colposuspension procedures, need to be documented and it should be remembered that irradiation to the pelvis can produce impaired bladder compliance.

Low oestrogen levels in postmenopausal women may lead to weakness of the bladder neck supports, so the age of onset of the menopause and use of HRT is useful to know, though the latter as therapy for urinary incontinence is controversial.

Urinary tract infections and history of sexually transmitted disease are important to document as those with a positive history should have additional investigations such as an midstream urine (MSU) and culture for chlamydia.

## Drug history

Many therapies in common use act on bladder or urethral function. Diuretics are obvious culprits, particularly as they are frequently needed by patients who find it less easy to reach a toilet quickly and can therefore precipitate urge incontinence. α-Adrenergic blockers such as doxazosin reduce urethral sphincter pressure and so increase stress incontinence. Tricyclic antidepressants can lead to voiding difficulties and occasionally retention of urine. Non-steroidal anti-inflammatory agents can induce cystitis-like symptoms. Drugs which cause constipation should be reduced or eliminated if possible.

## Social history

Social limitations may not be volunteered by the patient, so this aspect of the history requires sensitive probing. Frequently reported problems are lack of desire to leave the home, a worry about smelling of urine, a feeling of not being able to join in any sporting activity, and a fear of having sexual intercourse. This in turn can jeopardize relation- and friendships.

Going to work and on holiday may be tainted with fears of incontinence and the cost implications are considerable if frequent pad changing is necessary. Washing sheets and clothes can be onerous on the elderly and involve the use of the home care services. Sleep disturbance can lead to tiredness and so further damage ability to function during the day. Inevitably emotional problems emerge.

Women who completed the King's Health Questionnaire (mean age 51.4 years) showed that, despite good general health, those with detrusor instability noticed a greater detrimental effect on quality of social and emotional life than those with genuine stress incontinence. However, physical impairment was worse with the latter. Condition-specific quality of life questionnaires should be used more readily as they not only provide useful baseline information that might alter management but can be used post-treatment to assess the impact of different regimens on daily living. However, this may not be practical in a GP setting.

### Specific bladder history

#### Filling

A detailed history of fluid intake needs to focus not only on quantity but type of liquid consumed and at what times of day. Caffeine, which releases calcium from intracellular stores in the smooth muscle of the gut, can produce a hyper-active bladder with urge incontinence, presumably by facilitating calcium release within the cell. Add to this the diuretic effect of caffeine and it is not surprising that many patients notice a reduction in symptoms when they stop drinking it. Excess alcohol can also exacerbate urinary incontinence.

#### Voiding

This is the most tricky part of the history as by the end one needs to know the number of times, amount, and difficulties in the process of voiding. A urinary chart, with the time of day running vertically, and fluid volume in/output for each day of the week horizontally, is the most accurate way of gauging intake and output of fluid.

Frequency is defined as the passage of urine every 2 hours, or more than seven times during the day. Nocturia is the interruption of sleep on two or more occasions each night, on a regular basis, expressly to micturate. The number of voidings by day and by night should be recorded.

It is always difficult for the patient to estimate the *amount* of loss of urine but useful hints might be gained by asking:

- number of wet episodes per week or per day;
- number of events by night (more difficult to evaluate);
- pad use, and if so which 'strength' (most over-the-counter pad packets are marked with 'drip' symbols – one representing least absorbency and three most;
- the presence of soaked clothing despite pads;
- the presence of soaked bedclothes.

### Symptoms

#### Stress incontinence

This is the main symptom of urethral sphincter incompetence (USI), also known as genuine stress incontinence (GSI). It is important to note that stress incontinence is a symptom and *not* a diagnosis. It can also be a feature of detrusor instability.

Any activity that increases intra-abdominal pressure will provoke stress incontinence, so questioning should centre around coughing, sneezing, running, jumping, lifting heavy objects, or any sudden movement or change in posture.

## Urge incontinence

Urge incontinence and urgency of micturition are symptoms of detrusor instability. The need to hurry to reach the toilet day or night, and whether she makes it in time or not, are the hallmarks of these conditions. The presence of frequency, nocturia, urgency when putting the key in the door, giggle, and coital incontinence should all be ascertained as they too are symptoms of detrusor instability.

## Post-micturition dribbling

Post micturition dribbling, if present, might indicate a urethral diverticulum, but may also indicate overflow incontinence.

## Retention of urine

Retention of urine is marked by frequency, stress incontinence, and being continuously wet. The patient may have a recent history of needing to strain to pass urine and the feeling that voiding is incomplete.

## Unconscious incontinence

Unconscious incontinence is the involuntary loss of urine which is unaccompanied by urge or stress. The patient may be aware of the subsequent wetness. The most useful question is 'have you ever passed urine without realizing it?' Detrusor overactivity due to an underlying neurological condition is the most likely cause of this symptom.

## Continuous leakage

Continuous leakage is most distressing for the patient. Because they are wet all the time, the vulval skin becomes excoriated and infected and the added embarrassment of an unpleasant odour is difficult to eliminate. It is caused by sphincter incompetence, retention with overflow, or extraurethral incontinence.

# Examination

## General

A warm, relaxed environment, with a chaperone if appropriate, is crucial in securing the cooperation of the patient. In the first instance the body mass index (BMI) needs to be noted before she is asked to lie on the couch, and then her agility observed. Abdominal examination must focus on the kidney and bladder areas, as well as checking for a loaded bowel or masses arising from the pelvis.

The neurological examination needs to concentrate on the pupillary reflexes and a check for nystagmus, followed by lower limb examination with special attention paid to the S2–S4 nerve roots. The patient then ought to be turned over to look for evidence of spina bifida. Anal sphincter tone is assessed by rectal examination, and an intact sacral reflex, by stroking the surface of the skin adjacent to the anus, to elicit contraction.

### Specific

The vulva should be inspected for excoriation due to wetness. It is also necessary to look for evidence of atrophy, and the urethra examined for signs of discharge or caruncle. Bimanual examination can assess not only uterus and ovaries but also the bladder, urethra, and rectum. A residual volume of more than 200 ml can generally be detected. The presence of stress incontinence can be elicited by asking the patient, with a moderately filled bladder, to cough, whilst the doctor holds a small pad in contact with the urethra. A Cusco speculum examination will enable any intravaginal pathology to be seen, including any excess wetness from a fistula or ectopic ureter, while use of a Sims speculum helps to determine a prolapse. Anterior vaginal wall prolapse may be due to a cystocele or cystourethrocele and is important to note as its presence may affect management – earlier referral for instance. About 40% of patients with urethral sphincter incompetence will have significant anterior vaginal descent (Cardozo and Stanton 1980). Finally, the pelvic floor is evaluated for its ability to contract. It is important to look for rare causes of incontinence, for example congenital abnormalities such as epispadias and fistular openings might be seen in patients with other underlying pathologies such as Crohn's disease.

## Investigations done by the GP

### Midstream urine (MSU) culture and sensitivity and dipstick

A midstream urine dipstick should be performed looking for white blood cells and nitrites and if positive sent for culture and sensitivity.

### Blood biochemistry

If indicated, blood biochemistry should be done to exclude chronic renal disease, hypokalaemia or hyperparathyroidism.

## Investigations done in specialist centres

### Urodynamic studies

These tests are done at a specialist centre and are indicated in the following conditions:
- failure of conservative treatment;
- complex symptomatology;

- failed continence surgery;
- voiding difficulty;
- neuropathy.

### Pad test

A pad test is a simple, inexpensive and non-invasive method of demonstrating urinary loss when this is not proven on cystometry or videocystourethrography. The one hour pad test as recommended by the ICS is probably the most reliable (Abrams *et al.* 1988; Mayne and Hilton 1989). The pad test does not indicate the cause of the leakage, but gives a guide to the severity of involuntary urinary loss (Sutherst *et al.* 1981).

### Uroflowmetry

Uroflowmetry measures maximum flow rate, volume voided, average flow rate, flow time, and time to maximum flow and is used in women with voiding difficulties and before surgery for stress incontinence. A low preoperative flow rate indicates the likelihood of prolonged postoperative catheterization. A minimal of 15 ml/s when at least 150 ml is voided is quoted as normal. Measurement of urine flow provides objective evidence of voiding ability. It may predict urinary retention in a patient with detrusor instability and voiding difficulty which might be treated with antimuscarinics.

### Cystometry

Cystometry is the main urodynamic test to study bladder storage and emptying and to distinguish between detrusor instability, USI, and voiding difficulties. Simple cystometry measures the bladder pressure (vesical pressure or $P_{ves}$) in centimetres of water while subtracted cystometry or complex cystometry calculates the pressure in the bladder which originates from the bladder itself. This is obtained by subtraction of vesical pressure from intra-abdominal pressure. The intra-abdominal pressure may be measured in the rectum or vagina. When interpreting results, it must be borne in mind that the test is performed in artificial laboratory settings and will not represent real-life settings where the patient is incontinent. Many clinicians have demonstrated the discrepancy between clinical findings and urodynamic studies (Haylen and Frazer 1987; Ng and Murray 1989). In 800 consecutive women attending the urodynamic clinic, approximately 50% were diagnosed by urodynamic studies as having urethral sphincter incompetence. Of these, only 3% had the symptoms and signs of stress incontinence and 1.5% had the sole symptoms of stress incontinence. Of the total group, 85% had urgency, urge incontinence, and stress incontinence but only 25% had detrusor instability on testing (Haylen and Frazer 1987). Thus, during clinical evaluation one must take into consideration clinical findings and the urodynamic assessment.

### Urethral pressure profilometry

The role of urethral pressure profilometry in the diagnosis of stress incontinence is controversial and undecided as the overlap between normal and stress incontinence may make the accurate diagnosis impossible (Versi *et al.* 1986). A maximum urethral pressure of 20 cm $H_2O$ indicates likely intrinsic sphincter deficiency (Sand *et al.* 1987).

### Abdominal (Valsalva) leak point pressure (VLPP)

Abdominal leak point pressure has been suggested to evaluate the type and severity of stress incontinence (McGuire *et al.* 1993). At a standardized volume (200 ml in most reports), the patient is asked to Valsalva with progressively great effort. The lowest effort which produces incontinence is called abdominal leak point pressure. A low leak point pressure (less than 60 cm $H_2O$) is associated with intrinsic sphincter deficiency, a high leak point pressure (more than 90) with hypermobile-type stress incontinence and an intermediate value (60–90 cm $H_2O$) sometimes indicates combined type of stress urinary incontinence. Though some believe it helps to select patients for anti-incontinence procedures, e.g better outcome of sling procedures in women with low VLPP, this has been disputed.

### Ambulatory urodynamic monitoring

Ambulatory monitoring is assessment of bladder function by natural fill cystometry while the patient is ambulant. Catheter-mounted microtransducers are employed for pressure measurement in the bladder and leakage is recorded by a Urilos electronic nappy. The abdominal pressure is measured by transducer in the rectum or vagina. The woman is instructed to depress an event marker when significant events occur as she walks around. It is indicated when the patient complains of urgency, urge incontinence, and frequency and the conventional cystometrogram (CMG) is nornal. It has been shown that the rate of detection of detrusor instability increases by employing ambulatory urodynamics but 18% of normal bladders show uninhibited activity (Heslington and Hilton 1995).

### Videocystourethrography (VCU)

Videocystourethrography is a combination of cystometry and radiological screening and is used for more complicated cases, e.g neuropathic bladder disorders, voiding difficulties, previous failed continence surgery, suspected vesicovaginal fistula. Cystometry is performed with radio-opaque contrast as the filling medium and bladder and abdominal pressures are measured whilst observing bladder filling and emptying. Both the radiological image and the pressure tracing can be recorded simultaneously on videotape. Additional information is obtained on bladder morphology, the position of the bladder neck in relation to the pubic symphysis, whether or not it is closed during rest and stress, diverticuli of bladder or urethra, vesicoureteric reflux and voiding events. It is more costly, time consuming, is associated with irradiation and has not been shown to have many advantages over a CMG (Stanton *et al.* 1988).

# Treatment

## General

The emphasis must be placed on primary health care management for urinary incontinence which is shown to be effective in the short and long term and benefits secondary care by ensuring only patients who cannot be managed in primary care are referred (O'Brien and Long 1995; Seim *et al.* 1996). A cure or improvement rate of 70–80% has been observed in primary care (RCP 1995). A randomized controlled trial has shown that in treating mild and moderate incontinence, specialist nurses produce better results, with lower dropout rates and at 30% lower cost than urogynaecologists (Prasher *et al.* 1996). Where primary assessment indicates, or where primary interventions have failed to give significant improvement after 8–12 weeks of therapy, referral either to the continence advisor or to an appropriate consultant should be made.

According to the new NHS Guidance (Department of Health 2000), primary care teams should identify all people with incontinence, offer them a full 10-point assessment (Table 8.2), agree and copy to them a full management/ treatment plan; deliver first-line treatments; facilitate access to specialist services; and help carers understand the condition and its treatment. All incontinent women will benefit from simple advice regarding incontinent pads and garments. Women with high fluid intake will benefit from fluid restriction to a litre a day, particularly if frequency is a problem. Patients with chronic cough should be advised to stop smoking and constipation should be treated. Pelvic floor exercises may be helpful in the puerperium. Oestrogen replacement therapy may be beneficial in post-menopausal women (Fantl *et al.* 1994). Diuretics may have to be stopped or reduced. Women with chronic urinary incontinence, especially the elderly, may be better managed with an indwelling urethral or suprapubic catheter. Urinary incontinence may not always be cured but with an integrated care plan between the patient, continence adviser and the doctor, it is possible to improve the quality of life. Where the primary assessment indicates, or where primary interventions have failed to give significant improvement after 8–12 weeks of therapy, referral either to a continence adviser or to an appropriate consultant should be made.

**Table 8.2** Ten-point assessment of urinary incontinence

---

+ Review of symptoms and their effect on quality of life

+ Assessment of desire for treatment alternatives

+ Examination of the abdomen for palpable mass or bladder retention

+ Examination of the perineum to identify prolapse and excoriation and to assess pelvic floor contraction

+ Rectal examination to exclude faecal impaction (not to be carried out in children)

+ Urine analysis to exclude infection

+ Assessment of manual dexterity

+ Assessment of the environment, e.g. accessibility of toilet facilities

+ Use of an 'activities of daily living' diary

+ Identification of conditions that may exacerbate incontinence, e.g. chronic cough

---

Department of Health (2000). *Good practice in continence services*. DoH, London

## Urethral sphincter incompetence (USI)

USI is the most common cause of female incontinence. Conservative and surgical treatments are used depending on the patient's preference, condition, and urodynamic diagnosis.

### Conservative treatment

Conservative treatment is indicated when:

+ the patient refuses or is undecided about surgery;

+ the patient is physically or mentally unfit for surgery;

+ child-bearing is incomplete.

### *Devices*

*Electronic devices*   Electrical stimulation for incontinence has been applied with some success by stimulating the pudendal nerve using vaginal or anal electrodes at different frequencies. The woman adjusts the strength of the variable current and various regimens are available. Sand *et al.* (1995) in a prospective, multicentre, randomized, double-blind, placebo-controlled, 15-week trial found significant improvement when compared to controls in weekly and daily urinary leakage based on visual analogue scales, voiding diary analysis (48% vs 19%), pad testing (89% vs 32%) and vaginal muscle strength (15.2 vs 8.9 mm Hg).

*Elevating devices (Fig 8.2)*   For mild sphincter incompetence, a tampon, reusable foam pessary or bladder-neck support prosthesis may temporarily

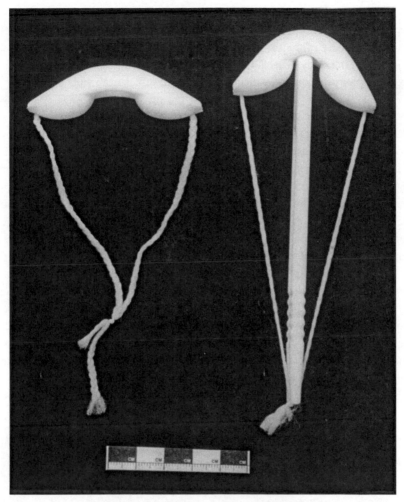

**Fig 8.2** The Conveen Continence Guard.

cure incontinence by elevating the bladder neck. This is recommended for incontinence at known times, i.e sports. A recent study of a bladder-neck prosthesis, a vaginal device designed to support the bladder neck (Introl, Uromed, Needham, MA) showed a mean reduction in urinary leakage from 59.8 to 22.8 episodes per week and this was confirmed on pad testing (78.5 to 23.4 g). Quality-of-life scores also improved. Side effects include urinary tract infections and vaginal mucosa soreness (Davilla *et al.* 1999).

*Occlusive devices* Urethral occlusive devices include urethral plugs and more recently, expandable urethral devices. Intraurethral devices have been shown to have an 80% continence cure with urinary tract infection in about

25% of women (Staskin *et al.* 1996). Published data on an external urethral occlusive device (Fem Assist, Insight Medical, Bolton, MA) reported low effectiveness and acceptability of the device with only 2 out of 31 (4.9%) patients recruited completing the study (Tincello *et al.* 2000). With all devices, compliance appears to be a major problem and patients need to have sufficient manual dexterity.

### Pelvic floor exercises

Pelvic floor exercises have been successfully used since 1948. Pelvic floor exercises concern re-education of the pelvic floor muscles by encouraging women voluntarily to contract their pelvic floor muscles. Visual or tactile biofeedback methods may be used to increase the strength of the contraction (Cammu and Van Nylen 1997). The overall cure/much improvement rate at 5 years is about 60% (Cammu and Van Nylen 1995; Bo and Talseth 1994). In a single blind, randomized study, Bo *et al.* (1999) found that pelvic floor exercises alone were superior to electrical stimulation and vaginal cones.

Vaginal cones (Fig 8.3) are useful adjuncts to pelvic floor exercises. These graduated cone-shaped vaginal weights between 20 and 100 g and are retained by passive and active contraction of the pelvic floor when individually introduced in the vagina. The cones are useful for making the women aware of their pelvic floor muscles, and graduation to the next weight lets the woman know she is making progress. A 70% cure and improvement rate was reported after one month's training in cone use, with a highly significant correlation between urine loss and increase in retained cone weight (Peattie *et al.* 1988). No important

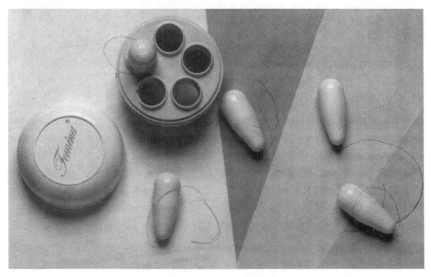

**Fig 8.3** Vaginal cones (Colgate Medical).

side effects have been found. In the only trial which has compared pelvic floor exercises with vaginal cones with pelvic floor exercises alone, the improvement rates in both groups were virtually identical (Pieber *et al.* 1995).

## Surgical treatment

Continence surgery is indicated when conservative treatment fails or the patient wants definitive treatment. The aims of continence surgery are to elevate the bladder neck or support the mid-urethra or increase urethral

**Table 8.3** Clinical, urodynamic features and complications

| Access | Operation | Cure | Clinical indications | Complications |
|---|---|---|---|---|
| Vaginal | Peri-/Transurethral bulking agents | 31–48%* (objective) | Mild stress incontinence, primary and failed surgery, physically frail | Transient urinary retention, urinary tract infection |
| Vaginal and suprapubic | Tension-free aginal tape | 86%** | Primary and secondary stress incontinence | Bladder perforation, retention, urgency |
| Suprapubic | Colposuspension | 60–90%* | Primary and secondary stress incontinence with cystocele | Voiding difficulty (10%), detrusor instability (17%), prolapse (14%) |
| | Sling | 85%* | Proximal urethra needs support; contracted vagina | Voiding difficulty (10%); urinary tract infection, sling erosion, detrusor instability (17%) |
| | Artificial urinary sphincter | 92%* (subjective) | Neurogenic, reconstructive surgery; failed conventional bladder neck surgery | Erosion, mechanical failure |
| | Laparoscopic colposuspension | 60–80%*[1] | Primary or secondary stress incontinence | Bladder injury, recurrent stress incontinence |

*Jarvis, G.J. (1994). Surgery for genuine stress incontinence. *British Journal of Obstetrics and Gynaecology*, **101**, 371–4.
**Ulmsten, U., Johnson, P. and Rezapour, M. (1999). A three-year follow-up of tension free vaginal tape for surgical treatment of female stress urinary incontinence. *British Journal of Obstetrics and Gynaecology*, **106**, 345–50.
*[1] Department of Health (2000). *Good practice in continence services*. Department of Health, London.

resistance. In general, the first attempt at continence surgery produces better results than repeat procedures (Jarvis 1999). Clinical features, urodynamic data and operation characteristics influence the choice of operation and the success rates vary (Table 8.3) (Jarvis 1999) The patient should be counselled that it is wise to avoid unnecessary heavy lifting or abnormal straining after continence surgery.

### Urethral bulking agents

These are indicated for mild stress incontinence and when the patient wants to defer or is unfit for surgery. The bulking agent is injected periurethrally or transurethrally under the submucosa to bulk the tissues around the bladder neck. Various bulking agents are available, e.g. GAX collagen (glutaraldehyde cross-linked bovine collagen), Macroplastique, fat, Durasphere. The procedure can be done as a day case under local or light general anaesthetic. Reinjection is often required and does not preclude future bladder-neck surgery. The success of the procedure detoriates with time (Gorton *et al.* 1999).

### Colposuspension

This procedure was described by Burch (1961) and nowadays is indicated for USI associated with a large (grade II) cystourethrocele. Two or three permanent sutures (Ethibond) are placed between the paravaginal fascia on either side of the bladder neck and the base of the bladder and attached to the ipsilateral iliopectineal ligament. The most distal suture is placed at the bladder neck and the most proximal suture is placed as far cephalad as possible to support the bladder base.

### Laparoscopic colposuspension

Laparoscopic colposuspension is a less invasive technique with minimal disruption to normal lifestyle but randomized controlled trials have shown there is 20% less success than an open procedure (Su *et al.* 1997; Burton 1999). Disadvantages for the surgeons include complications, cost of disposable equipment, a long operating time, and a steep learning curve.

### Sling operation

Various types of material have been used for sling operations which can be autologous (e.g. rectus sheath, vaginal wall graft) or synthetic (e.g. Silastic, nylon, Mersilene). When synthetic material is used there is a high incidence of erosion. Nonetheless, a success rate of more than 90% is claimed for primary surgery.

### Tension-free vaginal tape (TVT: gynecare)

Tension free-vaginal tape has gained increasing popularity for the treatment of USI. So far it has proven to be a safe and effective treatment. It is inserted under a local anaesthetic, regional block or general anaesthetic and involves a vaginal and two small suprapubic incisions. After minimal paraurethral dissection of the vaginal wall, a special prolene tape covered with a plastic sheath swaged on to a 5 mm needle attached to an introducer (or handle) is introduced from the vagina into the retropubic area. The tip of this needle first perforates the urogenital diaphragm and is then passed lateral to the mid-urethra, upward and behind the pubic bone to perforate the rectus sheath and then the abdominal wall. The procedure is repeated on the other side so as to place the tape in a U-shape around the mid-urethra. After cystoscopy to exclude bladder damage, the tape is adjusted without tension under the urethra. A 3-year follow-up study has shown an 86% cure rate and 11% improvement (Ulmsten *et al.* 1999). Results of a large randomized study comparing TVT and colposuspension showed no difference between these two procedures. However, the recovery was quicker after TVT (Ward *et al.* 2000).

### Artificial urinary sphincter (AUS)

The artificial urinary sphincter is used only in the most complex case of sphincter incompetence, where there is a total loss of urethral resistance and where conventional surgery has failed or for reconstructive procedures. The patient should be mentally alert and manually dextrous and have sterile urine. Currently, the American Medical Systems (AMS) 800 sphincter is used. Complications include recurrent urinary tract infections, mechanical failure, and erosion (Carson 1989; Elliott and Barrett 1998a). Elliott and Barrett reviewed their results and found at 5 years 90.4% had a properly functioning AUS (including results from male population) and overall 18% of these required reoperation to review the sphincter (Elliott and Barrett 1998b).

## The overactive bladder (OAB) (detrusor instability, unstable bladder)

The OAB, the second most common cause of urinary incontinence in women, affects 30% of incontinent women, the prevalence increasing with age (Sifo Research and Consulting AB 1998). The bladder is shown to objectively contract, spontaneously or on provocation, during the filling phase while the patient is attempting to inhibit micturition. It maybe due to hyperexcitability of detrusor muscle cells or a neuropathy involving the parasympathetic innervation. The symptoms include urgency, urge incontinence, frequency, and stress incontinence. OAB can only be diagnosed by subtracted filling cystometry. However, cystometry is not always necessary before treatment (Fig 8.4).

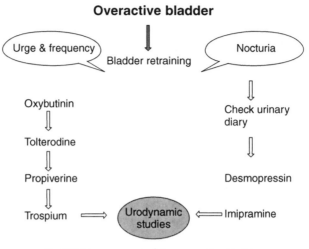

**Fig 8.4** Management of the overactive bladder.

## Conservative treatment

### Bladder retraining (behavioural therapy)

Bladder retraining should be the initial treatment for the vast majority of patients with the OAB, with or without stress incontinence. It is based on the assumption that conscious efforts to suppress sensory stimuli will re-establish cortical control over the OAB, thus re-establishing a normal voiding pattern. The aim is to reduce the voiding frequency until a 3–4-hourly pattern is achieved In a long-term study, the initial success rate was found to be 88% but declined to 38% after 6 months (Ferrie *et al.* 1984). A recent study showed that a biofeedback-assisted behavioural strategy was more effective and acceptable in women with urge and mixed incontinence than oxybutinin treatment (Burgio *et al.* 1998). Enthusiastic patient contact, reassurance, and long-term support are important. The degree of patient compliance determines the success.

### Biofeedback

Biofeedback is a form of learning or re-education in which the participant is retrained within a closed feedback loop by using visual, auditory, or tactile signals to inhibit consciously any bladder contraction. Objective responses are recorded on a polygraph trace. Cardozo *et al.* (1978) reported 81% subjective and objective improvement.

### Electrical stimulation

An initial 88% improvement or cure rate has been reported, with 77% still successful at one year (Eriksen *et al.* 1989). Recently, a cure rate of 49% at

8 weeks has been reported in a prospective, double-blind, randomized trial (Brubaker *et al.* 1997). The main difficulty is patient acceptance of the intravaginal or transanal stimulation for psychological or aesthetic reasons.

### Drugs

Drug therapy is the most popular mode of treatment for the OAB. In general, drugs help by inhibiting the contractile activity of the bladder and can broadly be classified into antimuscarinic drugs, calcium blockers, tricyclic antidepressants, musculotrophic drugs, and a variety of less commonly used drugs (Table 8.4). The majority have antimuscarinic activity and produce unwanted effects which must be balanced against the benefits. Patients become less alert and should be cautioned regarding driving or operating dangerous machinery. The optimal dose should produce beneficial effects with an acceptable level of adverse effects. Oxybutinin has for a number of years been the best drug therapy available for the OAB and is widely used as the first line of therapy. Tolterodine is a recently introduced antimuscarinic agent, which has a lower affinity for muscarinic receptors in the salivary glands. Data suggest that this drug is better tolerated, and associated with a higher compliance than oxybutinin (Appell 1997). For all antimuscarinic drugs, the dosage must be titrated depending on the subjective response and side effects and each should be given for at least 6 weeks. The patient should be warned that the OAB is a relapsing and remitting condition and treatment should be adjusted accordingly.

Recently, newer drugs have become available. Oxybutinin hydrochloride XL is now available in a once-daily controlled-release form and consists of the active component in an osmotically active bilayer. It has similar efficacy but lower side effects (Anderson *et al.* 1999). Trospium chloride is a new antimuscarinic drug with similar efficacy to other existing drugs with fewer side effects. Due to its hydrophilic nature, central anticholinergic side effects of the drug can not be detected as it does not cross the blood–brain barrier (Füsgen & Hauri 2000).

Tricyclic antidepressants, e.g imipramine hydrochloride, act by increasing the outlet resistance due to peripheral blockage of noradrenaline uptake and also as a sedative. Imipramine is particularly useful for the treatment of nocturia and nocturnal enuresis. Antidiuretic hormone analogues such as synthetic vasopressin (DDAVP) has been shown to reduce noctural urine production by 50%. It can be used for children or adults with nocturia or nocturnal enuresis but has to be avoided in patients with hypertension, ischaemic heart disease, or congestive cardiac failure (Hilton and Stanton 1982).

**Table 8.4** Pharmacological therapy for detrusor instability

| Name of drug | Minimum and maximum dose | Mechanism of action | Potential side effects | Contraindications |
|---|---|---|---|---|
| Oxybutinin hydrochloride | 2.5 mg b.i.d. to 5 mg q.i.d. | Antimuscarinic, smooth muscle relaxant, local anaesthetic | Dry mouth (78%), blurred vision, drowsiness, headache (11%), gastrointestinal symptoms (40%) | As above, bladder outflow obstruction |
| Tolterodine | 1 mg b.i.d. to 2 mg q.i.d. | Antimuscarinic | Dry mouth (40%), blurred vision, drowsiness, headache (7%), gastrointestinal symptoms (26%) | As above |
| Propiverine hydrochloride | 15 mg b.i.d. to 15 mg q.i.d. | Antimuscarinic | As above | As above |
| Propantheline bromide | 15 mg b.i.d. or 30 mg q.i.d. | Antimuscarinic | Dry mouth, blurred vision, drowsiness, constipation | Glaucoma, intestinal obstruction, myasthenia gravis |
| Dicyclomine hydrochloride | 10 mg b.i.d. to 40 mg q.i.d. | Smooth muscle relaxant | As above | As above |
| Imipramine hydrochloride | 25 mg q.i.d. to 75 mg q.i.d. | Tricyclic antidepressant, anticholinergic, α-adrenergic agonist, antihistaminic | As above, orthostatic hypertension, hepatic dysfunction, cardiovascular effects (especially in the elderly) | As above, cardiac dysrhythmia, monoamine oxidase inhibitors |
| DDAVP (synthetic vasopressin) | 20 mg, 40 µg intranasally at bed time | Antidiuretic | Transient headache, nausea, nasal congestion, rhinitis, flushing, mildabdominal cramps | Coronary artery disease, hypertension, epilepsy |

## Neuromodulation

During the 1990s, sacral neuromodulation began to develop as a new therapy. The exact mechanism of action is not known, but activation of the spinal interneurons or β-adrenergic neurons, which inhibit bladder activity, have been postulated. All patients must undergo a test of stimulation of the $S_3$ sacral nerve before they can be offered chronic sacral nerve stimulation with an implanted system. Approximately half the patients respond favourably to the test. Unfortunately, treatment fails in 20–33% within 1–1.5 years of a permanent implant (Bosch 1998). However, there is durable success in 60% of patients at 5 years (Bosch and Groen 1997). Chronic sacral nerve stimulation may be associated with surgical morbidity such as pain at the site of the electrodes or the neurostimulator, electrode migration, and implant infections. Hardware problems include broken electrodes, isolation defects, and battery exhausion.

## Surgery

The management of detrusor instability is mainly non-surgical. It is, however, a difficult condition to treat, and there are women who respond poorly to bladder retraining and pharmacological therapies. Surgery has a role in these women and should be done only as the last resort.

### Ileocystoplasty (clam cystoplasty)

This procedure involves anastomosis of approximately 25 cm of ileum on its vascular pedicle onto the bladder after the bladder has been cut along the coronal plane, thus increasing capacity with reduced activity during filling. A success rate of 53% has been reported (Awad *et al.* 1998). Because of the problems encountered with the use of gastrointestinal segments (e.g hyperchloraemic acidosis, calculi, failure to empty, infections, mucous production, and tumours) many investigators have tried alternative methods, materials and tissue for bladder repair or replacement. Amongst these are autoaugmentation, ureterocystoplasty, methods for tissue expansion, seromuscular grafts, matrices for tissue regeneration, and tissue engineering using cell transplantation (Atala 2000).

## Overflow incontinence

Chronic urinary retention with resultant overflow incontinence is uncommon in women. The causes include neurological, inflammation, antispasmodic drugs, continence surgery, obstruction, and psychosis. If there is outflow obstruction, urethral dilatation or urethrotomy may be required. Treatment includes clean intermittent self-catheterization or a suprapubic catheter and management of the underlying cause.

## Other causes of incontinence

Women with urinary fistulae (ureterovaginal, vesicovaginal, urethrovaginal) often complain of uncontrollable, continuous urinary leakage, usually occurring after pelvic surgery, advanced pelvic malignancy, or radiotherapy. A small recent fistula may well heal spontaneously if urine is diverted from the fistulous tract. If a fistula is diagnosed within 48 hours of surgery, and if there is no significant inflammatory reaction or necrosis about the fistula, immediate reoperation and repair should be considered. If associated with inflammation, treatment should be interim continuous bladder drainage.

# Conclusion

Incontinence causes distress, embarrassment, and inconvenience. It remains one of the last social taboos. Women should be encouraged to seek help earlier and discuss their problems openly. Recently, the NHS has issued guidance on the provision of continence services (Department of Health 2000). The document emphasizes the need for primary care to play a larger role in the efficient management of urinary incontinence.

# 10-minute consultation

A 35-year-old women presents to you with history of frequency, urgency, and mixed urinary incontinence which is increasingly getting worse. Her problems started after a forceps delivery 4 years ago.

## What issues you should cover

- Check how often she is voiding urine by day and night.
- Ask about urgency and how often and how severe is the incontinence.
- Ask about which activities create stress incontinence and ascertain the frequency with which they do so.
- Ask about any history of voiding difficulties so that treatment by surgery or antimuscarinics is not recommended inappropriately.
- It is crucial to understand the effect on her quality of life (QOL). A question like 'On a scale of 0 to 10, where 10 represents excellent QOL, what score would you give yourself in connection with your current symptoms?' can be useful in this context. The score can be recorded and, when treatment interventions are reviewed at subsequent consultations, it provides a benchmark for comparison.

- Any plans for further pregnancies need to be sought, as these will affect treatment plans, making physiotherapy and use of urethral bulking agents more appropriate than more major surgery.

- A brief look at her past history, particularly as regards continence surgery, is necessary to avoid a possibly unnecessary referral to a gynaecologist. The success rate of second operations for recurrent stress incontinence is lower than for primary surgery. Her drug history should be checked, looking, for example, for the use of diuretics and α-blockers which can affect both urgency and stress incontinence, respectively, as well as other drugs like tricyclic antidepressants, which may produce voiding difficulties. A quick check of her fluid intake, both quantity and type (thinking mainly of caffeine and alcohol), needs to be noted.

## What you should do

- Ask the nurse to check her urine with a 'Multistix' and weigh her. Watch her get onto the couch – it gives you a very rough idea of power and coordination in a consultation where a thorough neurological examination is not possible.

- Feel her abdomen for masses and any bladder enlargement, before examining the introitus and pelvis. A speculum examination, checking her pelvic sensation as you insert the instrument, should be carried out to look for local pathology and prolapse.

## What you should suggest

- Keep a fluid intake and output chart (have some already printed out to give her) for a week. She may then reduce excess liquid intake, especially late evening drinks, if it seems appropriate from the chart results. Give her leaflets describing how to carry out pelvic floor exercises and bladder drill.

- Offer to refer her to the local physiotherapist and/or district continence service.

- Drug treatment might be necessary: for urgency and urge incontinence, oxybutynin, tolterodine, and trospium chloride are all useful but evidence suggests that these agents are more effective when combined with bladder retraining. Nocturia may respond to imipramine and desmopressin should be reserved for more serious situations such as patients with multiple sclerosis.

- Drugs should be started in low dosage and titrated upwards to minimize side effects such as dry mouth, constipation, blurred vision, headache and gastrointestinal symptoms.

◆ Referral for more radical treatment will usually be deferred to the next consultation in 10–12 weeks' time (unless underlying pathology was found on examination). Tension-free vaginal tape insertion or colposuspension may then need to be considered for her urethral sphincter incompetence.

## Questions patients might raise

### Since you put me on those pills for my blood pressure the water has been just running away from me, especially when I am loading the shopping into the car. Can you do something to stop it?

It is important to remember that in some patients there may be an iatrogenic cause for a patients' worsening symptoms, and any new medication should be viewed with suspicion. In this particular situation, a patient had been changed on to doxazosin, and had never liked to mention her mild stress incontinence before, despite having been seen recently for a routine cervical smear. She now felt safer to discuss it because she could use the side effect of the medication as a tool to introduce the subject–her stress incontinence having been made significantly worse by the drug, with unpleasant social consequences.

There is a dilemma for the doctor in this sort of situation when a different antihypertensive agent needs to be chosen: diuretics are clearly inappropriate. An ACE inhibitor could be tried but if the side effect is cough, this could exacerbate incontinence. Calcium channel blockers can reduce frequency and urgency and would have no deleterious effect on stress incontinence and so perhaps represent the wisest choice.

Pelvic examination in this sort of situation will often reveal mild anterior vaginal wall prolapse and, provided urine analysis is negative and the patient is otherwise fit, pelvic floor exercises can be started and the use of vaginal cones advised. It may be appropriate to lose weight, to help both incontinence and hypertension, and to avoid constipation (an unlikely complication of class II calcium channel blockers). Finally, it is often helpful to probe patients' fears of surgery and brief them on alternatives such as vaginal devices, which have success rates approaching 70%.

### What do I do about getting pads because I can't afford them and I cannot go out? What if I run out of them?

Pads should be a last resort, but there are quite a few women with incontinence who have multiple pathologies which perhaps preclude them from benefiting further from exercises, bladder retraining, weight reduction, drug therapy and surgery and so have no choice but to start wearing pads.

The DOH 'Good practices in continence services' states that there should be pads available in all sizes and absorbencies and that consideration should be given to patient choice. Pads are free to all but the under-4s (NHS Act 1997 Section 1 EL(91) 129) and should be provided in quantities to suit the needs of the patient.

'Access to the service should not be *de facto* limited by the requirement to collect pads from a central point' is another tenet of the document and indeed, it should be possible to get a patient visited at home by the community continence adviser, who can fully assess the patient's needs, supply adequate quantities of pads, and reassess the situation annually to check for any change in requirements. Unfortunately, patients do not always get enough pads and need to supplement stocks privately.

Reusable pads are an option in cases where there is no faecal incontinence or menstruation involved, but many patients do not like the idea of them, they are less absorbent and the plastic pants can cause irritation of the skin. However, some women like the concept of the possible 'greener' image of reusable pads and are therefore prepared to try them. Hand-held female urinals are also worth considering.

### I'm like a sieve: I can't even go for a walk without leaking urine and as walking is my main exercise I don't want to stop so what can I do?

Women with this story often turn out to have urgency, urge incontinence, frequency, and some stress incontinence and need to be fully assessed. Taking shorter strides and walking on even ground to avoid sudden jolting may help. Bladder retraining should be reviewed and incorporated into their walking plan by making sure that they limit intake of fluid in the morning and void immediately before departure. They should consider using the same route each day, where toilets are available and their location known, and to use them regardless of whether they feel the need to or not. Distracting the mind when necessary with a particular preplanned thought or action can be useful.

As a supplementary issue, some women want to know about hypnotherapy. An objective cure rate of 50% has been reported in a non-randomized study (Freeman and Baxby, 1982) and though there is a high relapse rate, it is worth considering in willing patients. It is important to check for compliance with medication, as some women, who go out a lot, find the three times daily regimen of oxybutinin, for example, difficult to remember. A change onto the once-daily, slow-release version might be appropriate and improve symptom control.

## Useful information for patients

For confidential advice, information and help about the bladder and bowel:

The Helpline Nurse,
The Continence Foundation
307 Hatton Square
16 Baldwin Gardens
London EC1N 7RJ
Tel: 0845 345 0165
Website: www.continence-foundation.org.uk

### Self-help group for people with bladder and bowel problems

Incontact
Suite 2.7, Docklands Enterprise Centre
11 Marshalsea Road
London SE1 1EP
Tel: 0207 7717 1225

### Information about bed-wetting protection

PromoCon 2001
Redbank House
4 St Chad's Street
Cheetham
Manchester M8 9QA
Tel: 0161 834 2001

### Vaginal cones can be obtained from

Femina
Colgate Medical Ltd.
Unit 5, Burney Court
Wallis Park
Maidenhead SL6 7BZ
Tel: 01628 594 500

## References

Abrams, P.H., Blaivis, J.G., Stanton, S.L. and Anderson, J.T. (1988). Standardization of terminology of the lower urinary tract function. *Neurourology and Urodynamics*, 7, 403–27.

Anderson, R.U., Mobley, D., Blank, B., *et al.* (1999). Once daily controlled versus immediate release oxybutinin hydrochloride for urge urinary incontinence. *Journal of Urology*, **161**, 1809–12.

Appell, R.A. (1997). Clinical efficacy and safety of tolterodine in the treatment of overactive bladder: a pooled analysis. *Urology*, **50**, 90–9.

Atala, A. (2000). New methods of bladder augmentation. *British Journal of Urology International*, **85** (S3), 24–34.

Awad, S.A., Al-Zahrani, H.M., Gajewski, J.B. and Bourque-Kehoe, A.A. (1998). Long-term results and complications of augmentation ileocystoplasty for idiopathic urge incontinence in women. *British Journal of Urology*, **81**, 569–73.

Bo, K. and Talseth, T. (1994). Five year follow-up of pelvic floor exercises for treatment of stress incontinence. Clinical and Urodynamic assessment. *Neurourology and Urodynamics*, **13**, 374–75.

Bo, K., Talseth, T. and Holme, I. (1999). Single blind, randomised controlled trial of pelvic floor exercises, electrical stimulation, vaginal cones, and no treatment in management of genuine stress incontinence in women. *British Medical Journal*, **318**, 487–93.

Bosch, J.L.H.R. (1998). Sacral neuromodulation in the treatment of the unstable bladder. *Current Opinion in Urology*, **8**, 287–91.

Bosch, J.L.H.R. and Groen, J. (1997). Seven years experience with sacral ($S_3$) segmental nerve stimulation in patients with urge incontinence due to detrusor instability or hyperreflexia. *Neurourology and Urodynamics*, **16**, 426–27 (Abstract 56).

Brubaker, L., Benson, J.T., Bent, A., Clark, A. and Shott, S. (1997). Transvaginal electrical stimulation for female urinary incontinence. *American Journal of Obstetrics and Gynecology*, **177**, 536–40.

Burch, J.C. (1961). Urethro-vaginal fixation to Cooper's ligament for correction of stress incontinence, cystocele and prolapse. *American Journal of Obstetrics and Gynecology*, **81**, 281–90.

Burgio, K.L., Locher, J.L., Goode, P.S., *et al.* (1998). Behavioral vs drug treatment for urge urinary incontinence in older women: a randomized controlled trial. *Journal of the American Medical Association*, **280**, 1995–2000.

Burton, G. (1999). A five year prospective randomised urodynamic study comparing open and laparoscopic colposuspension. *Neurourology and Urodynamics* **18** (4), 295–6.

Cammu, H. and Van Nylen, M. (1995). Pelvic floor muscle exercises: 5 years later. *Urology* **38**, 332–7.

Cammu, H. and Van Nylen, M. (1997). Pelvic floor exercises in genuine stress incontinence. *International Urogynecology Journal and Pelvic Floor Dysfunction*, **8**, 297–300.

Cardozo, L. and Stanton, S.L. (1980) Genuine stress incontinence and detrusor instability: a review of 200 patients. *British Journal of Obstetrics and Gynaecology*, **87**, 184–90.

Cardozo, L.D., Abrams, P.D., Stanton, S.L. and Feneley, R.C. (1978). Idiopathic bladder instability treated by biofeedback. *British Journal of Urology*, **50**, 521–3.

Carson, C.C. (1989). Infections in genitourinary prostheses. *Urology Clinics of North America*, **16**, 139–47.

Chaliha, C., Kalia, V. and Stanton, S.L. (1999). Antenatal prediction of postpartum urinary and faecal incontinence. *Obstetrics and Gynecology*, **94**, 689–94.

Davilla, D.W., Neal, D., Horbach, N., Peacher, J., Doughtie, J.D. and Karram, M. (1999). A bladder-neck support prosthesis for women with stress and mixed incontinence. *Obstetrics and Gynecology*, **93** (6), 938–42.

Department of Health (2000). *Good practice in continence services*. Department of Health, London.

Elliott, D.S. and Barrett, D.M. (1998a). The artificial urinary sphincter in the female: indications for use, surgical approach and results. *International Urogynecology Journal and Pelvic Floor Dysfunction*, **9**, 409–15.

Elliott, D.S. and Barrett, D.M. (1998b). Mayo Clinic long-term analysis of the functional durability of the AMS 800 artificial urinary sphincter: a review of 323 cases. *Journal of Urology*, **159**, 1206–8.

Eriksen, B.C., Bergman, S. and Eiknes, S.H. (1989). Maximal electrical stimulation of the pelvic floor in female detrusor instability and urge incontinence. *Neurourology and Urodynamics*, **8**, 219–30.

Fantl, J.A., Cardozo, L. and McClish, D.K. (1994). Estrogen therapy in the management of urinary incontinence in postmenopausal women: a meta-analysis. First report of the Hormones and Urogenital Therapy Committee. *Obstetrics and Gynecology*, **83**, 12–18.

Ferrie, B.G., Smith, J.S., Logan, D., Lyle, R. and Paterson, P.J. (1984). Experience with bladder training in 65 patients. *British Journal of Urology*, **56**, 482–4.

Freeman, R.M. and Baxby, K. (1982) Hypnotherapy for incontinence caused by detrusor instability. *British Medical Journal*, **284**, 1831–2.

Füsgen, I. and Hauri, D. (2000). Trospium chloride: an effective option for medical treatment of bladder overactivity. *International Journal of Clinical Pharmacology and Therapeutics*, **38**, 23–234.

Gorton, E., Stanton, S.L., Monga, A., Wiskind, A., Lentz, G. and Bland, D. (1999). Periurethral collagen injections: long-term follow-up. *British Journal of Urology*, **84**, 966–71.

Haylen, B.T. and Frazer, M.I. (1987). Is the investigation of most stress incontinence really necessary? Proceedings of the 17th Annual Meeting of International Continence Society. *Neurourology and Urodynamics*, **6**, 188–9.

Heslington, K. and Hilton, P. (1995). Ambulatory monitoring and conventional cystometry in asymptomatic female volunteers. *British Journal of Obstetrics and Gynaecology*, **103**, 434–41.

Hilton, P. and Stanton, S.L. (1982) Use of desmopressin (DDAVP) in nocturnal urinary frequency in the females. *British Journal of Urology*, **54**, 919–33.

Jarvis, G.J. (1994). Surgery for genuine stress incontinence. *British Journal of Obstetrics and Gynaecology*, **101**, 371–4.

Jarvis, G.J. (1999) The surgery for genuine stress incontinence, In: Abrams, P., Saad, K. and Wein, A. (eds), *Incontinence*, pp. 637–56. Health Publications, St Heliar, NJ.

Lara, C. and Nacey, J. (1994). Ethnic differences between Maori, Pacific Island and European New Zealand women in prevalence and attitudes to urinary incontinence. New Zealand *Medical Journal*, **107**, 374–6.

Mayne, C.J. and Hilton, P. (1989). The short pad test: standardisation of method and comparison with the one hour pad test. *Neurourology and Urodynamics*, **7**, 443.

McGuire, E., Fitzpatrick, C., Wan, J., *et al.* (1993). Clinical assessment of urethral sphincter function. *Journal of Urology*, **150**, 1452–4.

Ng, R. and Murray, A. (1989). Place of routine urodynamics in the management of female GSI. *Neurourology and Urodynamics*, **8**, 307–8.

Norton, C. (1996). *Commissioning comprehensive continence services, guidance for purchasers.* The Continence Foundation, London.

Norton, P.A., Macdonald, L.D., Sedgwick, P.M. and Stanton, S.L. (1988). Distress and delay associated with urinary incontinence, frequency and urgency in women. *British Medical Journal*, **297**, 1187–9.

O'Brien, J. and Long, H. (1995). Urinary incontinence: long-term effectiveness nursing intervention in primary care. *British Medical Journal*, **311**, 1208.

Ouslander, J.G., Kane, R.L. and Abrass, I.B. (1982). Urinary incontinence in elderly nursing home patients. *Journal of the American Medical Association*, **248**, 1194–8.

Peattie, A.B., Plevnik, S. and Stanton, S.L. (1988). Vaginal cones: a conservative method of treating genuine stress incontinence. *British Journal of Obstetrics and Gynaecology*, **95**, 1049–53.

Perry, S., Assassa, R.P., Dallosso, H., *et al.* (2000). An epidemiological study to establish the prevalence of urinary symptoms and felt need in the community: the Leicestershire MRC Incontinence Study. *Journal of Public Health Medicine*, **22**, 3.

Pieber, D., Zivkovic, F., Tamussino, G., Ralph, G., Lippitt, G. and Fauland, B. (1995). Pelvic floor exercise alone or with vaginal cones in the treatment of mild to moderate stress urinary incontinence in pre-menopausal women. *International Urogynecology Journal and Pelvic Floor Dysfunction*, **6**, 14–17.

Prasher, S., Moore, K., Anderson, P., *et al.* (1998). A randomised controlled trial of nurse continence advisor management versus urogynaecology management of conservative continence therapy: benefits and costs. *Neurourology and Urodynamics*, **17**, 423–4.

Royal College of Physicians (1995). *Incontinence: causes, management and provision of services.* Report of working party. Royal College of Physicians, London.

Sand, P.K., Bowen, L.W., Panganiban, R. and Ostergard, D.R. (1987). The low pressure urethra as a factor in failed retropubic urethropexy. *Obstetrics and Gynecology*, **69**, 399.

Sand, P.K., Richardson, D.A., Staskin, D.R., *et al.* (1995). Pelvic floor electrical stimulation in the treatment of genuine stress incontinence: a multicenter, placebo-controlled trial. *American Journal of Obstetrics and Gynecology*, **173**, 72–9.

Seim, A., Silvertsen, B., Eriksen, B.C. and Hunkskaar, S. (1996). Treatment of urinary incontinence in women in general practice: observational study. *British Medical Journal*, **312**, 1459–62.

Sifo Research and Consulting AB. (1998) *A multinational tracking survey on overactive bladder problem.* Sifo Research and Consulting, Stockholm.

Snooks, S.J., Swash, M., Henry, M.M. and Setchell, M.E. (1984). Injury to innervation of pelvic floor sphincter musculature in childbirth. *Lancet*, **2**, 546–50.

Stanton, S., Krieger, M. and Ziv, E. (1988). Videocystourethrography: its role in the assessment of incontinence in the female. *Neurourology and Urodynamics*, **7**, 172–3.

Staskin, D., Bavemdam, T., Miller, J., A. *et al.* (1996). Effectiveness of a urethral control insert in the management of stress urinary incontinence. *Urology*, **47**, 629–36.

Su, T.H., Wang, K.G., Hsu, C.Y., Wei, H.J. and Hong, B.K. (1997). Prospective comparison of laparoscopic and traditional colposuspensions in the treatment of genuine stress incontinence. *Acta Obstetrica et Gynaecologica Scandinavica*, **76**, 576–82.

Sutherst, J., Brown, M. and Shawer, M. (1981). Assessing the severity of urinary incontinence in women by weighing perineal pads. *Lancet*, **1**, 1128–30.

The Continence Foundation (2000). *Making the case for investment in an integral continence service: a source book for continence services*. CF, London.

Tincello, D.G., Adams, E.J., Bolderson, J. and Richmond, D.H. (2000). A urinary control device for management of female stress incontinence. *Obstetrics and Gynecology*, **95**, 417–20.

Ulmsten, U., Johnson, P. and Rezapour, M. (1999). A three-year follow-up of tension-free vaginal tape for surgical treatment of female stress urinary incontinence. *British Journal of Obstetrics and Gynaecology*, **106**, 345–50.

Versi, E., Cardozo, L., Studd, J. and Cooper, D. (1986). Evaluation of urethal pressure profilometry for diagnosis of genuine stress incontinence. *World Journal of Urology*, **4**, 6–9.

Ward, K.L., Hilton, P. and Browning, J. (2000). A randomised trial of colposuspension and tension-free vaginal tape (TVT) for primary genuine stress incontinence. *Neurourology and Urodynamics*, **19**, 386 (7A).

# Chapter 9

# Vaginal discharge and sexually transmitted infections

Pippa Oakeshott

Good general practice management of women with vaginal discharge and sexually transmitted infections can make an important difference to their health. It may prevent the potentially devastating consequences of undiagnosed or inadequately treated cervical chlamydia infection. It can also help to reduce the discomfort, embarrassment, and anxiety often associated with genitourinary problems.

Not every woman needs investigation. If a woman in a long-term stable relationship develops symptoms of thrush after a course of antibiotics, blind treatment is perfectly reasonable. But in young women with abnormal vaginal discharge or suspected sexually transmitted infection, microbiological tests, especially for chlamydia and gonorrhoea, are essential for accurate diagnosis and management. It is totally unacceptable to reassure a woman that she has no serious infection merely on the basis of a normal high vaginal swab (Hopwood and Mallinson 1995). This chapter covers common genital and sexually transmitted infections seen in general practice, excluding HIV infection.

## Prevalence

Vaginal discharge is a common problem in general practice. The 1991–92 National Morbidity Survey found there were 421 general practice consultations annually for inflammatory disease of the cervix, vagina, or vulva per 10 000 women aged 16–44. Fig 9.1 shows the increase in diagnoses of sexually transmitted diseases seen in English and Welsh genitourinary clinics over the past decade. Between 1996 and 2001, diagnoses of genital chlamydia infection increased by 108% and of gonorrhoea by 87%. Although the rise in diagnoses of chlamydial infection partly reflects an increase in testing, it is likely that the overall rise in sexually transmitted infections is associated with increasing unsafe sexual behaviour, particularly among teenagers.

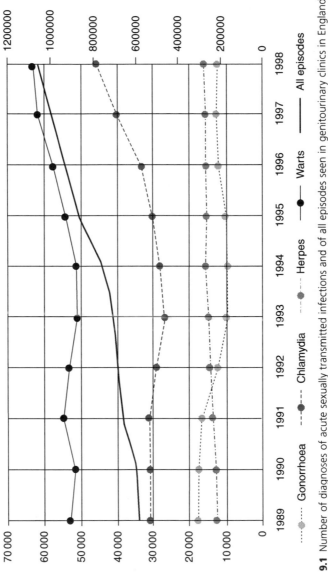

**Fig 9.1** Number of diagnoses of acute sexually transmitted infections and of all episodes seen in genitourinary clinics in England and Wales, 1989–98.

# Causes of vaginal discharge

Vaginal discharge may be physiological or pathological. Physiological vaginal discharge is white, becoming yellow on contact with air due to oxidation. The amount of discharge produced varies considerably between women. It may increase at ovulation, premenstrually, or when using oral contraception or an IUCD. What matters is that a woman is complaining of a change in her normal discharge.

Abnormal discharge is usually due to infection. Table 9.1 shows the organisms isolated from 386 consecutive women (mainly social classes 3 and 4) who presented with vaginal discharge, soreness, or vulval irritation in a suburban general practice in Cardiff (Owen *et al.* 1991). Bacterial vaginosis and *Candida albicans* are the commonest infections. They are relatively harmless and not generally regarded as sexually transmitted. The most important causes of vaginal discharge are *Chlamydia trachomatis* and *Neisseria gonorrhoeae*, since these sexually transmitted infections can cause pelvic inflammatory disease leading to tubal infertility, ectopic pregnancy, or chronic pelvic pain. *Trichomonas vaginalis* is also a vaginal pathogen. Its main significance is that it is sexually transmitted and a marker for other sexually transmitted diseases. *Streptococcus, Staphylococcus aureus* and *Haemophilus* species may be commensals in the vagina but should be treated if causing symptoms. Streptococci should always be treated in pregnant women near term or after delivery because of the risks

**Table 9.1** Organisms identified in 386 women aged 15–65 years presenting in general practice with lower genital tract symptoms

| Organism | Women infected (%) |
| --- | --- |
| Bacterial vaginosis | 56.5 |
| *Candida albicans* | 34.5 |
| *Chlamydia trachomatis* | 6.5 |
| *Trichomonas vaginalis* | 2.3 |
| *Streptococcus milleri* | 1.8 |
| *Haemophilus* species | 1.0 |
| *Staphylococcus aureus* | 0.5 |
| *Neisseria gonorrhoeae* | 0.3 |
| Herpes virus | 0.3 |

*Note*: some women had more than one infection.
No organism was identified in a third of women.

*Source*: By kind permission of the *British Journal of General Practice* (Owen *et al.* 1991).

of neonatal infection or post-partum endometritis. Herpes and genital warts are sexually transmitted viral infections, which can be distressing for the patient. Unfortunately, treatment for these infections is only suppressive and not curative.

Non-infective causes of vaginal discharge are usually diagnosed on clinical examination. They include cervical ectropion, polyp or carcinoma, retained products, and foreign bodies in the vagina, notably a 'lost' tampon. The latter should be disposed of in a self-sealing plastic bag before the smell in the surgery becomes intolerable. Fortunately, toxic shock syndrome is rare (see Chapter 1). Vulvovaginitis may also be due to dermatological problems such as eczema, or associated with irritants.

## Diagnosis of vaginal discharge

### History

Most causes of vaginal discharge will be elucidated by clinical examination and tests. However, if possible, a brief sexual history should be taken (Box 9.1). Finally, check if the patient has already treated herself unsuccessfully with an over-the-counter preparation such as clotrimazole cream or oral fluconazole.

---

### Box 9.1 **Taking a sexual history in general practice**

**Lifestyle**
- Are you in a relationship at the moment?
- When did you last have sex?
- When did you last have sex with someone other than your partner?

**Symptoms**
- When did you first notice this problem?
- Have you had it before?
- Do you know if your partner has any symptoms?
- Have you any idea what you think this might be?

---

If clinical history and prior knowledge of the patient suggest a sexually transmitted infection is likely, and the local genitourinary clinic is easily accessible and if the patient agrees to attend, it may be simpler to give the patient a letter and clinic leaflet and send her straight there. Otherwise appropriate swabs should be taken.

## Examination

The vulva should be examined for genital warts or herpetic ulcers. A bimanual examination may reveal adnexal tenderness or cervical motion pain suggestive of pelvic inflammatory disease. It is preferable to use warm water as a lubricant as other substances may interfere with cultures. A speculum should be passed and the appearance of the cervix and any discharge should be noted. However, as with symptoms, physical signs are not reliable in making a diagnosis.

## Tests

If these are to be done at all, they should be done properly. Although specimens taken will depend on arrangements with the local laboratory, minimum tests should include:

- Cervical swab for culture in Stuart's transport medium. The swab should be inserted in the endocervix to sample pus and discharge for gonorrhoea. This will also usually pick up vaginal infections such as bacterial vaginosis, candidiasis, and trichomoniasis.
- Opportunistic cervical smear if the patient has not had a normal routine smear, or there is some clinical indication.
- Endocervical swab for chlamydia.

Chlamydiae are intracellular bacteria, so specimens for chlamydia should contain cells from the endocervix or an ectropion if present, not pus or discharge. Sampling should be done *at the end* of a speculum examination after cleaning the cervix. (In practice, if a cervical smear or other swabs have been taken first, cleaning may not be necessary.) A cotton-tipped swab is rotated gently in the endocervix for at least 10 seconds to collect as much material as possible. Then it is placed in transport medium for ligase or polymerase chain reaction assay or enzyme immunoassay. Exact details will depend on the local laboratory. In future GPs will have access to urine screening.

If vulval or cervical ulcers are seen, a special viral swab should be taken for herpes simplex culture.

Box 9.2 **Basic investigations of a sexually active young woman complaining of abnormal vaginal discharge**

- Endocervical swab for *Neisseria gonorrhoeae* in Stuart's medium. May also diagnose *Candida albicans*, bacterial vaginosis, or *Trichomonas vaginalis*
- Cervical smear if not recently done
- Endocervical swab for *Chlamydia trachomatis* after cleaning the cervix

## Management

Ideally the patient should be asked to come back in a week when all the swab results will be available and appropriate treatment can be given. However, if she requests treatment for symptoms of possible thrush or bacterial vaginosis, it is not unreasonable to treat blind provided she returns for follow-up. Similarly, if pelvic inflammatory disease is suspected clinically, she should be given a 2-week course of doxycycline and metronidazole on the understanding that it is essential she returns for the swab results in case additional treatment or contact tracing is required. Detailed management in line with UK national guidelines (www.mssvd.org.uk/ceg.htm) will be discussed under the section for each infection and is summarized in Table 9.3.

## Infective causes of vaginal discharge

### Candidiasis

*Candida albicans* or thrush is an ubiquitous yeast-like fungus that is commonly carried as a commensal. It is present in the vaginas of 20% of women with no symptoms. Predisposing factors include diabetes (therefore exclude glycosuria), pregnancy, broad-spectrum antibiotic treatment, steroid treatment, and immunodeficiency as in AIDS. Contrary to popular opinion, the low-dose oral contraceptive pill is not a cause of thrush and the pill should not be discontinued for this reason alone. Although vaginal candidiasis in healthy women does not result in serious complications, it can cause considerable distress. In addition, in the lay press thrush has been blamed (with little scientific evidence) for a multitude of symptoms including those often attributed to irritable bowel syndrome.

#### Symptoms and signs

Candida may cause itching and soreness of vulva and vagina leading to dysuria and dyspareunia. However, it can improve spontaneously, and often causes no symptoms. On examination, the vagina and vulva may be inflamed and oedematous, and fissures can occur. The typical discharge is white or yellow, like cottage cheese, but clinical examination is notoriously unreliable for diagnosis.

## Diagnosis

This is by culture and microscopy of a high vaginal or cervical swab. Candida may occasionally be diagnosed on cervical cytology. However, most women in stable partnerships who have had microbiologically diagnosed thrush previously will not need swabs unless their symptoms fail to improve on treatment.

## Treatment

This is only required for symptomatic candida. Topical or oral treatments are both 80–90% effective in uncomplicated candida, but topical treatment is cheaper and less toxic. Common regimens are:

- clotrimazole pessaries 200 mg *per vaginam nocte* for 3 nights or 500 mg for one night; or
- fluconazole 150 mg orally as a single dose. This is contraindicated in pregnancy or lactation.

Additional creams containing steroid, e.g. clotrimazole with hydrocortisone, are useful for local irritation. All these treatments are available over the counter.

## Recurrent candida

Ideally 'thrush' should only be treated blind on one occasion before being investigated, and then only in low-risk women who will return if symptoms persist. Many women with so-called 'recurrent candida' do not have candida at all. Therefore clinical examination and full microbiological tests are essential. The patient may have bacterial vaginosis, herpes, or dermatological conditions such as eczema, lichen planus, or lichen sclerosis. There may be psychosexual problems and some women may use their symptoms as an excuse to avoid sexual intercourse (see Chapter 16).

Management of women with proven recurrent vaginal candidiasis can be difficult. They should be advised to use emollients, not to wash excessively, and to avoid vaginal deodorants, bubble baths, and other additives such as dettol and TCP. KY jelly can be used to reduce trauma during sexual intercourse. Loose clothing is recommended. Two-week courses of clotrimazole pessaries 100 mg *nocte* or oral fluconazole 50 mg daily may be effective. Unfortunately, oral treatment is no more likely than topical treatment to prevent relapse. If thrush occurs premenstrually, pessaries can be used prophylactically. Partners should be treated if symptomatic. There is little evidence that yoghourt, either orally or vaginally, is effective, but some patients find local application sooth-ing. Self-help books and complementary therapies may be useful.

## Bacterial vaginosis

Bacterial vaginosis is due to an overgrowth of *Gardnerella vaginalis* and mixed anaerobes. It is the commonest cause of abnormal vaginal discharge in women of child-bearing age. It is not generally regarded as a sexually transmitted infec-tion although its prevalence increases with increasing sexual activity.

### Symptoms and signs

Bacterial vaginosis has a characteristic fishy smell because of the production of diamines. The smell is worse after sexual intercourse and may be associated with a watery, grey, offensive discharge. It causes little irritation and up to 50% of women with bacterial vaginosis have no symptoms.

### Diagnosis

In general practice this is usually by culture and microscopy of a high vaginal or cervical swab. Clue cells – vaginal epitheliel cells covered with adherent bacteria – may be seen on a wet mount of vaginal fluid.

### Treatment

There is no absolute indication to treat healthy asymptomatic women with bacterial vaginosis. For those complaining of smelly vaginal discharge, a 90% cure rate is produced by:

- metronidazole orally 400 mg b.d. for 5 days or a single dose of 2 g orally. (Metronidazole is contraindicated in the first trimester of pregnancy, and patients should be advised to avoid alcohol because of the Antabuse-like effect.)
- alternatively, clindamycin 2% cream, one 5 g application may be inserted *per vaginam* nightly for 7 nights.

If initial treatment is unsuccessful, the alternative treatment may be tried. In resistant cases oral clindamycin 300 mg b.d. for one week is occasionally used. Treatment of the male partner has not been shown to increase cure rate or reduce recurrence, but is probably worthwhile in women with recurrent bacterial vaginosis.

### Bacterial vaginosis and adverse pregnancy outcome

Bacterial vaginosis (BV) is associated with second trimester miscarriage and preterm birth (Hay *et al.* 1994), although most pregnant women with BV will have a normal pregnancy. At present there is no clear evidence that treatment of BV in pregnancy prevents adverse outcomes (Carey *et al.* 2000). Until definitive studies are published, it would seem reasonable to consider pre-pregnancy screening and treatment of women with a history of late miscarriage or preterm birth.

## Trichomoniasis

*Trichomonas vaginalis* is a protozoon that is a relatively harmless sexually transmitted vaginal pathogen. It can cause severe vaginal inflammation, but may also be asymptomatic and diagnosed on a routine cervical smear. Although it may occasionally be linked to adverse pregnancy outcome or possibly pelvic inflammatory disease, its main importance is that it can be a marker for other sexually transmitted diseases and indicates the need for screening.

### Symptoms and signs

Women with trichomoniasis may complain of an intensely irritating, bubbly, purulent discharge and vaginal soreness (more than irritation). There may be a fishy smell due to associated bacterial vaginosis.

### Diagnosis

This is by culture and microscopy of a high vaginal or cervical swab, either in Stuart's medium or special *T. vaginalis* transport medium. *T. vaginalis* may also be seen on a cervical smear and associated with inflammatory changes.

### Treatment

Metronidazole 2 g stat or 400 mg b.d. for 5 days will cure 90% of women with trichomoniasis. Intravaginal 2% clindamycin cream may sometimes be used during pregnancy. Sexual partners should be treated. Ideally, both the woman and her partner should be screened for other sexually transmitted infections.

## Chlamydia

Cervical *Chlamydia trachomatis* infection is the commonest bacterial sexually transmitted disease in women, with prevalences in general practice populations of 2–12% (Table 9.2). In 2001, 38 248 women were diagnosed with genital chlamydia in English genitourinary clinics, and numbers are rising, especially in teenagers.

Untreated chlamydia can cause pelvic inflammatory disease, leading to tubal infertility, ectopic pregnancy, or chronic pelvic pain. Since many women with chlamydia infection are asymptomatic, the first sign that a woman has had

**Table 9.2** Prevalence of cervical chlamydial infection in UK general practices

| First author, year of publication | Location | No. of practices | Study populations | Age range (years) | Test used | No. infected/ no. tested | Prevalence (%) |
|---|---|---|---|---|---|---|---|
| Southgate, 1983 | East London | 3 | Women having speculum examination | 15–45 | Culture | 19/248 | 8 |
| Longhurst, 1987 | Central London | 1 | Women having speculum examination | Pre-menopausal | DFA | 18/169 | 11 |
| Southgate, 1989 | East London | 4 | Women requesting termination of pregnancy | 16–44 | DFA | 12/103 | 12 |
| Owen, 1991 | Cardiff | 1 | Women with lower genital tract symptoms. Mainly social classes III and IV | 15–65 | DFA | 25/386 | 6 |
| Smith, 1991 | Glasgow | 1 | Women attending for cervical smear. Mainly social class III | 19–58 | Culture | 24/197 | 12 |
| Oakeshott, 1992 | South-east London | 2 | Women having speculum examination. Mainly social classes IV and V | 17–45 | DFA | 36/409 | 9 |
| Thomson, 1994 | Fife | 10 | Women attending for cervical smear | 15–40 | DFA | 5/287 | 2 |
| Grun, 1997 | Central London | 4 | Women (asymptomatic) attending for cervical smear | 18–35 | LCR | 23/890 | 3 |
| Oakeshott, 1998 | South London | 30 | Women attending for cervical smear | 16–34 | EIA | 40/1382 | 3 |
| Pimenta, 2003 | Portsmouth | 77 | Women attending for any reason | 16–24 | LCR | 641/7546 | 8 |

DFA, direct fluorescent antibody test; EIA, enzyme immunoassay; LCR, ligase chain reaction on first-pass urine.

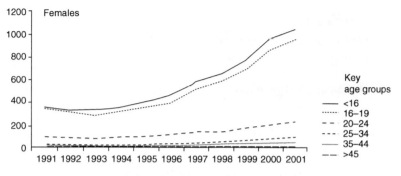

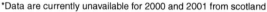

*Data are currently unavailable for 2000 and 2001 from scotland

**Fig 9.2** Rates of diagnoses of uncomplicated genital chlamydial infection made in GUM clinics by sex and age group, UK: 1991–2001* (Rates per 100,000 population). Source: PHLS, DHSS & PS and the Scottish ISD5 Collaborative Group. Sexually transmitted infections in the UK: new episodes seen at genitourinary medicine clinics 1991–2001 (2002). London, Public Health Laboratory Service. (Reproduced with permission)

chlamydia infection may be when she presents with infertility. Forty per cent of women thought to have uncomplicated chlamydial cervicitis have histological evidence of endometritis. Although the exact risk of infertility following cervical chlamydia infection is unkown, estimates suggest it may be 2–4% (Oakeshott and Hay 1995).

## Symptoms and signs

Up to 70% of women with cervical chlamydia infection have no symptoms. The remainder may have mild symptoms of vaginal discharge, intermenstrual or post coital bleeding, lower abdominal pain or dysuria. Occasionally, the first indication of infection in a mother may be chlamydial conjunctivitis in a neonate. Pelvic examination may be normal or show mucopurulent cervicitis or a friable cervix. Signs of pelvic inflammatory disease (see page 00) indicate the need to take endo-cervical swabs for *N. gonorrhoeae* as well as *C. trachomatis*. Since clinical findings in chlamydial infection are often variable or absent, opportunistic screening should also be performed on the basis of risk factors (Box 9.3). These have been established in two studies involving more than 2000 asymptomatic women attending UK general practices (Grun *et al.* 1997; Oakeshott *et al.* 1998).

## Diagnosis

The test used will depend on arrangements with the local laboratory. Previously, only antigen-detections tests – enzyme immunoassay or direct fluorescent antibody test – were available to most UK general practices. These are less than 80% sensitive (CMO's Expert Advisory Group 1998) and involve a speculum examination. GPs and their patients should demand access to

Box 9.3 **Indications for opportunistic chlamydia screening in sexually active young women attending general practice**

- Before termination of pregnancy
- Age <25, especially sexually active teenagers
- Two or more sexual partners in previous year
- Mucopurulent vaginal discharge
- Black African or Afro-Caribbean ethnic origin
- Friable cervix with contact bleeding

modern, sensitive, non-invasive DNA tests such as ligase chain reaction (LCR) or polymerase chain reaction (PCR) on first-pass urines or self-administered vaginal swabs. These are currently being introduced in primary care. These tests also allow the possibility of home testing.

The method of taking the endocervical swab is described on page 355. Specimens for chlamydia must contain endocervical cells, not pus or discharge.

### Treatment

- Doxycycline 100 mg b.d. for 7 days or azithromycin 1 g stat
- If pregnant or lactating: erythromycin 500 mg q.d.s. for 7 days or 250 mg q.d.s. for 14 days

It is vital that the woman's sexual partner is treated to prevent reinfection. She should be advised not to have sex with him until he can show her his empty bottle of tablets. In most cases, the patient should also be referred to the genitourinary clinic for follow-up and contact tracing and given a clinic leaflet.

A test of cure is only needed if there is a risk that the patient or her partner may not have complied with treatment, reinfection may have occurred, or a less effective antibiotic such as erythromycin was used. It should be done 2–4 weeks after completion of treatment. It also provides an opportunity for further patient education.

## Gonorrhoea

*Neisseria gonorrhoeae* is unusual in general practice (Table 9.1). Symptoms, signs and sequelae are similar to those of chlamydia infection, but patients with gonorrhoea are less likely to be asymptomatic. Rarely, gonococcal bacteraemia may produce skin lesions or septic arthritis.

## Diagnosis

An endocervical swab in Stuart's transport medium will diagnose 90% of cases. In genitourinary clinics, urethral and rectal swabs are also taken to increase sensitivity.

## Treatment

◆ Amoxicillin 3 g with probenecid 1 g in single oral dose, but the large number of tablets may cause problems with compliance

◆ Alternatively, ciprofloxacin 500 mg orally in a single dose may be used. This is contraindicated in women who are pregnant or have a history of fits.

In the UK the prevalence of penicillin-resistant infection is more than 5% (penicillinase-producing *Neissera gonorrhoeae*; PPNG), but imported infection should be presumed to be penicillin resistant when treated blind before anti-microbial sensitivity is known. The local laboratory should be consulted about appropriate antibiotic treatment.

If the patient has signs of pelvic inflammatory disease, longer treatment is required, for example an additional 10-day course of co-amoxiclav 375 mg t.d.s. (or erythromycin 500 mg q.d.s. in patients allergic to penicillin). Since contact tracing and screening and treatment for other sexually transmitted infections such as chlamydia are vital, referral to a genitourinary clinic is strongly recommended. A test of cure is advised (www.mssvd.org.uk/ceg.htm).

## Pelvic inflammatory disease

There is overwhelming evidence that sexually transmitted micro-organisms play a major role in the pathogenesis of pelvic inflammatory disease. Despite this, many women are still treated for pelvic inflammatory disease without their contacts being screened and treated. In England and Wales over the past decade, the increase in the number of new cases of uncomplicated sexually transmitted infections in women has been paralleled by a rise in the prevalence of pelvic inflammatory disease and ectopic pregnancy. Up to 50% of acute pelvic inflammatory disease has been shown to be due to chlamydia and many episodes are 'silent' or subclinical. More than 10% of women who have had one episode of pelvic inflammatory disease, and more than 50% of those who have had three episodes, develop tubal infertility. The risk of ectopic pregnancy is increased 10-fold after an episode of pelvic inflammatory disease.

### Symptoms and signs

Patients may have pelvic pain, dyspareunia, malaise, dysuria, purulent vaginal discharge, or be asymptomatic. In practice, pelvic inflammatory disease is

**Table 9.3** Diagnosis and management of infective causes of vaginal discharge

|  | Candida | Bacterial vaginosis | Trichomonas | Chlamydia | Gonorrhoea |
|---|---|---|---|---|---|
| Introduction | Test for glycosuria | Associated with preterm labour and late miscarriage | STD Screen for other STDs | STD Can cause PID, infertility, ectopic pregnancy | STD Can cause PID, infertility, ectopic pregnancy |
| Symptoms (unreliable for diagnosis) | Itchy discharge | OFTEN ASYMPTOMATIC — Fishy smell | Sore, frothy discharge IMB, pelvic pain, dysuria | Mucopurulent discharge, IMB, pelvic pain, dysuria | Mucopurulent discharge |
| Diagnosis | HVS or cervical swab | HVS or cervical swab | HVS or cervical swab | Special endocervical swab – need cells not discharge. Or LCR or PCR on first-pass urine | Cervical swab in Stuart's medium |
| Suggested treatment | If symptomatic: clotrimazole pessaries 200 mg PV *nocte* for 3 nights | If symptomatic: metronidazole 400 mg b.d. for 5 days. Avoid alcohol | Metronidazole 400 mg b.d. for 5 days. Avoid alcohol | Doxycycline 100 mg b.d. for 7 days or azithromycin l g stat. Additional Rx required for PID | Ask laboratory. Amoxicillin 3 g and probenecid 1 g stat. Additional Rx required for PID |
| Treat partner | If symptomatic | If recurrent infections | Yes | Treatment of partner vital. Refer to GUM for follow-up | Treatment of partner vital. Refer to GUM for follow-up |

*Note:* Microbiological tests are essential for effective diagnosis and management of vaginal discharge.
HVS, high vaginal swab; IMB, intermenstrual bleeding; PID, pelvic inflammatory disease; LCR, ligase chain reaction; PCR, polymerase chain reaction; Rx, treatment; GUM, genitourinary clinic.

notoriously difficult to diagnose clinically with any degree of accuracy. In a study of 147 women presenting with abdominal pain and clinical signs of acute salpin gitis (cervical motion pain, adnexal tenderness, and one of the following: pyrexia >38, ESR >15 mm/h, white cell count >10 000/ml), only 70% had acute pelvic inflammatory disease diagnosed at laparoscopy (Bevan *et al.* 1995). Of these, 45% had chlamydia infection, 14% had gonorrhoea and 8% had both.

## Diagnosis

Endocervical swabs for chlamydia and gonorrhoea are vital in all women with suspected pelvic inflammatory disease.

## Treatment

If the patient is ill, hospital admission may be considered. Otherwise treatment should be started immediately after swabs have been taken with a 2-week course of both metronidazole 400 mg b.d. and doxycycline 100 mg b.d. Erythromycin may be used instead of doxycycline if the patient is pregnant or lactating. If gonorrhoea is suspected, ciprofloxacin 500 mg stat may be given (or amoxicillin 3 g and probenecid 1 g if the patient is pregnant).

Rest and sexual abstinence are recommended. It is vital that the patient returns after one week for the swab results so that treatment for gonorrhoea and contact tracing can be arranged if required.

# Viral sexually transmitted infections

Genital warts and herpes are unpleasant viral sexually transmitted infections for which treatment is unsatisfactory. The infections can only be suppressed, not cured. Once infected, people may transmit the virus to others, even when they themselves are asymptomatic, and we do not know whether they remain infectious forever. Using condoms reduces the risk but does not always prevent infections.

Women with first attacks of either genital warts or herpes need screening for coexistent infections, especially chlamydia, and contact tracing. Therefore, in many cases the best option may be referral to the local genitourinary clinic.

## Genital warts

Genital warts are common, usually sexually transmitted, and difficult to treat. They are caused by human papilloma virus, and although most are benign, some types are associated with cervical cancer (see Chapter 13).

## Symptoms and signs

Genital warts are often asymptomatic, but may be associated with itching or discharge. They are usually noticed on the vulva or introitus. They may enlarge during pregnancy.

## Diagnosis

This is clinical. However, subclinical human papilloma virus infection is much commoner than clinical warts and is often diagnosed on a cervical smear or colposcopy. No treatment is required for subclinical infection but visible cervical warts are an indication for cytology and colposcopy.

## Treatment

As with commmon warts, this is laborious and not very effective. Patients find the fact that treatment is so inadequate very difficult to deal with. The aim is merely to remove obvious lesions as no therapy has been shown to eradicate the virus. Treatment is more effective for warts that are small and have been present for less than a year. Provided the patient is not pregnant, podophyllo-toxin 0.15% cream may be used for external warts. Treatment consists of twice daily application for 3 days followed by 4 days rest for 4 cycles. It can be used for home treatment but should be discontinued if there are side effects such as soreness or irritation. It is teratogenic.

If treatment is ineffective after 4 weeks, or the patient is pregnant and the warts are causing problems, patients may be referred to a genitourinary clinic for cryotherapy or electrocautery. Recurrence rates are at least 25% after 3 months. Warts may regress or reappear spontaneously and condoms should be used until at least 3 months after apparent cure.

Imiquimod 5% cream may be used for treatment failures but is not approved for use in pregnancy or internally. It is an immune response modifier. Cream is applied to lesions three times weekly and washed off 6–10 hours for up to 16 weeks. It costs £55 for a 4 week course and is normally prescribed by a geni-tourinary physician.

The NHS Cervical Screening Programme policy recommends that no changes are required to screening intervals in women with anogenital warts. However, this may change when we can routinely type human papilloma virus (see Chapter 3). Partner notification and screening for coexistent infections are recommended.

## Genital herpes

This is discussed in the '10-minute consultation' at the end of the chapter.

# Genitourinary clinics

These are much more user friendly than in the past. It is very helpful if there are good relations between general practitioners and local genitourinary physicians. A patient is much more likely to attend if the general practitioner gives her a clinic leaflet and letter and reassures her that the doctors are sympathetic and understanding.

Genitourinary clinics have positive advantages. Treatment is free and confidential. There are experienced health advisors with time for counselling and contact tracing (see below). The clinics will also screen for other sexually transmitted infections, including HIV if requested. Also the tests used may be more sensitive or investigations more extensive than those available in most general practices. Finally, they can review compliance with treatment and perform a test of cure if required.

## Contact tracing/partner notification

For each infected woman (index case) there are at least two people affected – her sexual contact and the person who infected her contact. Often it is more complicated. Thus, contact tracing requires time and sensitivity. In genitourinary clinics it is done with the assistance of health advisers. After discussion, the patient telephones or visits the partner and urges him to attend a genitourinary clinic for examination and treatment. The partner is given a contact slip, which includes the original patient's note number and a code for the diagnosis. When he goes to a genitourinary clinic for treatment, he hands in the contact slip which is then returned to the clinic of origin so that accurate contact tracing records can be kept. Health advisers prefer not to inform contacts themselves unless the patient is unable to do so. Confidentiality is paramount and no information will be given to anyone outside the clinic, including partners or other doctors, without the patient's permission.

In general practice, if a woman with a sexually transmitted infection is reluctant to attend a genitourinary clinic for contact tracing, she could be given a letter similar to a contact slip to give to her partner for him to take to a genitourinary clinic. The letter could state the woman's diagnosis and treatment given. If the partner hands this in at a clinic and gives consent for information to be released to the general practitioner, the clinic will reply with details of his diagnosis and treatment. Both partners should be advised not to have sexual intercourse until they have completed their courses of treatment.

## Sexual health promotion

Strategies to reduce the incidence of sexually transmitted infections include encouraging safer sex, increasing screening, and improving treatment and contact tracing among people found to be infected. For primary prevention, increasing condom use in women with multiple partners is likely to be beneficial. However, since barrier methods are unreliable in preventing pregnancy, the pill should also be used ('the double Dutch method').

Condom promotion schemes have been widely piloted in UK general practice. However, there is no clear evidence of their effectiveness. In the only randomized controlled trial of condom promotion in primary care, 37% of women with two or more partners in the previous year reported that their partner used a condom at the last sexual intercourse. But there was no difference between intervention and control groups (Oakeshott *et al.* 2000). Despite this, it would seem sensible to consider offering opportunistic advice about how to avoid sexually transmitted infections to all sexually active young women, especially when they attend for speculum examinations.

Secondary prevention of sexually transmitted diseases and their consequences is also important. Screening has been shown to reduce the prevalence of both chlamydial infection and pelvic inflammatory disease (CMO's Expert Advisory Group 1998). General practitioners and practice nurses have a vital role to play in screening women at risk of sexually transmitted infections, and ensuring that those found to be infected are managed appropriately.

## Key points

- All general practitioners and practice nurses performing speculum examinations should have appropriate equipment available and know how to take endocervical swabs for chlamydia and gonorrhoea.
- Women with chlamydia, gonorrhoea or a first attack of genital herpes or warts need:
  (a) appropriate treatment;
  (b) partner notification and no sex until both have been treated;
  (c) screening for other sexually transmitted infections;
  (d) referral to a genitourinary clinic.
- Good relationships with local genitourinary physicians are very helpful. The practice should have a supply of genitourinary clinic leaflets to hand to patients including the telephone number of the health advisers.

- The important bacterial causes of vaginal discharge which should not be missed are chlamydia and gonorrhoea because of their potential sequelae of pelvic inflammatory disease, tubal infertility, and ectopic pregnancy.
- All sexually transmitted infections can be asymptomatic.
- Opportunistic chlamydial testing on the basis of risk factors should be offered to sexually active young women who:
  - (a) request termination of pregnancy;
  - (b) are age <25, especially teenagers;
  - (c) had two or more sexual partners in the previous year;
  - (d) have mucopurulent cervicitis or a friable cervix.

# 10-Minute consultation: genital herpes

A young woman returns for a vulval swab result for 'cold sore virus'. She was seen a week ago complaining of being sore down below and had pain on passing urine for one week. A urine dipstick test was negative, but on examination she had two 1 mm red spots on her labia minor and a 0.5 cm linear fissure (scratch). There were no vesicles, ulcers or inguinal glands. After she had been told that this could be due to cold sore virus infection, the lesions were swabbed and sent for culture in viral transport medium. The laboratory report confirmed herpes simplex virus type 1.

## What issues you should cover

- *Sexual history* Has she had these symptoms before? Has she got other symptoms? When did she last have sexual intercourse? How long has she had a sexual relationship with her partner? Has he got symptoms? Has she had sex with anyone else in the past 6 months?
- *Implications of genital herpes* Explain that genital herpes is a sexually transmitted infection caused by the cold sore virus. It is common and relatively harmless. As it often causes few symptoms, she may have become infected some time ago. (Both herpes type 1 and 2 can cause genital ulceration; type 1 also causes facial cold sores.)
- *Partner notification* Advise her to be open with her partner about herpes. Often it is passed on by someone unaware of being infected. Both should be checked for other infections.
- *Screening for sexually transmitted infection* Screening is probably best done in a genitourinary clinic, where experts provide a thorough check-up, treatment is free and confidential, and health advisers offer information and support.

- *Reducing risk of transmission* Explain that she can have sex unless she has active sores or feels an outbreak coming on, when she should avoid sexual contact until the sores have healed. However, even when she is well a small risk of transmission remains. This can be reduced by consistent condom use. (Female-to-male infection rate is less than 5% a year.) Condoms also protect against other infections.

- *Treatment* Many infections are mild and symptomatic treatment usually suffices. Primary herpes may be severe, classically presenting up to 7 days after sexual contact with multiple, painful genital ulcers, often with inguinal lymphadenopathy. For the first acute episode, genitourinary referral is recommended, especially if tropical travel suggests other possible causes of ulcers. Aciclovir 200 mg five times daily for 5 days reduces pain, duration, and viral shedding. It is most effective if started within 6 days of onset. Later treatment or topical aciclovir has little effect.

- *Recurrences* Many patients never notice a recurrence. (Recurrences are more likely with type 2 or if the first episode is severe.) Symptoms are generally milder, and no specific treatment is needed. If she has six or more recurrences a year, referral for suppressive treatment should be considered. This prevents symptomatic recurrences in up to 80% of patients but is expensive.

- *Pregnancy* Herpes is rarely a problem unless the first ever episode is during pregnancy. She should be checked for signs of infection at the onset of labour. Risk of neonatal herpes in the UK is less than two per 100 000 live births.

## What you should do

- Advise dilute salt baths and paracetamol, with no sex until completely better.
- Refer her to the genitourinary clinic for partner notification and an infection screen. Alternatively, take endocervical swabs for chlamydia and gonorrhoea and ask her to advise her partner to get checked.
- Offer her a genital herpes leaflet and the telephone number of the local genitourinary clinic health advisers.

# Frequently asked questions

### I would know if I had a STD wouldn't I?

Not necessarily. All STDs may be asymptomatic. This particularly applies to chlamydia infection where the majority of infected women have few or no symptoms. This is why it is vital to be checked for chlamydia from time to time (evidence on frequency is unclear), and especially if you have a new partner. Similarly, warts and cold sore infections may be mild enough not to be noticed.

## Does this mean my partner has been with someone else?

It is a STD which means it is acquired by sexual intercourse with someone who is infected. It doesn't necessarily mean he's been with someone else recently. It is possible that either of you could have picked up the infection some time ago without knowing. But you do need to talk about it and both be checked and treated.

## How can I tell my partner?

Does your partner know there is a problem? If not, you could say you were concerned and went to the GP who did tests.

## Will someone be able to tell in future that I've had this?

If it is chlamydia infection, treatment should clear it up completely and it is of no concern to future partners. If it is herpes you might tell a future partner in due course: 'I've had cold sores down below in the past. I'm OK now, but the doctor says it can sometimes recur. To be on the safe side it would be better if we used condoms, especially if I feel a bit sore.' (You may find your partner says he's had it too and isn't bothered.)

## Do I really need to have a chlamydia check before my termination?

Women requesting termination of pregnancy have a high prevalence of chlamydia infection and up to 60% risk of developing post-abortal pelvic inflammatory disease if they have untreated chlamydia infection at the time of operation. For some women who then develop tubal infertility, this may be their only pregnancy. Despite these risks, many hospitals performing terminations still fail to screen or treat women for chlamydia infection. General practitioners should ensure that women awaiting termination are aware of the risks and the need for screening (which could be done either at the surgery or at the local genitourinary clinic).

## Does having chlamydia infection mean I can't have children?

Chlamydia infection is common and usually causes few problems. Provided you and your partner are treated, the risk of infertility due to blocked tubes is very low, probably <5%. If you've had pelvic inflammatory disease, the risk of infertility is higher, about 15%. I'm afraid you won't know about this until you try to get pregnant. But even after PID, the vast majority of women will be able to have children.

## Information for patients

There is an excellent series of booklets on sexually transmitted infections published by the former Health Education Authority and available from health promotion units and genitourinary clinics. These include: 'Vaginal infections', 'Thrush', 'Chlamydia and NSU', 'Genital herpes', 'Genital warts', and 'Guide to a healthy sex life'.

Practices should also have available a supply of local genitourinary clinic leaflets and the telephone number of the clinic health advisers.

There is an active self-help group for herpes sufferers: The Herpes Viruses Association, SPHERE, 42 North Rd, London N7 9DP; Tel 0207 6099061; website: www.herpes.org.uk. For reliable information on all health topics including STDs and women's health, contact: http://www.nlm.nih.gov/medlineplus. Select health topics. This website is also accessible via www.claphamhealth.org.uk.

Clinical effectiveness guidelines on the medical management of STDs are available from the Medical Society for the Study of Venereal Diseases: http://www.mssvd.org.uk/ceg.htm.

## Acknowledgements

My thanks are due to Dr Phillip Hay, Dr Ian Simms, Mrs Wendy Majewska, and Ms Lee-Ann Sallis.

## References and further reading

Bevan, C., Johal, B., Mumtaz, G., Ridgway, G. and Siddle, N. (1995). Clinical, laparoscopic and microbiological findings in acute salpingitis: report on a United Kingdom cohort. *British Journal of Obstetrics and Gynaecology*, **102**, 407–14.

Carey, J.C., Klebanoff, K., Hauth, J., *et al.* (2000). Metronidazole to prevent preterm delivery in pregnant women with asymptomatic bacterial vaginosis. *New England Journal of Medicine*, **342**, 534–40.

CMO's Expert Advisory Group (1998). *Chlamydia trachomatis*. Department of Health, London.

Drake, S., Taylor, S., Brown, D. and Pillay, D. (2000). Improving care of patients with genital herpes. *British Medical Journal*, **321**, 619–23.

Grun, L., Tassano-Smith, J., Carder, C., *et al.* (1997). Comparison of two methods of screening for genital chlamydial infection in women attending in general practice: cross sectional survey. *British Medical Journal*, **315**, 226–30.

Hay, P., Lamont, R., Taylor-Robinson, D., Morgan, D., Ison, C. and Pearson, J. (1994). Abnormal bacterial colonisation of the genital tract and subsequent preterm delivery and late miscarriage. *British Medical Journal*, **308**, 295–8.

Hopwood, J. and Mallinson, H. (1995). Chlamydia testing in community clinics – a focus for accurate sexual health care. *British Journal of Family Planning*, **21**, 87–90.

McCormack, S. (1999). The diagnoses and management of genital ulceration. In: Barton, S.E. and Hay, P.E. (eds), *Handbook of genitourinary medicine*, pp. 97–121. Arnold, London.

Oakeshott, P. and Hay, P. (1995). General practice update: chlamydia infection in women. *British Journal of General Practice*, **45**, 615–20.

Oakeshott, P., Kerry, S., Hay, S. and Hay, P. (1998). Opportunistic screening for chlamydial infection at time of cervical smear testing in general practice: prevalence study. *British Medical Journal*, **316**, 351–2.

Oakeshott, P., Kerry, S., Hay, S. and Hay, P. (2000). Condom promotion in women attending inner city general practices for cervical smears: a randomized controlled trial. *Family Practice*, **17**, 56–9.

Owen, P., Hughes, M. and Munro, J. (1991). Study of the management of chlamydial cervicitis in general practice. *British Journal of General Practice*, **41**, 279–81.

Chapter 10

# Vulval disorders
## Lois Eva

## Introduction

Vulval disease is a difficult area of women's health, and as a result is often neglected or overlooked. Assessment of vulval disease is particularly difficult in general practice where specialist equipment or even decent lighting may not be available and all too frequently examination of this area is omitted entirely from the consultation. A combination of factors including patient embarrassment or the assumption by both the woman and the clinician that all vulval symptoms are attributable to thrush can often lead to serious and potentially avoidable pathologies being missed. Vulval disease affects women of all ages and the golden rule is that if a woman has persistent symptoms that are not responding to antifungal medication, then it probably is not candida and she needs a proper examination.

Vulval disease has a major impact on women's lives and can have particular effect on sexual relationships. Early diagnosis and appropriate treatment or referral can alleviate suffering that otherwise may persist for many years.

## The normal vulva

The vulva comprises the mons pubis, labia majora, labia minora, clitoris, vestibule of the vagina, bulb of the vestibule, and the greater vestibular glands. Diseases of the vulva may involve all or part of the vulva but it is important to remember that certain pathologies may manifest themselves elsewhere in the body as well.

The appearance of the normal vulva changes throughout life and is affected by different physiological factors. Children with vulval problems are often assumed to be the victims of abuse, and although these problems may coexist, false accusations can easily be made without considering possible pathology. Pregnancy and subsequent childbirth will alter the appearance of the vulva and vulval varicosities are more common during this time. Episiotomy or birth trauma may lead to changes in the vulval appearance that are not necessarily pathological, although referral may be appropriate. The practice of female genital mutilation (female circumcision) in some countries of Africa is common and, depending on the extent of the mutilation, persistent vulval problems may occur. Atrophy of the tissues at the menopause is often attributed to many vulval symptoms described by older women; diagnosis prior to examination should be resisted.

## Clinical features of vulval disease

The two most common symptoms are itching or pain. Pruritus is probably the most common symptom and causes of vulval pruritus are found in Table 10.1. Pain is often described as soreness or a burning sensation and may or may not be related to intercourse. Often the initial presentation is prompted by difficulties with sexual intercourse. Pain at penetration, splitting of the vulval skin or postcoital burning are often described, as are problems with insertion or removal of tampons. Specific questions should be asked about these problems, as many women, and particularly older women, are often embarrassed and will not volunteer such information, or the clinician assumes the woman is not sexually active.

The woman may have discovered a lump or ulcer, or noticed changes in the colour of the vulva as pigmentation or pallor are common findings. Other skin conditions are relevant as is a smear history, as we know that certain conditions are related. A proportion of vulval lesions are asymptomatic and found incidentally at examination.

Adequate examination of the vulva may be difficult in general practice, especially in immobile patients and some lesions may not be seen with the naked eye. Examination should include the whole of the perineum extending up to the crural folds and posteriorly to the perianal area. The groin should be examined and lymph nodes palpated. Other areas of skin and the buccal mucosa may be involved and should also be examined, if appropriate.

Some of the physical changes seen in vulval disease are fairly obvious, whereas other changes may be more subtle. Commonly seen signs are changes in the pigmentation of the skin, either pallor or deposition of pigment. Lichenification or thickening of the skin may be part of the pathological process or as a result of scratch damage secondary to symptoms. Changes may be symmetrical (as in lichen sclerosus) or unilateral with a specific discrete lesion. Erythema may be generalized (in vulval candidiasis) or local (in vulval vestibulitis syndrome). Changes in the vulval architecture may be apparent and splitting or fusion of tissue is often visible. Tenderness may be elicited over different areas of the vulva and this should be noted.

Women who present with suspicious looking areas should be referred urgently.

**Table 10.1** Causes of vulval pruritus

| | Clinical features | Treatment |
|---|---|---|
| Fungal overgrowth | Red hot beefy vulva | Topical antifungals ± oral fluconazole |
| Lichen simplex | Thickened, flaky skin | Topical steroids and emollients |
| | Scratch damage or splitting | |
| Psoriasis | Symmetrical red scaly | Topical steroids, avoid tar products |
| Eczema | Scaly thickened skin | Topical steroids |
| Dermatitis (allergic or contact) | Erythematous, oedematous skin | Remove offending irritant |
| | May blister | May need patch testing |
| | | Topical steroids |
| Lichen planus | Erosive or hypertrophic lesions | Topical or systemic steroids |
| | Desquamative vaginitis, ulceration or stenosis | Retinoids |
| | | Immunosuppression |
| | Wickham's striae in mouth | |
| Hygiene | Excoriated, erythematous, oedematous tissue | Improve hygiene |
| | | Emollients for symptomatic relief |
| Atrophy | Loss of glycogenated tissue | Hormone replacement therapy |
| | Dry vagina | |
| Medical disorders | Varied: e.g. in association with diabetes, chronic renal failure | Treat underlying condition |

**Table 10.1** (*continued*)

| | Clinical features | Treatment |
|---|---|---|
| Lichen sclerosus | Atrophic or hypertrophied skin | Topical steroids |
| | Symmetrical pallor, loss of architecture. Ecchymosis | Biopsy suspicious areas |
| | | Surgery only for adhesions or malignancy |
| Vulval intraepithelial neoplasia | Warty lesions | Excision and regular surveillance |
| | Unifocal or multifocal | |
| | May involve anus | |
| Vulval carcinoma | Ulcerated lesion | Surgery |
| | Hypertrophic lesion | |
| | May coexist with lichen sclerosus or VIN | |
| Paget's disease | Erythematous, scaly lesions | Surgery |

## Psychological features of vulval disease

Vulval disease can have a massive impact on women's lives, both physically and psychologically. Many vulval patients, particularly those with vulval pain syndromes, are labelled 'mad' as there are no obvious physical signs, and although there is no doubt that psychological factors play a large role in the understanding and treatment of these conditions, many of these are a result of the physical condition and not the cause.

The vulva is a sexual organ and conditions that affect physical appearance and function will have detrimental effects on sexual relationships, leading to other relationship difficulties. Both disease and treatment, be it surgical or radiotherapy, can be disfiguring and/or impair sexual function. Studies have looked at psychosexual dysfunction in women undergoing vulvectomy for vulval cancer and found distress levels compatible with other cancer sufferers; dysfunction was both physical and psychological and manifested itself more severely in younger and single women (Corney et al. 1993).

Non-malignant conditions can be equally distressing and destructive. Adhesion formation and fusion of the labia with lichen sclerosus and obliteration of the vagina with lichen planus severely affect sexual function. Often this aspect is overlooked, as these conditions tend to affect the older population, who are often assumed not to be sexually active. It is therefore vital to explore this avenue in consultation.

Work looking at the psychological aspects of vulval pain has confirmed the need for a prompt diagnosis, as labelling the problem is often the first step to resolution. Women with vulval pain syndromes have significantly increased psychological morbidity compared with asymptomatic controls and within the category of vulval pain, women with dysaesthetic vulvodynia (where there are no physical findings) have the greatest levels of psychological stress, compared with women with other vulval diseases. These women are highly aware of their body image, are more likely to consult their doctor about other symptoms, and have increased levels of somatization (Schover et al. 1992; Stewart et al. 1994; Jantos and White 1997).

Often these women have had symptoms for many years and are trapped in a vicious circle to the extent that even when the physical problem is resolved, they are unable to resume a normal life. Vaginismus is commonly secondary to the initial disorder and the role of psychosexual counsellors and physiotherapists with an interest in the pelvic floor is important. In women with persistent symptoms, coping mechanisms, pain management strategies, and support groups may help (Nunns 2000).

Because of the potential long-term problems that vulval disease may cause, referral to a multidisciplinary vulval clinic is ideal, although not always available, rather than to routine gynaecology or dermatology out-patients.

# The vulva clinic

Vulval disease overlaps the areas of gynaecology, dermatology, and genitourinary medicine. Ideally, referral of patients from primary care should be to a specialist vulval clinic that is multidisciplinary.

Prior to referral it is important that the primary care doctor has examined the patient. Often vulval clinics have long waiting times for first appointments, but if a potential malignancy is suspected, then urgent referral is paramount. High vaginal and endocervical swabs may be performed prior to referral to eliminate any infective cause that can be treated easily. Blood tests generally are of no value.

Examination of the vulva should be conducted in a private area, preferably a separate room and not a curtained-off area. Adequate lighting should be available. Optimum examination is in the lithotomy position and a tilting chair is ideal to achieve this.

Colposcopy is increasingly being used in the assessment of vulval disease and closed circuit television to be attached so the patient can identify problem areas. KY jelly may be used to minimize the reflection of light in hair-bearing areas. As in cervical colposcopy, acetic acid may be used to identify lesions. Toludine blue may also be used to define areas of abnormality. Swabs may be taken to exclude infective causes of acute vulvovaginitis, e.g. *Candida*, gonorrhoea, *Trichomonas*, bacterial vaginosis.

Biopsy is easily performed in an out-patient setting. Local anaesthetic is injected using a dental syringe and punch biopsy may be obtained using a 4 mm Stiefel punch. Haemostasis is achieved using silver nitrate sticks or Monsel's solution and sutures are rarely required.

# Diseases of the vulva

The classification of vulval disease has long been disputed and is regularly updated (Ridley and Neill 1999). The International Society for the Study of Vulval Disease (ISSVD) was founded to address these problems and to give clinicians the opportunity to meet and share knowledge.

In 1998 the ISSVD updated its classification of non-neoplastic vulval disorders (Table 10.2). GPs may find this comprehensive classification useful as a reference once a specialist dermatological diagnosis has been made; in particular, it may help the GP to explain to the patient where her condition lies within the spectrum of vulval disease. Classification of vulval pain (Table 10.3) is currently under review.

A simple overview of vulval disease would be to divide it into three categories: non-neoplastic disease, neoplastic disease, and vulval pain

**Table 10.2** Revised ISSVD classification of vulvar disease (1998)

1. INFECTIONS

Parasitic: e.g.. pediculosis, scabies

Protozoal: e.g.. amoebiasis

Viral: e.g.. herpes virus infection, condyloma acuminata

Bacterial

Fungal: e.g.. candidosis, dermatophytosis

Others

2. INFLAMMATORY SKIN DISEASE

Spongiotic disorders

    Contact dermatitis

      Irritant

      Allergic

    Atopic dermatitis (acute and chronic)

    Seborrhoeic dermatitis

    Others

Psoriasiform disorders

    Lichenification (lichen simplex)

    Atopic dermatitis (chronic)

    Seborrhoeic dermatitis

    Others

Lichenoid disorders

    Lichen sclerosus

    Lichen planus

    Fixed drug eruption

    Plasma cell vulvitis

    Lichenoid reaction, not otherwise specified (focal or diffuse)

    Lupus erythematosus

    Others

Vesicobullous disorders

    Pemphigoid

    Pemphigus

    Erythema multiforme

    Stevens–Johnson syndrome

    Others

**Table 10.2** (*continued*)

---

Granulomatous disorders

    Non-infectious

        Sarcoidosis

        Crohn's disease (hidradenitis suppuritiva)

        Others

    Infectious

        Tuberculosis

        Granuloma inguinale

Vasculitis or related inflammatory disorders

    Leucocytoclastic

    Urticaria

    Aphthous ulcer

    Lymphoedema

    Behcet's disease

    Pyoderma gangrenosa

    (Fixed drug eruption)

    (Erythema multiforme)

    (Stevens–Johnson syndrome)

3. SKIN APPENDAGES DISORDERS

Hidradenitis suppuritiva

Fox–Fordyce disease

Disorders of sweating

4. HORMONAL DISORDERS

Oestrogen

    Excess

        Precocious puberty

        Others

    Deficiency

        Physiological

            Lactation

            Postmenopausal

            Others

        Iatrogenic

**Table 10.2** (*continued*)

---

Androgen

  Excess

    Physiological

    Iatrogenic

5. ULCERS AND EROSIONS (diseases that ulcerate and/or erode are listed according to histological findings)

Trauma

  Obstetric

  Surgical

  Sexual

  Accidental

Others (include fissures of the fossa navicularis)

6. DISORDERS OF PIGMENTATION

Hyperpigmentation

  Melanin

    Lentigo

    Melanosis vulvae (post-inflammatory pigmentation)

  Haemosiderin (post-inflammatory pigmentation)

  Vitiligo

Hypopigmentation

  Vitiligo

  Post-inflammatory pigmentation

---

syndromes. The prevalence of vulval disease in the general population is largely unknown. The most commonly referred pathology from general practice is lichen sclerosus, but recent years have seen an increase in vulvodynia. Fig 10.1 shows the referral patterns from a study of 1000 women attending two specialist vulval clinics (MacLean *et al.* 1998).

## Non-neoplastic disease

### Lichen sclerosus

Lichen sclerosus is a condition of unknown aetiology. Previously known as lichen sclerosus et atrophicus, leukoplakia or vulval kraurosis, it may occur in any age group. It may present from childhood (where it may be mistaken for

**Table 10.3** The International Federation of Gynaecology and Obstretrics (FIGO) staging of vulval carcinoma (1995)

| | |
|---|---|
| Ia | Confined to vulva, <1 mm invasion |
| Ib | Confined to vulva, <2 cm diameter |
| | No lymph node involvement |
| II | Confined to vulva, >2 cm diameter |
| | No lymph node involvement |
| III | Local spread to vagina, urethra, perineum or anus but no lymph node involvement |
| | *or* |
| | Any size confined to the vulva and unilateral lymph node involvement |
| IVA | Any size involving bladder or rectal mucosal or bone |
| | *or* |
| | Any size with bilateral lymph node involvement |
| IVB | Distant metastases |

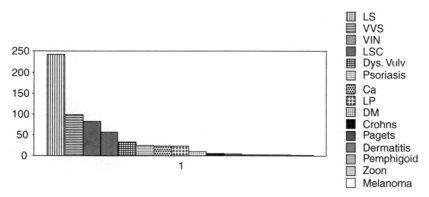

**Fig 10.1** Review of 1000 women seen in a vulval clinic.

sexual abuse) to old age and although the incidence increases with age, the mean age of onset is the fifth and sixth decades. It is more common in Caucasians although the appearance is more dramatic in dark skin, due to loss of pigment.

It has been suggested that lichen sclerosus could be an autoimmune disease and studies have reported associations with other autoimmune conditions, including thyrotoxicosis and hypothyroidism, diabetes mellitus, vitiligo, systemic lupus erythematosus, bullous pemphigoid, primary biliary cirrhosis, and pernicious anaemia (Meyrick Thomas *et al.* 1988).

It involves the vulva and perianal region but never the vagina. Lichen sclerosus will also affect other areas such as the limbs or trunk in approximately 11% of patients (Thomas *et al.* 1996). Large studies have not found an association with class I HLA antigens, although they did find a link with the class II antigen DQ7 (Marren *et al.* 1995).

There is an association between lichen sclerosus and vulval malignancy and these two conditions are often found coexisting in specimens containing squamous cell carcinoma of the vulva. The exact mechanism is unknown and it is not certain whether lichen sclerosus itself is a premalignant condition or whether other pathways are involved. However, the associated risk of malignancy appears to be 4–5% (Wallace 1971) and therefore long-term follow-up and regular surveillance, normally annually, is important. Initially follow-up is normally in hospital, but if a patient is well controlled she can then be seen by the general practitioner. If, however, her symptoms flare again, then re-referral is recommended.

### Clinical features

Lichen sclerosus often presents as vulval pruritus, which may be intense. The itching is often worse at night and it has been known for a woman to use a kitchen scrubbing brush to try to alleviate the intense irritation. As a result of this scratch, damage and trauma are not unusual. Soreness and splitting of the skin are also often reported and this may lead to superficial dyspareunia. However, some women are asymptomatic and present due to changes in physical appearance.

The classical appearance is of thin papery white skin in a symmetrical figure-of-eight pattern around the vulva and anus. Loss of architecture is common and the labia minora may be completely absorbed. Fusion of the labia and burying of the clitoris may also be seen. Ecchymosis and haemosiderin deposits are often seen secondary to scratch damage due to the intense vulval pruritus. The Koebner phenomenon occurs in lichen sclerosus – scarring or trauma may induce typical skin lesions of the disorder, and extragenital lesions commonly occur in pre-existing scars and damaged sites.

Clinical diagnosis is confirmed by biopsy showing characteristic histology. The classic features are hydropic degeneration of the basal cells and a pale staining homogeneous zone in the upper dermis, below which is a band of inflammatory cells that are mainly monocytic (Powell and Wojnarowska 1999).

### Treatment

There is no cure for lichen sclerosus. Treatment is aimed at controlling the symptoms and monitoring the disease to prevent progression to malignant change. Treatment is initially twice daily with a potent topical steroid such as clobetasol for 2–3 months (Dalziel *et al.* 1991) followed by maintenance with potent steroid less frequently or with a moderately potent steroid. Use of weak steroids such as hydrocortisone is not appropriate. Patients are often concerned about using steroids on the genital area as there may be instructions not to do so on the packaging, so it should be explained that the skin in lichen sclerosus is abnormal and, providing use is supervised and not excessive (e.g. less than 30 g in 3 months, as maintenance), then long-term use is acceptable. If symptoms are not controlled during maintenance therapy, then referral to an appropriate clinic should be made to exclude malignant change. Topical testosterone, progesterone and oestrogen creams are no longer considered to be effective treatment of lichen sclerosus and should not be used.

There is no place for surgery in the treatment of uncomplicated lichen sclerosus. Vulvectomy was used in the past but we know that even after removal of the vulva, lichen sclerosus will recur. Surgery is reserved for treatment of adhesions or for excision of suspicious areas. Surgery is far more conservative than previously practised and wide local excision for atypical areas is used as opposed to more radical surgical intervention.

Once asymptomatic, patients should be kept under review and seen annually. Lichen sclerosus, like any scarring vulval disease, can have psychological effects and some patients may benefit from support groups.

## Lichen simplex chronicus (LSC)

Previously known as neurodermatitis, this condition occurs in normal skin in response to scratch damage.

### Clinical features
The presenting symptom is pruritus. The vulval skin is thickened, dry, and flaky. Splitting may occur.

### Treatment
Underlying pathology should be excluded. Topical steroid and emollients are used to alleviate symptoms. Oral antihistamines may be used at night as a sedative if the itching is intense.

## Contact dermatitis

This may occur as a result of an irritant or allergen. Allergic contact dermatitis is a type IV hypersensitivity reaction and usually occurs 1–2 days after exposure to the allergen. Common allergens are washing powder, lubricants, latex, and perfumes.

### Clinical features

Acute reactions present with pruritus and/or soreness. The vulva is diffusely erythematous and may be oedematous or blistered. Secondary bacterial infection may be superimposed. Chronic reactions usually lead to lichenification of the skin.

### Treatment

The offending allergen should be isolated and removed. Patch testing may be of use in isolating the allergen. Moderate potency topical steroids are usually effective.

## Eczema

Vulval eczema is a dermatitis without an allergen or irritant aetiology. Vulval atopic eczema is rare but should be considered if there are lesions elsewhere on the body. Treatment is with topical steroids.

## Psoriasis

Psoriasis may present solely affecting the vulva but often there is evidence of the disease elsewhere on the body.

### Clinical features

Vulval psoriasis does not present with the classical pearly scaling appearance seen in flexural psoriasis. It appears as sharply demarcated erythematous plaques and may have satellite lesions. It mainly affects hair-bearing areas and is rarely seen in mucous membranes. It may extend into the natal cleft where it may fissure.

### Treatment

Treatment is with moderately potent or potent topical steroids. Tar preparations used to treat psoriasis elsewhere on the body should be avoided on the genital area, as they are highly irritant. In severe cases that do not respond, referral to a dermatologist for PUVA or systemic treatment may be required.

## Lichen planus

Unlike lichen sclerosus, which only affects the vulva, lichen planus is a condition of the vulva and the vagina. It is most common in women over the age of 40 and unusual in children. It presents in two different forms, erosive and hypertrophic. The prevalence of vulval lichen planus is unknown but it is less common than many other vulval conditions.

### Clinical features

Lichen planus may present as pruritus, pain, or a combination of both. Erosive lesions are more likely to be painful. Contact bleeding or dyspareunia are also common symptoms. The hypertrophic lesions are hyperkeratotic and elevated.

If these areas become infected or ulcerate, they may be confused with malignancy. Erosive lesions are red and raw, affect the vestibule, and often extend up into the vagina where they may cause a desquamative vaginitis and ulceration. In time these lesions will cause severe scarring and may progress to vaginal stenosis or obliteration.

The appearance of a white lacy reticular pattern of Wickham's striae may be visible on the buccal mucosa and therefore oral inspection should be included in the examination.

### Treatment

Suspected lichen planus should be referred as treatment is often difficult and may be prolonged. Diagnosis is confirmed by histology and although some may respond to potent topical steroids, systemic steroids, immunosuppresion, or retinoids may be indicated if the condition is severe (Lewis 1998).

## Neoplastic disease

### Vulval intraepithelial neoplasia

Previously known as Bowen's disease, carcinoma *in situ*, dystrophy with squamous atypia, vulval intraepithelial neoplasia (VIN) is a premalignant condition of unknown aetiology, although there are strong associations with smoking and human papillomavirus (HPV). VIN affects a wide age range with the peak incidence in women in their forties. There is an association with cervical intra epithelial neoplasia (CIN) in 20–50% of cases.

VIN is recognized as a premalignant condition; however, there is debate as to the risk of progression. Originally thought to be around 5%, but greater in older women, it has now been suggested that the rate may be much higher (Jones and Rowan 1994). Equally, VIN may regress in a similar fashion to CIN. For these reasons patients need careful surveillance and regular follow-up, usually under hospital care.

### Clinical features

VIN has variable presentation and is often mistaken for vulval warts. The most common symptom is pruritus, but patients may present with bleeding, dyspareunia, or have noticed skin changes. Lesions may vary in colour, ranging from white to pigmented red-brown. There may be a discrete lesion or multifocal areas extending over the vulva and perianal area. Abnormal areas may be visualized more easily under colposcopic examination with the application of acetic acid or toludine blue. It is important to exclude multifocal intraepithelial neoplasia and therefore the cervix and vagina should be examined carefully. Persistent pruritus despite treatment should always be treated with suspicion.

### Treatment

Regular surveillance of these patients is important, even after surgical treatment, as recurrence may occur. Symptoms may be controlled with potent topical steroids. VIN 3 is treated by wide local excision, or, in the case of extensive disease, skinning vulvectomy using a laser may be appropriate.

## Vulval cancer

Vulval carcinoma is a relatively uncommon cancer of the female genital tract, accounting for less than 5% of genital tract malignancies. It most commonly affects older women. Ninety per cent of tumours are squamous cell carcinomas, the remainder being malignant melanomas or basal cell carcinomas.

### Squamous cell carcinoma

Vulval cancer may occur spontaneously, but is often associated with a pre-existing condition such as VIN or lichen sclerosus. Spread is local and then to the lymphatics with late spread to the lungs and liver. Prognosis depends on the depth of invasion and nodal involvement (Hacker *et al.* 1983). Overall 5-year survival is 75%. If there is no nodal involvement, this increases to 90–100%; if there is inguinal node involvement, survival is 30–70%; the involvement of pelvic lymph nodes significantly reduces 5-year survival to less than 25%.

The International Federation of Gynaecology and Obstetrics (FIGO) (staging of squamous cell carcinoma is shown in Table 10.3).

### Clinical features

Vulval cancers are often not discovered until they are advanced. This is either due to late presentation by the patient, often due to embarrassment, or by failure of the clinician to examine an older woman with persistent vulval pruritus and blind treatment, assuming the symptoms are due to candida infection. Therefore it is imperative to examine any woman with persistent symptoms. The most common symptom is pruritus, although vulval carcinoma may present with bleeding, ulceration, lump, pain, or abnormal discharge.

### Treatment

Histological diagnosis should be obtained prior to treatment. It is now generally agreed that stage I and II cancers can be treated with wide local excision and do not need radical surgery (Hacker and van der Velden 1993). Lateralized tumours initially only need dissection of ipsilateral lymph nodes; the contralateral nodes are taken only if the initial nodes prove positive (Royal

College of Obstetricians and Gynaecologists 1999). Stages III and IV are treated with radical vulvectomy with lymph node dissection; this is normally now performed through separate incisions and the traditional 'butterfly' incision is seldom used. If there is lymph node involvement, then external beam radiotherapy is used. Chemotherapy is not routinely used.

## Other vulval malignancies

### Malignant melanoma

Melanoma accounts for approximately 10% of vulval malignancies and has a poor prognosis, as it has often spread before presentation. Peak incidence is in the sixth and seventh decades of life.

It usually presents as a pigmented lump that is growing rapidly. There is a move to treating with local surgery, as more radical surgery does not appear to improve survival. Five-year survival is 8–50% and, as with other melanomas, a Breslow depth of more than 0.76 mm worsens prognosis. Metastases may occur years after treatment.

### Basal cell carcinoma

Basal cell carcinoma accounts for 2–4% of vulval malignancies and is usually found on the anterior labia majora, although they may occur elsewhere. Metastasis is unusual and treatment is by local excision, although about 20% may recur.

### Adenocarcinoma

Adenocarcinoma of the vulva is very rare.

### Paget's disease

Extramammary vulval Paget's is usually found in postmenopausal women. Unlike breast disease, there is only underlying adenocarcinoma in about a quarter of cases. About 10% will have carcinoma elsewhere, e.g. breast.

Again the most common symptom is pruritus, which may take years to develop and so a large proportion will be asymptomatic. Lesions are usually erythematous and scaly with sharp demarcation and raised edges. Management involves wide excision, as progression to invasive carcinoma is rare, although recurrence may occur.

# Vulval pain

Vulval pain is a complex and poorly understood area of vulval disease, which as a result is often inadequately managed, or not even recognized. The majority of women who have some form of vulval pain may be labelled as chronic

**Table 10.4** ISSVD classification of vulval pain (1991)

- Vulvar dermatoses
- Cyclic vulvodynia
- Vestibular papillomatosis
- Vulval vestibulitis
- Essential vulvodynia
- Idiopathic vulvodynia

thrush sufferers for many years or be labelled as mad as they don't have any obvious physical signs. Assessment of vulval pain is particularly difficult in primary care, as any physical changes are often subtle and not easily seen with a naked eye. The term vulvodynia is defined as chronic vulval discomfort, especially that characterized by the patient's complaint of burning, stinging, irritation or rawness (McKay).

In 1991 the ISSVD classified vulvodynia in six categories, as shown in Table 10.4. This classification is currently under review and a revised classification is expected.

As the vulval dermatoses have already been discussed earlier in this chapter and vestibular papillomatosis refers to the papillae present on the labia minora, which are now considered to be a normal variant, we will consider a simplified, broader classification of vulval pain. In general terms, vulval pain can be divided into three categories:

- infective causes
- dysaesthetic vulvodynia
- vulval vestibulitis syndrome.

Vaginal infections and sexually transmitted infections are covered separately (Chapter 9) and so will not be dealt with in great detail. Less common causes of vulval pain include Behçet's syndrome, Crohn's disease of the vulva, benign mucous membrane pemphegoid, Stevens–Johnson syndrome, and pemphigus, but these will not be covered in detail in this chapter.

It is important to take a thorough history. As previously mentioned, the majority of vulval disease will either present with pruritus or pain as the primary complaint. True vulvodynia does not have a pruritic component. It is a persistent raw, burning sensation that throbs, and may last for many hours, if not days. Vulval pain has been compared to glossodynia or post-herpetic neuralgia and the similarities persist in some of the treatments available.

## Infective causes of vulval pain

### Candida

Vulval candidiasis does not usually present with the classic curd-like discharge and itching of vaginal candida, although it is probably the most common mis-diagnosis within vulval disease.

It is more common in older women, often in those who are using a steroid-based preparation for a vulval dermatosis. Immunocompromised patients are prone to this infection, as are diabetics. The management at initial consultation should include urine analysis for glucose.

#### Clinical features

The classic presentation is symmetrical erythematous, swollen labia majora, with sharply demarcated borders. The area is hot to touch and has a beefy appearance. Vaginal swabs will not always yield a positive result as laboratories usually look for *Candida albicans* and not for other subgroups of the *Candida* species.

#### Treatment

The treatment of choice is oral fluconazole 150 mg twice, at weekly intervals, plus vaginal nystatin pessaries and topical nystatin cream. If the patient were using a steroid-based preparation and experiencing fungal overgrowth, it would be advisable to change to a preparation which has a combination of steroid and antifungal, e.g. Dermovate NN.

Candida may be a cause of cyclic vulvodynia where episodes of pain are related to a point in the menstrual cycle. If such a relationship can be identified, then prophylactic treatment can be implemented before symptoms occur.

Herpes simplex virus (especially a primary attack), syphilis, chancroid, and *Trichomonas vaginalis* may also present with severe vulval pain.

## Dysaesthetic vulvodynia

### Clinical features

This condition classically affects older women. It presents with a persistent burning of the genital area, which is unremitting and often worse at night. In patients who are sexually active, coitus does not have any effect on the symptoms and is not a precipitating factor.

Multiple topical creams do not cause relief and many resort to applying ice to the vulval area. On examination, there is no physical abnormality and even under detailed colposcopic examination the vulva has a normal appearance.

## Treatment

First-line treatment is usually tricyclic antidepressants as, although they act centrally, they also have a modifying effect on peripheral nerves, which may relieve the burning. Amitryptiline is commonly used but as the affected population tends to be older women, it is prudent to start with a low dose of 10 mg at night, and increase as necessary up to maximum doses of 100–150 mg. This regimen minimizes the antimuscarinic side effects, although the patient should be warned that these might occur.

The pain is often compared to post-herpetic neuralgia and carbamazepine may be of use with a starting dose of 100 mg/day, which may be increased sequentially as with the tricyclic antidepressants (McKay 1993).

## Vulval vestibulitis syndrome

Vulval vestibulitis syndrome (VVS) was described by Friedrich in 1987, although the condition appears to have existed under a variety of different names for over a century. It is defined by a triad of signs and symptoms:

- severe pain on vestibular touch or attempted vaginal entry;
- tenderness to pressure localized within the vestibule;
- physical findings confined to vestibular erythema of varying degrees.

Even among gynaecologists this is a little known condition, but its incidence, or certainly its recognition, is increasing and now accounts for 10–15% of referrals to specialist vulval clinics (Goetsch 1991).

The diagnosis is particularly difficult in general practice as often there does not appear to be any abnormality to the naked eye. Even under colposcopic examination, the changes seen within the vestibule may be subtle. Classically this condition affects young Caucasian women in the twenties and thirties, although it has been observed in postmenopausal women. It never appears to affect the black population. The aetiology of this condition is still unknown, but is now thought not to be an infective cause (Bergeron 1997).

### Clinical features

The history is of sudden onset vulval pain precipitated by intercourse. Prior to this the woman has been able to achieve penetration, often for many years without difficulty. The pain is superficial dyspareunia, often so severe that it leads to cessation of sexual activity. It is not unusual to experience difficulty with tampon insertion and removal. The pain caused is burning in nature and may persist postcoitally for hours, if not for days. Some women find this discomfort sufficient that it has stopped them from wearing tight jeans or participating in activities such as horse riding or cycling. Occasionally, the woman may be able to identify a precipitating event, such as a particularly nasty bout of thrush, but more usually there is no particular event that can be recalled. Often these women will have self-treated for candida, but obviously with no effect.

As previously mentioned, physical examination is difficult, but on close inspection erythema of the openings of the vestibular glands can be identified. If any pressure is applied to these areas, the patient will experience reproduction of the pain felt at attempted intercourse. Traditionally this 'Q-tip tenderness' was achieved by rolling a cotton bud over the entrance to the glands (Goetsch 1991), but more recently other methods have been developed to quantify the tenderness and record this level more accurately (Eva *et al.* 1999).

Treatment of this condition is still difficult and treatment strategies vary throughout the world. Topical steroid preparation such as Trimovate can be first-line treatment (Sonnex 1997). This is applied over the affected area nightly for 2 months. Some women do not respond to steroid and a proportion respond to topical oestrogen cream. Use of local lignocaine gel may be of use short term to allow penetrative intercourse and may be used prior to surgery. About 80–90% of women will respond to medical treatment; however, a small proportion require surgical management in the form of vestibulectomy, which involves removal of the skin of the vestibule. Success of this procedure is usually quoted at about 85% (Marinoff and Turner 1991), but success rates can be increased by careful selection of patients suitable for surgery, which should only be used as a last resort if all medical treatment fails.

# 10-Minute consultation

## The patient

A 30-year-old woman comes to see you with vulval itching. She has previously been told it was due to thrush infection and so has treated herself with anti-fungals intermittently over the last year but her symptoms have remained.

## What issues you should cover

- Ask about the duration of the pruritus and whether it is inside the vagina or outside on the vulva. Is there any irritation around the anus?
- It is important to establish whether the primary symptom is itching or pain. Often a patient will have initial pruritus but develops pain secondary

to skin damage caused by scratching, or if the skin has split. Vulvodynia tends to be intense burning that affects the vulval area and is difficult to localize. Pain secondary to splitting of the skin may be more specific in location.

- Ask whether she has noticed any change in the appearance of the vulval skin. This may be change in colour or texture or appearance of discrete lesions.

- Ask whether she has had any bleeding or abnormal discharge.

- Ask whether any event has precipitated the symptoms and whether there are any exacerbating or relieving factors. Enquire as to whether new washing powder has recently been used or whether she has changed her soap or perfume.

- Ask about previous treatment. It is not unusual for multiple topical treatments to have been used without success.

- Ask whether her symptoms are affecting intercourse and whether her partner has any symptoms. Never assume that a woman is not sexually active because of her age.

- Ask whether she has any itching elsewhere on the body and whether she has any known skin disorders.

- Smear history and whether the patient smokes are important details as risk factors for VIN, particularly in younger women are HPV infection and smoking.

## What you should do

- Examine the patient. Examine the entire vulval region, including the perianal region and crural folds. Look for changes in pigmentation, loss of architecture, fusion of labia, discrete lesions, ecchymosis, hyperkeratosis, scratch damage, and symmetry of lesions.

- A speculum examination should be performed and swabs taken to exclude infection. This also allows examination of the vaginal skin.

- Examination of the buccal membranes and other areas of abnormal skin should be performed.

- If there is no evidence of thrush, it is worth a 6-week trial of topical steroids (e.g. Dermovate) to see if the condition resolves.

- If lichen sclerosus is suspected clinically or if symptoms persist despite a trial of topical steroids, then referral is appropriate.

- Biopsy of abnormal areas may be indicated and any suspicious areas warrant immediate referral.

# Frequently asked questions

## What causes vulval disease?

Most vulval conditions still do not have an identifiable cause. There are associations between VIN and smoking and human papillomavirus infection, but they are not caused by these factors. Vulval vestibulitis syndrome is often reported as being precipitated by a bout of thrush but a causative link has not been established. Dermatoses such as allergic or contact dermatitis, however, do have specific causal agents that may be easily identifiable, although sometimes patch testing is needed to establish a cause. Lichen sclerosus has an association with autoimmune disorders but again this is not identifiable in all cases and not considered to be a cause.

## How did I catch it?

With the exception of vulval infections, vulval disorders cannot be caught. Vulval skin disease is like any other form of skin disease elsewhere in the body but it is often assumed that any changes in the genital area have been acquired by sexual contact. As a result women are often embarrassed or reticent about seeking help and advice. The difference between vulval skin and skin elsewhere in the body is that is often moist and poor hygiene may exacerbate symptoms.

## Will it affect my partner?

No. Apart from the sexually transmitted diseases mentioned earlier in the chapter, vulval disorders are not infectious. They cannot be passed on through sexual contact and other members of the family will not be affected. Therefore it is not necessary to treat your partner.

Some conditions will have an effect on a partner or relationship as intercourse becomes painful or impossible. Equally, some woman lose interest in sex as they are self-conscious about the changes in the genital area and this can be particularly difficult after vulval surgery. There are patient support groups that can help overcome these difficulties and the majority of women are able to resume sexual relationships.

## Do I need any tests?

Your GP may perform swab tests to exclude any infections. These are done by passing a speculum in the same way as when having a smear test performed. Generally these tests are negative as the problem is with the skin of the vulva. If referred to a vulval clinic, a biopsy is often performed at this visit. This is done by removing a very small piece of vulval skin under local anaesthetic.

Stitches are not usually necessary. You may be a little sore for a couple of days but this soon passes. A biopsy is important as many vulval conditions are difficult to diagnose just by looking at the skin.

### Can I buy treatment over the counter?

No. Many women assume that if they have itching it is due to thrush and often will have self-medicated with over-the-counter medication. Although anti-fungal creams in general may have a soothing emollient effect, they will not treat the underlying condition. In general, moderately potent or potent steroids are needed and these are only available on prescription.

### Is it safe to use steroid cream?

Often manufacturers' information leaflets with steroid cream contain instructions to avoid use on the genital area. This can lead to poor patient compliance or undertreatment. It is safe to use potent steroids to treat vulval dermatoses. Overuse can lead to fungal overgrowth, particularly in older patients, and the general recommendation is that a 30 g tube should last about 3 months. Long-term use as maintenance in conditions such as lichen sclerosus does not appear to have harmful effects, although some practitioners prefer to reduce the potency. Weakly potent steroids such as hydrocortisone are not effective on vulval skin.

### Will it come back?

This depends on the condition that has been diagnosed. Simple conditions such as allergic dermatitis will not recur unless re-exposed to the allergen. Other conditions such as eczema or psoriasis may be intermittent. However, there is no cure for conditions such as lichen sclerosus and treatment revolves around control of symptoms and monitoring for potential malignant change.

## Websites

- British Society for the Study of Vulval Disease (BSSVD): www.BSSVD.fsnet.co.uk
- Vulval Pain Society: www.vul-pain.dircon.co.uk
- National Lichen Sclerosus Support Group: www.hiway.co.uk/lichensclerosus
- BACUP: www.cancerbacup.org.uk/info/vulva/vulva-4.htm
- National Vulvodynia Association (US): www.nva.org
- Vulvar Pain Foundation (US): www.vulvarpainfoundation.org

- Support/discussion groups
  www.egroups.com/group/UKVulvalPain
  www.egroups.com/group/VulvarDisorders
  www.egroups.com/group/vulvodynia

# References and further reading

Bergeron, S. (1997). Vulvar vestibulitis syndrome: a critical review. *Clinical Journal of Pain*, **13**, 27–42.

Corney, R.H., Crowther, M.E., Everett, H., Howells, A. and Shepherd, J.H. (1993). Psychosexual dysfunction in women with gynaecological cancer following radical surgery. *British Journal of Obstetrics and Gynaecology*, **100**, 73–8.

Dalziel, K., Wojnarowska, F. and Millard, P. (1991). The treatment of lichen sclerosus with a very potent topical steroid. *British Journal of Dermatology*, **124**, 461–4.

Eva, L.J., Reid, W.M.N., Morrison, G. and MacLean, A.B. (1999). Assessment of response to treatment in vulvar vestibulitis syndrome by means of the vulvar algesiometer. *American Journal of Obstetrics and Gynecology*, **181**, 99–102.

Friedrich, E.G. Jr (1987). Vulvar vestibulitis syndrome *Journal of Reproductive Medicine*, **32**, 110–14.

Goetsch, M.F. (1991). Vulvar vestibulitis: prevalence and historic features in a general gynaecologic population. *American Journal of Obstetrics and Gynecology*, **164**, 1609–16.

Hacker, N.F. and van der Velden, J. (1993). Conservative management of early vulval carcinoma *Cancer*, **71**, 1673–7.

Hacker, N.F., Nieberg, R.K. and Berek, J.S. (1983). Superficially invasive vulval carcinoma with nodal metastases. *Gynecologic Oncology*, **15**, 65–77.

Jantos, M. and White, G. (1997). The vestibulitis syndrome: medical and psychosexual assessment of a cohort of patients. *Journal of Reproductive Medicine*, **42**, 145–52.

Jones, R. and Rowan, D. (1994). Vulval intraepithelial neoplasia III: a clinical study of the outcome in 113 cases with relation to the later development of invasive vulval carcinoma. *Obstetrics and Gynecology*, **8**, 741–5.

Lewis, F.M. (1998). Vulval lichen planus. *British Journal of Dermatology*, **138**, 569–75.

Luesley, D. (1999). Malignant disease of the vulva and vagina. In: Edmonds, D.K. (ed.), *Dewhurst's textbook of obstetrics and gynaecology for postgraduates*. Blackwell Science, London.

MacLean, A.B. (1999). Benign disease of the vulva. In: Edmonds, D.K. (ed.) *Dewhurst's textbook of obstetrics and gynaecology for postgraduates*. Blackwell Science, London.

MacLean, A.B., Roberts, D.T. and Reid, W.M.N. (1998). Review of 1000 women seen at two specially designated vulval clinics. *Current Obstetrics and Gynaecology*, **8**, 159–62.

Marinoff, S.C. and Turner, M.L.C. (1991). Vulvar vestibulitis syndrome: An overview. *American Journal of Obstetrics and Gynecology*, **165**, 1228–31.

Marren, P., Yell, J., Charnock, M. and Wojnarowska, F. (1995). The association between lichen sclerosus and antigens of the HLA system. *British Journal of Dermatology*, **132**, 197–203.

McKay, M. (1991). Vulvar vestibulitis and vestibular papillomatosis. Report of the ISSVD Committee on vulvodynia. *Journal of Reproductive Medicine*, **36**, 413–15.

McKay, M. (1993). Dysaesthetic vulvodynia: treatment with amitriptyline. *Journal of Reproductive Medicine*, **38**, 9–13.

Meyrick Thomas, R.H., Ridley, C.M., McGibbon, D.H. and Black, M.M. (1988). Lichen sclerosus et atrophicus and autoimmunity – a study of 350 women. *British Journal of Dermatology*, **118**, 41–6.

Nunns, D. (2000). Vulval pain syndromes. *British Journal of Obstetrics and Gynaecology*, **107**, 1185–93.

Powell, J.J. and Wojnarowska, F. (1999). Lichen sclerosus. *Lancet*, **353**, 1777–83.

Ridley, C.M. and Neill, S. (eds) (1999). *The vulva*. Blackwell Science, London.

Royal College of Obstetricians and Gynaecologists (1999). *Clinical recommendations for the management of vulval cancer*. RCOG, London.

Schover, L.R., Youngs, D.D. and Cannata, R. (1992). Psychosexual aspects of the evaluation and management of vulvar vestibulitis. *American Journal of Obstetrics and Gynecology*, **167**, 630–6.

Sonnex, C. (1997). Vulval vestibulitis syndrome: a descriptive study and assessment of response to local steroid and topical clindamycin treatment. *Obstetrics and Gynecology*, **89**, 291–6.

Stewart, D.E., Reicher, A.E., Gerulath, A.H. and Boydell, K.M. (1994). Vulvodynia and psychological stress. *Obstetrics and Gynecology*, **84**, 587–90.

Thomas, R.H., Ridley, C.M., McGibbon, D.H. and Black, M.M. (1996). Anogenital lichen sclerosus in women. *Journal of the Royal Society of Medicine*, **89**, 694–8.

Wallace, H.J. (1971). Lichen sclerosus et atrophicus. *Transactions of the St. Johns Hospital Dermatological Society*, **57**, 9–30.

Chapter 11

# Chronic pelvic pain
## Stephen Kennedy and Jane Moore

## Epidemiology of chronic pelvic pain in UK

Chronic pelvic pain (CPP) is most commonly defined for research purposes as 'constant or recurrent pain in the lower abdominal region lasting for at least 6 months, excluding pain related to pregnancy or malignancy, or pain that occurs only with menstruation or intercourse'. Clearly, however, women usually present with a much shorter history than 6 months and the causes described in this chapter must be considered from the time of first presentation. The major causes are endometriosis, irritable bowel syndrome (IBS), and pelvic inflammatory disease (PID), but CPP often appears to have no apparent cause despite extensive investigation.

CPP is commonly seen in a primary care setting: its annual prevalence amongst women aged 15–73 in the UK was recently estimated to be 38/1000, based upon an analysis of the general practice records of approximately 280 000 women (Zondervan *et al.* 1999a). This figure was higher than that reported elsewhere for migraine (21/1000), but comparable to figures for asthma (37/1000) and back pain (41/1000). In a subsequent follow-up study, Zondervan *et al.* (1999b) reported that a quarter of women with CPP received no diagnostic label, and only 40% had evidence of referral to secondary care. The majority of women received one of two diagnoses only, the most common being IBS or cystitis in all age groups; PID was common in women aged up to 40, and other gastrointestinal diagnoses in women above 50.

These prevalence figures must have underestimated general population rates, since they only provided information on women with CPP seeking health care. To investigate the true community prevalence, the Oxfordshire Women's Health Study was conducted. This was a postal questionnaire survey among 4000 women, randomly selected from 141 400 women aged 18–49 on the Oxfordshire Health Authority register. A semiquantitative questionnaire was developed for the study, collecting information on a wide range of issues related to women's health (see www.medicine.ox.ac.uk/ndog/cppr/frame.html). CPP in the last 3 months was reported by 24% of the women; the lowest rate (20%) was found in the age groups 18–25 and 31–35, and the highest (28%) in 36–40 year olds (Zondervan *et al.* 2001a). Prevalence did not vary with social class, marital status, or employment status; 41% of the women with CPP had never consulted a doctor for pelvic pain. Last, a third of the women with CPP reported that they were anxious about their pain, particularly its cause. This symptom-related anxiety was as common in non-consulters as in consulters (Zondervan *et al.* 2001b).

# History

To make an accurate diagnosis, it is necessary to listen carefully to the patient's story at the first consultation as it may give valuable clues as to the source of the pain, and provide an opportunity for the patient to feel that she has been heard and her pain accepted as real. Pain is by definition an emotional experience and does not have to have identifiable organic pathology to be experienced as real pain. Allowing the woman to tell her story may in itself be therapeutic, particularly if she makes connections in her own mind as to the origin of the pain. We appreciate that this takes time but it may be worthwhile in the long run.

Some of the causes of CPP and contributing factors are shown in Box 11.1. The main gynaecological diagnoses include endometriosis, chronic PID, and adhesions; the most common gastrointestinal diagnosis is IBS; possible genitourinary diagnoses include interstitial cystitis and the urethral syndrome. However, CPP is notoriously difficult to diagnose and treat due to our poor understanding of the condition and the wide range of possible causes with overlapping symptomatology. In the Oxford community survey, half the women with CPP also had genitourinary symptoms and/or IBS (Zondervan *et al.* 2001b).

To try to distinguish between these conditions, it is important to take a detailed history from the woman to assess the severity of the pain, its characteristics and association with the menstrual cycle, and to estimate the effect of the problem on the physical and emotional well-being of the woman. Despite the obvious need to take a detailed history, there are few studies in the literature that give predictive values for diagnoses based upon clusters of these symptoms, which inevitably makes the clinician's task difficult. Mahmood *et al.* (1991) investigated the prevalence of menstrual symptoms in women with endometriosis in a prospective study of 1200 women undergoing laparoscopy or laparotomy. Although dysmenorrhoea, dyspareunia, and pelvic pain were reported more frequently in women with endometriosis than in those without the disease, dysmenorrhoea, the most commonly reported

> ## Box 11.1 **Contributory factors in CPP**
>
> - Endometriosis
> - Pelvic inflammatory disease
> - Adhesions
> - Irritable bowel syndrome
> - Constipation
> - Interstitial cystitis
> - Urethral syndrome
> - Mechanical pelvic pain
> - Muscle imbalance or trigger points
> - Pelvic pain posture
> - Nerve entrapment
> - Referred pain
> - Neuropathic pain
> - Moderation by the nervous system
> - Psychosocial factors
> - Psychogenic pain
> - Physical and sexual abuse

symptom, had a positive predictive value (PPV) for the diagnosis of endometriosis of only 28%, with a negative predictive value (NPV) of 85% (sensitivity 68% and specificity 50%).

If allowed to tell her story, the patient is likely to include many important pieces of information. Nevertheless the doctor may need to ask some of the following specific questions. In addition, enquiries should be made about her social circumstances, including factors such as her work environment and the attitude of her partner.

- How long has she had the pain?
- Has she ever had pain like this in the past?
- Is there any association with the menstrual cycle?
- Does the pain vary with the time of day?
- Where is the pain maximally located?
- Where does it radiate, i.e. into the back, down the thighs?

- Is the pain exacerbated by movement (including sexual intercourse) or particular postures?
- Do simple remedies provide any relief, for example herbal teas, painkillers, local heat?
- Is there deep pain on intercourse, and if so, in all or only some positions?
- Is there pain in the 24 hours following intercourse?

- Are her periods also painful?
- If so, how incapacitated is she by the pain?
- How many days of dysmenorrhoea does she have?
- Is the pain similar to her CPP?
- Is the pain relieved by simple remedies?
- How severe is the pain in terms of emotional and functional disability?

- Does the woman perceive that she has gynaecological disease or some other disease?
- If not, what does she perceive to be the cause?
- Does she associate her symptoms with any specific event, such as a traumatic vaginal delivery?
- Does she wish to conceive?

- Does she have a relevant family history, for example malignancy or endometriosis?
- Has she had gynaecological surgery in the past, such as a hysterectomy with ovarian conservation?

- Has she taken hormonal contraception in the past and, if so, was she asymptomatic then?
- Is she currently taking a hormonal contraceptive?
- Has she taken hormonal medication in the past, for example danazol, which has relieved the pain?
- What side effects were experienced on hormonal medication/contraception?
- Has she ever used an IUCD?
- Has she had vaginal discharge?
- Has her partner been symptomatic?
- Does she or her partner have a past history of a sexually transmitted disease?
- Does she suspect that her partner has been unfaithful?

◆ Has she had episodes of acute pelvic pain in the past, associated with fever?

◆ Has the pain successfully been treated with antibiotics in the past?

◆ Has she had problems conceiving?

◆ What effect have any pregnancies had upon the pain?

◆ Does she have any urinary symptoms?

◆ Has her bowel habit changed?

◆ Are the stools well-formed?

◆ Is there pain associated with or relieved by defecation?

◆ If so, is the pain worse around the time of a period?

◆ Does she have abdominal bloating?

◆ Does she pass mucus or blood per rectum?

## Examination

It is essential to pass a speculum and perform a bimanual examination if acceptable to the woman. There may be tenderness that is generalized or localized to one anatomical position. There may be vaginal discharge (Chapter 9) and cervical excitation, suggestive of infection. Taking swabs for *Chlamydia* may be appropriate. The uterus may feel enlarged, as is sometimes the case in adenomyosis; it may be retroverted and fixed, especially if the pouch of Douglas has become obliterated by severe endometriosis. It may be possible to palpate adnexal masses, such as ovarian endometriomas or tubo-ovarian masses. There may be thickening of the uterosacral ligaments due to endometriosis, or a tender nodule due to deeply infiltrating endometriosis in the posterior fornix or rectovaginal septum. There is evidence to suggest that such lesions are most easily detected at menstruation because they are larger and more tender than at other stages of the menstrual cycle; understandably, however, many women object to having a vaginal examination when they are menstruating. Last, abdominal and pelvic examination may be entirely normal in many cases. Nevertheless, it may well be worth trying to recreate the pain, not least to establish with the patient that you believe that her pain is real and you understand what she is talking about.

The vaginal examination is a potentially difficult and painful time for the patient but it may also be very revealing. It is an opportunity to demonstrate respect and sympathy for her. It should be remembered that a significant proportion of women suffering from CPP will have been abused or have had negative experiences of doctors examining them. The patient may have feelings about the vaginal examination of which the doctor is unaware. Being sensitive to her issues may lead the doctor much nearer to the true origin of the pain.

# Common causes of chronic pelvic pain

Some specific causes are highlighted in the sections below. There may well be more than one contributory factor. For example, constipation, poor posture, or depression, although not the original source of pain, may now be adding to the overall pain burden. Teasing these out and addressing at least some of them may give the patient confidence that the pain may be controllable.

## Endometriosis

The pain associated with endometriosis is traditionally described in characteristic ways. Dysmenorrhoea commences 1–2 days before the onset of, and lasts throughout, the menstrual flow. It tends to be bilateral lower abdominal pain that radiates to the lower back and down the thighs. Pain on intercourse is common, especially on deep penetration: the pain is caused, it is believed, by pressure on endometriotic nodules in the uterosacral ligaments, pouch of Douglas, or rectovaginal septum. Pain may also be experienced up to 24 hours after intercourse has occurred. The pain of intercourse may be very intense as this quote from a sufferer demonstrates:

> It is intense pain at first and then you get a dull pain that goes right across your abdomen. You are sore afterwards but sometimes it will grab you in the night and you can't move, you get this pain in the pelvis area and you are doubled and you try to move and it is such a spasm that you literally can't move. You think god this can't be endometriosis, this has to be something more serious, this can't surely be this painful, but then it eases off and it is like cramp, real intense cramp, that is probably what it is, I don't know.

If the rectum or sigmoid colon is involved, women may complain of rectal pressure, an urgency to defecate and pain on defecation, especially during menses; suprapubic discomfort and dysuria may occur with bladder involvement. Haematuria and pain in the flanks or iliac fossae may occur secondary to ureteric involvement. The pain of endometriosis should be cyclical in nature, although many women describe the gradual onset of symptoms throughout the menstrual cycle, which may progress to constant pain. Not surprisingly, this often causes a state of emotional despair and anxiety. There may be a family history of endometriosis: first-degree relatives have a 6–9 times increased risk compared with the general population and current research aims to identify genes conferring susceptibility to the disease. There is no evidence that endometriosis has a predilection for middle-aged, upper class, ambitious, white women, as suggested in many gynaecology textbooks; this stereotype probably only demonstrates that such women have greater access to medical care and a laparoscopic diagnosis. *Current* use of the combined oral contraceptive (COC) is believed to be protective. Possible risk factors include heavy and frequent periods, *past* use of the COC, Müllerian anomalies, tampon use and sexual intercourse during menses.

The occurrence of any one of the above symptoms should alert health-care professionals to the possibility of endometriosis. If a woman has all three of the major symptoms (CPP, dysmenorrhoea, and dyspareunia) she is 3.1 (95% confidence interval 1.5–6.5) times as likely to have endometriosis found at laparoscopy as a woman with no symptoms.

Patient self-help groups emphasize how frequently doctors in both primary and secondary care delay making the diagnosis, either because they fail to consider endometriosis as a diagnostic possibility or because there are insufficient resources in the health service to allow all symptomatic women to be laparoscoped. Sociocultural issues also contribute to the delay in diagnosis given that women in many societies are led to believe that pain is an experience they simply have to endure without complaining. Even in the USA, where women have arguably greater access to laparoscopy, 27% of women with endometriosis in a retrospective study had been symptomatic for at least 6 years before a diagnosis was finally made. Not surprisingly, many women believe that a delayed diagnosis leads to increased personal suffering, more prolonged ill-health and a disease state that is more difficult to treat. We feel therefore that it is unreasonable to allow a woman to suffer from CPP without offering some intervention.

## Chronic PID

Inadequately treated acute PID, leading to hydrosalpinges, pelvic adhesions, tubo-ovarian abscesses and anatomical distortion, is one of the major causes of infertility throughout the world. The term chronic PID is used loosely to mean either recurrent episodes of acute PID, or the damage caused by past episodes of pelvic infection including a possible effect upon the nerves supplying the pelvis. Either of these mechanisms may cause or contribute to chronic pain, as may recurrent or inadequately treated infection.

PID is usually diagnosed clinically on the basis of:

- symptoms, such as unilateral or bilateral pain and dyspareunia;
- the sexual history;
- the pelvic findings, which may include generalized tenderness, cervical excitation, and an adnexal mass, with or without tenderness.

Infection screening tests of the woman and her partner(s) should be performed ideally in a genitourinary medicine clinic (see Chapter 9), but negative results do not exclude the diagnosis.

Many women who are found at laparoscopy to have chronic PID do not give a history of previous acute episodes, presumably because they have had *Chlamydia* infections, which are frequently asymptomatic: this highlights the difficulty of managing the condition. Nevertheless, given the disastrous consequences of not making the diagnosis and not treating PID adequately, there is a strong case for empirically treating all patients with a suspected diagnosis of PID. Provided that the treatment has been adequate, this may be the only way of excluding PID as a component of the problem. Aside from possible side effects associated with antibiotic treatment, the only potential disadvantage is the anxiety and anger that can be generated between doctor and patient and between the woman and her partner(s) by making this diagnosis inappropriately. Unfortunately, resolution of the pain following a course of antibiotics does not prove that the pain was due to infection, because CPP of whatever cause tends to wax and wane over time. Some antibiotics, such as tetracycline, are known to have an anti-inflammatory effect in their own right, which may explain why some patients experience a transient relief of symptoms during the antibiotic course.

## Irritable bowel syndrome

Irritable bowel syndrome (IBS) has been defined as a 'functional bowel disorder in which abdominal pain is associated with defecation or a change in bowel habit, with additional features of disordered defecation and abdominal distension'. It is a functional disease, meaning that pain and changes in bowel habit arise from abnormal behaviour of the bowel, or abnormal perception of physiological events, rather than from any structural abnormality. Other conditions such as inflammatory bowel disease may present with pain, but additional features, such as bloody diarrhoea, are usually present.

Using well-established diagnostic criteria (Box 11.2), the prevalence of IBS in the general population is estimated to be 10–20%. Not surprisingly, the prevalence is greater in women with CPP: in a survey of 798 women aged 18–70 attending out-patients for a variety of gynaecological problems, the prevalence of IBS was 37%, but IBS was present in 50% of the women referred with abdominal pain, dysmenorrhoea, or dyspareunia (Prior *et al.* 1989). The diagnosis of IBS is based entirely on pain and bowel symptoms, but these symptoms are known to vary with the menstrual cycle: 50% of women with IBS have a perimenstrual increase in symptoms, which may lead to confusion with gynaecological diagnoses such as endometriosis. The degree of symptom overlap extends into urological diagnoses, as women with IBS tend to have increased bladder dysfunction. As women with idiopathic detrusor instability have an increased prevalence of bowel symptoms, it has been suggested that these overlapping complaints indicate a common underlying dysfunction, perhaps in the autonomic nervous system.

---

## Box 11.2 **Diagnostic criteria for IBS**

### At least 3 months of continuous or recurrent symptoms of:

Abdominal pain or discomfort which is:

- relieved by defecation, and/or
- associated with change in frequency of stool, and/or
- associated with a change in consistency of stool

### Two or more of the following on at least a quarter of occasions or days:

- altered bowel frequency (>3 bowel movements per day or <3 per week)
- altered form of stool (lumpy/hard or loose/watery stool)
- altered passage of stool (straining, urgency or feeling of incomplete evacuation)
- passage of mucus
- bloating or feeling of abdominal distension

There may or may not be an association with the menstrual cycle.

---

## Trapped ovary and ovarian remnant syndromes

Trapped ovary syndrome occurs in 1–3% of women who have had a hysterectomy with ovarian conservation. Women typically present with pelvic pain, dyspareunia and a fixed, tender ovary at the vaginal vault. At laparoscopy, the residual ovary or ovaries are found adherent to the vaginal vault and are usually covered by extensive adhesions. Ovarian remnant syndrome is defined as the presence of functioning ovarian tissue despite an apparently complete bilateral oophorectomy. It usually occurs following surgery for severe endometriosis or PID. The ovarian remnant may be difficult to locate at laparoscopy, but the diagnosis should be suspected if the FSH level is in the premenopausal range. Surgery remains the most effective treatment for both these conditions; ovarian remnants must be removed by an experienced surgeon because of the high risk of ureteric damage.

## Pelvic congestion syndrome

The existence of a syndrome characterized by CPP associated with dilated pelvic veins and venous congestion is still disputed. Women thought to have the condition are typically in the reproductive years and complain of a dull ache in one or both iliac fossae that may have acute exacerbations. The pain is often relieved on lying down and made worse on standing or bending forwards. It is usually accompanied by dysmenorrhoea, backache, vaginal discharge, headache, urinary symptoms, deep dyspareunia, and postcoital ache. On abdominal examination, deep pressure over the ovarian point (the junction of the upper and middle third of a line drawn from the umbilicus to the anterior-superior iliac spine) is said commonly to elicit pain in the iliac fossa. The vagina may appear congested and the whole pelvis may be tender. At laparoscopy, large dilated pelvic veins may be seen in the absence of other pathology; although pelvic venography is supposed to be the definitive diagnostic test, it is still only employed as a research tool.

## Musculoskeletal and nerve-related pain

Pregnancy or trauma can lead to skeletal malalignment, for example pubic symphysis separation or sacroiliac dysfunction – so-called mechanical pelvic pain. Pain may arise from associated muscle spasm or from the joints themselves, perceived either locally or in a referred site such as from the sacroiliac joints to the ipsilateral iliac fossa. The original insult may have occurred many years previously, and only comes to light with a change in circumstances, for example carrying a baby. Such pain varies characteristically with movement and posture, and may get worse towards the end of the day. Confusingly, pain may vary with the menstrual cycle although the reason is unknown. Dyspareunia may occur in some positions. Pain can usually be elicited by manoeuvres, which stress the affected joints or ligaments, such as straight leg raising, standing on one leg, or touching toes.

Pain may also arise from primary muscle dysfunction perhaps due to imbalance between muscle groups secondary to poor posture. The term 'pelvic pain posture' has been coined to describe the posture of a person permanently hunched up due to CPP. The existence of myofascial trigger points (a hyperirritable spot, within a taut band of muscle or fascia) is a subject of some controversy, but increasing emphasis is being placed on their role in the genesis of chronic pain syndromes. It has been suggested that up to three-quarters of patients with unexplained CPP may have myofascial trigger points in the abdominal wall.

When nerves become trapped in scar tissue (for example, in a Pfannenstiel incision or fascia), they may give rise to pain, typically at or beneath the scar, or in the distribution of the nerve. Pain is usually highly localized and may be exacerbated by particular movements. Nerves may also become trapped as they pass through narrow foramina. This may lead to visceral dysfunction, as well as disordered sensation and possibly motor function. It has been suggested that the compression of the sacral nerve roots as they leave the lumbar spine may lead to bladder, bowel, and sexual dysfunction.

It is well established that visceral pain may be perceived in a distant cutaneous site. Little is known about how pain is referred from the pelvis, although it has been shown during conscious pelvic pain mapping performed at laparoscopy that stimulation of the pelvic peritoneum can induce referred pain in areas such as the iliac fossae and perineum. The uterus is innervated by T11 to L1 and it is likely that pain arising from the uterus will be referred to the corresponding dermatomes on the lower abdomen and upper thighs. It has also been suggested that tenderness and hyperalgesia (increased sensitivity to pain) may be generated in the 'referred' area. Tenderness may be caused by antidromic transmission of pain producing substances via the afferent nerves, or by secondary muscle spasm.

When nerves themselves are damaged, for example by a fibrotic disease process such as endometriosis, they may behave abnormally, leading to altered sensation or motor dysfunction. The term for pain arising from a damaged nerve, rather than ongoing tissue damage, is neuropathic pain. Little is known, however, about the role of neuropathic pain in the genesis of CPP.

## Psychosocial factors

It is clear that CPP is an experience which has a number of contributory physical, psychological, and social factors; the balance between these factors is likely to vary from woman to woman and over time in individuals. Research in other chronic pain syndromes such as low back pain suggests that certain personality traits, coping strategies, or health beliefs may predispose an individual to the development of chronic pain and disability. The factors which have been found to correlate most closely with outcome include a tendency to 'catastrophize', use of negative coping strategies, feeling no control over the pain, and a belief that pain represents ongoing tissue damage. Psychosexual problems may also be contributory factors or may alter the perception of chronic pain: a history of childhood sexual abuse is perhaps the best example. However, it is very difficult to dissect out such problems and deep offence may be caused in the process. There are no simple solutions and specialized counselling skills may be helpful. However, every health-care professional should have the skills to listen respectfully to a patient's complaints and accept the validity of her symptoms, whatever their origin. Unfortunately, health-care professionals may misinterpret women or give the impression that they do not believe the pain is real, particularly in the absence of pathology, and it is not uncommon to hear comments such as:

> One of the problems is doctors' attitudes towards women complaining of this sort of pain – they always seem to think: 'She is neurotic, therefore she says she *is* in pain.' They never think: 'She is anxious because she is in pain.'

## Who should be referred to hospital?

It would seem sensible to refer any woman who has:

* pelvic findings, i.e. pelvic mass, tender uterosacral nodule;
* failed to respond to a course of antibiotics and/or simple therapies, i.e. painkillers or COC;
* infertility as well as pelvic pain;
* pain sufficient to restrict her daily activities;
* extreme concerns and anxiety herself about the possibility of pelvic pathology.

A pelvic ultrasound scan is frequently performed although its usefulness in the management of CPP in primary care has not been formally assessed. Our feeling is that there is little need to arrange a scan 'just in case something might be detected' unless, on bimanual palpation, pathology is actually detected or it is not possible to assess the pelvis adequately. We accept that it is common practice in secondary care to organize an ultrasound scan but we feel that even in that context there is little evidence that the test has more clinical value than a well-performed bimanual examination.

It is also important to remember that pelvic pain in young women in the absence of other ominous symptoms is unlikely to be due to life-threatening disease.

Ultimately, the decision to refer for a hospital opinion will depend upon the severity of the woman's symptoms, her own personal wishes, and the general practitioner's philosophy of medicine. There are two equally valid points of view:

- the primary objective is to treat the woman's pain and if that is successfully achieved then the diagnosis is irrelevant;
- it is essential to establish a diagnosis in every woman with CPP and then treat the pathology that is found.

Whether the woman is referred to a gynaecologist, gastroenterologist or genitourinary medicine clinic will depend entirely upon which symptoms are predominant. As there is so much overlap between these disciplines, there is a strong argument for a 'one-stop' pelvic pain clinic where patients can be counselled by doctors from all three specialities and from pain-relief services and liaison psychiatry.

## Laparoscopy

Laparoscopy is considered by gynaecologists to be the 'gold standard' diagnostic tool in the management of CPP; in fact, more than 40% of all diagnostic laparoscopies worldwide are performed to investigate the cause of CPP. However, the operation is associated with significant morbidity and mortality; there is a strong possibility that the pelvis will look normal, and it is increasingly recognized that the relationship between 'pathology' found at laparoscopy and pain symptoms may not always be causal. It seems reasonable therefore that laparoscopy should only be offered if diagnoses such as IBS have first been excluded and if the woman:

- is fully informed about the possible risks (see Box 11.3, below);
- understands the purpose of the investigation;
- appreciates the possibility that the findings might be normal.

Recent qualitative research in our department highlights the importance of conveying this kind of information to patients (Moore *et al.*, submitted). Women in particular want to be told about the risks of laparoscopy such as bowel perforation leading to a laparotomy:

> I think it's important that you should know everything about what's happening and all of the risks attached because it's then up to you whether you want to have this

operation or not, I would probably have been a little bit more apprehensive had I known that but nevertheless I think that's just part of the risk, I mean you weigh up the pros and cons and if it is 1 in 200 I think perhaps well, OK if I'm that 1 in 200 hey I'm unfortunate but it's one of those things . . . I'd have been extremely cross if I'd woken up and had found that I had a 6 inch scar across my tummy and had a perforated bowel or something, I'd have been extremely annoyed and probably have taken further action . . . because there was nothing in the literature that I'd signed to say that it was OK to go ahead with the operation, that that particular accident could happen.

Some women would not have had the investigation if they had known that the findings were normal in as many as one in three laparoscopies. Others were so desperate to find a cause for their pain that knowing this information would not have changed their decision to proceed. Many patients saw laparoscopy as the 'perfect assessment' of the pelvis, the best and quickest way of detecting pathology:

I think in one sense I got the impression that if they were going to find anything this would be the operation that would find out what was causing it and I think I was more hopeful that they would find something this time round.

---

## Box 11.3 **Risks of diagnostic laparoscopy (see Jansen *et al.* 1997)**

- The risk of trauma is approximately 2.7 per 1000 diagnostic laparoscopies.
- Bowel, bladder, or blood vessels are the most commonly damaged structures.
- The damage may be recognized intraoperatively. If the damage is minor, the patient may simply need to be observed in hospital for 24–48 hours. If major, a laparotomy may be necessary to repair the damage.
- The risk of laparotomy is approximately 1.6 per 1000 diagnostic laparoscopies.
- The damage may not be recognized intraoperatively, particularly if bowel has been damaged. In such circumstances, the patient may present with an acute abdomen a few days after the laparoscopy. In such circumstances, a laparotomy is usually required and there is a risk that the patient will need a temporary colostomy.

Unfortunately, however, the test may not be the gold standard it is perceived to be. First, the accuracy of diagnostic laparoscopy depends greatly upon the experience of the gynaecologist, and upon other factors such as the quality of the equipment, the thoroughness of the examination, and the presence of coexisting pelvic adhesions. Laparoscopy will fail to identify physical causes of pain such as adenomyosis and nerve entrapment and a negative laparoscopy may lead the gynaecologist to draw the unjustifiable conclusion that the pain is 'non-organic'. Second, laparoscopy provides an assessment of a woman's pelvis for only a few minutes in her life; the appearance may therefore change in subsequent months or years, or at different phases of the menstrual cycle. Last, although endometriosis, chronic PID, or adhesions may be found, there is little correlation between the degree of pathology and the severity of symptoms, which has led many researchers to question whether such conditions are genuinely causal.

# Treatment

It is beyond the scope of this chapter to consider the treatments available for IBS and chronic PID, but some general measures in the management of CPP and the principles underlying the treatment of endometriosis and other gynaecological conditions are outlined below.

## General measures

There are a number of measures provided by the general practitioner that may produce pain relief and reassurance, without necessarily establishing a definitive diagnosis; for example:

- simple remedies such as herbal teas, or alternative practices such as acupuncture (although a systematic review of the effectiveness of such approaches has not been conducted);
- regular analgesia particularly with NSAIDs with or without paracetamol;
- respectfully listening to the patient's complaint and taking it seriously;
- joining a self-help group such as the Endometriosis Society;
- the use of the COC taken continuously (see below);
- exploring relevant past events such as a traumatic vaginal delivery or a termination;
- addressing problems associated with infertility;
- dispelling fears about malignancy, especially if there is a family history.

## Endometriosis (surgical treatment)

General guidelines for the management of endometriosis in secondary care have recently been produced and are available on the website of the Royal College of Obstetricians amd Gynaecologists (RCOG) (www.rcog.org.uk). The management depends upon factors such as the severity of the disease; the nature and severity of the woman's symptoms; her age and previous treatment; and whether she wishes to conceive or not. It will also be influenced by an individual gynaecologist's experience and the facilities available in that hospital (Table 11.1).

Radical surgery is the best advice for a symptomatic woman over the age of 40 who wants a permanent cure for the pain associated with endometriosis. This implies resection of all endometriotic tissue, a total abdominal hysterectomy and bilateral salpingo-oophorectomy, as there is a 50% likelihood of further surgery being needed if endometriotic ovaries are conserved at hysterectomy. Most cases, however, involve much more complex management decisions, especially in young symptomatic women with severe disease. If radical surgery is being considered in a young woman, it is imperative that the decision should only be taken after lengthy discussion as years after a surgical cure, some women forget their past pain and deeply regret the decision to have their pelvic organs removed. In such circumstances, it may be beneficial to attempt a therapeutic trial of a gonadotrophin-releasing hormone (GnRH) agonist before a final decision about surgery is made (see medical treatment section below).

**Table 11.1** Five key points in the management of endometriosis from the RCOG Guidelines

---

1. The choice between the combined oral contraceptive, progestogens, danazol, and GnRH agonists depends principally upon their side-effect profiles because they relieve pain associated with endometriosis equally well.

2. GnRH agonist therapy given for 3 months may be as effective as treatment given for 6 months in relieving endometriosis-associated pain. If longer treatment is required, GnRH agonist use can be extended safely with 'add-back' therapy.

3. Laparoscopic ablation of minimal-moderate endometriosis appears to relieve pain, although it is unclear whether uterine nerve ablation is required as well.

4. There is no role for medical therapy with hormonal drugs in the treatment of endometriosis-associated infertility and laparoscopic ablation of minimal-mild endometriosis may improve fertility rates.

5. Severe cases of endometriosis should be referred to centres of excellence where relevant clinical expertise is available.

---

For most young women, conservative surgery performed laparoscopically, with or without adjuvant medical treatment, is a better option. This implies resection of all endometriotic tissue and restoration of normal anatomy. The role of surgery in the management of endometriosis-associated pain has been assessed in a recent systematic review. One double-blind, randomized, controlled trial was identified which compared the effects of laser ablation of minimal-moderate endometriosis plus uterine nerve ablation with diagnostic laparoscopy alone for pain relief (Sutton *et al.* 1994). At 6 months' follow-up, 62.5% of the treated patients reported improvement or resolution of symptoms compared with 22.6% in the no-treatment group. Outcome was poorest in patients with minimal endometriosis; however, 73.7% of women with mild-moderate disease experienced pain relief. Symptom relief continued at 1 year follow-up in 90% of those who initially responded. The effect of the denervation component of such surgery has been assessed in a separate systematic review: Vercellini *et al.* (2000) concluded that there was insufficient high-quality evidence to recommend the technique as a routine procedure.

There is some evidence to suggest that postoperative medical treatment with GnRH agonists may prolong the pain-free interval after conservative surgery in symptomatic women. Although these limited data suggest that conservative surgery relieves pain, there are clearly some women who fail to respond, possibly because of incomplete excision or postoperative disease recurrence. Treatment failure may also arise because endometriosis was not the cause of the woman's pain.

## Endometriosis (medical treatment)

Hormonal treatments for endometriosis have traditionally attempted to mimic pregnancy or the menopause, based upon the clinical impression that the disease regresses during these physiological states. There is scanty evidence of a therapeutic effect for pregnancy; however, the hypo-oestrogenic state induced by lactation may, like the menopause, be beneficial.

The modern aim of hormonal treatment is still to induce ovarian suppression in the hope this will lead to atrophy of endometriotic implants, and there are Cochrane reviews dealing with all the major hormonal treatments available. Thus, Prentice *et al.* (2001a) reported that the limited data available suggest that the use of a continuous progestogen such as medroxy-progesterone acetate (Provera) or an anti-progestogen such as gestrinone (Dimetriose) is effective in treating endometriosis-associated pain, although progestogens given in the luteal phase are not effective. Moore *et al.* (2001) showed that there are very few data regarding the use of the COC, although the data available support the common practice of using it as a first-line therapy. Thus, the RCOG Guidelines include the following Good Practice Point:

> If a woman is not trying to conceive and there is no evidence of a pelvic mass on examination, there may be a role for a therapeutic trial of a combined oral contraceptive (monthly or tricycling) or a progestagen to treat pain symptoms suggestive of endometriosis without performing a diagnostic laparoscopy first.

The drugs most commonly used to treat endometriosis-associated pain, danazol and GnRH agonists, are both effective (Prentice *et al.* 2001b; Selak *et al.* 2001) but they are associated with numerous side effects and should ideally not be used until laparoscopy has been performed. Danazol is a testosterone derivative that can have marked androgenic side effects (including permanent voice changes), and barrier forms of contraception are advisable as there are case reports of female pseudohermaphroditism in fetuses conceived on the drug. Despite low oestrogen levels during treatment, danazol does not induce bone loss because its androgenic properties are bone sparing. GnRH agonists induce hypo-oestrogenism by reversible suppression of gonadotrophin secretion – a form of medical oophorectomy. They are taken by nasal spray or by subcutaneous/intramuscular injection; the choice depends upon the patient's own wishes and cost considerations. Some women will notice an exacerbation of their symptoms caused by an initial rise in gonadotrophin levels that results in high oestradiol levels for the first few days of treatment – the so-called flare effect, about which women should be warned. Prentice *et al.* (2001b) concluded that there is little or no difference in the effectiveness of GnRH agonists in comparison with other medical treatments for endometriosis-associated pain but their side-effect profiles differ (Table 11.2); in general, GnRH agonists tend to be associated with more hot flushes and headaches, and danazol with greater weight gain. The major considerations therefore that influence decision-making are the preferred side-effect profile, route of administration, cost (Table 11.3) and planned duration of treatment.

Treatment is usually given for 6 months, after which most patients would expect to have their first period within 6–8 weeks. Menopausal side effects and the additional problem of bone loss can be resolved by the use of 'add-back therapy', an androgenic progestogen such as norethisterone at a dose of 5 mg daily with or without low-dose oestrogen (in the form of continuous combined HRT) during GnRH agonist treatment. Some women feel so much better on treatment that they have no desire to stop taking the medication for fear of the pain returning. The use of GnRH agonists beyond the licensed period of 6 months has been advocated with the use of 'add-back

**Table 11.2** Side effects associated with danazol and GnRH agonists

| Danazol | GnRH agonists |
| --- | --- |
| Weight gain | Hot flushes |
| Bloating | Headaches |
| Hirsutism | Vaginal dryness |
| Acne | Decreased libido |
| Deepened voice | Irritability |
| Oily skin | Depression |
| Muscle cramps | Palpitations |
| Headaches | Joint stiffness |
| Hot flushes | Insomnia |
| Irritability | Bone loss |
| Depression | |
| Decreased libido | |

therapy', but the practice is not common, principally because of the cost involved. Danazol can be taken beyond the manufacturer's recommended duration of 6 months but it is important to counsel patients about the small risk of developing hepatic tumours with long-term use. Long-term therapy is also theoretically inadvisable as danazol reduces high-density lipoprotein levels. The current practice in Oxford for such patients is to recommend 6 months' treatment with a GnRH agonist followed by a COC taken using a tricycle regimen. We recommend that therapy beyond this duration with drugs such as Provera, danazol, and GnRH agonists should not be initiated in primary care because of the uncertainties regarding long-term effects.

The limitations of medical therapy, for example the side effects and the possibility of symptoms returning off treatment, should be communicated to the patient. Women with endometriosis frequently complain that doctors provide them with insufficient information about the nature of the disease and the implications of treatment. Complementary treatments include selenium, magnesium, calcium, vitamin E, zinc, and evening primrose oil, a rich source of $\gamma$-linolenic acid, which blocks leukotriene production and is said by endometriosis sufferers to be effective treatment for pelvic pain. There are also anecdotal accounts of pain relief from acupuncture, homeopathy, hypnosis, and aromatherapy.

**Table 11.3** Costs of treatments for endometriosis (2001 BNF data)

| | Dose | Unit cost | Total cost |
|---|---|---|---|
| *Combined oral contraceptives* | | | |
| EE 35/NET 0.5 (Brevinor) | Continuously | £1.67 (63 tablets) | £5.01* |
| EE 30/LNG 250 (Eugynon 30) | Continuously | £2.07 (63 tablets) | £6.21* |
| EE 30/GEST 75 (Minulet) | Continuously | £5.70 (63 tablets) | £17.10* |
| EE 20/DSG 150 (Mercilon) | Continuously | £8.57 (63 tablets) | £25.71* |
| *Progestogens* | | | |
| Norethisterone (Primolut N) | 5 mg t.d.s. | £2.16 (30 tablets) | £38.88* |
| Norethisterone (Utovlan) | 5 mg t.d.s. | £6.48 (90 tablets) | £38.88* |
| Dydrogesterone (Duphaston) | 10 mg t.d.s. | £4.49 (60 tablets) | £40.41* |
| Medroxyprogesterone (Provera) | 10 mg t.d.s. | £22.16 (90 tablets) | £132.96* |
| *Testosterone derivatives* | | | |
| Danazol (Danol) | 200 mg t.d.s. | £33.75 (60 tablets) | £303.75* |
| Gestrinone (Dimetriose) | 1 twice weekly | £111.73 (8 tablets) | £782.11† |
| *GnRH agonists* | | | |
| Nafarelin (Synarel) | 1 sniff b.d. | £53.01 (60 doses) | £318.06* |
| Buserelin (Suprecur) | 2 sniffs t.d.s. | £75.43 (200 doses) | £377.15‡ |
| Triptorelin (Decapeptyl) | Monthly injection | £105.05 | £630.30 |
| Goserelin (Zoladex) | Monthly depot | £122.27 | £733.62¶ |
| Leuprorelin (Prostap SR) | Monthly injection | £125.40 | £752.40¶ |

*180 days; †28 weeks; ‡166–8 days; ¶6 months.
DSG, desogestrel; EE, ethinyl estradiol; GEST, gestodene; LNG, levonorgestrel; NET, norethisterone.

## Treatment of CPP due to other causes

A Cochrane review (Stones and Mountfield 2001) assessed the effectiveness of therapies such as progestogens, psychotherapy, ultrasound scanning, a multidisciplinary approach, and adhesiolysis for women with CPP associated with conditions other than endometriosis, chronic PID, and IBS – such as pelvic congestion syndrome and adhesions. There is some evidence to support the use of medroxyprogesterone acetate (Provera) with or without psychotherapy in such patients although benefit is not maintained 9 months after treatment. The only women who may benefit from adhesiolysis appear to be those with severe adhesions. Hysterectomy remains the last resort for many women, particularly those with CPP that is associated with pelvic varicosities or believed to be uterine in origin, and a recent systematic review provides encouraging data regarding the long-term consequences (Vercellini *et al.* 2000). The findings of the five studies identified showed that 83–97% of the women reported pain relief or symptomatic improvement one year following surgery. A therapeutic trial of a GnRH agonist before surgery may be useful for women with an uncertain diagnosis, particularly those requesting bilateral oophorectomy as well as a hysterectomy.

## Conclusion

It is easy to forget that CPP is a chronic condition and to ignore its full impact upon the lives of affected women. Pain impinges upon every aspect of a woman's life. For example, sex becomes unenjoyable and something to be avoided, which may not be appreciated by a partner; a boss may not relish constant absenteeism because of symptoms or visits to the doctor. Many women feel embittered by the lack of understanding they receive from the medical profession, without realizing the difficulties inherent in making an accurate diagnosis and in treating the condition. An acknowledgement of these difficulties and an unequivocal acceptance of the pain as real is a good starting point in the management of CPP. Careful listening to the history at the outset not only emphasizes that the problem is being taken seriously but may also help to avoid the problem of women being shunted from one speciality to the next in search of a diagnosis. Some women may benefit from a multi-disciplinary approach involving anaesthetists specializing in pain relief, gastroenterologists, liaison psychiatrists, and specialized nursing staff, but such resources are in limited supply.

## References

Jansen, F.W., Kapiteyn, K., Trimbos-Kemper, T., Hermans, J. and Trimbos, J.B. (1997). Complications of laparoscopy: a prospective multicentre observational study. *British Journal of Obstetrics and Gynaecology*, **104**, 595–600.

Mahmood, T.A., Templeton, A.A., Thomson, L. and Fraser, C. (1991). Menstrual symptoms in women with pelvic endometriosis. *British Journal of Obstetrics and Gynaecology*, **98**, 558–63.

Moore, J. and Kennedy, S.H. (2000). Causes of chronic pelvic pain. *Baillière's Clinical Obstetrics and Gynaecology*, **14**, 389–402.

Moore, J., Kennedy, S.H. and Prentice, A. (2001). Modern combined oral contraceptives for pain associated with endometriosis (Cochrane Review). In: *The Cochrane Library*, Issue 2. Update Software, Oxford.

Moore, J., Ziebland, S. and Kennedy, S.H. (2002). 'People sometimes react funny if they're not told enough' Women's views about communicating the risks of diagnostic laparoscopy. *Health Expectations*, 5, 302–9.

Prentice, A., Deary, A.J. and Bland, E. (2001a). Progestagens and anti-progestagens for pain associated with endometriosis (Cochrane Review). In: *The Cochrane Library*, Issue 2. Update Software, Oxford.

Prentice, A., Deary, A.J., Goldbeck-Wood, S., Farquhar, C. and Smith, S.K. (2001b). Gonadotrophin-releasing hormone analogues for pain associated with endometriosis (Cochrane Review). In: *The Cochrane Library*, Issue 2. Update Software, Oxford.

Prior, A., Wilson, K., Whorwell, P.J. and Faragher, E.B. (1989). Irritable bowel syndrome in the gynecological clinic. Survey of 798 new referrals. *Digestive Diseases and Sciences*, 34, 1820–4.

Selak, V., Farquhar, C., Prentice, A. and Singla, A. (2001). Danazol for pelvic pain associated with endometriosis (Cochrane Review). In: *The Cochrane Library*, Issue 2. Update Software, Oxford.

Stones, R.W. and Mountfield, J. (2001). Interventions for treating chronic pelvic pain in women (Cochrane Review). In: *The Cochrane Library*, Issue 2. Update Software, Oxford.

Sutton, C.J., Ewen, S.P., Whitelaw, N. and Haines, P. (1994). Prospective, randomized, double-blind, controlled trial of laser laparoscopy in the treatment of pelvic pain associated with minimal, mild, and moderate endometriosis. *Fertility and Sterility*, 62, 696–700.

Vercellini, P., De Giorgi, O., Pisacreta, A., Pesole, A.P., Vicentini, S. and Crosignani, P.G. (2000). Surgical management of endometriosis. *Baillière's Clinical Obstetrics and Gynaecology*, 14, 501–23.

Zondervan, K.T., Yudkin, P.L., Vessey, M.P., Dawes, M.G., Barlow, D.H. and Kennedy, S.H. (1999a). Prevalence and incidence in primary care of chronic pelvic pain in women: evidence from a national general practice database. *British Journal of Obstetrics and Gynaecology*, 106, 1149–55.

Zondervan, K.T., Yudkin, P.L., Vessey, M.P., Dawes, M.G., Barlow, D.H. and Kennedy, S.H. (1999b). Patterns of diagnosis and referral in women consulting for chronic pelvic pain in UK primary care. *British Journal of Obstetrics and Gynaecology*, 106, 1156–61.

Zondervan, K.T., Yudkin, P.L., Vessey, M.P., *et al.* (2001a). The community prevalence of chronic pelvic pain in women and associated illness behaviour. *British Journal of General Practice*, 51, 541–7.

Zondervan, K.T., Yudkin, P.L., Vessey, M.P., *et al.* (2001b). Chronic pelvic pain in the community: symptomatology, investigations and diagnoses. *American Journal of Obstetrics and Gynecology*, 184, 1149–55.

Chapter 12

# Breast disorders
## Danielle Power and Jane Maher*

*Updated from the original chapter by Joan Austoker, Ann McPherson, Jane Clarke, and Anneke Lucassen in *Women's Health*, 4th edition

Breast diseases are an increasing issue for general practitioners, who can expect 30 presentations per 1000 women per year, ranging from mild breast pain to breast lumps, but overall only 6% are found to have breast cancer (RCGP and OPCS 1995). Most women referred to specialist services will be reassured that the breast abnormality is due to a benign process. Nevertheless, breast cancer remains a major health issue. The lifetime risk of breast cancer is 11% (1 in 10 women in their lifetime), representing almost 30% of all cancers in women. In 1997 there were 36 100 new registrations of breast cancer in the United Kingdom (Office of National Statistics 2001), with an overall increase of one to two per annum, particularly in the elderly. Breast cancer remains the leading cause of death from malignancy in women, accounting for almost 20% of these deaths in the UK (13 198 deaths in 1998). The UK has had one of the highest mortality rates from breast cancer in the world, but there has been a substantial decline in mortality since the late 1980s (just over 20% overall). Death rates have improved in all ages, with the fall being largest for the 55–69 years age group. This marked decrease is not due to the implementation of the National Screening Programme alone, but reflects overall improvements in the way breast cancer is diagnosed and treated.

This overview covers both benign and malignant breast diseases. Indications for referral and the consultation process for patients presenting with a history of a breast disorder are reviewed. The path to diagnosis of malignancy, with particular reference to the National Screening Programme, are outlined. Treatment options, both of primary and metastatic disease, are discussed. Despite the wealth of clinical trials in the area of breast cancer treatment, controversies and uncertainties remain. This overview highlights some of these areas of uncertainty, particularly those in which trials are ongoing.

The short reference list includes both seminal papers and broad overviews. Some Internet sites are listed, particularly those of cancer and self-help organizations, which provide important support for patients diagnosed with cancer.

# Benign breast disease

About 50% of women in the UK experience symptoms of benign breast disease during their reproductive years. Compared with breast cancer there has been relatively little work on the epidemiology of benign breast disease. While hormonal imbalances are thought to contribute to its development, oral contraceptive use decreases the risk of fibrocystic breast changes, presumably by providing a balanced source of oestrogen and progesterone.

## The four major symptoms

The four major symptoms with which women present are:

- lumps
- nipple discharge
- nipple retraction
- pain.

### General principles of management and referral

Having taken a history and examined the patient, the key issue is whether a breast mass is indeed present. Lumps may be within the skin (for example, sebaceous cysts or lipomas), or deep to the breast (for example, costochondral junctions). Some women experience a lump or lumpiness as part of the menstrual cycle or in association with pregnancy. If on examination there is no discrete lump present, or the symptoms can be explained by a history of trauma or hormonal fluctuations, reassurance should suffice, even if no clear diagnosis has been made.

It is important to elicit particular fears of breast cancer, either due to family history or personal exposure. The patient may be reassured by counselling, but specialist referral may be indicated, even if there is no significant abnormality, in order to alleviate her concerns. Advice should always be given about breast awareness, and the woman should be invited to re-consult should there be further problems or persisting symptoms. For many women complaining of lumpy breasts, particularly in their thirties and forties, it can be very difficult to make a definite diagnosis. It can be helpful to ask a woman to return for repeat examination at a different time in the menstrual cycle, especially after a period. If at presentation or at second examination there is some abnormality, nodularity, or thickening, then referral to a specialist is the safest course of action. The act of referral induces anxiety and so the general practitioner (GP) should advise her about what is likely to happen when she attends hospital.

## Box 12.1 **Summary of conditions requiring referral to a surgeon with a special interest in breast disease**

### Lump

- Any new discrete lump
- New lump in pre-existing nodularity
- Asymmetrical nodularity that persists at review after menstruation
- Cyst persistently refilling or recurrent

### Pain

- If associated with a lump
- Intractable pain, not responding to reassurance, simple measures such as wearing well-supporting bra and simple analgesics
- Unilateral pain in postmenopausal women

### Nipple discharge

- All women over the age of 50 years
- Women under 50 with:

  bilateral discharge sufficient to stain clothes

  blood-stained discharge

  persistent single duct

### Nipple retraction or distortion, nipple eczema

### Change in skin contour

### Family history

- Request for assessment by a woman with a strong family history of breast cancer (refer to a family cancer genetics clinic if possible) – see 'genetic testing' for further discussion

Source: Austoker *et al.* (1999).

There is evidence that delay of over 3 months in breast cancer diagnosis has a significant impact on overall survival from breast cancer (Richards *et al.* 1999). Clearly, total delay in the diagnostic pathway should be kept to a minimum, and has medicolegal implications. Referral without delay for specialist assessment should be made as clinically indicated. Conditions requiring referral to a specialist for further assessment are summarized in Box 12.1. Conditions that initially can be managed by the GP are shown in

Box 12.2. There is clear evidence that the outcome for women with breast cancer is improved if they are treated in specialist centres in a multidisciplinary team setting, and by surgeons with a special interest in breast disease.

---

### Box 12.2 **Women who can initially be managed by their GP**

◆ Young women with tender lumpy breast and older women with symmetrical nodularity, provided that they have no localized abnormality

◆ Women with minor and moderate degrees of breast pain who do not have a discrete palpable lesion

◆ Women aged under 50 who have nipple discharge that is from more than one duct or is intermittent and is neither blood-stained nor troublesome

Source: Austoker *et al.* (1999).

---

## Breast lumps

Benign discrete breast masses are most commonly fibroadenomas or breast cysts. Fibroadenomas are most common in the 15–30 years age group; they account for about 12% of all palpable, symptomatic breast lumps, but for about 60% of mass lesions in women under the age of 20 years. They tend to be smooth and spherical, with a rubbery consistency, and are very mobile within the skin (hence the alternative name of 'breast mouse'). About 5% will grow in size and 20% will spontaneously regress. Most will remain unchanged, becoming less distinct after the menopause. They arise from a whole breast lobule rather than single cells and are under the same hormonal control as the rest of the breast tissue. The diagnosis is made by a combination of clinical examination, ultrasound, and aspiration cytology. These lesions are benign without malignant potential and can be safely left *in situ*, but women may request surgical excision.

Breast cysts are the most common benign breast abnormality, affecting 7% of women in Western countries. They occur in an older age group (40–50 years) and are multiple in more than 50% of women, occurring most often in the upper outer quadrant. They are frequently asymptomatic and found incidentally by the patient, but may be painful if they are tense or rapidly accumulating fluid. A cyst may be completely missed if soft, or misdiagnosed as cancer if hard.

Clinical diagnosis is confirmed by needle aspiration of the fluid, followed by re-examination to ensure that no residual mass exists. Cyst aspiration in primary care is not encouraged, as it may make subsequent assessment of a mass lesion difficult, but it may be used for relief in women with a history of multiple breast cysts. If the fluid is blood-stained, the aspirate should be sent for cytology and further investigation is required. If the mass persists following aspiration, full diagnostic assessment is necessary. Ultrasound is a sensitive and specific test for cyst diagnosis, but usually not necessary if needle aspiration is diagnostic. Mammography is important to exclude secondary pathology, but is not appropriate as the sole or initial diagnostic test for symptomatic breast disease. About 10% of cysts refill to become palpable again and approximately 50% of women will develop another cyst elsewhere in the breast. Cysts usually disappear following the menopause, but they will continue if women are on HRT.

In the absence of proliferative breast disease, cystic change *per se* does not increase the risk of breast cancer, but they can be mistaken for carcinoma and may make clinical detection of breast cancer more difficult. Women with multiple breast cysts are considered to have a slightly higher risk of cancer when compared with the general population, but this is not at a rate sufficient to warrant increased screening.

## Breast pain and nodularity

Breast pain (mastalgia), alone or in combination with breast nodularity, is reported in up to half of women attending breast clinics. Cyclical (related to menstrual cycle) pain and nodularity are so common as to be regarded as physiological. As a rule, symptoms are not severe, and resolve following menstruation. A small proportion of women experience cyclical breast pain that is clinically significant. Non-cyclical breast pain tends to occur in an older age group. The symptoms last for a shorter time and tend to resolve spontaneously. The pain is also well localized to an area of the breast and may be associated with an area on the chest wall that 'triggers' the pain. Nodularity is less common than with cyclical pain. Injection of the painful area with steroid and lignocaine may relieve symptoms. Occasionally breast pain may be mistaken for inflammation of the costochondral junction (Tietze's syndrome). Typically this pain worsens on pressure on the affected cartilage, and responds to non-steroidal anti-inflammatory drugs.

Breast pain may also be caused by infection (periductal mastitis) or abscess formation, which is particularly associated with lactation.

### Treatment

Reassurance that the pain they are experiencing is not related to cancer, together with an explanation of the hormonal basis of the symptoms, helps in the majority of women. In about 15% of women, the pain is so severe as to affect their quality of life and to require active treatment. Some women find that stopping the oral contraceptive pill helps. Pre- and postmenopausal women who start hormone replacement therapy (HRT) may also experience an increase in cyclical breast pain and nodularity, and this is treated by stopping the HRT or changing to a low-dose, combined preparation for a short time only. Simple measures such as wearing a soft support sleep bra may help. Antibiotics should not be prescribed, unless there is evidence of infection.

Medical treatments effective in controlled studies for breast pain include:

- Danazol (200 mg once daily) is the most effective treatment, with a response in about 70% of women. However, side effects of weight gain and hirsuitism limit its usefulness.
- LHRH analogues are effective treatments, but again the side effect profiles may be unacceptable.
- Bromocriptine at a dose of 2.5 mg twice daily reduces the secretion of prolactin. It may be useful for cyclical mastalgia, but not for non-cyclical breast pain. However, 20% of women experience side effects, such as nausea, vomiting, and dizziness on bromocriptine, which are severe enough to require that treatment be stopped.
- Tamoxifen has been found to reduce mastalgia, but is not licensed for this use and its prescription is best restricted to specialist clinics.

Vitamin B6, diuretics, and progestogens are not effective in the management of breast pain.

## Nipple discharge

Nipple discharge alone tends to be a relatively uncommon presenting complaint, but it may be associated with a breast lump and requires prompt assessment. Discharge may be bloody, coloured opalescent, or milky. Duct ectasia or epithelial hyperplasia are the commonest benign causes of nipple discharge.

The major subareolar ducts dilate and shorten during involution, and by the age of 70, 40% of women have substantial duct dilation or duct ectasia. Some women with excessive shortening and dilation develop nipple discharge, nipple retraction, or a palpable mass or abscess formation. Typically the discharge arises from multiple rather than single ducts. Although the appearances may be mistaken for cancer, duct ectasia *per se* is not associated with increased risk of malignancy.

Epithelial duct hyperplasia is a benign condition where there is an increase in the number of cells that line the lobular duct unit of the breast.

If the cells also appear abnormal, the condition is called atypical hyperplasia and is associated with an increased risk of breast cancer, of the order of 8% at 10 years, if there is no family history. Epithelial hyperplasia may also be associated with benign polyp-like growth called papilloma, which can present with bloody nipple discharge arising from a single duct of the breast. There may also be a palpable nodule below the skin, which, upon pressure, results in the release of discharge. Benign papillomas are very common and are of low malignant potential. However, the risk of these disorders being associated with an invasive cancer increases with age, particularly in postmenopausal women, and invasive malignancy should be excluded.

Galactorrhoea is the production of milk from the breast, which is unrelated to breast-feeding. The cause of this is usually physiological, but it may be related to the intake of certain drugs, such as the phenothiazines, or metoclopramide. Rarely, galactorrhoea is due to increased production of prolactin from a pituitary tumour.

## Treatment

The management of nipple discharge depends on the underlying cause and age of the patient. Galactorrhoea can be treated with bromocriptine if it is excessive and the underlying cause has been identified and managed appropriately. Blood-stained discharge in women under the age of 40 years is rarely associated with cancer, but malignancy should be excluded. In older women, the risk of malignancy is much higher and the affected ducts should be excised. Sometimes antibiotics can help in duct ectasia, particularly if there is an inflammatory component. Occasionally surgery is required if the volume of discharge is sufficient to require the use of pads for symptom relief, once a more serious underlying cause has been excluded.

## Infection of the breast

The commonest cause of breast abscess is infection associated with lactation, although the incidence of this problem appears to be decreasing. The commonest infectious agent is *Staphylococcus aureus*. The early symptoms of non-infectious mastitis may be identical to an infectious cause: namely, a painful, red, and swollen breast often with some constitutional upset. It is extremely important to empty the breast, either by continuing suckling or expression. An antipyretic/anti-inflammatory drug is recommended. In non-infective

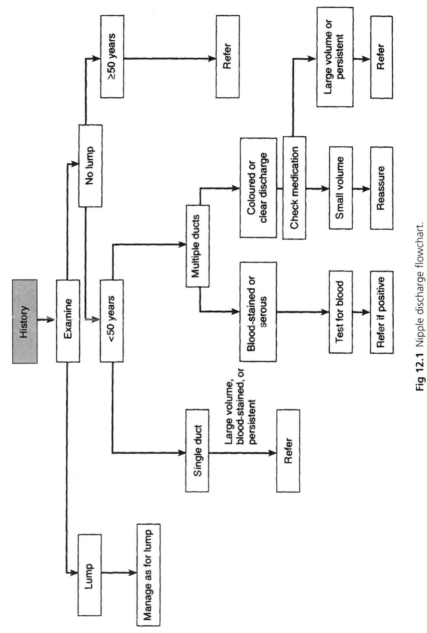

**Fig 12.1** Nipple discharge flowchart.
*Source: Austoker et al.* 1995.

mastitis, symptoms will resolve quickly. If the cause is infective, treatment with flucloxacillin is usually adequate to resolve the infection. However, a small number of women (5–10%) go on to develop an abscess requiring surgical drainage. In older women, periductal mastitis and duct ectasia, sometimes associated with inverted nipples and a chronic nipple discharge, is the commonest cause of infection. The causative organism in this scenario is more likely to be anaerobic.

# Malignant breast disease

## Risk factors for breast cancer

### Age, reproductive factors, and the menstrual cycle

The main risk factor for breast cancer is increasing age, with breast cancer being relatively rare under the age of 50 years, unless there is a family history. Length of exposure to female reproductive hormones is also important, with early onset of menstruation, late menopause, and nulliparity increasing the risk of breast cancer. Women who have a natural menopause at the age of 55 years, compared to menopause before the age of 45 years, are twice as likely to develop breast cancer. Artificially induced menopause has a similar protective effect to that of the natural menopause. Full-term pregnancy at an early age has a protective effect, halving the risk of breast cancer compared to nulliparous women, or women whose first full-term pregnancy is after 35 years of age.

### Geographical variation

There is marked geographical variation worldwide, with a fivefold difference in incidence between the Far Eastern and Western countries. The incidence of breast cancer in migrants assumes that of the host country within a few generations, emphasizing that environmental factors are also important in breast cancer development.

### Previous breast disease

The risk of developing a second primary breast cancer after the first is reported to be up to five times the general risk. Primary ovarian or endometrial cancer is also associated with a slightly higher risk compared to the general population. The cancer risk associated with benign breast disease is in general low, but women with atypical epithelial hyperplasia have a four or five times risk of primary breast cancer. This risk increases further if there is also a family history.

## Exogenous hormones

There has been ongoing concern regarding the use of oral contraception and hormone replacement therapy and the risk of breast cancer. Even if increased risk with use is small, the effect on breast cancer rates could be substantial, as breast cancer itself is common and both oral contraceptives and HRT are widely used.

- *Oral contraceptive pill (OCP)*

A systematic review by the Collaborative Group on Hormonal Factors in Breast Cancer, 1996, pooled the results from 54 case-controlled studies involving 53 297 women with breast cancer and 100 239 without. Overall, there appears to be no increased risk of breast cancer with OCP use. However, there is a 24% increased risk in those women currently using the Pill or who have recently stopped. This risk appears to decline over 10 years from stopping. The risk of breast cancer in young women is very small, so the 24% increased risk is not actually large. In women aged 40 or more, the increased risk becomes more relevant. As yet there are no clear data whether long-term use of the OCP prior to first pregnancy or the use of hormone replacement therapy following previous use of the OCP increases the risk of developing breast cancer later in life. The meta-analysis does suggest that those cancers occurring while on the OCP appear to be clinically less advanced, although this could be due to earlier detection through surveillance.

- *Hormone replacement therapy (HRT)*

HRT is associated with a slight increase in the risk of breast cancer, which is restricted to current and recent users, the risk increasing with duration of use. HRT does appear to increase the fibroglandular tissue of the breast in a significant proportion of women (25–30%), the risk being higher with combined oestrogen/progesterone HRT. This results in an increase in the breast density, making mammograms harder to interpret radiologically. This potentially reduces the sensitivity of the mammogram in detecting significant abnormalities, as reflected by an increased interval cancer rate if on HRT (Litherlang et al. 1999). However, it is also recognized that HRT-associated breast cancers tend to have favourable prognostic features. By 5 years after stopping HRT, the effect on breast cancer risk has essentially disappeared. Among 1000 women who use HRT continuously for 20 years starting at the age of 50 years, it is estimated that there will be an additional 12 breast cancer cases by the age of 70. Balanced against this are the short-term benefits to quality of life by relief of menopausal symptoms, and long-term beneficial effects of HRT on bone density. For a 50-year-old woman, the baseline lifetime risk of coronary artery disease is 45%, of hip fracture is 15%, and breast cancer is 8% (Clinical Synthesis Panel on HRT 1999).

## Ionizing radiation

There is direct evidence of carcinogenic effect of radiation on breast cancer risk from atomic bomb survivors and women exposed previously to radiation in the management of benign conditions. This relationship has led to anxiety about the use of mammographic screening. However, the probability of a woman developing breast cancer as a consequence of radiological examination as part of breast screening is extremely low – perhaps one extra cancer for 2 million women screened for 10 years!

## Weight, diet, and alcohol

Postmenopausal women who are obese have a 1.5–2-fold risk of breast cancer. This is thought to be due to the peripheral conversion of sex steroids to oestrogen in fatty tissue, resulting in an increased oestrogen state. Certainly, countries with high fat diets tend to have higher incidences of breast cancer, but large prospective studies have failed to show any clear relationship between fat intake or alcohol intake and breast cancer. Smoking is not a risk factor. There has been much interest in the possibility that phyto-oestrogens, found in high concentrations in soya and other foods, may block the action of endogenous oestrogens and have a protective effect against breast cancer. The results of studies to date have been inconclusive.

## Family history

Familial breast and ovarian cancer have received much publicity following the identification of specific predisposing genes. Only 5–10% of breast cancer in Western countries is associated with an identifiable genetic abnormality. When present, it is inherited in an autosomal dominant pattern with limited penetrance. This means that the gene can be transmitted through either sex, and that some family members may transmit the gene without developing breast cancer themselves. *BRCA1* (breast cancer 1) and *BRCA2* are the two major breast cancer genes identified to date, carriage of which is associated with a 50–85% lifetime risk of breast cancer. Certain ethnic groups such as Jewish women and Ashkenazi Jews have a much higher incidence of specific mutations. The *BRCA1* and *BRCA2* genes are very large and many mutations have been reported to date. Some families affected by breast cancer also show an excess of other malignancies – specifically ovarian, colon, and prostate cancer. A variety of specific inherited syndromes are also associated with increased risk of breast cancer, such as Li–Fraumeni syndrome (mutation of *p53* gene and a greater than 50% risk of breast cancer by the age of 50 years), ataxia telangiectasia, Cowden's and Gorlin's syndromes.

## Genetic testing

Identifying women at high risk of breast cancer begins by taking an accurate family history, but large families may have several sporadic breast cancers by chance, and in small families, the absence of a family history does not rule out the mutation. See Box 12.3 for clinical indicators of the presence of a predisposing breast cancer mutation.

---

### Box 12.3 **History that may indicate genetic susceptibility**

- Multiple episodes of breast cancer within a single family (for example, 2 cancers below the age of 50 years, 3 cases below the age of 60 years, 4+ cases at any age)
- Early-onset breast cancer – not all genetically determined cancers occur in young women, but the earlier the onset the greater the risk
- Bilateral breast cancer
- Breast and ovarian cancer combined
- Colon and prostate cancers in male relatives

---

Routine genetic testing for *BRCA* mutations in women without a strong family history is not practicable due to the size of the genes involved ('like looking for a needle in a haystack'). For high-risk women, referral to a clinical geneticist should be made as per local guidelines. Full counselling will occur prior to genetic testing, with discussion of the consequences of testing positive including the risk of genetic discrimination. Genetic testing is a complex, lengthy process and may not provide useful information. The testing of an affected relative greatly improves the chance of identifying a mutation in an unaffected woman. If the affected relative does not have an identified mutation of *BRCA1* or *BRCA2*, a negative test in an unaffected individual may mean that she is not at increased risk or simply has an unidentified predisposing gene in her family. The management of a woman at increased risk of breast cancer has yet to be clearly defined, and entry into clinical trials should be offered if possible. Options include prophylactic mastectomy, oophorectomy (reducing the risk of ovarian cancer and breast cancer), or careful surveillance, clinically and radiologically. Bilateral prophylactic mastectomy is known to be effective in preventing breast cancer in recent prospective studies, but remains controversial, due to concerns regarding the personal effects of the surgery and no proven survival benefit compared to intensive screening as yet.

# Breast cancer screening

Generally speaking, the earlier breast cancers are detected, the better the chances of survival. This is the basis of the National Breast Screening Programme. It was introduced in England and Wales in 1988, as a result of several large, randomized controlled trials of screening, suggesting that mammography significantly reduces mortality from breast cancer by 20–40%, particularly in women aged 50 years and over.

The best screening tool currently available is mammography, which has a sensitivity of 95% alone, but many lesions identified will be benign. Compared with cancers presenting symptomatically, breast carcinomas detected at screening are more likely to be small (50% of cancers being less than 15 mm in size) and non-invasive (*in situ*). Those cancers that are invasive are more likely to be well differentiated or of special histological type, which itself confers better prognosis. Screen-detected cancers are more likely to be node negative compared with symptomatic cancers of equivalent size. Approximately 20% of cancers are *in situ* and up to 70% of cancers detected by screening are impalpable clinically.

## The UK screening programme

### General guidelines

- Age
  - (a) All women aged 50–64 years
  - (b) Women aged 65 years and over may be screened on request at 3-yearly intervals
  - (c) Women aged under 50 years are not offered routine screening
- Frequency: 3-yearly
- Views: two views (mediolateral oblique and craniocaudal) for first and subsequent screening. Studies have shown that two views are associated with significant improvements in cancer-detection rates and lower rates of recall, and should be standard for screening.

### Screening over the age of 70 years

The National Screening Programme has been extended to include all women up to the age of 70 years, but as yet there is no indication for screening over this age, unless there is a prior history of breast cancer. Breast cancer incidence continues to rise in this age group, and yet this is also the group with the smallest decline in overall mortality. The EUROCARE

Study highlights the poor UK performance in terms of survival from breast cancer (Berrino *et al.* 1999). The lack of screening and differences in management of early and advanced disease in the elderly may be contributory factors.

## Screening under the age of 50 years

Because the incidence of breast cancer under the age of 50 years is significantly lower, the number of cancers identified in any screening programme will be less. There is also difficulty in interpreting mammograms in premenopausal women as increased breast density makes radiological interpretation harder, reducing the test sensitivity. Despite these factors, there does appear to be a significant reduction in mortality achievable by screening women aged 40–50 years. However, the cost-effectiveness of introducing a screening programme in this age group is under debate and in Europe, the consensus view is that mammographic screening of younger women on a population basis cannot be justified currently.

## Interval of screening

Three-yearly screening of women aged 50–64 years appears to be the most cost-effective screening policy. An interval cancer is one which arises within 3 years of a negative screen. The interval cancer rate rises quickly between the second and third year after the initial screen and UK rates are higher than in the Swedish screening mammogram studies upon which our screening policy is modelled. This suggests that the 3-yearly interval may be too long and should be reduced. A recent UKCCCR trial comparing annual with standard 3-yearly mammograms has shown a non-significant advantage to the yearly mammogram programme. The current UK 'Health of the Nation' targets for breast cancer mortality reduction due to screening are unlikely to be met if current trends in interval cancer rates continue (Baum and Spittle 1999).

## Guidelines for special groups

### A strong family history

Women with a strong family history of breast cancer may be offered mammography under the age of 50 years outside the screening programme, depending on local policies. In practice it is recommended that mammographic screening starts at an age 5–10 years younger than the age at which the youngest relative developed the disease. After the age of 50 years, high-risk women are screened as part of the National Screening Programme, unless there is another clinical indication. Alternative imaging techniques such as ultrasound or magnetic resonance imaging (MRI) in the younger age group are currently being investigated.

### Previous history of breast cancer

Ongoing mammographic follow-up is important because of the increased risk of contralateral breast cancer and for early detection of local recurrence following conservative breast surgery. There is no clear consensus as to frequency of screening, but a typical protocol would be yearly for 5 years and 3-yearly thereafter.

### Hormone replacement therapy

There is no indication for routine mammography prior to starting hormone replacement therapy, although all women should have a full clinical examination. The majority of women will automatically fall into the age range of the screening programme. There is no evidence that younger women should commence screening earlier if they are on HRT. However, HRT does appear to increase the fibroglandular tissue of the breast in a significant proportion of women (25–30%), the risk being higher with combined oestrogen/progesterone HRT. This results in an increase in the breast density, making mammograms harder to interpret radiologically. This potentially reduces the sensitivity of the mammogram in detecting significant abnormalities.

## Potential adverse effects of screening

- Discomfort and pain of mammography.
- Compression of the breast against the x-ray plate causes discomfort for the majority of women, usually short lived.
- Reassurance to those with a false-negative result.
- Anxiety and psychological morbidity of false-positive results. Nine of ten women recalled following abnormality at mammogram do not have cancer. Yet the recall process itself is associated with heightened levels of anxiety, which can occasionally persist despite reassurance.
- Overdiagnosis of minor abnormalities.
- Unnecessary biopsies. A proportion of women who undergo biopsy following the screening process will not have cancer, but in the UK this number is small.
- Risks of radiation. The overall risk of inducing malignancy by screening is extremely small, particularly in view of the high incidence of breast cancer in the population being screened.

## Organization of breast cancer screening

For the screening programme to be effective at significantly reducing mortality, more than 70% of the target population must accept the invitation to screening. In 1999–2000, 1.3 million women of all ages were screened (Department of Health 2001). The overall acceptance rate of invitation to screen currently is 76%. Women eligible for the screening programme are identified through the health authorities and contacted via their general practitioners. GPs should be informed of non-attendance to the screening programme. Several studies have shown that uptake of the screening programme is strongly influenced by general practice staff, with women being 4–12 times more likely to attend after a discussion with their GP, however brief.

Mammograms detect stellate opacification in the breast or areas of microcalcification reflecting areas of high cellular proliferation. Stellate lesions may represent a benign scarring lesion such as a radial scar, complex sclerosing lesion, or sclerosing adenosis. Alternatively, opacification could represent an invasive or non-invasive cancer. Of 10 000 women who have a mammographic abnormality, 500 (5%) will be recalled, of whom 80 will require an operation (0.8%) and 60 will have invasive cancer (0.6%). Further assessment may involve further mammographic views, ultrasound scan, and/or image-guided fine-needle aspirate or core biopsy. A biopsy should be performed if there is a suspicion of malignancy on radiological or clinical grounds, even if the cytology is benign. To achieve this, impalpable lesions may be localized under ultrasound or mammographic guidance by placing a guidewire prior to definitive surgery.

## The role of breast self-examination

In the past, breast self-examination has been promoted as a means of detecting early breast cancer. The UK Trial of Early Detection of Breast Cancer invited women aged between 45 and 64 years to an educational programme on breast self-examination. After 10 years of follow-up there was no difference in mortality rates from breast cancer in the 'educated' group compared with the control group. Therefore there is no evidence to support breast self-examination as a primary screening technique. However, the majority of women detect their breast cancer themselves, therefore breast awareness is important and is encouraged. Education should be given as to the importance of recognizing what is normal for the individual, awareness of the cyclical changes which occur in the premenopausal breast, and what changes to look out for. Leaflets such as 'Be Breast Aware', the media, GPs, and practice nurses play an important role in raising the issue of breast awareness. It is important for medical professionals to address individuals' concerns raised by breast self-examination, either by reassurance or secondary referral for further assessment as appropriate.

## Non-invasive breast cancer

Ductal and lobular carcinoma *in situ* (DCIS and LCIS) involve the epithelial cells lining the ductal lobular system of the breast undergoing malignant differentiation, without invasion through the myoepithelial layer. Progression to an invasive tumour occurs in approximately 40% if untreated. Clinically, DCIS may present as a mass, nipple discharge, or Paget's disease. In the past, DCIS constituted 3% of new breast cancer presentations, but now it accounts for 20–30% of all malignant lesions identified at screening. It is almost impossible to predict the 40% of women with DCIS who will go on to develop invasive cancer and consequently a group of women may receive unnecessary treatment.

The mainstay of DCIS management is surgery and, paradoxically, women with this non-invasive lesion may be offered more extensive surgery than those with invasive breast cancer. Risk of local recurrence following surgery is associated with the size of the lesion, adequacy of excision, and histological features of the DCIS. Extensive DCIS (>4 cm) and multifocal disease is associated with high risk of relapse and is best treated with mastectomy. The management of a small area of screen detected DCIS is more controversial. Two large clinical studies, the National Surgical Adjuvant Breast and Bowel Project (NSABP-17) and the European Organization for Research and Treatment of Cancer (EORTC-10853) have reported that radiotherapy after local excision of DCIS reduces local recurrence of preinvasive and invasive disease significantly. However, the EORTC study had an increased incidence of contralateral breast cancer in the study group receiving radiotherapy, offsetting this benefit (Fisher *et al.* 1998; Julien *et al.* 2000). Therefore the indications for irradiation post-lumpectomy for DCIS remain under debate and depend on local policies.

Tamoxifen reduces both recurrence and second primary breast tumours when used in invasive breast cancer treatment. It is hypothesized that a benefit would also be seen in DCIS. The NSAPB-24 study looking at this issue demonstrated additional benefit from tamoxifen, but balanced against this are potential life-threatening side effects of tamoxifen usage (thromboembolic disease and endometrial carcinoma), in addition to quality of life issues. The FDA (USA) has approved tamoxifen for the treatment of DCIS, but it is not yet standard practice in the UK due to concerns regarding long-term toxicity, with no proven survival benefit as yet. Further studies are awaited.

# Diagnosis of malignant breast disease

Diagnosis breast cancer should involve 'triple assessment', performed in a specialist unit with immediate access to diagnostic facilities and psychological support services for the woman undergoing assessment. Breast clinical nurse specialists provide an important source of information and emotional support, consolidate information given by medical staff and guide the women through the diagnostic process. Practically, the triple assessment involves clinical examination, radiology, and pathological confirmation. Information obtained should be reviewed in a multidisciplinary team meeting with specialist input.

### Clinical examination

- Inspection: looking for skin dimpling, new inversion of the nipple or change of breast shape/symmetry.
- Breast palpation: the breast tissue is examined systematically with the flat of the hand with the woman's arms held above her head, causing deep muscles to tense. Any lump is assessed with fingertips for size, position, and for fixation to the deep muscles.
- Assessment of axillary nodes: 40% of women who have no palpable nodes may have axillary nodal metastases, and it is not uncommon for clinically palpable nodes not to be associated with significant breast or other disease. It is important to check the supraclavicular fossa.

## Radiology

Mammography and ultrasonography are the commonest radiological modalities used. Impalpable screen-detected lesions need to be localized and skilled radiologists and radiographers are an important part of the diagnostic team. Newer imaging techniques are being used more frequently, such as magnetic resonance imaging, which may be useful in the evaluation of impalpable abnormalities. Nuclear medicine scans will also be increasingly used.

## Pathological diagnosis

Preoperative diagnosis is important to allow for discussion on the various treatment options. The two main methods are fine-needle aspiration (FNA) cytology and core biopsy. FNA has the advantage of being simple and quick, and it can give a diagnosis as part of the one-stop evaluation process, thereby avoiding delay and reducing patient anxiety. As a test it has a sensitivity (i.e. true positive detection rate) for malignancy of 95%. Core biopsy has the advantage of providing structural as well as cytological information, differentiating true invasive from *in situ* cancer. It can also provide information regarding grade and hormone receptor status. Occasionally an 'open' surgical biopsy is required if the FNA or core biopsy is inconclusive, and this can be done under local or general anaesthetic.

# Management of breast cancer

There are two major aims influencing the clinicians' treatment decisions. The first is to eradicate disease from the breast and prevent local and regional recurrence (achieved mainly by a combination of surgery and radiotherapy). The second is to prolong overall survival from the disease by the use of adjuvant local and systemic treatments. The choice of treatment combinations for an individual depends on the characteristics of the tumour, breast size and shape, the presence or absence of nodal metastases and, of course, patient preference.

## Staging and prognostic factors

There are many factors to consider when deciding on the management of a particular tumour. Staging is the assessment of disease extent and is based on the TNM classification (International Union Against Cancer) system (Table 12.1). The tumour stage, together with other important prognostic factors, guides the decision-making process and provides predictive information for overall survival (Table 12.2).

**Table 12.1** Modified TNM classification for breast cancer (UICC 1997)

| | |
|---|---|
| Tis | *In situ* carcinoma – preinvasive changes |
| T1 | Tumour ≤2 cm |
| T2 | Tumour >2 cm and ≤5 cm in size |
| T3 | Tumour >5 cm |
| T4 | Any size tumour with direct extension into chest wall or skin |
| N0 | No evidence of metastases |
| N1 | Axillary metastases – mobile (same side as tumour) |
| N2 | Axillary metastases – fixed (same side as tumour) |
| M0 | No distant metastases |
| M1 | Distant metastases |

**Table 12.2** Prognostic groups in early breast cancer

| Risk group | Tumour stage | Nodes involved | 5-year disease-free survival (%) |
|---|---|---|---|
| Low risk | T1 grade 1 or 2 | 0 nodes | 90–95 |
| | T2 grade 1 or 2 | 0 nodes | 80–90 |
| | T3 grade 1 or 2 | 0 nodes | 70–80 |
| Intermediate risk | T1–3 grade 3 | 0 nodes | 50–60 |
| | Any stage | 1–3 nodes | 40–50 |
| High risk | Any stage | >4 nodes | 20–30 |

Source: Royal College of Radiologists (2000).

## Prognostic factors

*Tumour size* correlates directly with survival. Tumours less than 2 cm in size have 5-year survival rates of between 84 and 90% compared with 60% for tumours 2–5 cm.

*Axillary node* involvement is the single most important prognostic factor. Overall survival depends on the level and number of axillary nodes involved.

*Grade* is assessed by looking at the differentiation and mitotic activity of cells microscopically. Tumour is graded 1–3, with grade 3 associated with the worst prognosis.

*Tumour histology* is another important consideration. The commonest type of breast cancer is ductal carcinoma, no specific type. Other types of breast cancer, for example lobular, medullary, mucinous, or tubular, generally have better prognoses. Tubular carcinoma is recognized to behave less aggressively with better overall survival, even if lymph-node positive.

*Vascular and lymphatic invasion* by tumour cells is found in one in four patients with breast cancer. The presence of this increases the risk of locoregional and systemic relapse.

*Hormone and growth factor receptors* are found in many breast cancer cells. The presence of oestrogen receptors (ER status) and progesterone receptors (PR status) on cancer cells determines whether the cancer is likely to respond to hormonal manipulation. In general terms, postmenopausal women are more likely to have ER-positive tumours. The development of new hormonal treatments has made the receptor status relevant and positivity is a good prognostic feature. Up to 30% of tumours will be ER negative, but if there is expression of PR, there may still be a response to hormone therapy. However, the presence of epidermal growth factor receptors (also known as *HER2* or c-*erbB2* receptors) on the cancer cells is known to be associated with reduced overall survival, chemotherapy resistance, and more aggressive tumours. This influences treatment decisions, particularly as there are new treatments such as 'herceptin', a monoclonal antibody, which targets the cells expressing these growth factor receptors. There is much interest in other epidermal growth factors in breast cancer, and future therapeutic developments may include molecular-based treatments targeting these receptors.

Although individual factors are useful, the formation of an index allows identification of groups of patients at different risks of relapse, which can guide advice as to management – one commonly used index is the Nottingham prognostic index, based on tumour size, grade, and lymph node status (Table 12.3).

# Early stage breast cancer treatment

The following treatment modalities are used in the management of localized breast cancer:

- Surgery
- Radiotherapy
- Systemic treatments:
  (a) chemotherapy
  (b) hormone manipulation

## Surgery

Over the last 20 years there has been a move from radical to more conservative surgical techniques. The two main aims of surgery are, first, to remove the tumour from the breast to achieve local control of primary disease and, second, to provide information as to prognosis and tumour stage by performing a regional lymph node dissection, which will simultaneously provide disease control within the axilla. Surgical options include wide local excision around the

**Table 12.3** Nottingham Prognostic Index (NPI)* and survival

| Prognosis | NPI score | Survival (15 years) |
| --- | --- | --- |
| Good | <3.4 | 80% |
| Moderate | 3.4–5.4 | 40% |
| Poor | >5.4 | 15% |

*NPI = (0.2 × tumour size) + lymph node stage (1 = no nodes, 2 = 1–3 nodes, 3 = ≥4 nodes) + grade (1, 2 or 3).

tumour, or removal of part (quadrantectomy) or whole breast (mastectomy). A mastectomy is usually offered if the tumour involves multiple areas in the breast, is very large (>4 cm), centrally placed, or occurs within a small breast. The presence of extensive non-invasive (*in situ*) disease may be a contraindication to conservative surgery. Adequate discussion, counselling, and psychological support throughout the decision-making process in the choice of best surgical technique is important.

Axillary dissection may be either limited to 'sampling' of representative nodes, without treating an involved axilla, or a 'clearance' of nodal tissue giving both prognostic information and treatment to the involved nodes, but will overtreat the node-negative axilla. The 'sentinel node' biopsy is increasingly being used to try to judge more accurately who needs formal axillary surgery. This identifies the first node to which lymph drains from the breast by injecting a radioactively labelled or blue dye below the nipple, followed by surgical removal of the node that takes up the dye/tracer. Theoretically, no tumour involvement of this node implies the rest of the lymph nodes will be clear and surgical resection of the axilla is not required. Trials are still underway to assess whether this can be used in routine practice. Currently, the technique is limited to certain specialists, as there is a learning curve in terms of technical expertise.

### Breast reconstruction

Breast reconstructive techniques are continually improving, and immediate or delayed reconstruction post-mastectomy is an alternative approach if breast conservation is not appropriate or if the patient prefers it. Replacement can be by use of an implant (usually saline) or flap of muscle and skin (myocutaneous flap). The easiest approach is to place a prosthesis behind the pectoral muscle. If the nipple has been maintained and minimal skin removed (a subcutaneous mastectomy), then the correct-sized implant can be placed at the time of operation. Alternatively, a tissue expander can be used, which is inflated gradually by injecting saline through a 'port', stretching the overlying skin until the desired size is achieved. Although a simple procedure, the natural shape of the breast can be difficult to mimic. In the long term there may be formation of a capsule of scar tissue around the prosthesis, which can cause pain and distortion of the breast shape. This may not be possible if the chest wall has been irradiated, due to loss of skin elasticity.

The main tissue flaps used are the 'latissimus dorsi flap' from the back and the 'TRAM flap' from the lower abdomen. The latissimus dorsi flap is probably the simpler procedure with good flap survival, but usually also requires an implant to achieve sufficient tissue bulk. The TRAM flap is a lengthy operation with a higher complication rate and a longer recovery period, without the need for implant. Both types of reconstructions can give good cosmesis in correctly selected patients, performed by experienced surgeons. The main side effects of flap techniques are infection and flap necrosis. Careful preoperative counselling is essential in achieving a satisfactory outcome psychologically as well as physically. Involving a partner in these discussions may help to diminish fears and dispel myths about the final cosmetic results.

## Silicone implants

Silicone implants have been used in the past for breast reconstruction. There is widespread concern regarding the safety of silicone implants. Fatigue and rupture can lead to leakage of silicone gel. There is no convincing evidence that rupture causes damage to other organs, and in particular, connective tissue diseases. An independent review group on silicone gel implants reported in October 2000, commissioned by the Department of Health. There is no indication for routine removal, unless there are particular problems related to the silicone implants.

## Adverse effects of surgery

Infection and collections of fluid (seroma) within the surgical area can occur. Surgery involving axillary dissection may result in damage to the intercosto-brachial nerve, causing numbness, paraesthesia or pain on the inner aspect of the upper arm. Usually this is self-limiting as the nerve regenerates, but it may be permanent. Physiotherapy and arm mobility exercises are essential in the immediate postoperative period and thereafter to reduce postoperative arm swelling and prevent/reduce debilitating axillary fibrosis. Lymphoedema (chronic arm swelling) can occur postoperatively, following axilla radiotherapy or as a result of disease recurrence. Discomfort can be lessened by the use of elasticated arm stockings, and referral to a lymphoedema nurse specialist should be made. There is a significant risk of cellulitis in the lymphoedematous arm, and long-term prophylactic antibiotics may be recommended.

The breast care nurse frequently has a key role in providing information and psychological support for women following diagnosis, through the surgical process and beyond. The impact of surgery on body image is important and the provision of appropriate prostheses is essential.

## Radiotherapy

Radiotherapy following conservative surgery for breast cancer will reduce the risk of local tumour recurrence to a level comparable to that following mastectomy. Completely excised, good-prognosis tumours or preinvasive (ductal carcinoma *in situ*) changes alone may be treated with surgery alone. The Early Breast Cancer Trialists' Collaborative Group have reviewed the evidence for radiotherapy, the latest update being in 2000. In summary, there were three times fewer recurrences when radiotherapy was added to surgery. Positive surgical margins, high-grade tumour with lymphovascular invasion, large tumour associated with carcinoma *in situ*, and node involvement all increased the risk of local recurrence, even after radiotherapy is given. Postoperative chest wall and regional lymph node radiotherapy is also indicated post-mastectomy for a selected group of patients at high risk of local relapse. The axilla is not routinely irradiated following surgery to the axilla because of a high risk of morbidity, particularly lymphoedema.

Does radiotherapy actually improve survival from breast cancer, or does it just improve local control? A review of patients treated in the 1970s revealed an increase in cardiovascular mortality thought to be due to induction of ischaemic heart disease by the radiotherapy treatment, offsetting any survival advantage. Modern improved radiotherapy techniques are reducing treatment-related morbidity and recent Danish studies have shown that loco-regional radiotherapy has improved survival rates in appropriately treated high-risk patients, with no increase in cardiovascular events. The debate is ongoing.

## Radiotherapy side effects

Radiotherapy typically involves daily treatment over several weeks to the whole breast followed by a short boost of treatment to the original tumour site in selected patients. A number of studies worldwide, including the 'START' trial in the UK, are investigating the optimum treatment schedule.

The side effects of radiotherapy vary from patient to patient. Immediate side effects are fatigue and tiredness, almost universally experienced. This may continue for several months following treatment completion. Early side effects are acute skin reactions, varying from a slight reddening of the skin to severe erythema and blistering, which can be mistaken for cellulitis, particularly in women of larger breast size. Antibiotics are rarely required and the erythema and blistering improves with conservative management. Breast pain and discomfort may occur, particularly in the areolar area. Women are advised regarding skin care to minimize the acute toxicity. E45 or aqueous cream can be used. At the end of treatment, the skin can remain thickened and hyper-pigmented. It may take up to 6 months for the skin to settle, although the worst effects improve usually within 6 weeks. Late effects of radiotherapy can include breast pain, breast shrinkage or induration, and rib pain (costochondritis), which usually respond to simple painkillers such as ibuprofen. The incidence of lymphoedema ranges from 5 to 25%, depending on extent of axillary irradiation and surgery. Symptomatic pneumonitis, characterized by cough, fever, and shortness of breath, may occur 2–9 months after radiotherapy in less than 1% of women. Symptoms usually resolve with conservative management. Brachial plexus damage is now very rare (1–2%) with modern planning and avoidance of axillary radiotherapy, but in patients treated with older regimens, symptoms of neuropathic pain, paraesthesia, or weakness should be fully investigated.

## Systemic therapy

Systemic treatments are given in addition to surgery and radiotherapy in early breast cancer to reduce the risk of recurrence and improve survival, by targeting 'micrometastatic' disease. Choice of treatments depends on prognostic factors related to the tumour and on the patient's general health and preferences. (Table 12.4).

### Chemotherapy

Chemotherapy can be given before surgery ('neoadjuvant') for large, high-grade tumours. By reducing the tumour size preoperatively, it may allow breast conservation, whereas previously the only option was a mastectomy. Neoadjuvant chemotherapy does not alter overall survival from breast cancer compared to adjuvant chemotherapy.

Adjuvant chemotherapy involves the use of cytotoxic drugs following definitive surgical management, in the hope of eradicating microscopic

**Table 12.4** Improvements in 10-year survival of node-positive women associated with different treatments

| Treatment | Number of extra survivors at 10 years per 100 women treated (best estimate) |
|---|:---:|
| *Women aged >50 years* | |
| Chemotherapy only | 5 |
| Tamoxifen only | 8 |
| Chemotherapy and tamoxifen | 12 |
| *Women aged <50 years* | |
| Chemotherapy only | 10 |
| Ovarian ablation only | 11 |
| Chemotherapy and ovarian ablation | +12 |

*Note*: proportional reduction in mortality would be less for earlier node-negative disease.

residual disease. An overview by the Early Breast Cancer Trialists' Collaborative Group showed moderate improvements in overall survival with benefits greater in younger women and women who are at high risk of future relapse as predicted by pathological features of the tumour. The smaller the risk of relapse for the individual patient, the smaller the absolute benefit of chemotherapy and it is not always easy to balance advantages of chemotherapy against the potential toxicity and inconvenience of treatment.

In general terms, adjuvant chemotherapy involves giving combinations of cytotoxic drugs cyclically over several months. Various combinations exist, the previous 'gold standard' being CMF regimens (cyclophosphamide, methotrexate and 5-fluorouracil). Increasingly it is felt that regimens containing anthracyclines (typically doxorubicin- and epirubicin-containing, such as 'FEC' or 'AC' or 'EC') offer a survival advantage (2–4%) over CMF, and should be offered first line for all women, but particularly the young. Unfortunately, anthracyclines can be associated with cardiac toxicity in the long term, increased alopecia, and significant bone marrow suppression. No single regimen has emerged as treatment of choice for all women (Table 12.5). There is no evidence that continuing adjuvant therapy longer than 6 months, or that using very high-dose therapy has any advantage over standard practice. The efficacy of high-dose chemotherapy with stem cell transplantation is a controversial issue. Historically controlled studies suggested a survival benefit in the metastatic and high-risk adjuvant setting. Two randomized controlled trials in South Africa appeared to confirm this, until the research was discredited following scientific misconduct. At this time, there is no role for these treatments outside the clinical trial setting. Newer chemotherapy agents, such as the taxanes, have not yet been shown to be more effective than currently available drugs in the adjuvant setting, although early studies from the USA are encouraging, and UK and international trials are ongoing. Molecular developments, such as the monoclonal antibody herceptin, are likely to change the pattern of adjuvant treatment in the future.

**Table 12.5** Absolute survival advantage from adjuvant chemotherapy (EBTCG overview 1998)

| | |
|---|---|
| *Women <50 years* | |
| Node negative | 11% |
| Node positive | 7% |
| *Women >50 years* | |
| Node negative | 2.4% |
| Node positive | 3.4% |

## Adverse effects of chemotherapy

Chemotherapy has a frightening reputation, yet with improved symptom control management, many potential side effects can be ameliorated. Morbidity varies from woman to woman and is difficult to predict in advance. Fatigue, weight gain, sore mouth, nausea, and vomiting are common side effects. Nausea and vomiting are usually controlled with prophylactic use of a variety of antiemetic agents, including small doses of steroids. Alternative routes of administrating antiemetics, such as subcutaneous pumps or suppositories, can be effective if nausea control is difficult. Rarely, women may develop anticipatory vomiting before their chemotherapy treatment, which can respond to short-acting anxiolytics such as lorazepam or visualization/relaxation techniques.

Hair loss is not inevitable and regrowth occurs within a few months of completing treatment. Its extent depends on the chemotherapy agents used. CMF chemotherapy has the advantage that most women do not experience complete alopecia. 'Ice-caps' to reduce the blood supply to hair follicles during the period of chemotherapy administration may be an effective preventive measure in a small proportion of women. Hair loss can cause considerable psychological distress, which can be lessened by information, hair care advice, stylish head coverings, and wigs.

The most serious short-term risk of chemotherapy is neutropenic sepsis, a consequence of the action of cytotoxics on bone marrow. It is important women are informed as to the need to report immediately any symptoms of infection. Urgent assessment and admission to hospital for a blood check and antibiotic therapy is required, as potentially life-threatening infection may occur.

Anthracyclines (epirubicin and doxorubicin) may affect myocardial function, although in current regimens, significant cardiac toxicity is extremely rare. One study documented a reduction in left ventricular ejection fraction in 8% of women receiving doxorubicin (compared with 1% on CMF). It is not known in the long term whether this subclinical reduction in systolic function will have long-term sequelae.

In premenopausal women, cytotoxics are teratogenic and contraception must be used. There is a significant risk of ovarian failure following chemotherapy and the closer you are to your natural menopause, the more likely this is to occur. Six months of CMF chemotherapy induces ovarian failure in 70% of women aged over 40 years, and 40% of younger women. The risk of permanent infertility increases with age, and may be an important issue for an individual. Successful conception post-adjuvant chemotherapy does occur, but it is recommended that pregnancy be avoided for at least 2 years following treatment, as aggressive cancers are most likely to recur early in the natural history. The probability of successful pregnancy following chemotherapy if ovarian failure has been induced is low, and women must be fully informed as to this risk. New techniques such as ovarian storage have not been successful in preserving fertility yet, but can be offered on a trial basis.

Early menopause due to ovarian failure has potential short- and long-term consequences on health and quality of life. It increases the risk of cardiovascular disease and osteoporosis. Long-term follow-up data on the significance and impact of early menopause in this group is lacking. Adequate dietary intake of vitamin D and calcium and regular exercise are advised, with monitoring of bone density long term. Menopausal symptoms of hot flushes, vaginal dryness, dyspareunia, and sleep disturbances can be debilitating. The use of oestrogen to alleviate menopausal symptoms and for the long-term prevention of osteoporosis and cardiovascular disease is controversial. There is increasing evidence of the benefit of HRT, without an adverse effect on breast cancer risk of recurrence, particularly in oestrogen-receptor-negative tumours and there is currently a national study looking at the use of HRT in people with a prior history of breast cancer, which will hopefully address this issue.

It is increasingly recognized that there may be long-term subtle effects on cognitive function following adjuvant chemotherapy, the mechanism of which is unknown. Psychological support is critical in helping women to cope with side effects of treatments, and relaxation therapy and complementary techniques may have a role to play.

## Adjuvant hormone therapy

Routine use of hormonal manipulation has had a major impact on survival from breast cancer. Treatments include:

- systemic agents, e.g. tamoxifen;
- ovarian ablation – surgical or chemical.

It has long been recognized that some breast cancers are hormone sensitive. It is possible to identify the presence of oestrogen (ER) and progesterone (PR) receptors on breast cancer cells, predicting the responsiveness of the tumour to hormone manipulation.

### Tamoxifen

Clinical trials have shown that tamoxifen, which is an anti-oestrogen, significantly improves overall survival and reduces the risk of recurrence and contralateral breast cancer in patients that express ER or PR receptors. It is estimated that half a million women are taking tamoxifen in the UK currently. It is taken as a tablet, at a dose of 20 mg daily. Current results suggest that 5 years of tamoxifen therapy is better than 2 years of treatment, after which potential side effects outweigh benefits. Optimum duration of treatment is being evaluated in the aTTom study (adjuvant tamoxifen treatment offer more?).

Tamoxifen is generally well tolerated, with only 3% of patients needing to stop the drug due to side effects, although more than 50% of women experience hot flushes, which can have an impact on quality of life. These symptoms are particularly marked in pre- and perimenopausal patients. They often improve with time, but there are other measures that can improve symptoms (see questions). Vaginal dryness and discharge, and loss of libido may occur. Lubricating ointments and topical oestrogens may be helpful. Rarer side effects can be hair thinning or visual disturbances due to retinopathy and an increased risk of thromboembolic events. The main side effect of concern with tamoxifen use is the increased incidence of endometrial carcinoma due to a pro-oestrogenic action on the endometrium. It has been estimated that for 1000 women treated for 5 years, 160 cases of breast cancer are prevented, which can be balanced against 5–10 new endometrial cancers. Women are advised to report any abnormal vaginal bleeding and prompt referral should be made for gynaecological assessment. Early-stage endometrial cancer is amenable to treatment with hysterectomy. There is an ongoing debate as to the degree to which tamoxifen has additional benefits of cardiovascular disease protection (by lowering cholesterol) and protection against bone mineral loss.

## Aromatase inhibitors

Aromatase inhibitors (for example letrozole, anastrazole, exemestane), developed in the 1980s, act by preventing peripheral conversion of androgen substrates to oestrogen, thereby lowering the level of oestrogen in the body. The main source of oestrogen in postmenopausal women is by peripheral conversion. In premenopausal women the natural source of oestrogen is predominantly from the ovaries, and aromatase inhibitors are not effective in this group. Trials comparing tamoxifen with aromatase inhibitors in the setting of metastatic breast cancer have shown modest superiority of the new agents over tamoxifen, without major toxicity, and are increasingly being used. Based on this, major studies have been undertaken in the adjuvant setting. The ATAC study (anastrozole alone or in combination with tamoxifen versus tamoxifen for the adjuvant treatment of postmenopausal women with early breast cancer) is a large study of 9366 patients, which reported in 2002, arousing much media and patient interest. The early results appear to show a benefit for the aromatase inhibitor compared with tamoxifen both in disease recurrence and the incidence of contralateral breast cancer, translating to a disease-free survival at 3 years of 91% compared with 89%. The study showed no advantage to combining tamoxifen with an aromatase inhibitor. Aromatase inhibitors have a similar side-effect profile to tamoxifen, with lower risk of thromboembolic complications, endometrial carcinoma, and retinopathy, but with an increased risk of gastrointestinal disturbance. Other quality of life toxicities of treatment such as hot flushes do not appear to be significantly different between the two agents based on preliminary unpublished quality of life data (presented at the American Society of Clinical Oncology meeting 2002). However, the rate of bone fractures in the group receiving the aromatase inhibitor was relatively high, whereas tamoxifen is known to be osteoprotective. This may have important long-term consequences on health, and the long-term safety data for the new aramotase inhibitors is currently not available. So despite early encouraging results of adjuvant trials, tamoxifen remains the gold standard in this setting, as recommended in guidance issued in 2002 by the American Society of Clinical Oncology. In the adjuvant setting, where women will hopefully be cured of their cancer long term, we must be cautious about the late effects of new treatments. Time will tell.

### Ovarian ablation

Ovarian ablation is the oldest form of systemic treatment for breast cancer. Ablation can be surgical (oophorectomy – removal of ovaries), by radiotherapy (less common now), or medically with subcutaneous injections of LHRH agonists, which has the potential advantage of reversibility and is usually given for 2 years. Clinical trials in premenopausal women with early breast cancer who have hormone-sensitive disease, show improvements in overall survival equivalent in magnitude to the benefits of chemotherapy. Ovarian ablation may be used instead of chemotherapy in a low-risk, node-negative subgroup of premenopausal, ER-positive women. Randomized trials are underway to examine the contribution of ovarian ablation in the adjuvant setting when combined with chemotherapy. It is also increasingly being offered to high-risk premenopausal, ER-positive women who fail to go into menopause following chemotherapy, although the magnitude of benefit is uncertain. Ovarian ablation is associated with marked vasomotor disturbance (hot flushes), vaginal dryness, and loss of libido, which can have significantly consequences on quality of life. Long-term impact on cardiovascular disease and bone density also needs to be considered when offering this treatment to young women. Hopefully further trials will help clarify the risk–benefit.

## Follow-up, recurrence, and metastatic breast cancer

### Follow-up

Completion of primary treatment for breast cancer is a difficult time for women. There is uncertainty as to what the future holds, and concern relating to disease recurrence. Regular long-term hospital review has been a well-established practice, to provide psychological support and detect locoregional recurrence or distant metastases. However, there is no evidence that intensive follow-up improves quality of life related to health or overall survival from breast cancer. In the majority of women, recurrence is detected between routine follow-up appointments, or when patients present with signs or symptoms of disease, frequently first to their general practitioner. Studies have shown that general practice follow-up is a possible and acceptable alternative for both patients and general practitioners (Grunfeld *et al.* 1995). Women should be fully informed as to symptoms and signs (Box 12.4), which may alert them to potential problems, and are advised to attend for regular mammograms. All women who have undergone treatment for primary breast cancer should have open access to a follow-up clinic, should they have concerns.

---

Box 12.4 **Signs and symptoms to alert patients to**

♦ Pain in the back, hips or neck – no obvious cause, present >2 weeks, waking at night, pain not responding to simple analgesics

♦ Lumps – breast, neck or axilla masses

♦ Swelling – arm or hand

♦ Shortness of breath, haemoptysis, or cough

♦ Abdominal pain (particularly right upper quadrant), bloating, nausea, diarrhoea or unexplained weight loss

---

## Recurrence and metastatic disease

Although early diagnosis and new treatments have improved the outlook for breast cancer patients, up to 60% will have some form of recurrence. This may be local or distant.

### Locoregional recurrence

Locoregional recurrence ($\approx$10%) manifests as breast or chest wall infiltration and ulceration, excematous skin changes, new lymphoedema, or nodal mass. Local disease recurrence may be treated with curative intent, depending on pattern of recurrence, for example, by mastectomy if recurrence follows wide local excision.

### Metastases

Metastases occur most commonly to bone (70%), lungs (10%), and liver (10%). They may occur to any organ. Metastatic breast cancer is incurable. Treatments are aimed primarily at maintaining quality of life by symptom relief and prevention. There may be an additional benefit of prolonging survival. Community palliative care nurses provide an invaluable support network for the patient and relatives and contact should be initiated as early as possible.

### Endocrine therapies

As first line, endocrine treatments are generally preferred for hormone sensitive symptomatic advanced disease, because they are better tolerated and produce a longer response. Most patients who are hormone sensitive will have been on tamoxifen previously, in which case, aromatase inhibitors or ovarian ablation can be used. Changing aromatase inhibitor may also have an effect. As a class, they have been shown to be more effective and better tolerated than progestins, which were previously used as a second-line hormone therapy after tamoxifen. Ovarian ablation should be considered in premenopausal women.

### Chemotherapy and biological therapies

For patients who have visceral metastases, with short disease-free interval, or ER-negative tumours, palliative chemotherapy is considered. Median disease response is 40–70%, depending on the criteria used. There is no particular chemotherapy regimen that is more effective with respect to survival, although anthracyclines have the best response rates as single agents in breast cancer. Participation in clinical trials is encouraged. Choice will depend on the extent of the disease, patient fitness, and wishes. Re-challenge with previously used chemotherapy regimens may also be effective, if there has been a prolonged symptom-free period. The chance of disease response becomes significantly less with second- and third-line chemotherapy regimens. Recent chemotherapy developments in advanced breast cancer include the introduction of taxanes (docetaxel and paclitaxel) and vinorelbine. National Institute of Clinical Excellence (NICE) recommends that taxanes be used in fit patients who have life-threatening anthracycline-resistant disease. Approximately 20% of patients expressing the epidermal growth factor receptor 'c-*erbB2*' ('*neu*' or '*HER2*') may respond to the monoclonal antibody, herceptin. It is important to accept the limitations and potential complications of chemotherapy. Treatment should be discontinued if no further benefit, which for the patient can be psychologically very difficult. Concentrating on supportive care should be viewed as an equal, if not a more important treatment option rather than as a failure.

### Effective supportive care

Supportive care is carried out in a multidisciplinary setting with involvement of the primary care team, palliative care specialists, district and community

Macmillan nurses. Key factors in successful supportive care are assessment, communication, and symptom control. Physical signs and treatment-related symptoms are more readily assessed than psychosocial and spiritual issues. Common symptoms include fatigue, pain, nausea, shortness of breath, and anorexia, not all of which are reversible. Short-term steroid therapy may be effective for appetite and mood, with progestogens being used longer term. Supportive care is patient focused, accepting and addressing limitations of medical care and the emotional needs of the patient.

## Common symptoms in advanced disease

Bone is the commonest site for metastatic disease. Bone metastases may be present for several years before the development of visceral metastases, with a median survival of 2 years. Sometimes only simple analgesia is required, bone pain being particularly responsive to non-steroidal anti-inflammatory agents. For more persistent, localized pain, a single treatment with radiotherapy can be very effective. If there are lytic bone metastases in weight-bearing bones, prophylactic surgical intervention is recommended as there is a high risk of fracture and surgery provides symptom relief. Systemic treatment with oral or intravenous bisphosphonates reduces skeletal complications by 30–40%, relieves bone pain, improves bone healing, and is used to treat malignancy-related hypercalcaemia. Oral absorption tends to be poor and is associated with gastrointestinal upset in many patients. Newer bisphosphonates are being developed, which may overcome this problem. Trials are currently evaluating their use in an adjuvant setting, where they may reduce the development of bone metastases.

Breathlessness can be distressing and it is important to identify whether there is a potentially treatable cause. Pleural effusion symptomatically responds to drainage by pleural aspiration or chest drain followed by pleurodesis. There is an increased risk of thromboembolic disease associated with malignancy and immobility, which should also be considered. Systemic treatments may provide relief for pulmonary metastases or lymphangitis carcinomatosis.

## Medical emergencies

In advanced disease, a variety of medical conditions may occur requiring urgent intervention to reduce the chance of potentially debilitating or immediately life-threatening complications.

*Spinal cord compression* presents with weakness, possibly associated with sphincter and sensory disturbance. Development of neurological deficit requires urgent investigation with spinal MRI, and commencement of high-dose steroid therapy, as rapid intervention may prevent permanent disability.

**Table 12.6** World Health Organization score of performance status

| | |
|---|---|
| 0 | Fully active, able to carry on all pre-disease performance without restriction |
| 1 | Restricted in physically strenuous activity but ambulatory and able to carry out work of a light or sedentary nature, e.g. light housework, office work |
| 2 | Ambulatory and capable of self-care but unable to carry out any work activities. Up and about more than 50% of waking hours |
| 3 | Capable of only limited self-care, confined to bed or chair more than 50% of waking hours |
| 4 | Completely disabled. Cannot carry out any self-care. Totally confined to bed or chair |

*Superior vena caval obstruction* symptomatically causes breathlessness, particularly on lying flat, headache, arm and facial oedema. Local radiotherapy or mechanical stenting may be beneficial.

*Cerebral or choroidal metastases* can occur and treatment is steroid therapy followed by radiotherapy. Main side effects of whole brain radiotherapy are alopecia, and somnolence syndrome, which may occur about 6 weeks post-treatment. This is a time of profound tiredness, which resolves without further intervention. Isolated cerebral metastases may be managed neurosurgically if there is good performance status (Table 12.6) and otherwise limited metastatic disease.

*Thromboembolic disease* is common in advanced malignancy. Pulmonary embolism and deep venous thrombosis may present as emergencies.

*Development of immobility associated with pain* may be due to pathological fracture, which may require surgical intervention, if in weight-bearing bones.

*Brachial plexopathy* can present with hand and arm weakness, clumsiness, and loss of sensation. Referral for urgent investigation may prevent progression of neurological deficit.

## Psychosocial aspects

Thirty per cent of women with breast cancer experience an anxiety state or depressive illness within a year of diagnosis, which is three times higher than expected in the community at large. Significantly more women will experience non-pathological distress associated with her diagnosis and its treatment. Much can be done to reduce this distress. Most women do appreciate the significance of finding a breast lump, but a significant minority delay seeking medical attention. Once referral has been made, there is considerable anxiety while awaiting biopsy results, and the development of multidisciplinary one-stop diagnostic clinics in many breast units has helped to reduce this.

Individual reactions to the diagnosis will vary and be influenced by personal experience of cancer in friends or family members. Fears can be alleviated with a thorough knowledge of these factors. Frequently very little information is absorbed at the time of first diagnosis apart from the word 'cancer' and it is important to repeat information as required. The presence of close friends or relatives, or taping of consultations, can help in the recall of facts and reduce subsequent anxiety. The majority of patients want as much information as possible about their illness, but the nature and flow of information should be given at a pace suited to the individual. The primary care physician, with the specialist breast care nurses, are in an ideal position to support the patient and her family. They can check the patient's understanding of and reaction to a consultation, particularly if bad news has been given. They can offer information as well as practical and emotional support. A good professional working relationship with the hospital team, with rapid dissemination of information regarding management plans or treatment dilemmas, will facilitate this support and ensure that a coordinated approach to patient care is achieved. It is important that consistent messages are given by the health professionals involved to avoid confusion, which can increase anxiety.

With the move to conservative breast surgery, the anxiety related to loss of the breast has been replaced by anxiety about recurrence. Since there is no clear advantage in terms of survival or psychological functioning between different surgical treatments, women's personal choices are important. Whatever treatment is given, there are certain risk factors predisposing to significant psychological morbidity: inadequate information, adjuvant chemotherapy, complications of treatment, pre-existing psychological problems, lack of social support (particularly a close confiding relationship), and poor coping strategies. It is important to acknowledge the patient's pyschological, social, and spiritual well-being, as well as addressing her physical needs. Simple counselling relieves many women's anxieties, whereas others may require more intensive psychological support or specialized therapy. Access to high-quality information about local services, patterns of disease and available treatments, and sources of emotional support for the patient (such as self-help groups and resource centres) are known to reduce anxiety. It helps the woman to understand her illness and the treatment and adjust to living with, or coping with the terminal phase of her disease.

# Frequently asked questions

### How can I treat breast pain?

A comfortable support bra may provide relief. There may be particular stimuli for pain to avoid, such as caffeine or chocolate. Evening primrose oil, a natural source of gamolenic acid (GLA), can reduce pain and nodularity (dose of 300 mg daily). If that fails, there are other drugs that can be used, but they tend to have significant side effects, and are held in reserve.

### Do breast cysts increase my chance of breast cancer?

The cancer risk associated with benign breast disease is in general very low. There appears to be a slightly increased risk (1.5–2 × the general population risk) in women with a history of fibrocystic breast disease. If the diagnosis of atypical epithelial hyperplasia has been made, the risk is higher (4–5 ×), increasing still further if there is also a family history (up to 9 × the risk). Cystic breast disease alone is not an indication for routine mammographic screening, outside of the National Breast Screening Programme.

### I have completed my treatment for cancer – am I cured?

Everything has been done at this time to prevent the cancer coming back. However, despite this, there is a chance of the cancer returning. The probability of this depends on the characteristics of your cancer. There is no test that can be done at this time to say that all the abnormal cancer cells have gone and that you have been cured. Two-thirds of all recurrences occur within the first 5 years after treatment. Thereafter, the probability of recurrence decreases exponentially with time, although late recurrences may still occur. It is important to have initial yearly imaging with mammograms following treatment, looking for local recurrence or problems in the other breast. Alternative imaging techniques may be used for certain clinical indications. Whole body scans or bone scans have no role in breast cancer follow-up, unless there are particular symptoms requiring further investigation.

### I had breast cancer when I was 50 years of age. Is my daughter at increased risk?

Only a very small number (5–10%) of all breast cancers are associated with an identifiable genetic abnormality. It is important to obtain an accurate family history, not only of breast cancer but also of ovarian cancer and other epithelial malignancies such as prostate and bowel cancer in male family members. If there is no other family history, then the lifetime risk of your daughter having breast cancer will be no different to the general population. Your daughter should be 'breast aware', and enter the National Breast Screening Programme at an appropriate age. If there is a strong family history (see Box 12.3), then you should be referred to a family history clinic/genetic clinic for further assessment, counselling, and the opportunity to take part in screening or prevention studies.

## I have a strong family history of breast cancer, can I prevent breast cancer?

The NSABP-P1 prevention study (13 388 women) randomized women at high risk of developing breast cancer into receiving tamoxifen or not. The study was halted early due to a 45% reduction in the incidence of breast cancer in the tamoxifen arm (85 cases in the tamoxifen arm versus 154 cases in the placebo arm) and the FDA has approved tamoxifen for prevention. However, there was also a significant incidence of toxic side effects of tamoxifen such as endometrial carcinoma (33 in tamoxifen group, 14 in placebo) and thromboembolic complications (17 cases of pulmonary embolism, 6 in the placebo), in addition to quality of life issues. The majority of side effects occurred in patients more than 50 years old, who also experience the most benefit. A British and Italian study of women at high risk (mainly due to family history rather than age) failed to demonstrate significant reduction in breast cancer incidence with tamoxifen. There is evidence that women at increased risk due to genetic mutation are less likely to benefit from tamoxifen because their tumours are more likely to be hormone insensitive. For some women it is an alternative to prophylactic mastectomy or a watch and wait policy, but the jury is still out as to the overall benefit. The use of tamoxifen should be an individual decision, balancing probability of benefit and potential side effects of treatment.

## Does tamoxifen cause me to go into the menopause?

Menopausal symptoms may occur during the treatment for breast cancer and can be due to a variety of factors:

- You may have reached the menopause naturally at about the same time as you developed breast cancer.
- You may have stopped taking hormone replacement therapy at the time of diagnosis, bringing on the symptoms.
- Chemotherapy treatment may cause your ovaries to stop working, causing an early menopause. Sometimes the ovaries start working again, depending on your age and other factors.
- Tamoxifen can cause similar symptoms to the menopause, such as hot flushes and night sweats. It does not cause the menopause to occur – indeed, tamoxifen was developed initially as a fertility agent.

## Will I still be able to have a successful pregnancy following chemotherapy?

It is possible to have a successful pregnancy following chemotherapy. However, chemotherapy does affect ovarian function and may cause permanent ovarian failure and early menopause. The older you are, the more likely this is to occur, and infertility may be a consequence of treatment. Once chemotherapy has started, periods may stop or be irregular. It may be possible to become pregnant, even if experiencing menopausal symptoms. Therefore it is important to continue using contraception, particularly as chemotherapy agents could damage the fetus. It is best to avoid pregnancy for a period of time (2 years usually recommended) following treatment. The oral contraceptive pill is typically avoided. Periods may still return many months following breast cancer treatment. Ovarian storage is highly experimental, and there is no evidence that it can overcome ovarian failure and result in successful pregnancy.

## What are the side effects of early menopause?

Menopause causes a reduction in oestrogen levels, which can in the long term have adverse effects on bone density and cholesterol control. Tamoxifen slows bone loss in postmenopausal women, and other drugs may be used to reduce the risk of osteoporosis. A bone density study should be performed to assess baseline bone characteristics and family history should also be taken into account. Weight-bearing exercise such as walking can help prevent bone loss. Other drugs, for example, the selective oestrogen receptor modulators (e.g. raloxifene), may have a role in preventing osteoporosis, if you are not on tamoxifen. HRT prevents the long-term complications of early menopause, but is not recommended routinely in breast cancer patients (see below).

## Can I use HRT for my menopausal symptoms, if I have had breast cancer?

Because breast cancer is, in the majority of cases, a hormone-sensitive disease, the administration of hormone replacement therapy for the relief of menopausal symptoms and prevention of other medical complications of menopause, such as osteoporosis, is controversial. In general, HRT is not recommended. However, for some women, the magnitude of their symptoms is such that they are willing to accept a possible increase in breast cancer recurrence for the potential benefits of the treatment. It may also be that the risk is not increased in hormone-negative tumours. There are recent non-randomized studies that have shown HRT can be used without adverse effects on breast cancer recurrence rates. HRT may be prescribed, if the patient is fully aware that complete data are still outstanding as to the risk–benefit ratio. Randomized controlled trials addressing these questions are underway and hope to give us more information as to whether it is safe to prescribe HRT to breast cancer patients.

## What can I do about hot flushes on tamoxifen?

The majority of women experience hot flushes on treatment, which can be very debilitating. Sometimes changing the brand of tamoxifen can help or taking 10 mg twice daily. A variety of agents have been used to treat these symptoms in clinical trials. Vitamin E (800 IU/day) is a reasonable first-line therapy, as it is safe and inexpensive, with demonstrated benefit. Clonidine has traditionally been used, but is generally not well tolerated. Venlafaxine (37.5 mg/day), one of the new antidepressants, has been shown in clinical trials to alleviate hot flushes in about 40% of patients (compared with 27% in placebo). Finally, a progestational agent such as megestrol acetate can be used (40 mg/day for one month, decreasing to 20 mg/day thereafter). Traditional hormone replacement therapy is the most effective treatment, but there remains concern over its use following breast cancer (see above).

## Can I take complementary medicine with my treatment?

Women who have tried complementary approaches have found them helpful, although in most cases there is no evidence from clinical trials that they work. It is important to go to a recognized, qualified practitioner for advice if you wish to do this. Complementary therapies such as aromatherapy, relaxation therapy, and acupuncture may help with coping with chemotherapy or menopausal symptoms. There is little clinical evidence for homeopathy or traditional Chinese medicines, although there are anecdotal reports of their use in controlling menopausal symptoms. It is important to tell your specialist if you are taking additional herbal remedies, in case there may be a recognized interaction with the treatment you are having.

## I have completed my treatment – what follow-up will I have following treatment and how do I know my cancer hasn't come back?

Follow-up will depend on the local services, and there is no clear follow-up strategy that is 'the best'. It is increasingly recognized that many hospital visits can increase anxiety regarding the diagnosis, and regular follow-up does not appear to affect overall survival if a recurrence does occur. Some centres will see you regularly following treatment for a period of time. It is important to have regular mammographic follow-up, to detect local problems within the treated breast or contralateral breast problems. Sometimes the GP will see you on a regular basis, or you will be given written information as to symptoms or signs that you should see your GP or specialist about (see Box 12.4).

The initial period following completion of treatment can often be a difficult time, as the 'active treatment' is over with. It is often the time to adjust to having had a potentially life-threatening illness, with no guarantees possible as to the future outcome. It is important to talk about these fears and anxieties, either to your breast care nurse, general practitioner, self-help groups, or others who support you.

## 10-Minute consultation: breast lump

A 48-year-old woman comes to see you complaining of a 'swelling' in her breast, which is uncomfortable.

### What issues you should cover

◆ The concern is whether there is an abnormality requiring referral for specialist assessment, to exclude malignancy. Ask about the duration and nature of symptoms. Is there nipple discharge and if so, volume and nature. Blood-stained or clear discharge should be referred for further assessment. Breast pain alone is an uncommon presentation of breast cancer, but examination is essential to exclude an underlying breast lump. Does the lump fluctuate with the menstrual cycle and is she pre-, peri-, or post-menopausal? The use of oral contraceptive pill or hormone replacement therapy should be documented. Other symptoms, such as significant weight loss, or severe skeletal pain, may indicate advanced cancer, but is uncommon at presentation.

◆ Is there a past history of benign breast disease or previous investigations for breast abnormality? There may be a particular anxiety regarding the diagnosis breast cancer precipitating the referral. Is there a family history of breast cancer and if so, how old were the relatives at time of diagnosis: 5–10% of breast cancer cases have an underlying identifiable genetic abnormality. Patients with a strong family history according to local guidelines, should be referred for specialist genetic counselling, once significant underlying pathology has been excluded.

### What should you do?

◆ On breast examination, look for change in breast contour, puckering or dimpling of the skin, cutaneous oedema (*peau d'orange*), and nipple changes. If nipple inversion present, is it of recent onset? Skin involvement or nipple changes are strong indicators of malignancy and urgent referral is recommended.

◆ Clinically determine if there is a discrete, definable lump, or an area of nodularity. If an abnormality is found, does it appear to be within the breast substance or related to the chest wall? If within the breast, clarify clinically whether this is a smooth, rounded mobile mass or irregular and fixed within the breast substance. Irregular lumps are highly suspicious and urgent referral should be arranged. If there is a possible lump or nodularity, it is helpful to ask the women to attend again after her next period for repeat examination and if abnormality persists, referral is recommended.

◆ Benign causes of breast lumps include cysts or fibroadenomas. Breast cysts are most common in the 40–50 years age group, and are frequently multiple. Cysts constitute 17% of all discrete breast masses, and referral should be made to establish the diagnosis. They are readily diagnosed at ultrasonography and typically resolve following fine-needle aspiration. Fibroadenomas are typically mobile, smooth, and well defined, but an unlikely cause of this woman's symptoms, as they occur most commonly in the 15–30 years age group. Breast nodularity is ill defined, may be bilateral, and tends to fluctuate with the menstrual cycle. Again, it can be helpful to re-examine following menstruation, when nodularity typically decreases.

◆ Also check for axillary and supraclavicular fossa lymphadenopathy. Palpable lymph nodes may be found in up to 30% of patients who, with further assessment, have no evidence of malignancy. But if present, urgent referral is indicated.

◆ Specialist assessment is likely to induce anxiety, although most women will be relieved by the act of referral. Explain to the woman the reasons for the referral and the likely diagnostic tests that will be undertaken. Diagnosis will be achieved by the triple assessment of clinical assessment, imaging (mammography and ultrasound), and cytology (fine-needle aspirate or core biopsy).

◆ Indications for hospital referral are given in Box 12.1.

## Useful reading and information for patients

Sampson, V. and Fenlon, D. (2000). *The breast cancer book*. Vermilion, London.
   *A comprehensive overview of breast cancer and treatments from a patient and her breast care nurse.*
Farrell Yelland, T. (2000). *All woman*. Metro, London.
   *Thirty women who have had breast cancer tell their stories, including personal tips. Also has a guide to treatment and a list of resources.*

Daniel, R. (2000). *Living with cancer*. Robinson, London.
   *A positive, self-help guide for people with cancer, based around the holistic approach of the Bristol Cancer Help Centre.*

## Advisory groups, useful addresses and websites

BACUP (British Association for Cancer United Patients)
3 Bath Place, Rivington Street, London EC2 A3JR
Tel: 020 7613 2121
www.cancerbacup.org.uk

Breast Care Campaign
Blythe Hall, 100 Blythe Road, London W14 0HB
www.bcc.uk.org
   *The UK's leading source of information on benign breast disorders for health professionals and the public*

Breast Cancer Care
Kiln House, 210 New Kings Road, London SW6 4NZ
Nationwide Freeline: 0500 245 345
www.breastcare.co.uk

Breast Care and Mastectomy Association (BCMA)
7–26 Harrison Street, kings Cross, London WC1H GJG
Tel: 020 7837 0908

CancerLink
17 Britannia Street, London WC1X 9JN
Tel: 020 7833 2451
www.cancerlink.org

Cancer Research UK
10 Cambridge Terrace, London NW1 4JL
Tel: 020 7224 1333
www.crc.org.uk

CR UK Primary Care Education Group,
Institute of Health Sciences, University of Oxford
Old Road, Headington, Oxford OX3 7LF
www.dphpc.ox.ac.uk/crcpcerg

DIPEx, Institute of Health Sciences
University of Oxford, Old Road, Headington, Oxford OX3 7LF
www.dipex.org

*A database of patients' experiences of illness: stories from over 40 patients with breast cancer linked with evidence-based information and details about support groups*

The Royal London Homeopathic Hospital
Great Ormond Street, London WC1N 3HR
Tel: 020 7837 8833
*General practitioner referral required. Out-patient menopause and cancer clinics*

The Women's Health Concern (WHC)
PO Box 429, Addlestone, Surrey KT15 1DZ
*A registered medical charity offering advice and information on gynaecological conditions, HRT and hormonal problems*

The Women's Nationwide Cancer Control Campaign
First Floor, Charity House, 14–15 Perseverance Walks, London E28 8DD
Tel: 020 7729 4688
www.wnccc.org.uk

# References and further reading

ATAC (the Arimidex, Tamoxifen Alone or in Combination) Trialists' Group (2002). Anastrazole alone or in combination with tamoxifen *vs* tamoxifen alone for the adjuvant treatment of postmenopausal woman with early breast cancer: first results of the ATAC randomized trial. *Lancet*, **359**, 2131–9.

Austoker, J. *et al.* (1999). *Guidelines for referral of patients with breast problems*. NHS Breast Screening Programme. Cancer Research UK.

Baum, M. and Spittle, M. (1999). *Key advances in the effective management of breast cancer*. Royal Society of Medicine Press, London.

Berrino, F., Capocaccia, R., Esteve, J., Gatta, G., Hakulinen, T., Micheli, A., and others (1999). *Survival of cancer patients in Europe- the EUROCARE-2 Study*. IARC Scientific Publications. OUP.

Blanks, R., Moss, S., McGahan, C., Quinn, M. and Babb, P. (2000). Effect of NHS breast screening programme on mortality from breast cancer in England and Wales, 1990–8 comparison of observed with predicted mortality. *British Medical Journal*, **321**, 665–9.

Breast Surgeons Group of the British association of Surgical Oncology (1998). Guidelines for surgeons in the management of symptomatic breast disease in the United Kingdom. *European Journal of Surgical Oncology*, **21**, 1–13.

Clinical Synthesis Panel on HRT (1999). Hormone replacement therapy. Review. *Lancet*, **354**, 152–5.

Collaborative Group on Hormonal Factors in Breast Cancer (1996). Breast cancer and hormonal contraceptives: collaborative reanalysis of individual data on 53,297 women with breast cancer and 100,239 women without breast cancer from 54 epidemiological studies. *Lancet*, **347**, 1713–27.

Crown, J. and O'Leary, M. (2000). The taxanes: an update. *Lancet*, **355**, 1176–8.

Cuzick, J., (2001). Editorial: is hormone replacement therapy safe for breast cancer patients? *Journal of the National Cancer Institute*, **93**, 733–4.

Dixon, M. and Morrow M. (1999). *Breast disease: a problem-based approach.* W.B. Saunders, London.

Dixon, M. (2000). *ABC of breast diseases.* BMJ Publishing Group, London.

Early Breast Cancer Trialists' Collaborative Group (1998a). Polychemotherapy for early breast cancer; an overview of the randomised trials. *Lancet*, **352**, 930–42.

Early Breast Cancer Trialists' Collaborative Group (1998b). Tamoxifen for early breast cancer: an overview of the randomised trials. *Lancet*, **351**, 1451–67.

Early Breast Cancer Trialists' Collaborative Group (2000). Favourable and unfavourable effects on long term survival of radiotherapy for early breast cancer: an overview of randomised controlled trials. *Lancet*, **355**, 1757–70.

Fisher, B., Dignam, J., Wolmark, N., *et al.* (1998). Lumpectomy and radiation therapy for the treatment of intraductal breast cancer: findings from National Surgical Adjuvant Breast and Bowel Project B-17. *Journal of Clinical Oncology*, **16**, 441–52.

Fisher, B., Dignam, J., Wolmark, N., *et al.* (1999). Tamoxifen in treatment of intraductal breast cancer: National Surgical Adjuvant Breast and Bowel Project B-24 randomised controlled trial. *Lancet*, **353**, 1993–2000.

Grunfeld, E., Mant, D., Vessey, M. and Yudkin, P. (1995). Evaluating primary care follow-up of breast cancer: methods and prelimary results of three studies. *Annals of Oncology*, **6**(S2), 47–52.

Hojris, I., Overgaard, M., Christensen, J. and Overgaard, J. (1999). Morbidity and mortality of ischaemic heart disease in high-risk breast cancer patients after adjuvant postmastectomy systemic treatment with or without radiotherapy; analysis of DBCG 82b and 82c randomised trials. *Lancet*, **254**, 1425–30.

Hortobagyi, G.N. (1998). Treatment of breast cancer. Review. *New England Journal of Medicine*, **14**, 974–84.

Jones, G. (2001). Review: radiotherapy decreases death and recurrence of breast cancer, but increases death from other causes. *Evidence Based Medicine*, **6**, 53.

Julien, J., Bijker, N., Fentiman, I., *et al.* (2000). Radiotherapy in breast conserving treatment for ductal carcinoma in situ: first results of the EORTC randomised phase III trial 10853. *Lancet*, **355**, 528–33.

Kauff, N.D., Satagopan, J.M., Robson, M.E., *et al.* (2002). Risk-reducing salpingo-oophorectomy in women with BRAC1 or BRAC2 mutation. *New England Journal of Medicine*, **346**, 1609–15.

Litherlang, J.C. (1999). The effect of hormone replacement therapy on the sensitivity of screening mammograms. *Clinical Radiology*, **54**(5), 285–8.

Loprinzi, C., Barton, D. and Rhodes, D. (2001). Management of hot flashes in breast cancer survivors. Review. *Lancet Oncology* **2**(4), 199–204.

Meijers-Hoijboer, van Geel B., van Putten W.L.J., *et al.* (2001). Breast cancer after prophylactic bilateral mastectomy in women with BRCA1 or BRCA2 mutation. *New England Journal of Medicine*, **345**, 159–64.

Osborne, K. (1998). Tamoxifen in the management of breast cancer. Review. *New England Journal of Medicine*, **339**, 1609–18.

Quinn, M., Babb, P., Jones, J., *et al.* (1999). CD-ROM *Cancer 1971–97: registration of cancer cases and deaths in England and Wales by sex, age, year, health region and type of cancer.* Office of National Statistics, London.

RCGP and OPCS (1995). *Morbidity statistics from general practice 1991–92.* Fourth national study. HMSO, London.

Richards, M.A., Westcombc, A.M., Ramirez, A.J., *et al.* (1999). *A systematic review of the delay in diagnosis/treatment of symptomatic breast cancer, 1999: a report commissioned by the NHS Cancer Research and Development Programme.* Department of Health, London.

Royal College of Radiologists (1999). COIN guidelines: breast cancer management. *Clinical Oncology,* **11**(Supplement).

Whelan, T.J., Julian, J., Wright, J., Jadad, A.R. and Levine, M.L. (2000). Does locoregional radiotherapy improve survival in breast cancer; a meta-analysis. *Journal of Clinical Oncology,* **18**, 1220–9.

# Chapter 13

# Women's cancer screening: cervical, breast, and ovarian screening

## Clare Bankhead and Joan Austoker

A screening programme invites asymptomatic people in a population at risk to be tested for a disease for which there is an effective treatment. Screening does not diagnose illness. Those who (screen) test positive are sent on for further diagnostic tests to determine whether they do have the disease. Ideally, screening should be able to detect a precursor condition so that the disease can be stopped before it even starts. A good example of this is cervical screening that aims to detect a precancerous lesion called cervical intraepithelial neoplasia (CIN). If this condition is detected and treated, cervical carcinoma is very unlikely to develop. Breast screening, however, can detect very early stage breast cancer when the tumour is too small to be felt. Around half the cancers found at screening are still small enough to allow breast-saving surgery and most breast cancers are found at an early stage when there is a good chance of a successful recovery. Screening for ovarian cancer is not routinely offered as it has not yet been demonstrated to reduce mortality. However, a very large, randomized, controlled trial of screening using transvaginal ultrasound and CA125 testing as the basic screening tests has recently started to evaluate the effectiveness of ovarian cancer screening in postmenopausal women. Further details are given in the section on ovarian cancer screening.

## Definition of screening terms

A screening test does not diagnose a particular condition, but merely sorts the population into test-positive and test-negative groups.

The *sensitivity* of a screening test is the ability to detect disease. It is the proportion of all those with disease that test positive. A sensitivity of 70% means that for every ten participants with the disease, seven of them will test positive, the other three will be false negatives. If the test has a poor sensitivity, a large number of those with the condition will escape detection, will be falsely reassured and could possibly delay presenting important symptoms.

The *specificity* of a test is the ability to exclude people who do not have the condition. It is the proportion of all those who are disease free who test negative. A specificity of 90% means that nine out of ten people who do not have the disease will give a negative result. One out of ten will be false positive and require further assessment before the possibility of disease can be ruled out. A test with poor specificity will have important consequences for the individual, including anxiety and unnecessary further investigations.

An ideal screening test should have a high sensitivity (to reduce the number of false negatives) and a high specificity (in order to reduce the number of false positives). However, it is often not possible to achieve this as there is a trade-off between between the two measures; tightening the criteria for one will result in a decrease in the other.

Another feature of a screening test is the *predictive value* and there are two aspects to this. The positive predictive value of a test is the proportion of those who test positive, who actually have the disease. The negative predictive value is the proportion of those who test negative, who are truly disease free (or the proportion of those who are healthy among those with a negative test). The predictive value is influenced by both the sensitivity and specificity of the test, and also the population prevalence of the condition being screened for. The relationships between specificity, sensitivity, and predictive value are shown in Table 13.1.

**Table 13.1** Definitions: sensitivity, specificity, predictive value

|  |  |  | **Disease** | |
|---|---|---|---|---|
|  |  |  | **Present** | **Absent** |
| **Screening** | **Positive** | | a | b |
| **test** | **Negative** | | c | d |

$$a = \text{true positive} \qquad b = \text{false positive}$$
$$c = \text{false negative} \qquad d = \text{true negative.}$$

| Term | Definition | Formula |
|---|---|---|
| Sensitivity | Proportion with condition who test positive | $a/(a + c)$ |
| Specificity | Proportion without condition who test negative | $d/(b + d)$ |
| Positive predictive value | Proportion with positive test who have the condition | $a/(a + b)$ |
| Negative predictive value | Proportion with negative test who do not have the condition | $d/(c + d)$ |

## Cervical screening

In 1996, approximately 2600 new cases of invasive cervical cancer were registered in England and Wales (based on provisional data), making it the tenth most common cancer in women (Quinn *et al.* 1999b). Since 1990, the incidence of invasive disease has been steadily decreasing from a standardized incident rate of 15.4/100 000 women to only 8.9/100 000 women in 1996 (Quinn *et al.* 1999b). Mortality rates have also been declining and currently the reduction is around 7% per year, whereas previously the decline in mortality had been around 1% per year. This sudden fall coincided with the improvements in the call–recall system.

The purpose of cervical screening is to reduce the incidence of malignant carcinoma of the cervix by detecting and treating cervical intraepithelial neoplasia (CIN), which is a necessary precursor lesion. This will lead to a decreased incidence of cervical carcinoma and ultimately to decreased mortality. Cervical screening uses cytology to detect areas of nuclear abnormalities, which are described as dyskaryotic. Dyskaryosis ranges from borderline through to severe. Depending on the severity of dyskaryosis, women may undergo colposcopy to provide a histological diagnosis of CIN.

There have been no randomized controlled trials to assess the effectiveness of cervical screening, although early evidence from the Nordic countries showed a beneficial effect of screening. Organized screening was introduced in Iceland, Finland, Sweden, and Denmark soon after 1960. All these countries obtained nationwide coverage, except for Denmark, which only covered 45% of the eligible population by 1991 (Sigurdsson 1999). Reductions in both mortality and incidence of cervical cancer between 1986 and 1995 have been greatest in Iceland (mortality reduced by 76% and incidence 67%), and Finland (73% mortality, 75% incidence reduction) and lowest in Norway (43% and 34% reduction, respectively), where systematic cervical screening was only introduced in 1994 (Sigurdsson 1999), indicating that organized screening is an important determinant of risk reduction.

A cervical screening programme was introduced in the UK in the 1960s, but for two decades it was chaotic and the proportion of women over the age of 40 who were not receiving screening was extremely high. As a result, the programme made no impact on incidence or mortality. In 1988, the National Health Service Cervical Screening Programme (NHSCSP) was reorganized and a computerized call–recall system was introduced. All women aged 20–64 (25–64 in Scotland) are invited for screening every 3–5 years depending on the local primary care trust (and previously the local health authority). In 1996–97, 60% of health authorities were operating a 3-year screening interval, compared with 39% in 1991 (National Audit Office 1992, 1998). The majority of cervical smears (86%) are taken in general practice. The NHSCSP recommends that all women should receive their results in writing. More than 80% should receive their results within 4 weeks of the smear and 100% within 6 weeks (Austoker *et al.* 1997). Data on this aspect were collected for the first time in 1999–2000. Currently, only 65% of women are being sent result letters by the responsible primary care trust or their GP and of those, only 32% are received within 4 weeks and a further 27% by 6 weeks (Government Statistical Service 2000). This is obviously an area that needs improvement.

Recent evidence is now demonstrating a clear reduction in mortality from cervical cancer that can be attributed to screening (see section on potential effects of screening for more details).

Target payments for cervical screening were introduced in the UK in 1990 as part of the general practitioner's contract. Payments are triggered on reaching 50% or 80% coverage over the last 5 years, with a differential of 3:1 in favour of the latter. This has led to a considerable increase in screening activity. At the time that the targets were introduced, 53% of GPs were achieving the 80% target. This proportion has increased steadily and since 1993 more than 80% of GPs have been meeting this target. A very small proportion of GPs are failing to achieve even the 50% target.

Whilst this is good news in increasing the proportion of the population that receive screening and therefore achieve the public health aim of decreasing mortality from the condition, it has largely been achieved by providing a 'positive spin' on screening. Criticisms have been made that general patient information emphasizes the benefits of interventions whilst glossing over the risks and side effects (Coulter 1998) and certainly cancer screening has been offered as a service that will do good and implicitly will do no harm. One of the major problems with cervical screening is that of overdiagnosis. A report of cervical screening from Bristol showed that new abnormalities were found in 15 551 of 225 974 women tested: 6000 were referred for colposcopy (Raffle *et al.* 1995). The numbers were excessively high compared with the incidence of malignancy that could possibly be prevented. The study concluded that, despite being well organized, much of the effort was devoted to limiting the harm done to healthy women (Raffle *et al.* 1995).

The climate is now changing, and a move to provide fuller information was made in 1999 when the General Medical Council issued guidance for ensuring informed consent by users of medical services (General Medical Council 1999). Following this guidance, the National Screening Committee recommended that new patient information leaflets should be produced, that now for the first time provide both advantages and disadvantages of screening. These leaflets (National Screening Programme 2001b) were first circulated in November 2001, and will be fully evaluated and revised accordingly (Austoker *et al.* 2001). However, it has been reported that a tension exists between those wanting 'more honest' information to be available to women invited for screening and the medical experts running the screening programmes, who were worried that such information would discourage people from attending and that target payments for GPs work against the spirit of enabling women to make an informed choice on whether or not they want to be screened (Anderson and Nottingham 1999). It is not known how the provision of detailed, full information will affect the uptake of screening or whether the targets set for GP payments may need to be reviewed to reduce any conflicts.

## Results of the NHS Cervical Screening Programme, 2000–2001 (Government Statistical Service 2001)

The total number of cervical smears examined in England during 2000–2001 was 4 089 440. This figure includes smear tests taken from well women for screening purposes, repeat surveillance smears, and symptomatic smears. The total represents the results for approximately 3.6 million women. About 67% of these women (2.4 million) were screened as a result of an invitation from the health authority. The remaining 1.2 million women were screened either opportunistically or as a result of a GP invitation.

### Smear results

Of the 4.1 million smears examined in England in 2000–2001, 9.7% were inadequate. Of the adequate smears, 92.2% were negative and 7.7% were abnormal (Table 13.2).

Fig 13.1 shows the proportion of adequate smears that are abnormal by age. It can clearly be seen that younger women have a higher proportion of

**Table 13.2** Percentage of results of smear tests from GP and Community Clinics*, women aged 20–64, England 2000–2001

| Result of test | Mean (%) | Range (between RHAs) (%) |
|---|---|---|
| Inadequate | 9.7 | 8.0–11.4 |
| Adequate | | |
| Negative† | 92.2 | 90.7–93.4 |
| Borderline changes† | 4.2 | 3.5–5.2 |
| Mild dyskaryosis† | 2.2 | 1.5–2.9 |
| Moderate dyskaryosis† | 0.7 | 0.6–0.9 |
| Severe dyskaryosis or worse† | 0.6 | 0.5–0.7 |

*Smears from GP practices and community clinics reflect the results from the NHSCSP.
†Percentage of all adequate smears.

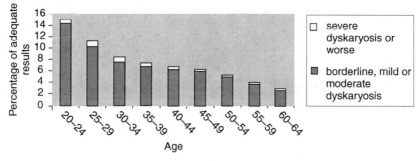

**Fig 13.1** Abnormal test results by age, England 2000–2001.

abnormal smears and this proportion declines with increasing age. The majority of abnormal smears are due to borderline changes, mild and moderate dyskaryosis: only 0.6% of smears show severe abnormalities.

## Outcome of referrals for smears

Between April and June 2000, in England 27 880 women were referred to gynaecology; 15 536 (56%) of these were following persistent non-negative smears and 12 344 (44%) were as a result of a smear test showing a potentially significant abnormality (moderate dyskaryosis or worse). The outcomes for the two types of referrals are quite different; the cancer detection rate in the persistent abnormalities group was only 0.1% compared with 2.6% in those with a smear test indicative of moderate dyskaryosis or worse. Seventeen per cent of referrals for persistent nuclear changes were found to have CIN2 or CIN3/carcinoma *in situ*, whereas the corresponding proportion in referrals after a single occurrence of a potentially significant abnormality was 71%.

## Potential effect of screening

If screening for premalignant cervical lesions is effective, we could expect to see an increase in carcinoma *in situ* rates, a progressive decrease in cancer registrations and, finally, a reduction in mortality due to cervical cancer. This is demonstrated below.

### Registrations of carcinoma *in situ*

Trends in new cases of carcinoma *in situ* (CIS) need to be treated with caution for the following reasons. Registration rates for CIS are not true incidence rates (defined as number of new cases arising per head of population per year). As women are not screened annually, registration rates are a mixture of prevalence rates (for women being screened for the first time) and cumulative

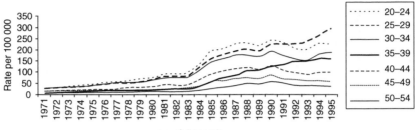

**Fig 13.2** Age-specific registrations of *in situ* cervical cancer in women aged 20–54, England and Wales 1971–95.

incidence rates from the date of last screen for women who have previously attended for cervical screening.

Also, CIS is asymptomatic and therefore cases can only be detected by screening. An increase in screening activity would then lead to an increase in registrations.

It has been shown that the registrations of CIS have broadly increased in line with the increase in the number of smears being undertaken (Quinn *et al.* 1999a). However, it can be seen from Fig 13.2 that since 1987 there has been a steady rise in CIS registrations in women aged 20–24 and 25–29, with no corresponding increase in the other age bands. The large increase in registrations that is visible in 1984 is due to the inclusion of CIN3 in the CIS registrations for the first time.

### Invasive cancer

The incidence of invasive cancer in England was 35% lower in 1995 than it was in 1990 (Quinn *et al.* 1999a). Fig 13.3 shows the age-specific incidence rates of invasive cervical cancer. Prior to 1990 there was little change in the rates in women aged over 55. However, the incidence in the 45–54 age group decreased from 388 per million in 1971 to 223 per million in 1989. During the same period, there was an increase in incidence from 89 to 142 per million in women

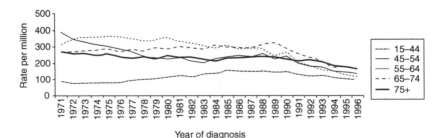

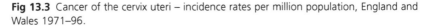

**Fig 13.3** Cancer of the cervix uteri – incidence rates per million population, England and Wales 1971–96.

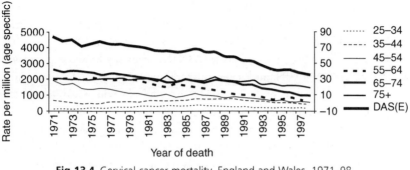

**Fig 13.4** Cervical cancer mortality, England and Wales, 1971–98.

aged 15–44. After 1990, the incidence in all age groups have shown a decrease. This could correspond to the increased number of women that were found to have CIN3 or CIS in the late 1980s and were successfully treated and subsequent development of invasive disease was prevented.

## Mortality

Age-standardized mortality from cervical cancer has been falling since the 1950s. However, the rate of the decrease was around 1% a year until 1988 and then it accelerated to around 7% a year. This sudden fall coincided with the improvements in the call–recall system (Sasieni *et al.* 1995).

The age-standardized mortality hides differing patterns of age-specific mortality. As shown in Fig 13.4, in all groups except the youngest group, mortality was lower in 1998 than it was in 1971. The largest decreases since 1988 have occurred in women aged 55–64 and 65–74.

A recent paper estimated that cervical screening has saved more than 8000 lives between the introduction of the computerized call–recall system (1988) and 1997. It also showed that prior to the mid-1980s there were no significant mortality trends that could not be explained in terms of a birth cohort effect, but since then, mortality had significantly fallen each year (Sasieni and Adams 1999).

## Recent news and future possibilities

### The role of human papillomavirus testing

Infection with certain types of human papillomavirus (HPV), in particular HPV 16 and HPV 18, have been shown to be associated with development of cervical cancer and also cervical intraepithelial neoplasia (CIN). Recently it has been shown that 99.7% of cervical cancers contain HPV DNA (Walboomers *et al.* 1999) and it is currently being debated whether any HPV-negative carcinomas exist (Herrington 1999). All grades of CIN have also been shown to be associated with HPV infection with at least 76% of CIN being attributable to

HPV (Schiffman *et al.* 1993). Women who have an HPV infection have odds ratios of about 70 for the development of high-grade cervical abnormalities, and higher odds ratios if infected with HPV 16 (Olson *et al.* 1995).

HPV testing has a higher sensitivity for CIN than cytology, 86% compared with 60% for all grades of CIN, and 93% compared with 73% for CIN2 and CIN3 (Cox *et al.* 1995), but a lower specificity, especially in young women (under 30 years old) who tend to have transient HPV infections. A recent review (Cuzick *et al.* 1999) of the role of HPV testing within cervical screening has concluded that the most plausible role of HPV testing in the NHSCSP may be to guide the management of women with borderline or mildly dyskaryotic smears as currently it is unclear which are likely to progress. HPV testing to triage women with low-grade abnormalities is currently being piloted in a few areas by the NHSCSP.

HPV testing may also be used to indicate situations where screening may be undertaken less frequently or be stopped early for older women.

## Liquid-based cytology

Technologies are being developed to improve cervical screening, including improved methods of sampling and preparing the smear, such as liquid-based cytology. Using this technique, the cells collected from the cervix are placed in a preservative fluid that is then sent to the laboratory. At the laboratory the sample is mixed and treated to remove unwanted material, and then a thin layer of the cell suspension is placed on a slide for inspection. This method should reduce the number of inadequate smears by producing clearer slides. The three pilots of liquid-based cytology in the UK have now reported that the rate of inadequate smears has decreased from 9% to 1–2%. There was no overall impact on the rates of borderline results, mild, moderate, or severe dyskaryosis, but there was a worrying reduction in the rate of reporting of glandular neoplasia. The report concludes that liquid-based cytology is cost saving, although there is uncertainty about the extent of any time-savings in primary care (Moss *et al.* 2003). Disappointingly, a further French study has also concluded that liquid-based cytology is less reliable and more likely to give false positive and false negative results than the conventional smear test (Coste *et al.* 2003).

## Frequently asked questions about cervical screening

### How likely am I to be recalled for further/repeat tests?

About 1 in 10 tests the cells cannot be seen properly under the microscope and the smear test must be taken again. In addition, another 1 in 10 tests will need to be investigated further due to an abnormality being found.

### If I'm recalled, what are my chances of having cancer?

Over half (58%) of women who are invited for further investigations were invited after having persistent non-negative smears. The cancer detection rate in this group is very low at only 0.2% and 22% of referrals for persistent nuclear changes were found to have CIN2 or CIN3/carcinoma *in situ*.

The 42% of referrals that were as a result of a smear test showing a potentially significant abnormality (moderate dyskaryosis or worse), showed a quite different pattern of outcomes. The cancer detection rate in this group was 3.0% and CIN2 or CIN3/carcinoma *in situ* was found in 72% of these women.

### Could a cancer be missed by screening?

Cervical screening does not pick up every abnormality of the cervix. Although regular screening can prevent about 8 out of every 10 cervical cancers developing, it does not prevent every case. If you have any abnormal symptoms, such as bleeding after sex or between periods, you should see your doctor.

### Should younger women be screened more frequently?

For younger women, particularly those aged 25–34, there was a significant increase in cervical cancer incidence and mortality, though the mortality rates are now starting to decline. Some health authorities screen women under 35 at 3-year intervals, and women over 35 at 5-year intervals. There is no good evidence to support this decision one way or another. Further research on the natural history of the disease is necessary, for example, to clarify whether the disease is more aggressive in younger women or not.

### Should high-risk women be screened more frequently?

Although there are several risk factors associated with increased risk of invasive cancer, it is not possible to use these factors reliably to predict which women will develop CIN. Moreover, there is no evidence that these risk factors affect the rate of progression of CIN. Thus it has been argued that there is little value in targeting these women for screening or selecting them for more frequent screening.

### Is screening teenagers worthwhile?

The prevalence of invasive carcinoma of the cervix does not justify including women under the age of 20 in the routine screening programme, provided there is good uptake in women aged 20–25. While CIN does exist in teenagers, invasive cancer is extremely rare. There is no rational basis for routinely screening teenagers, regardless of whether that are 'promiscuous' or not;

a smear is not needed for at least 2–3 years after becoming sexually active. In particular cases, an approach could be to take a smear where a teenage girl has had multiple sexual partners for more than 3 years. This is *not* screening, but a matter of responding to individual cases on merit.

### When in my menstrual cycle should I have my smear?

You cannot have your smear during your period, so it is best to make an appointment for another time.

### What is HPV?

HPV is a virus (called human papillomavirus). It is thought to be a cause of cervical cancer. More information is given in the section entitled 'the role of human papillomavirus testing' in this chapter.

### I've been told I've got dyskaryosis – what does this mean?

Dsykaryosis is a term for areas of nuclear abnormalities which can be seen in your smear. There are different degrees of severity of dyskaryosis, and some women may undergo colposcopy to provide a histological diagnosis of cervical intraepithelial neoplasia (CIN). The management options are outlined in Table 13.3.


## Breast screening

Breast cancer is the most common cancer in women, with more than 30 000 new cases being diagnosed in England and Wales every year (Quinn *et al.* 1999b). It also accounts for almost 12 000 deaths each year (Office of National Statistics 2001), which is a 14% reduction from the late 1980s when about 14 000 women were dying each year (Office of Population 1989).

The value of breast screening by mammography has been demonstrated in rigorous randomized trials. In all randomized trials of women aged 50 and over who have been offered screening compared with unscreened controls, mortality from breast cancer is reduced, although not significantly in all cases. Further details are given in the section on 'potential effects of screening'.

In 1986, the Forrest Report (Forrest 1986) recommended the provision of a National Health Service Breast Screening Programme (NHSBSP) offering 3-yearly mammography to women aged 50–64. It was estimated from the Swedish Two County Study that if 70% of eligible women attended for screening, a reduction in mortality of 25% from breast cancer in those invited for screening could be expected. This uptake target was first incorporated into the Health of the Nation white paper in 1992 and remains the minimum standard for the NHSBSP.

**Table 13.3** Summary of smear results and management options

| Smear results | Normal | Inadequate | Borderline dyskaryosis | Mild dyskaryosis | Moderate dyskaryosis | Severe dyskaryosis or worse |
|---|---|---|---|---|---|---|
| What it means | No nuclear abnormalities identified | Insufficient material present or poorly spread/fixed. Vision of cells obscured by debris (9% of all smears) | Nuclear changes that are not normal are present. Unsure whether the changes represent dyskaryosis (5–10% of all smears are borderline or mild) | Nuclear abnormalities that are indicative of low-grade cervical intra-epithelial neoplasia (CIN1)* (5–10% of all smears are borderline or mild) | Nuclear abnormalities reflecting probable CIN2* (~1% of all smears) | Nuclear abnormalities reflecting probable CIN3 (~0.6% of all smears) |
| Action | Place on routine recall | Repeat the smear immediately. Consistently inadequate, refer for colposcopy. | Repeat smear in 6–12 months. Most smears will have reverted to normal. After 3 consecutive normal smears, return to routine recall. If abnormality persists or worsens, refer for colposcopy. Management options not clear (currently being investigated in a randomized controlled trial) | Repeat smear at 6 months. Many will have returned to normal. After 3 consecutive normal results, return to routine recall. Refer for colposcopy if changes persist. Management options not clear (currently being investigated in an RCT) | Refer for colposcopy | Refer for colposcopy or (rarely) make urgent referral to gynaecological oncologist (if invasive carcinoma is suspected) |

**Table 13.3** (continued)

| | Normal | Inadequate | Borderline dyskaryosis | Mild dyskaryosis | Moderate dyskaryosis | Severe dyskaryosis or worse |
|---|---|---|---|---|---|---|
| Colposcopy results | | | | CIN1 confirmed histologically | CIN stage confirmed histologically | CIN3 confirmed histologically |
| Action | | | | Management options not clear (continue to watch and wait, or treat?) | Treat to remove area containing abnormal cells | Treat to remove area containing abnormal cells |

*Mild and moderate dyskaryosis do not always correlate well with the presence of CIN1 and CIN2. The difference is more the quantity of CIN rather than the quality. It is possible to detect CIN3 after a mildly or moderately dyskaryotic smear, but the size of the abnormality is usually smaller. Adapted from Austoker and Davey (1997).

The NHSBSP began in 1988 and full coverage of the population was achieved by 1994. All eligible women registered with GPs (those aged 50–64) are called for screening once every 3 years, mainly on a practice-by-practice basis. Women aged over 64 may request mammography once every 3 years, as they are no longer routinely invited. However, following feasibility studies, routine screening will be offered to women up to the age of 70 by the year 2004.

The screening process is organized by dedicated professionals at special screening sites (either fixed or mobile units). Unlike cervical screening, there is no financial incentive for practices that achieve a high uptake rate.

Currently, women are offered two-view mammography at their prevalent screen (first screen) and a single oblique view mammogram in subsequent screens (incident screens). From 2003, two views will be taken at each screening appointment. All women are sent written results. For some women, the mammography will be inconclusive and they will be invited for further investigations at dedicated assessment centres that are run by multidisciplinary teams. All women undergoing further investigations will have a further mammogram and a clinical breast examination, some may have ultrasound, fine-needle aspiration (cytology), or proceed to surgical biopsy.

The NHS Breast Screening Programme is the first programme in the NHS to be based on rigorous quality standards, both for the programme as a whole plus each specialist group has its own standards (e.g. surgeons and radiologists). An adherence to these standards has led to the high reputation of the breast screening programme.

As with the Cervical Screening Programme, a new patient information leaflet has been designed to facilitate informed choice in the Breast Screening Programme. The leaflet outlines what breast screening can and cannot achieve, including an explanation about false-positive and false-negative results (National Screening Programme 2001a).

### Results of the NHS Breast Screening Programme, 2000–2001 (Government Statistical Service 2002)

Approximately 1.5 million women aged 50–64 were invited for breast screening in the year 2000–2001 and 1 148 811 were screened. This figure includes almost 31 000 women who were screened after GP or self-referral. Therefore the estimated uptake rate in women who were routinely invited as part of the screening programme was 75.3%. This figure ranges between 45.7% and 87.9%, depending on breast screening unit, so in some areas there is the potential to improve screening uptake rates. It has been shown that a cost-effective and effective way of improving uptake of breast screening is to send personalized letters to the women from the GPs (Bankhead *et al.* 2001; Richards *et al.* 2001).

**Table 13.4** Outcome of screening in women aged 50–64, by type of invitation, England 2000–2001

| Type of invitation | Percentage referred for assessment | Numbers of women |
|---|---|---|
| First invitation for routine screening | 8.3% | 19 233/230 418 |
| Routine invitation to previous non-attenders | 8.2% | 3026/36 861 |
| Routine invitation to previous attenders, but last screen more than 5 years ago | 5.3% | 2256/42 554 |
| Routine invitation to previous attenders, with last screen within 5 years (regularly screened women) | 3.9% | 31 061/804 788 |
| Early recalls | 85.9% | 2780/3235 |
| Self/GP referral (with no previous screen) | 7.4% | 970/13 023 |
| Self/GP referral (screened at least 5 years ago) | 5.7% | 90/1570 |
| Self/GP referral (screened within 5 years) | 4.9% | 797/16 372 |
| **Total** | 5.2% | 60 213/1 148 811 |

## Outcome of screening (women aged 50–64)

Of the 1.2 million women screened in England in 2000–2001, 5.2% were referred for further investigations (approximately 60 000 women). After further investigation, a woman may be diagnosed with cancer or a precancerous lesion (ductal carcinoma *in situ*, DCIS), be given the all clear, or be placed on 'early recall'. 'Early recall' occurs when a woman is not given a result but asked to reattend for further tests before the 3-yearly examination is due, most frequently after 6 or 12 months. The rates of referral for further tests varies dramatically according to the type of invitation that women receive. The rate is much higher in women who have never been invited before or have never attended for screening (8.3%) compared with 3.9% in women who have undergone routine screening (Table 13.4).

## Outcome after referral for further investigation (women aged 50–64)

Of the women aged 50–64 who were referred for further tests, 7009 were found to have cancer (cancer detection rate of 6.1/1000 women screened). This equates to 11.6% of those women who went on for further tests. In other words, women have approximately 5% chance of being recalled and of those, just over 1 in 10 have cancer and the remaining 9 out of 10 women are given an 'all clear' result.

The majority of cancers detected by screening are non-invasive or microinvasive (1514/7009 = 22%) or small (<15 mm) in size (2911/7009 = 42%). When cancers are small enough, they can most often be removed without removing the whole breast (a lumpectomy), but this depends on the position of the cancer.

## Potential effect of screening on mortality from breast cancer

A meta-analysis of nine randomized, controlled trials and four observational studies showed that mortality from breast cancer is reduced by 26% in women aged 50–74 who are offered screening mammography [relative risk (RR) 0.74, 95% confidence interval (CI) 0.66–0.83] (Kerlikowske *et al.* 1995). The same meta-analysis did not show a mortality reduction for women aged under 50 (RR 0.93, 95% CI 0.76–1.13).

Another systematic review, which was published in 2000, concluded that screening for breast cancer with mammography is unjustified (Gotzsche and Olsen 2000). However, this review has been widely criticized (de Koning, 2000; Woolf, 2000; Duffy, 2001) because it has been accused of taking critical appraisal techniques to far too stringent lengths. The reviewers excluded six out of the eight randomized controlled trials that were found by the search strategy on the basis of potential age imbalances between intervention and control groups. However, on inspection, the age differences are very small (the largest difference observed was 5 months), and this greatest difference was likely to be due to the cluster design of the trial (Swedish Two County). The authors of the original trial adjusted for the differences in age and observed a significant reduction in breast cancer mortality associated with breast screening of 30%.

Further support for a beneficial effect of breast screening are outlined below: a recent analysis of mortality from breast cancer showed a 21.3% absolute reduction in death rates from breast cancer by 1998, although it was estimated that breast screening resulted in a 6.4% reduction, the rest being due to improved treatment and earlier diagnosis independent of screening (Blanks *et al.* 2000).

The controversy surrounding the effectiveness of breast screening has continued with the publication of an adapted version of the 2000 review (Olsen and Gotzsche 2001), which reported that they have strengthened and confirmed the findings of the previous review (Gotzsche and Olsen, 2000), questioning the impact of breast screening on all-cause mortality. However, the International

Agency for Research on Cancer (IARC) have more recently evaluated the available evidence regarding breast screening, including the quality of the previous trials. The working group found that many of the earlier criticisms were unsubstantiated, and the remaining deficiencies were judged not to invalidate the findings from the trial. They concluded that organized breast screening of women aged 50–69 results in a 35% reduction in breast cancer mortality (IARC Working Group 2002).

## Recent news and potential changes

### Frequency of screening

As stated earlier, mammography is routinely offered to eligible women every 3 years. A recent randomized controlled trial to evaluate the optimum screening interval compared annual mammography with 3-yearly mammography for a period of 7 years. More than 76 000 women were involved and the mortality rates in the two groups have now been compared. The results of the trial showed that shortening the screening interval from the current 3 years did not produce a statistically significant decrease in the predicted mortality from breast cancer (Breast Screening Frequency Trial Group 2002).

### Age of women screened

Recent research has examined the effectiveness and cost-effectiveness of providing screening routinely to both younger (40–49 years) (Moss, for the Trial Steering Group 1999) and older women (>64 years). The results of screening women aged under 50 are not yet available, but pilot studies of screening in older women have indicated that it is feasible to increase the upper age limit and has led to the screening programme being extended so that routine invitations are also sent to women aged 65–70. This is gradually being phased in and will be fully operational by 2004.

### Numbers of views taken at prevalent (repeat) screens

Originally the breast screening programme took one view of each breast at every appointment but two-view mammography was introduced for incident (first) screens following a randomized controlled trial that resulted in a 24% increase in cancer detection rates as a result of two-view mammography at the first appointment (Wald *et al.* 1995). Recent epidemiological evidence has confirmed this result and has shown that there has been an increase of 45% of small invasive cancers being detected when double-view mammography is used at prevalent screens and about 42% increase at incident (subsequent) screens (Blanks *et al.* 1997). The programme will be extended in 2003 to include two-view mammography at every screen.

# Frequently asked questions about breast screening

## How likely am I to be recalled for further/repeat tests?

About 1 in 20 women who undergo breast screening are asked to go back for further investigations.

## If I'm recalled, what are my chances of having cancer?

Even if you are recalled, you are quite likely not to have cancer. About 1 in 10 women who are recalled are found to have cancer.

## Could a cancer be missed by screening?

Mammography, like other screening tests, is not 100% accurate and a cancer could be missed. If you have any symptoms, such as a breast lump, after you have been screened, it is important that you visit your doctor.

## What is DCIS?

DCIS (ductal carcinoma *in situ*) is an area of cancer cells that are located within the milk ducts and have not spread into the surrounding tissue. This type of cancer is called non-invasive. However, without treatment, some of these cancers will become invasive, although it is not clear which ones, and therefore treatment is always offered. Treatment may be a wide area excision (lumpectomy) with or without radiotherapy, or a mastectomy may be more appropriate, depending on the size and stage of DCIS.

## Does HRT affect breast screening?

A systematic review of the relationship between use of HRT and the effectiveness of mammography has recently been published (Banks 2001) and concluded that women using HRT are more likely to experience reduced sensitivity (more likely to get false-negative screening results) and reduced specificity (more likely to be recalled for further investigations that results in no cancer being diagnosed, a false-positive recall) than women who do not take HRT. However, the results of the studies had not been adjusted for crucial confounding factors such as age of the woman and menopausal status and therefore the author concluded that the size of the effect could not be estimated with confidence.

# Ovarian cancer screening

Ovarian cancer is the fourth commonest female cancer, accounting for more than 5000 new cases per year with an annual incidence rate of 20.3/100 000 women (Office of National Statistics 1999a) and is responsible for just over 4000 deaths a year. It is therefore the fourth commonest cause of cancer mortality in women (CRC 2000). Diagnosis at an early stage of disease is associated with a 5-year survival rate of about 75–80%. This decreases dramatically with increasing disease stage with 5-year survival rates of 59% for stage II disease, 23% for stage III disease and only 14% for stage IV diseases (metastatic disease) (CRC 1997). Most ovarian carcinomas (65–75%) are discovered at a late stage when there is widespread disease. Correspondingly, there is a poor overall survival rate, with only 28% surviving for 5 years. Only stomach, lung, and pancreas cancers have worse 5-year survival rates (CRC 1999).

Currently, there is no national screening programme for ovarian cancer, although a very large, randomized, controlled trial has recently started in the UK, which aims to recruit 200 000 women. The screening modalities being tested are annual CA125 testing and transvaginal ultrasound as the primary tests (UKCTOCS 2001). The key issues with this trial is that transvaginal ultrasound is a costly process as it required expertise to interpret the image at the time of screening and whether this method as a primary screening tool is acceptable to women is not yet known. In addition, this trial is not due to be completed until 2010, by which time a better screening test may have been developed. In the meantime, it is important that potential symptoms are better recognized by both women and health professionals. In order to facilitate this process, a study is commencing. This study will attempt to understand the way in which symptoms suggestive of ovarian cancer are expressed, interpreted, and acted upon by patients and general practitioners and identify potentially significant modifiable diagnostic factors in order to improve the referral and diagnostic pathways.

## Frequently asked questions about ovarian screening

### I've heard there is a screening trial – can I be included?

Only women who are invited to participate in the trial can take part. This is to eliminate all bias so that at the end of the study it is not claimed that screening saved more lives in the trial than it would in reality because the women who volunteered were more informed, had a healthier lifestyle, etc.

### I've had IVF three times and I understand it might increase the risk of ovarian cancer. Should I be screened?

A recent pooled analysis of studies that have investigated the relationship between ovarian cancer and fertility treatment concluded that fertility drug use was not associated with ovarian cancer. The same review showed an increased risk among women who had attempted to get pregnant for more than 5 years (Ness *et al.* 2002).

---

## Box 13.1 **Summary**

The ultimate aim of screening for cancer is to reduce cancer-specific mortality

### Cervical screening

- Cervical screening is coordinated by primary care trusts.
- Most of cervical screening is conducted in primary care.
- Women aged 20–64 are invited for cervical screening every 3–5 years.
- Screening is currently undertaken using Pap smears.
- New technologies are being tested which may improve cervical cytology.
- Approximately 10% of women are recalled for further investigation after screening (and another 10% have to have repeated smears due to poor quality).

### Breast screening

- Breast screening is organized and conducted by dedicated breast screening units.
- Women aged 50–64 are eligible for breast screening every 3 years.
- Women aged over 64 may request breast screening at 3-yearly intervals.
- The upper age limit will be extended to 70 in the next few years.
- At the first mammography, two images are taken. At subsequent mammography, only one view is taken.
- From 2003, two views will be taken at each screening appointment.
- Approximately 5% of women are recalled for further investigation after screening. Of these, around 90% do not have cancer.

### Ovarian screening

- There is no national organized screening programme.
- A randomized controlled trial to evaluate ovarian screening started in 2001. It aims to recruit 200 000 postmenopausal women.
- Screening is by transvaginal ultrasound or by CA125 testing.
- Results of the trial will be available sometime after 2010.

# References

Anderson, C.M. and Nottingham, J. (1999). Bridging the knowledge gap and communicating uncertainties for informed consent in cervical cytology screening; we need unbiased information and a culture change. *Cytopathology*, **10**, 221–8.

Austoker, J. and Davey, C. (1997). *Cervical smear results explained: a guide for primary care*. NHSCSP, Sheffield.

Austoker, J., Davey, C. and Jansen, C. (1997). *Improving the quality of the written information sent to women about cervical screening. Part 1: Evidence-based criteria for the content of letters and leaflets. Part 2: Evaluation of the content of current letters and leaflets*. No. 6. NHSCSP, Sheffield.

Austoker, J., Bankhead, C. and Webster, P. (2001). Enabling informed choice in cancer screening: the development and evaluation of statements giving information on the advantages and disadvantages of breast and cervical screening. A report prepared for the Department of Health at the request of the Advisory Committees on Breast and Cervical Screening. Oxford, CRC Primary Care Education Research Group.

Bankhead, C., Richards, S.H., Peters, T.J., *et al.* (2001). Improving attendance for breast screening among recent non-attenders: a randomized controlled trial of two interventions in primary care. *Journal of Medical Screening*, **8**, 99–105.

Banks, E. (2001). Hormone replacement therapy and the sensitivity and specificity of breast cancer screening: a review. *Journal of Medical Screening*, **8**, 29–35.

Blanks, R.G., Moss, S.M. and Wallis, M.G. (1997). Use of two view mammography compared with one view in the detection of small invasive cancers: further results from the National Health Service breast screening programme. *Journal of Medical Screening*, **4**, 98–101.

Blanks, R.G., Moss, S.M., McGahan, C., Quinn, M. and Babb, P. (2000). Effect of NHS breast screening programme on mortality from breast cancer in England and Wales, 1990–8: comparison of observed with predicted mortality. *British Medical Journal*, **321**, 665–9.

Breast Screening Frequency Trial Group (2002). The frequency of breast cancer screening: results from the UKCCCR Randomised Trial. *European Journal of Cancer*, **38**, 1458–64.

Coste, J., Cochand-Priollet, B., de Cremoux, P., *et al.* for the French Society of Clinical Cytology Study Group (2003). Cross sectional study of conventional cervical smear, monolayer cytology, and human papillomavirus DNA testing for cervical cancer screening. *British Medical Journal*, **326**, 733–6.

Coulter, A. (1998). Evidence based patient information. is important, so there needs to be a national strategy to ensure it [editorial; comment] [see comments]. *British Medical Journal*, **317**, 225–6.

Cox, J., Lorincz, A.T., Schiffman, M., Sherman, M.E., Cullen, A. and Kurman, R.J. (1995). Human papillomavirus testing by hybrid capture appears to be useful in triaging women with a cytologic diagnosis of atypical squamous cells of undetermined significance. *American Journal of Obstetrics and Gynecology*, **172**, 946–54.

CRC (1997). *Factsheet 17: Ovarian cancer – UK*. CRC, London.

CRC (1999). *CancerStats: Survival – England and Wales 1971–1995*. CRC, London.

CRC (2000). *CancerStats: Mortality – UK*. CRC, London.

Cuzick, J., Sasieni, P., Davies, P., *et al* (1999). A systematic review of the role of human papillomavirus testing within a cervical screening programme. *Health Technology Assessment*, **3**.

de Koning, H.J. (2000). Assessment of nationwide cancer-screening programmes. *Lancet*, **355**, 80–1.

Duffy, S.W. (2001). Interpretation of the breast screening trials: a commentary on the recent paper by Gotzsche and Olsen. *Breast*, **10**, 209–12.

Forrest, A.P.M. (1986). *Breast cancer screening: report to the Health Minister of England, Wales, Scotland and Northern Ireland.* HMSO, London.

General Medical Council (1999). *Seeking patients' consent: the ethical considerations.* General Medical Council, London.

Gotzsche, P.C. and Olsen, O. (2000). Is screening for breast cancer with mammography justifiable? *Lancet*, **355**, 129–34.

Government Statistical Service (2000). *Cervical screening programme, England: 1999–2000.* HMSO, London.

Government Statistical Service (2001). *Cervical screening programme, England: 2000–2001.* HMSO, London.

Government Statistical Service (2002). *Breast screening programme, England: 2000–2001.* HMSO, London.

Herrington, C. (1999). Do HPV-negative cervical carcinomas exist? – revisited. *Journal of Pathology*, **189**, 1–3.

IARC Working Group (2002). Mammography screening can reduce deaths from breast cancer. http://www.iarc.fr/pageroot/PRELEASE/pr139a.html, accessed 5–7/2002.

Kerlikowske, K., Grady, D., Rubin, S. M., Sandrock, C. and Ernster, V.L. (1995). Efficacy of screening mammography. A meta-analysis. *Journal of the American Medical Association*, **273**, 149–54.

Moss, S., for the Trial Steering Group (1999). A trial to study the effect on breast cancer mortality of annual mammographic screening in women starting at age 40. *Journal of Medical Screening*, **6**, 144–8.

Moss, S.M., Gray, A., Legood, R. and Henstock, E. (2003). *Evaluation of HPV/LBC cervival screening pilot studies. First report to the Department of Health on evaluation of LBC (December 2002, revised January 2003).* Cancer Screening Evaluation Unit, Sutton.

National Audit Office (1992). *Cervical and breast screening in England: a report by the Comptroller and Auditor General.* HMSO, London.

National Audit Office (1998). *The performance of the NHS cervical screening programme in England: a report by the Comptroller and Auditor General.* The Stationary Office, London.

National Screening Programme (2001a). *Breast screening: the facts.* http://www.cancer-screening.nhs.uk/breastscreen/publications/ia-02.html.

National Screening Programme (2001b). *Cervical screening: the facts.* http://www.cancerscreening.nhs.uk/cervical/publications/in-04.html.

Ness, R., Cramer, D., Goodman, M., *et al.* (2002). Infertility, fertility drugs and ovarian cancer: a pooled analysis of case-control studies. *American Journal of Epidemiology*, **155**, 217–24.

NICE (2000). Guidance on the use of liquid-based cytology for cervical screening.[www available from: http:/ /server1.nice.org.uk/article.asp?a = 1864].

Office of National Statistics. (1999). *Cancer statistics: registrations. England and Wales 1993.* MB1 no. 26. The Stationery Office, London.

Office of National Statistics. (2001). *Mortality statistics: cause. England and Wales 1999.* DH2 No. 26. The Stationery Office, London.

Office of Population, CAS. (1989). *Mortality statistics: cause. England and Wales 1988.* DH2 no. 15. HMSO, London.

Olsen, O. and Gotzsche, P. C. (2001). Cochrane review on screening for breast cancer with mammography. *Lancet,* **358,** 1340–2.

Olson, A., Gjoen, K., Sauer, T., *et al.* (1995). Human papillomavirus and cervical intraepithelial neoplasia grade II-III: a population-based case control study. *International Journal of Cancer,* **61,** 312–15.

Quinn, M., Babb, P., Jones, J. and Allen, E. on behalf of the United Kingdom Association of Cancer Registries (1999a). Effect of screening on incidence of a mortality from cancer of cervix in England: evaluation based on routinely collected statistics. *British Medical Journal,* **318,** 904–908 (full version: www.bmj.com/cgi/content/full/318/188/904).

Quinn, M., Babb, P., Jones, J. and Brock, A. (1999b). Report: registrations of cancer diagnosed in 1993–1996, England and Wales. *Health Statistics Quarterly,* **4,** 59–70.

Raffle, A.E., Alden, B. and Mackenzie, E.F. (1995). Detection rates for abnormal cervical smears: what are we screening for? *Lancet,* **345,** 1469–73.

Richards, S.H., Bankhead, C., Peters, T.J., *et al.* (2001). Cluster randomised controlled trial comparing the effectiveness and cost-effectiveness of two primary care interventions aimed at improving attendance for breast screening. *Journal of Medical Screening,* **8,** 91–8.

Sasieni, P. and Adams, J. (1999). Effect of screening on cervical cancer mortality in England and Wales: analysis of trends with an age period cohort model. *British Medical Journal,* **318,** 1244–5.

Sasieni, P., Cuzick, J. and Farmery, E. (1995). Accelerated decline in cervical cancer mortality in England and Wales. *Lancet,* **346,** 1566–7.

Schiffman, M., Bauer, H., Hoover, R., *et al.* (1993). Epidemiological evidence showing that human papillomavirus infection causes most cervical intrapithelial neoplasia. *Journal of the National Cancer Institute,* **85,** 958–64.

Sigurdsson, K. (1999). The Icelandic and Nordic cervical screening programs: trends in incidence and mortality rates through 1995. *Acta Obstetrica et Gynaecologica Scandinavica* **78,** 478–85.

UKCTOCS (2001). *UK Collaborative Trial of Ovarian Cancer Screening.* http://www.mds.qmw.ac.uk/gynaeonc/UKCTOCS/welcome.htm.

Walboomers, J.M., Jacobs, M., Manos, M., *et al.* (1999). Human papillomavirus is a necessary cause of invasive cervical cancer worldwide. *Journal of Pathology,* **189,** 12–19.

Wald, N.J., Murphy, P., Major, P., Parkes, C., Townsend, J. and Frost, C. (1995). UKCCCR multicentre randomised controlled trial of one and two view mammography in breast cancer screening. *British Medical Journal,* **311,** 1189–93.

Woolf, S. (2000). Taking critical appraisals to extremes: the need for balance in the evaluation of evidence (editorial). *Journal of Family Practice,* **49,** 1081–5.

Chapter 14

# Familial cancers and women's health

Anneke Lucassen and Eila Watson

## Introduction

There have been many recent advances in research into genetic diseases and conditions. More and more genetic tests are becoming available which can provide information about a woman's health. Although individually many genetic conditions are rare, collectively they account for a significant proportion of the general practitioner's (GP) workload. This chapter focuses on the genetic aspects of a family history of cancer, as this is the area of genetics influencing women's health that the GP is most likely to face today (2002). In particular breast, ovarian, endometrial, and colorectal cancers are discussed, each of which can occur in the context of a strong inherited predisposition.

If GPs can acquire the basic skills in determining which cancers are likely to have an hereditary component, they will be able to reassure the many patients who are at no or low additional risk. Because perceived risks of cancer often far outweigh the actual risks of cancer, there is much scope for reassurance in this area.

## Susceptibility to cancer

Research developments in genetics have received increasing public and media attention over the last decade and, partly as a result of this, more and more people are worried that their family history of cancer may imply they have themselves inherited a factor that increases their risk of cancer. However, it is important to remember that faulty (or mutant) genes are not the only explanation for a family history of cancer. Shared lifestyles within a family; for example, smoking habits or diet can also contribute to a family history. In fact, susceptibility to cancer is usually multifactorial, that is to say, it involves the interaction of environmental predisposing factors (e.g. smoking, radiation, hormones) with genetic predisposing factors (Fig 14.1). Genetic factors can be alterations in either 'high-risk' or 'low-risk' genes. The majority of genetic

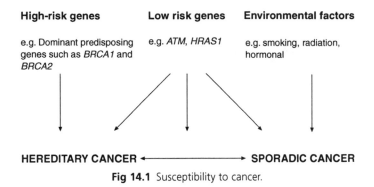

**Fig 14.1** Susceptibility to cancer.

predisposing factors to cancer come in the form of 'low-risk' genes, that is, the presence of a particular genetic variant may increase the chance of cancer in a lifetime by, say, 1 or 2%. Whilst the total public health burden of such genes may be large, for each individual woman the increase in risk is small. Predictive genetic testing that could tell a woman that her lifetime risk of breast cancer is increased by 1 or 2% is at present deemed to be of little practical benefit, especially when it is not clear how this risk factor interacts with other risk factors. In any case, insufficient details are currently known about the nature of such low-risk genes to undertake prognostic genetic testing. Only a small proportion of cancers (approximately 5%) can be attributed to a clear hereditary component.

## Dominant 'high-risk' genes

Much attention has focused on the discovery of high-risk genes, which when altered or mutated result in a high lifetime risk of cancer. For example, two genes, *BRCA1* and *BRCA2*, are known to confer a lifetime risk of breast cancer of up to 80% and of ovarian cancer of up to 60%. Mutations in several different so-called 'mismatch repair' genes can result in a high lifetime risk of colorectal cancer and/or endometrial cancer. These genes are inherited in a dominant fashion. All genes come in pairs with children inheriting one gene in each pair from each parent. For a dominantly inherited gene such as *BRCA1* or *BRCA2*, an affected person will have one normal copy of the gene and one mutated copy of the gene. Each child of an affected person will have a 50% (1 in 2) chance of inheriting the mutated copy of the gene from their parent (Fig 14.2).

Many women are surprised to hear that even if they have an extremely strong family history, they still have a 50% chance that they have *not* inherited the causative factor; they feel that if they have such a strong family history, they too must have inevitably inherited this tendency. Even if such a 'high-risk' gene

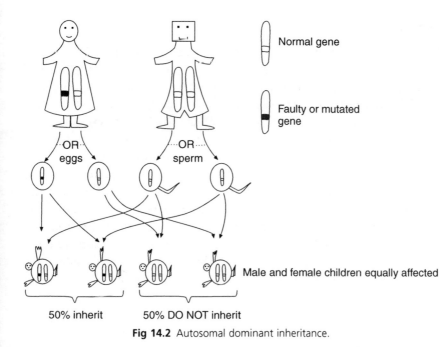

**Fig 14.2** Autosomal dominant inheritance.

has been inherited, this does not inevitably lead to cancer and the interaction of other genes and/or environmental factors is probably required before a cancer develops. The percentage of women who have such a faulty gene and develop cancer in their lifetime reflects the *penetrance* of the gene. Thus if the faulty gene is 80% penetrant in women, then 20% of women who have inherited it will not develop cancer in their lifetime.

This is best understood in terms of the development of cancer being a multi-stage process; several steps are required before a cancer arises and in most cases these steps take many years to accumulate. In women who have inherited a dominant cancer-predisposing gene mutation, they have inherited one of these steps and started off life at a disadvantage. In effect, they need to acquire fewer steps for a cancer to develop, which explains why often these cancers arise at a younger age on average than sporadic cancers, but it is not inevitable that they will acquire these steps in a lifetime.

It is important to put these high-risk genes in perspective. For example, out of every 100 women with breast cancer, only approximately 5 are caused by high-risk genes. Similarly, out of every 100 colorectal cancer cases, only about 5 can be attributed to a high-risk gene. However, it is these genes that many people seek advice about or request testing for. This chapter outlines which features of a family history suggest the presence of such a high-risk gene and conversely, which features of a family history are likely to exclude the presence of such a gene.

## Taking a family history (FH)

This is the most important tool in assessing the chance that there is a particular cancer-predisposing genetic factor segregating through a family. The age of onset of the cancer, the number of relatives, the types of cancer, and the degree of relatedness to the concerned patient should all be noted. Start with the patient in front of you and mark her with an arrow to indicate she is the *consultand.* Note ages and sexes of children and siblings (circle for females and squares for males) and note the age at diagnosis of any cancers. Colour in an affected individual and make a key for colours or patterns to denote different types of cancer. Next note the age or age and cause of death of both parents. Work out from there; ask how many siblings each parent has/had – note ages, ages of death, or ages of diagnoses of cancer, whether they themselves had children, what sex, age, and whether or not have had cancer. If the exact age is not known, indicate an approximate age. Three generations (including the proband) will usually suffice to be able to make basic assessment of risk, but if more is known make a record of this also.

Age at diagnosis of any cancer is much more important than age of death, but note the age of death of any unaffected female relatives (this is because many female relatives who lived into their latter life – seventies or eighties – without being affected by cancer, is more exclusive of an inherited cancer risk than few female relatives who died of other causes at a young age). Ask especially if there are other cancers in the family. Certain cancers such as lung cancers – especially in smokers – and cervical cancer are much more likely to be sporadic cancers than due to an inherited faulty gene. However, the presence of other cancers may be suggestive of such an inherited factor. For example, a FH of both breast and ovarian cancer or of both colon cancer and endometrial cancer may be suggestive (see below). Remember that even though a family history may be of female cancers, predisposing genes are transmitted through the paternal and maternal lines equally.

If details of FH are unclear, ask the patient to find out more from relatives or death certificates and come back with gathered information. Often 'family stories' of cancer turn out to be a different type of cancer on closer investigation (e.g. reported ovarian cancer may turn out to be cervical cancer or even stomach cancer).

Fig 14.3 shows how this information can be recorded in pedigree form

## Making a referral decision

Consensus referral guidelines for breast and ovarian cancer have recently been published to indicate which family histories warrant referral and those

NAME & ADDRESS          REF DR.          GP
Mrs.Breast              SPEC.            ADDRESS


POST CODE               DATE REF.        PHONE NO.
PHONE NO.                                HV


DIAGNOSIS: FH breast cancer    DATED      SIGNED        G NO.

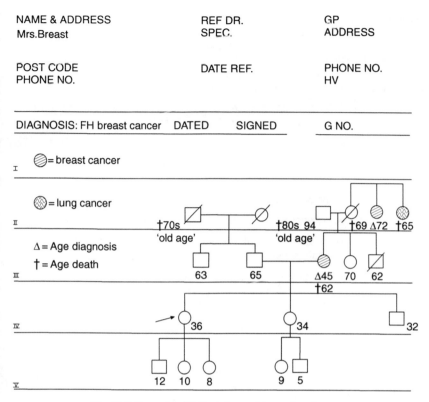

**Fig 14.3** Example of Patient form picture of pedigree.

where reassurance in primary care is appropriate. These guidelines are given in Table 14.1. There are no consensus guidelines as yet for colorectal cancer FH, but an example of a local guideline is also given in Table 14.1. Different regional genetics centres do operate slightly different referral guidelines and in some areas funding levels may determine which patients can be seen in clinic. In general, the greater the number of relatives with cancer, the younger their age of onset, the closer they are related to the woman concerned, then the higher the risk that she has inherited a strong genetic factor predisposing her to cancer. A head count of affected relatives is not enough for risk assessment.

The majority of women presenting to their GP with a worry about their family history are likely to fall into the lower-risk group. This group can then be reassured whilst the higher-risk group can be referred on to secondary care. The guidelines in Table 14.1 were designed to be sensitive rather than specific so that high-risk patients would not be missed. However, on more detailed analysis of the family history in secondary care, some women who fulfilled the referral criteria may be assessed as low additional risk.

**Table 14.1** Family history of cancer – referral guidelines

If a patient's family history fits within any of those listed below, then this may indicate a higher risk of developing an inherited form of cancer and the patient may benefit from referral for more detailed assessment. If you are unsure about whether or not to refer an individual, please contact your local genetics service for advice.

It is important to remember that these are simply guidelines and that some of the patients who fit the referral criteria will be considered low additional risk following assessment.

| | |
|---|---|
| *Breast cancer* | ◆ 3 close relatives from the same side of the family diagnosed at any age |
| | ◆ 2 close relatives from the same side of the family with an average age of diagnosis under 60 years |
| | ◆ mother or sister diagnosed under 40 years |
| | ◆ father or brother with breast cancer diagnosed under 60 years |
| | ◆ 1 close relative with bilateral breast cancer, with the first cancer diagnosed under 50 years |
| *Breast and ovarian cancer* | ◆ 1 close relative diagnosed with ovarian cancer at any age *and* at least 2 close relatives with breast cancer with an average age of diagnosis under 60 years, from the same side of the family |
| | ◆ 1 close relative diagnosed with ovarian cancer at any age *and* at least one close relative diagnosed with breast cancer under 50 years from the same side of the family |
| | ◆ 1 close relative diagnosed with breast cancer under 50 years *and* ovarian cancer at any age |
| *Ovarian cancer* | ◆ 2 close relatives from the same side of the family, at least one of whom is either a mother or sister, diagnosed at any age with ovarian cancer |
| *Colorectal cancer* | ◆ Parent or sibling diagnosed with colorectal cancer below the age of 45 |
| | ◆ 2 close relatives from the same side of the family with an average age of diagnosis under 60 years |
| *Colorectal and endometrial cancer* | ◆ Family history of both endometrial and colorectal cancer (+/− ovarian cancer) with an average age of diagnosis under 60 years |

A close relative means a parent, brother, sister, child, grandparent, aunt, uncle, nephew, or niece. Individuals of Ashkenazi Jewish origin are at higher risk and family histories which do not meet the guidelines may still warrant referral – please contact your local genetics service for further advice. Inherited forms of breast, ovarian, and endometrial cancer can also be passed down through the father's side of the family.

# Family history of breast (±ovarian) cancer

To many women, having one or possibly more relatives with breast cancer implies an hereditary tendency. Remember that only a small proportion of cancers (approximately 5%) can be attributed to a clear hereditary component.

Since breast cancer is a common cancer (one in nine women in the UK are diagnosed with breast cancer at some point in their lives), it is quite possible to have a family history of the condition just through chance alone. Taking a careful FH is an important first step in the management of a woman concerned about her risk of developing breast cancer. Using the referral guidelines (Table 14.1) or local guidelines, a decision whether referral to secondary care is indicated can be made.

## Lower- (average) risk women

For women whose family history does not meet the referral guideline criteria, the GP has an important role to play in providing reassurance and advice. These women need to understand that their risk of developing breast/ovarian cancer is similar to, or only slightly higher than, a woman of a similar age in the general population who has no affected relatives. There are no available clinical interventions thought likely to be of benefit and hence further hospital follow-up is not needed. It is important these women understand the importance of breast awareness (leaflet available from the NHS Breast Screening Programme and Cancer Research Campaign 1999) and that they need to report any suspicious signs or symptoms immediately. It is also important that they tell the GP if there are any further changes to their family history as this could change their level of risk. Women should also be encouraged to participate in the National Breast Screening Programme (NHSBSP) from the age of 50.

## Higher-risk women

For women whose family history falls within the referral guidelines, referral to secondary care is usually recommended. This may be either a regional genetics centre or a breast unit, or both, depending on local circumstances. Management would usually include discussion of the topics outlined below. Fig 14.4 illustrates a FH of breast cancer, that seemed strong to the patient, but since the affected relatives were not all closely related to the woman concerned and the ages of onset were relatively late, the chance that this FH is due to a breast cancer-predisposing gene is very small indeed. Conversely, Fig 14.5 shows a pedigree where there is a strong FH of both breast and ovarian cancer, of young onset in close relatives, so that there is a high chance the cancers in this family can be attributed to a high-risk faulty gene.

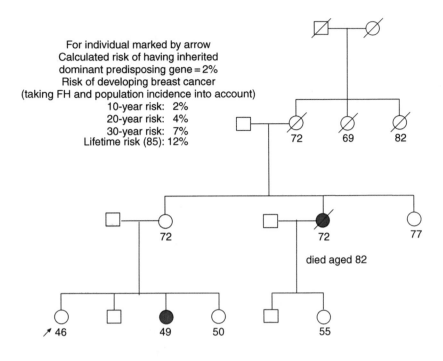

For individual marked by arrow
Calculated risk of having inherited
dominant predisposing gene = 2%
Risk of developing breast cancer
(taking FH and population incidence into account)
10-year risk: 2%
20-year risk: 4%
30-year risk: 7%
Lifetime risk (85): 12%

● Breast cancer

**Fig 14.4** Family history of breast cancer – low risk of dominant predisposing gene.

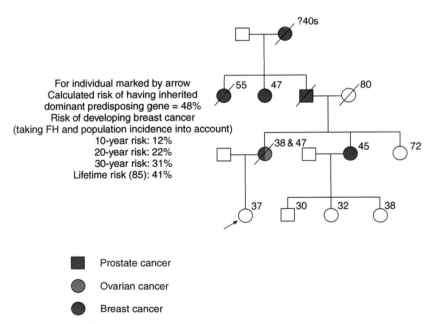

For individual marked by arrow
Calculated risk of having inherited
dominant predisposing gene = 48%
Risk of developing breast cancer
(taking FH and population incidence into account)
10-year risk: 12%
20-year risk: 22%
30-year risk: 31%
Lifetime risk (85): 41%

■ Prostate cancer

● Ovarian cancer

● Breast cancer

**Fig 14.5** Family history of breast cancer – high risk of dominant predisposing gene.

# Management of the higher-risk woman

## Detailed risk assessment

There is a considerable degree of variation in secondary care in exactly how this is done, but computerized risk programs are increasingly popular. Such programs enable the pedigree to be drawn by computer and then tend to use an algorithm derived from a large epidemiological dataset to calculate the probability that the consultand has inherited a high-risk predisposing gene. This calculation takes into account the numbers of affected relatives, their age at diagnosis, their relationship to the consultand, and the number and ages of unaffected female relatives. The presence of ovarian cancer family history or of bilateral breast cancer is also taken into account. The program can then calculate for any marked person in the pedigree the chance that they carry a high-risk predisposing gene, and using the penetrance (see above) of the gene and the background population risk, a probability of developing cancer over the next few decades (see text in Figs 14.4 and 14.5).

### Mammographic screening

For women with a significant family history (higher risk) and who are under 50 and therefore not eligible for the national breast screening programme (NHSBSP), some form of screening is usually recommended. Whilst it is widely accepted that breast screening reduces mortality in women aged 50–64, screening women below the age of 50 is much more controversial. Although the consensus view is that the benefits of screening are likely to outweigh the harm in younger women with a family history (and therefore higher risk), there is as yet no firm evidence that screening will reduce deaths from breast cancer in this group. Several observational studies have been conducted, although most have only small sample sizes (Lucassen *et al.* 2001). One large recent American study compared cancer detection rates in screened women with and without a family history. The study found that the cancer detection rate for women under 50 with a family history is comparable to that seen in women over 50 in a screening programme (Kerlikowske *et al.* 2000). A different, smaller study reported more cancers detected in higher-risk groups than lower-risk groups (Chart and Franssen 1997). It is noteworthy that most of these studies combined mammographic screening with clinical breast examination and in one case with self-breast examination. Furthermore, details of the type of mammography (e.g. one or two views) used varied.

Of the studies that investigated the pathological features of the detected tumours, it appeared that screening the young family history group will detect cancers at an earlier stage than if they presented symptomatically, suggesting that a survival benefit may be expected.

### Limitations of mammography

The potential limitations of mammography need to be considered as well as the potential benefits. The younger breast is more dense and hence more radio-opaque and studies have shown that the sensitivity and specificity of mammography is lower for women below the age of 50 and also for women with a family history of breast cancer. This results in a greater number of false negatives and false positives, which in turn may lead to false reassurance or unnecessary further tests with associated anxiety/adverse psychological consequences (Christiansen *et al.* 2000).

Furthermore, regular mammography carries a cumulative radiation risk. Dose and age of exposure are the two most important determinants of radiation risk and hence the risk is theoretically greater for younger women. In addition, those who have an inherited cancer predisposition may be more susceptible to environmental carcinogens such as radiation.

Several studies have attempted to estimate the number of breast cancer deaths induced by breast screening for women under 50 compared with the number of deaths prevented. Bearing in mind the uncertainties inherent in modelling studies of this nature, these studies all show that the benefit-to-risk ratio is considerably less favourable for women under 50 compared with older women. Some authors conclude that the benefits of mammography still clearly outweigh the theoretical risks of radiation in younger women, whilst others appear to support this conclusion but more cautiously (Mettler *et al.* 1996; Beemsterboer *et al.* 1998). Some of these concerns may be resolved if the trials of MRI breast screening for high-risk women prove successful (see below).

In summary, there does appear to be growing, albeit indirect, evidence to support the widespread pragmatic approach of mammographic screening below the age of 50 if there is a significant family history. However, it is important the younger woman understands no mortality benefit has yet been proven and that there are also potential downsides to consider. This is of course especially true for the woman whose family history falls into the lower-risk category, but who may request mammography.

### Breast examination

This is a useful adjunct to mammography in diagnosing breast cancer, especially in the young breast where mammography is less sensitive: more than 90% of breast cancers are found by women themselves (Austoker 1994). However, the effectiveness of breast self-examination in reducing mortality from breast cancer has never been consistently demonstrated. Although teaching women to be 'breast aware' is widely accepted, self-examination or examination by practice nurses in well-women clinics should not be recommended (Department of Health, February 1998). Where there is a strong family history, many authorities recommend some form of regular examination in a breast clinic.

## MRI screening

This technique does not involve ionizing radiation. Sensitivity for detecting *invasive* cancer is reported to be >90% and it is suggested that MRI has additional value for patients with dense breast tissue and in detecting lesions that are clinically and mammographically occult. Sensitivity of detection of *pre-invasive* lesions requires further evaluation. Encouraging early results show higher sensitivity and specificity than mammography (Kuhl *et al.* 2000), but larger trials are awaited. A national trial of MRI as a screening measure for women with a strong family history is in progress.

## Chemoprevention

Tamoxifen has been shown to reduce the occurrence of contralateral tumours by 40–50%, when taken for more than 2 years by women with breast cancer.The use of this drug as *primary* breast cancer prevention is still experimental and several large, randomized, controlled trials are investigating prophylactic tamoxifen for women at increased risk of breast cancer. In 1998, the large US Breast Cancer Prevention Trial (BCPT) was stopped early after finding a 49% reduction in the incidence of breast cancer among those on tamoxifen (Fisher *et al.* 1998). However, this decision was criticized by the UK study leaders as premature and interim findings from the Royal Marsden tamoxifen trial found no effect of tamoxifen on the incidence of breast cancer (Powles *et al.* 1998) – final data are awaited. Furthermore, the Italian tamoxifen trial has recently reported that tamoxifen did not *significantly* protect against breast cancer in women at usual or slightly decreased risk (hysterectomized women) (Veronesi *et al.* 2002).

The International Breast Cancer Intervention Studies (IBIS 1 and 2) in Europe should provide evidence to help clarify the risk–benefit ratio of tamoxifen in preventing familial breast cancer. A recent case–control study suggested that the risk of further cancer was reduced by 75% in *BRCA1* or *BRCA2* gene mutation carriers taking tamoxifen (Narod *et al.* 2000). Tamoxifen is known to be associated with an increase in the risk of endometrial cancer and thromboembolism. Continuing follow-up and pooling of data from the various tamoxifen intervention trials is required to assess the long-term risks and benefits of tamoxifen use, and the effect the drug has on mortality from breast cancer.

A trial in postmenopausal women with osteoporosis demonstrated a 76% reduction in incidence of breast cancer during 3 years of treatment with raloxifene, a selective oestrogen-receptor modulator (SERM). The efficacy and safety profile of raloxifene in women at increased risk of breast cancer should be clarified by the Prevention Study of Tamoxifen and Raloxifene (STAR) currently in progress (Cummings *et al.* 1999). New trials in the chemoprevention of breast cancer are focusing on luteinizing hormone releasing hormone analogues, aromatase inhibitors, and other SERMs.

## Prophylactic surgery

### Prophylactic mastectomy (PM)

Reductions in the incidence of recurrent breast cancer have been observed in women who had contralateral mastectomy because of breast cancer in the other breast and a reduced incidence of breast cancer in women from the general population who had reduction mammoplasty has also been observed (Baasch *et al.* 1996). Prophylactic surgery to women at high genetic risk has therefore been recommended by some surgeons for many years. Recently there has been greater study of the effect on risk that such surgery has in women with a strong family history. A retrospective cohort study showed that there was a greater than 90% reduction in expected number of breast cancers in women at moderate or high risk of breast cancer because of a family history (Hartmann *et al.* 1999). There have as yet been no long-term prospective studies that demonstrate a reduced mortality from breast cancer following PM. Bilateral mastectomy does not remove all breast tissue even with the most radical operation, hence there is a risk that cancer may develop within the remaining tissue. A recent prospective study (Meijers-Heijboer *et al.* 2001) studied a strong FH group and showed that over a 3-year follow-up there was a significant reduction in breast cancer cases in the PM group compared with those screened regularly. However, even with advances in reconstructive surgery, this option may be unacceptable for some women.

### Prophylactic oophorectomy (PO)

Similarly, whilst there is evidence for the value of oophorectomy in prevention of ovarian cancer, there remains the possibility of primary peritoneal cancer development in cells derived from remnants of the mullerian duct in the abdominal cavity. However, studies that have addressed this issue suggest that only 1% of women who have PO because of a family history of this cancer will develop such cancer (Haber 2002). This residual risk needs to be contrasted with the risk that such women have with their ovaries *in situ* – up to 60% lifetime risk for *BRCA1* carriers – see below.

Premenopausal PO has been associated with a lower than expected incidence of breast cancer as well as ovarian cancer. In a prospective study of *BRCA1* and *BRCA2* patients, those with PO had significant reduction in breast cancer risk compared with aged-matched controls (Haber 2002). Whilst oophorectomy is a relatively straightforward procedure in the postmenopausal woman, clearly a younger woman may not have completed her family and would require several decades of hormone replacement therapy (HRT). Encouragingly, however, premenopausal HRT does not seem to have the same effect on the risk of breast cancer as postmenopausal HRT, presumably because it is a replacement therapy rather than a supplement. A study of PO in *BRCA1* carriers showed that oestrogen replacement therapy in doses sufficient to protect against osteoporosis did not negate the risk reduction (Rebbeck 2000).

## Hormonal therapies

The interaction between genetic and other risk factors, e.g. oral contraception (OC), hormone replacement therapy (HRT), is not well understood. However, this is a frequent concern and a commonly held belief is that both HRT and OC may be contraindicated in women with a family history of breast cancer.

### HRT

A number of studies have shown an increased risk of breast cancer in women currently taking HRT. A large collaborative study found a 2.3% increased risk with every year of use, although the effect reduced as soon as HRT is stopped and wholly disappeared after about 5 years (Collaborative Group on Hormonal Factors in Breast Cancer 1997). However, most studies in the collaborative group were on oestrogen-only types of HRT. Before stopping such treatment in women with a family history of cancer, it is important to consider the original indications for prescribing these drugs (see Chapter 3). Furthermore, a study of the cancers detected in women taking HRT suggests that the increase in risk is composed almost entirely of cancers with a favourable prognosis (Gapstur *et al.* 1999). Thus, in practice, the GP should make women aware of a slight increase in risk, but the advantages of HRT will usually outweigh this risk even in women with a strong family history.

### OC

A meta-analysis (Collaborative Group on Hormonal Factors in Breast Cancer 1996) of oral contraceptive studies concluded that there is a slight increase in the risk of having breast cancer diagnosed during combined oral contraceptive use and in the following 10 years, but the excess disappears 10 years or more after cessation of use and the absolute risk is small. (In the period between starting use and up to 10 years after stopping OC use, an additional 0.5–5 cancers were diagnosed per 10 000 women in OC users compared to non-users). Evaluation of the effects are continuing. However, the risk of breast cancer associated with the OC may be greater in women with a family history of breast cancer, particularly those with a strong family history (Grabrick *et al.* 2000). Conversely, long-term OC use will significantly *reduce* the risk of ovarian cancer. A case–control study of OC use in *BRCA1* and *BRCA2* mutation carriers showed a 60% reduction in incidence of ovarian cancer after 6 years of use (Narod *et al.* 1998). For many women, the benefits of being on the Pill outweigh the potential risks.

## Lifestyle factors

Lifestyle factors are also believed to play a part in the development of breast cancer. There is some evidence to suggest a high fat diet (Huang *et al.* 1997) and regular alcohol consumption (Smith-Warner *et al.* 1998) increase risk, whereas possible preventive factors include high levels of physical activity, breast-feeding, high-fibre diets and a high intake of fresh fruit and vegetables. Again, it is not yet known how these risk factors are influenced by a FH of breast cancer. Given the known additional health benefits, adopting a general healthy lifestyle is recommended, but may not necessarily protect against breast cancer.

## Genetic testing for breast cancer

The two genes that have received the most publicity are the *Breast Cancer* genes 1 and 2 (*BRCA1* and *BRCA2*), which confer a lifetime risk of breast cancer of up to 80%. Although called breast cancer genes, these genes are present in all individuals and it is only when they are altered or mutated that there is an increased risk of breast cancer. Everyone has two copies of both the *BRCA1* and *2* genes; it is only when the mutated form is inherited that they carry a predisposition to cancer. Conversely, mutations in these genes can occur in sporadic cancers, but these cannot then be inherited.

Mutations in these genes also carry a risk of other cancers, for example of the ovary and prostate, although the degree of increased risk for the latter is not yet clear. The lifetime risk of ovarian cancer in someone with a *BRCA1* mutation is up to 40–60%, but lower (10–20%) in *BRCA2* gene mutation carriers. The risk figures vary between different ethnic populations and certain *BRCA1* mutations have a lower penetrance in, for example, the Ashkenazi Jewish population (Levy Lahad *et al.* 1997). Mutations in these genes account for approximately 5% of all breast cancer cases, but a greater proportion of young onset cases (35% of cancers diagnosed below age of 35 are thought to be due to a dominant gene mutation).

*BRCA1* mutations are more likely to result in high-grade tumours of medullary histology that are oestrogen-receptor negative, but *BRCA2* tumours cannot be distinguished from sporadic tumours by such features. In general, women who have a *BRCA* gene mutation have an increased risk of multifocal tumours and of second primaries.

Since the genes are inherited in a dominant fashion, the maximum risk of inheriting a mutated copy from an affected parent is 50%. Transmission occurs equally through men and women, although the *penetrance* for breast cancer is much lower in men (men are much less likely to develop breast cancer). Thus family history should be taken from both sides of the family since men can pass on the genes without developing breast cancer themselves.

Box 14.1 **Factors in the family history which suggest the presence of a dominant breast cancer-predisposing gene**

- A large number of affected family members in several generations (usually at least 3 or 4)
- The pattern of inheritance within the family (consistent with autosomal dominant)
- A young age of onset of breast cancer, particularly premenopausal cancer
- Occurrence of bilateral breast cancer or of multiple primaries
- Occurrence of male breast cancer
- The clustering of other cancers within the family, e.g.
  - ovarian cancer
  - prostate cancer
  - (rarely) malignant melanoma, thyroid cancer, pancreatic cancer, child hood sarcomas

It is thought that between 1 in 500–800 people in the general population carry mutations in the *BRCA1* or *BRCA2* genes (up to 1 in 50 in some ethnic populations such as Ashkenazi Jews), although the true population prevalence is not yet known. The average GP's list may include between 5 and 10 such women, and several more that are at risk of having inherited such a gene. At the genetics clinic, the geneticist will assess the likelihood of an individual's FH being due to a *BRCA* gene mutation and, if the risk is sufficiently high, testing will be offered.

## Predictive and diagnostic genetic testing

There are two steps to genetic testing:
- diagnostic testing (mutation searching)
- predictive testing.

### Diagnostic testing

There are many different known mutations (faults) in the *BRCA* genes. To offer genetic testing to an individual at increased risk, first a blood sample must be available from an affected relative in order to determine which mutation (if any) is running in their family. The genes are large, and testing is technically difficult and time-consuming – mutation searching may take anything up to one year or more.

If no mutation in the *BRCA* gene(s) is found in the affected relative, then either the test may have missed the fault (current tests can pick up at best 60–80% of all possible mutations in the gene) or a different, as yet unknown gene may be running in that family. Alternatively, it may reflect that there is no mutation present in the family, but this would be less likely if the family has been selected on the basis of a very strong FH. In this situation, the test has provided no new information. Testing can not then be offered to the unaffected relative and their risk of developing breast cancer is not significantly altered.

## Predictive testing

If a mutation in the *BRCA* genes is found in the affected relative, then the laboratory knows exactly which change to look for in the unaffected individual and predictive testing is technically straightforward and much quicker than mutation searching.

If the 'family' mutation is *not found* in the individual being tested, then he/she has *no increased risk* of developing breast cancer. This does not mean he/she has no risk of developing breast cancer – rather he/she has the same risk as any individual of the same sex and a similar age in the general population.

If the 'family' mutation *has* been inherited, then for women the lifetime risk of developing breast cancer is very high (up to 80%) and the lifetime risk of developing ovarian cancer is up to 60%. The risks for male breast cancer are highest with a *BRCA2* mutation, the lifetime risk is thought to be approximately 10%. It is not possible to determine exactly how likely it is that any given woman will develop cancer if she carries a faulty gene, or indeed when she will develop cancer, but she is more likely to do so at a young age ($<50$).

The sensitivity of current genetic tests depends on clinical circumstances and laboratory methods. If families are selected on the basis of a very strong family history, approximately 40% of these families will have breast cancer linked to the *BRCA1* gene and approximately 35% of families will have breast cancer linked to the *BRCA2* gene. The remainder are thought to be linked to an as yet unidentified gene or genes.

Even with a very strong family history, a mutation will only be detected in approximately 60% of cases because of the sensitivity of the diagnostic test. Many different mutations have been described in both *BRCA1* and *BRCA2*, and the search for such mutations therefore needs to be systematic throughout these genes, which is technically difficult. Interpretation of the clinical significance of detected mutations can also be problematic since there is as yet no reliable functional test of the protein. This is the reason for the two-stage process outlined above. Predictive testing of an unaffected person is not possible with the low sensitivity of the test since a negative result would not distinguish between a true negative and a false negative. However, if predictive testing is done in the context of a positive diagnostic test in a relative, the sensitivity is close to 100% and technically more straightforward.

### Advantages and disadvantages of predictive genetic testing

If a woman tests negative, she can be reassured that her risk of developing breast cancer is no different than for someone without a family history. Furthermore, if she has not inherited the mutation, she cannot pass it on to her children. Women with a strong family history are normally enrolled in early screening programmes, thus a negative test will allow these resources to be allocated elsewhere. Women with very strong FHs often also consider prophylactic surgery, and predictive testing will allow these choices to be more informed.

Knowing whether or not a person has inherited a breast cancer gene mutation will end some of the uncertainty that many women with a family history have lived with and, if positive, appropriate screening programmes can be implemented. However, there is as yet insufficient evidence to suggest that screening by examination and mammography are effective tools in reducing *mortality* from breast cancer among *BRCA* gene carriers (Burke *et al.* 1997a). Furthermore, whilst evidence from chemoprevention trials is still accumulating, the only preventative option is prophylactic surgery (either mastectomy and/or oophorectomy) and this does not completely eliminate the risk of cancer (see above).

Some uncertainty will remain despite gene testing since at least 20% of women carrying a mutation will never develop breast cancer and at least 40% will not develop ovarian cancer. Evidence is emerging that the risks of developing cancer may be much lower with certain mutations or in certain families (for example, in Ashkenazi Jewish populations). Further research is needed before we can predict with accuracy the chances of a woman developing cancer. Uncertainty about *when* a cancer will develop also remains. Thus a woman in her late twenties finding she carries a breast cancer gene mutation may not develop the cancer for another 20 years (if at all).

## Familial ovarian cancer

As has already been outlined is the discussion of familial breast cancer, the *BRCA1* and *BRCA2* genes also predispose to ovarian cancer to varying degrees. Because the frequency of ovarian cancer is much lower than breast cancer (approximately 1 in 80 women will develop ovarian cancer at some point in their lives), a family history of the disease is much more likely to imply hereditary factors. Approximately 50% of families with two cases of ovarian cancer in close relatives will have a dominant predisposing gene.

## Dominant ovarian cancer genes

+ *BRCA1* and *BRCA2* (*BRCA1* has a relatively greater contribution than *BRCA2*) – see above.

+ Genes that predispose only to ovarian cancer (site-specific ovarian cancer genes). These are known to exist from epidemiological studies of families with only ovarian cancer, but they have yet to be localized.

+ Mismatch repair genes which also predispose to hereditary non-polyposis colorectal cancer (HNPCC) (see below in discussion of familial colorectal cancer).

## Ovarian cancer screening

Pelvic examination, ultrasound imaging, and serum tumour markers have all been suggested as screening strategies for individuals with a family history of ovarian cancer. Unfortunately, none of these strategies has been proven as a screening modality. Small trials have demonstrated that the combination of ultrasound with CA125 can find stage 1 ovarian cancers. However, the positive predictive value of the test in this study was 1 in 6, meaning that 6 women required a laparotomy to detect one cancer (laparoscopy is not sufficient and a laparotomy with the attendant risks is required to follow up a positive scan). Further studies are ongoing in the UK and current recommendations are that women with a family history that includes ovarian cancer should be offered entry into these studies where possible. Local clinical genetics centres will be able to inform on the latest protocols. Screening should not be offered to women with a weaker family history because of its poor predictive value and the considerable morbidity involved in following up screen-positive results with laparotomies.

## Prophylactic surgery, oral contraception, and gene testing

See under breast cancer.

# Familial colorectal cancer (CRC)

As for breast cancer, the great majority of colorectal cancers are sporadic and/or due to weakly penetrant or low-risk genes. Nevertheless, a family history of colorectal cancer is a major risk factor for developing cancer and a number of dominantly inherited cancer syndromes causing colorectal cancer are recognized. This chapter concentrates on one such cancer syndrome, hereditary non-polyposis colorectal cancer (HNPPC), since it is the commonest of these syndromes but also because it confers a significant risk of gynaecological cancer to women who have inherited this syndrome. Both men and women are at risk of colorectal cancer, but women have the additional risk of ovarian cancer, and especially endometrial cancer. As for breast cancer, a family history need not necessarily imply the presence of an *HNPCC* gene (only 5–10% of all bowel cancer cases will be attributable to such a gene mutation) and again there is therefore scope for reassurance for many patients who are concerned about their family history.

## Hereditary non-polyposis colorectal cancer (HNPCC)

This is also known as Lynch syndromes 1 and 2. This syndrome predisposes to bowel cancer, endometrial cancer, and, to a lesser extent, ovarian cancer. Its unelegant name derives from the fact that the characteristic profuse polyposis of familial adenomatous polyposis (FAP or Gardner's syndrome) is absent. The true prevalence of *HNPCC* gene mutation carriers is not yet known but may be up to 1 in 500 people. Whilst the profuse polyposis of FAP provides a characteristic premalignant stage, polyps in HNPCC are rare or absent and thus identification of at-risk individuals relies on careful interpretation of the family history and confirmation of histology. Similar to the identification of families at risk of hereditary breast cancer, families are identified by a combination of family history of colorectal cancer, with a young age at onset, and the presence of endometrial, ovarian, or, rarely, urinary tract malignancies in the FH. Colorectal cancers tend to be right-sided or proximal and there is an increased risk of synchronous cancers (several tumours presenting at the same time) and metachronous tumours (multiple tumours at different times).

HNPCC arises from mutations in any one of at least five genes normally involved in repair of faulty DNA, known as *mismatch repair genes (MMR)* or DNA damage-response genes. These genes play an important role in the repair of DNA damage acquired during normal daily life. Mutations in these genes cause accumulation of such damage and a susceptibility to particular cancers.

As for breast cancer genes, the different HNPCC genes are located on different chromosomes and within each gene several different mutations are possible. Thus different mutations in different families may each have a different degree of cancer risk. Mutations in the genes *MSH2* and *MLH1* are the most frequent causes of HNPCC.

## Management of familial colorectal cancer

As for breast and ovarian cancer, local referral guidelines exist to describe which families may benefit from referral to secondary care (see Table 14.1 for example of referral guidelines).

## Low (average) risk

As for breast cancer, a FH of colon or endometrial cancer does not necessarily imply a hereditary factor. One in 25 people will develop CRC in their lifetime and, especially if this has a late age of onset (>60), it is less likely to be hereditary. Local referral guidelines will vary slightly depending on local circumstances; national guidelines have not yet been agreed upon. However, as a rule of thumb, if a person has just one relative with CRC diagnosed >45 or two relatives >60 they can be reassured that their own risk is not greatly increased above the general population risk. Similarly, one relative with endometrial cancer is more likely to be sporadic.

## Higher risk

As for breast cancer, this group can be divided into a moderate-risk group where some form of screening is probably indicated and a higher-risk group where a mutation in a *MMR* gene is likely to be responsible. Such high-risk families have traditionally been defined by FH criteria ('Amsterdam criteria' or more recently 'modified Amsterdam criteria' – see Table 14.2). Genetic testing may be an option for such high-risk families – see below.

## Early detection

Retrospective observational studies suggest an increased frequency of adenomas and early onset of cancer in HNPCC and thus colonoscopy every 1–3 years from the age of 25 is generally recommended. The optimal interval is not yet clear and follow-up studies are still ongoing. In a controlled trial, 3-yearly colonoscopy and removal of polyps reduced incidence of colorectal cancer by 62% and total mortality at 15 years by 65% (Jarvinen *et al.* 2000). Colonoscopy is the screening method of choice, because of the high frequency of proximal or right-sided colonic disease.

The value of endometrial cancer screening through transvaginal ultrasound and endometrial biopsy is uncertain, especially for premenopausal for women with HNPCC. Ovarian screening is discussed above.

For those individuals who fall into the higher-risk group, but whose family history is not strong enough to suggest HNPCC, some form of surveillance

**Table 14.2** Modified Amsterdam criteria

| | |
|---|---|
| 1 | At least three relatives with an hereditary non-polyposis colorectal cancer (HNPCC) |
| 2 | One of these must be a first-degree relative of the other two relatives |
| 3 | At least one case diagnosed below the age of 50 |
| 4 | At least two generations involved |

**Table 14.3** Empiric lifetime risk figures for familial colorectal cancer (CRC)

| | |
|---|---|
| Population risk | 1 in 25 |
| One first-degree relative affected diagnosed after age 45 | 1 in 17 |
| One first- and one second-degree relative affected, diagnosed after age 45 | 1 in 12 |
| One first-degree relative affected, diagnosed before age 45 | 1 in 10 |
| Two first-degree relatives affected | 1 in 6 |
| Dominant pedigree (50% risk of inheriting gene but risk of CRC less due to ~75% penetrance) | ≤1 in 3 |

may also be recommended. Local policies vary. Many surgeons will screen if the lifetime risk of CRC is thought to be greater than 1 in 10. Table 14.3 outlines lifetime risks according to FH.

## Lifestyle modification

There is some evidence that modification of the starch content of the diet and certain forms of chemoprevention (e.g. non-steroidal anti-inflammatory agents) may protect against the progression of the adenoma–carcinoma sequence. Double-blind, controlled trials evaluating the effect of aspirin and or digestion-resistant starch on the incidence of CRC are currently in progress (CAPP2 study). Research has implicated a number of adverse lifestyle factors in the aetiology of sporadic CRC; for example, high-fat, low-fibre, low-folate diets, little exercise, smoking, and excess alcohol (Janne and Mayer 2000). How much these factors contribute to hereditary cancer remains unclear, but few GPs would argue the overall benefits of eating lots of fresh fruit and vegetables, regular exercise and cessation of smoking.

## Genetic testing

Current techniques can identify a mutation in approximately 60% of cases with a strong family history. As discussed under breast cancer gene testing, different families carry different mutations; thus a mutation must first be found in an affected relative before predictive testing can be offered to family members. Those who test positive should be counselled regarding the 70–75% risk of CRC by the age of 65. The average age of diagnosis is 45 years, though the range extends to the early 20s. The lifetime risk of endometrial cancer in women who have a mutant *HNPCC* gene has been reported as 20% in the Netherlands and USA (Watson and Lynch 1994), but studies from Finland suggest a lifetime risk of 60% and a cumulative 12% incidence of ovarian cancer (Aarnio *et al.* 1999).

Uncertainty will therefore remain before research gives more definitive figures, but predictive testing where a family mutation is known may allow screening measures to be directed at those truly at risk whilst reassuring those found not to carry the gene (see under genetic testing for breast cancer genes).

### Prophylactic surgery

Prophylactic surgery should be discussed with individuals found to carry an *HNPCC* mutation, but evidence that this reduces mortality from the disease is lacking (Burke *et al.* 1997b). Perhaps surprisingly, far fewer people consider prophylactic colectomy as a practical option than those who consider prophylactic mastectomy. However, prophylactic hysterectomy and bilateral salpingo-oophorectomy should be discussed with women who have an *HNPCC* mutation and who are approaching or have passed the age of the menopause (Lynch and Casey 2001).

## The role of primary care in familial cancers

Professional and government bodies have recommended that primary care play a role in the delivery of genetic services. Whilst the impact of genetics on primary care is currently still relatively small, it is likely this will increase significantly in the coming years as more genetic tests become available and patients increasingly request information and advice.

Currently, the main impact of genetics on GPs is with regard to familial cancers. A GP with 2000 patients will have 40–50 patients with at least one first-degree relative affected by either breast, ovarian, colorectal, or endometrial cancer and studies in the UK and Holland have shown that approximately one to two patients per month per GP discuss their family history of cancer or other common disease. This is similar to the consultation rates for other 'common' diseases in primary care, such as diabetes (Emery *et al.* 1999).

In terms of managing familial cancers, the primary care team has an important role to play in performing an initial assessment of risk and making appropriate referral decisions (Fig 14.6). This requires some knowledge and skill in taking an adequate family tree and being aware of factors that indicate a significant genetic risk. Referral guidelines are now widely available to assist in this process. Women whose family history is not indicative of high genetic risk can be provided with information and reassurance in primary care, and spared the possibly anxiety of referral to secondary care. For women whose family history is suggestive of increased genetic risk, the GP has a role to play

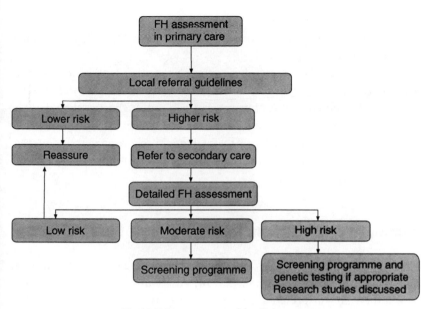

**Fig 14.6** Management of familial cancer.

in ensuring the woman has realistic expectations of the referral process and understands that genetic testing is only relevant for a small minority of women who have a very strong family history. They are also likely to be involved in the follow-up care.

Research is currently examining the effectiveness of computerized pedigree drawing and decision support for GPs in this area and, increasingly, online resources will be useful both for primary health care professionals and their patients. In the future, GPs may play a greater role in the delivery of genetic counselling services.

There are still many uncertainties in the management of inherited cancers, but over the next decade we can expect to see many of these clarified by research findings and it will be possible to provide patients with clearer choices between prophylactic surgery, screening, or chemoprevention.

Routine family history screening of *asymptomatic* patients is currently performed by many primary care practitioners, although often without a management plan if a family history is identified. Routine family history screening does not meet accepted criteria for a screening test given the limited evidence for interventions to manage increased risk of most cancers. Formal screening in primary care for a family history of breast or ovarian cancer may be appropriate once stronger evidence exists for *at least one* intervention for that specific cancer, be it chemoprevention, screening, or prophylactic surgery. We may never have evidence from randomized controlled trials for all such interventions, so physicians will need to discuss the uncertainties about other management options with patients whom they identify through family history screening.

In the meantime, GPs must advise people presenting with concerns about their family history, or when family history is discussed in relation to specific symptoms. The potential role of primary care in cancer genetics should not be understated. Many patients overestimate the risk associated with their family history. Appropriate reassurance by their GP might relieve anxiety and prevent falsely raising a patient's fears and expectations through unnecessary referral, screening, or genetic testing.

## 10-Minute consultation: family history of breast cancer

A woman comes to see you because she is approaching the age at which her sister developed breast cancer. She is worried about her risk and is keen to know if there are any preventative measures she can take.

### What issues should you cover?

- Take a family history going back for at least two generations on BOTH sides of the family.

- Start with the patient in front of you and mark her with an arrow to indicate she is the consultand. Note ages and sex of children and siblings (circle for females and square for males) and note the age of diagnosis of any cancers. Colour in an affected individual and clearly indicate the type of cancer (by a colour/pattern code).

- Next note the age or age and cause of death of both parents, and note the age of diagnosis of cancer, if affected. Work out from there; ask how many siblings each parent has/had – note ages, ages of death or ages of diagnoses of cancer, whether they themselves had children, what sex, age, and whether or not have had cancer.

- Finally ask about grandparents. Three generations will usually suffice to be able to make a basic assessment of risk.

- When noting cancer diagnosis, make sure to note age at diagnosis as this is more important than age of death.

- If relatives have not had cancer but have died, age at death should be recorded (if women died when young from other causes, then the risk of an inherited tendency to breast cancer cannot be excluded as thoroughly as when many female relatives have lived into their seventies or eighties without being affected).

- Ask especially if there are other cancers in the family such as ovarian cancer.
- Make sure to enquire about paternal family history as well, since cancer-predisposing genes can be inherited from either parent.
- If details of FH are unclear, ask patient to find out more from relatives or death certificates and come back with gathered information. Often 'family stories' of cancer turn out to be a different type of cancer on closer investigation (e.g. reported ovarian cancer may turn out to be cervical cancer or even stomach cancer).
- Establish if anyone else in the family obtained advice about FH? Is anyone else receiving screening, or have any genetic studies been done in relatives?
- Ask about hormonal risk factors – age of menarche/menopause, use of OC or HRT. Long-term HRT or OC use increases risk of breast cancer, OC may protect against ovarian cancer. Enquire about number of children and ages at which pregnant.
- Ask about ethnic origin. Certain groups such as Ashkenazi Jews have a higher frequency of genetic breast cancers.
- Find out what the main worries about cancer are. For many women, the options they want to explore depend on their experience of cancer in the family. For example, women who have seen all their relatives die rather than be successfully treated may be more likely to consider options such as prophylactic mastectomy.

## What should you do?

Refer to local guidelines. Consensus national guidelines exist (Watson and Lucassen 1999), but there may be local variation (see also Fig 14.3).

- If the patient does not meet guideline referral criteria, then reassure that the risk of carrying a breast cancer gene is very low and the risk of developing breast cancer is similar to any women of a similar age in the general population.
  (a) Explain no additional screening required.
  (b) Make sure patient knows about NHS Breast Screening Programme from age 50.
  (c) Make sure patient knows about breast awareness.
  (d) Make sure patient understands they need to advise you of any change to family history.

[*As a rule of thumb*: if your patient has just one first-degree relative (mother, sister, or daughter) with breast cancer diagnosed over the age of 40 you can reassure. Similarly, if she has two close relatives (first- or second-degree) diagnosed >60, you can reassure.]

- If patient meets guideline referral criteria, refer to secondary care (either breast unit or genetics unit, depending on local circumstances). If unsure whether referral is warranted, contact local service for advice.

- Explain secondary care will make a detailed assessment of FH and attempt to confirm cancers in the family through histology reports. Ensure woman understands that a detailed risk assessment can be time consuming and that genetic testing is only possible in a minority of women who have a very strong FH.

## Frequently asked questions

### My mother had cancer of the ovaries when she was 45. What are my chances of getting it?

As you have only one close relative with ovarian cancer and if you have no close relatives with young onset (<50) breast cancer, it is unlikely there is a strong genetic factor running in your family, and your chances of developing the disease are only slightly higher than someone of a similar age with no family history. If any other close relatives develop the disease, it is important you seek further advice as your risk may then change.

### There is a history of breast and ovarian cancer in my family. Am I at greater risk of developing these cancers? Should I have my ovaries out?

Depending on how many close relatives have been diagnosed with breast and/or ovarian cancer, and the ages at which they were diagnosed, it is possible that you are at increased risk of developing these cancers. The first step would be for you to receive genetic counselling to accurately assess your risk and to discuss the available options. Some women found to be at high risk do opt to have their ovaries removed to reduce the risk of ovarian cancer. However, a full discussion of the benefits and limitations of this procedure should take place before such a decision is made.

### My sister had breast cancer when she was 42. I am now at that age but have been told I cannot have a mammogram until I am 50. Why is this?

Your family history does not suggest you are at a greatly increased risk of breast cancer and therefore a mammogram would not be recommended. You may be aware that there is a National Breast Screening Programme for women aged 50 and over. For women in this age group, research has convincingly shown that mammographic screening will reduce the death rate from breast cancer.

However, for women under 50, to date there is no strong research evidence to show that women will benefit in the same way from mammography. Therefore a mammogram may do more harm than good. If you notice any changes in your breasts or if your family history of cancer alters, you should of course report these to your doctor.

### My mother had womb cancer in her sixties and I was told this did not increase my risk, but now my sister has had cancer of the cervix. Does that alter the original advice?

Probably not. Cervical cancer is unlikely to be due to a strong inherited factor and there is no known genetic link between endometrial (womb) and cervical cancer. It is more likely that these two cancers have arisen together in your family through unlucky chance.

### My mother and sister developed breast cancer at a young age. Should I consider an operation to remove my breasts?

The first step would be for you to receive genetic counselling to accurately assess your risk and to discuss the available options. Depending on your family details, genetic testing *might* be possible. Even if the cancers in your mother and sister were found to be due to a strong genetic factor, genetic testing could show that you have not inherited this genetic factor from your mother, in which case an operation would be unnecessary. If you were found to be at high risk, preventive surgery would be a potential option to reduce your risk of breast cancer. However, a full discussion of the benefits and limitations of this procedure should take place before such a decision is made.

### My mother and aunt have both had breast cancer in their sixties. Am I at increased risk?

Only a small proportion of all breast cancers can be explained by the inheritance of a strong genetic factor. Most breast cancers are thought to be more influenced by lifestyle, environmental, and weak genetic factors. Since the ages of onset of your relative's breast cancer is not suggestive of a strong genetic predisposing factor, your own risk is probably only slightly raised above the general population lifetime risk of 1 in 9.

## Further reading

Hodgson, S.V. and Maher, E.R. (1998). *A practical guide to human cancer genetics.* Cambridge University Press, Cambridge.

Offit, K. (1998). *Clinical cancer genetics: risk counselling and management.* Wiley-Liss, New York.

Rose, P. and Lucassen, A. (1999). *Practical genetics and primary care.* Oxford University Press, Oxford.

# References

Aarnio, M., Sankila, R., Pukkala, E., *et al.* (1999). Cancer risk in mutation carriers of DNA-mismatch-repair genes. *International Journal of Cancer*, **81**(2), 214–18.

Austoker, J. (1994). Screening and self examination for breast cancer. *British Medical Journal*, **309**, 168–74.

Baasch, M., Nielsen, S.F., Engholm, G. and Lund, K. (1996). Breast cancer incidence subsequent to surgical reduction of the female breast. *British Journal of Cancer*, **73**, 961–3.

Beemsterboer, P.M., Warmerdam, P.G., Boer, R. and de Koning, H. J. (1998). Radiation risk of mammography related to benefit in screening programmes: a favourable balance? *Journal of Medical Screening*, **5**, 81–7.

Burke, W., Daly, M., Garber, J., *et al.* (1997a). Recommendations for follow-up care of individuals with an inherited predisposition to cancer. II. BRCA1 and BRCA2. Cancer Genetics Studies Consortium. *Journal of the American Medical Association*, **277**, 997–1003.

Burke, W., Petersen, G., Lynch, P., *et al.* (1997b). Recommendations for follow-up care of individuals with an inherited predisposition to cancer. I. Hereditary nonpolyposis colon cancer. Cancer Genetics Studies Consortium. *Journal of the American Medical Association*, **277**, 915–19.

Chart, P.L. and Franssen, E. (1997). Management of women at increased risk for breast cancer: preliminary results from a new program. *Canadian Medical Association Journal*, **157**, 1235–42.

Christiansen, C.L., Wang, F., Barton, M.B., *et al.* (2000). Predicting the cumulative risk of false-positive mammograms [In Process Citation]. *Journal of the National Cancer Institute*, **92**, 165–6.

Collaborative Group on Hormonal Factors in Breast Cancer (1996). Breast cancer and hormonal contraceptives: collaborative reanalysis of individual data on 53 297 women with breast cancer and 100 239 women without breast cancer from 54 epidemiological studies. *Lancet*, **347**, 1713–27.

Collaborative Group on Hormonal Factors in Breast Cancer (1997). Breast cancer and hormone replacement therapy: collaborative reanalysis of data from 51 epidemiological studies of 52,705 women with breast cancer and 108,411 women without breast cancer. *Lancet*, **350**, 1047–59.

Cummings, S.R., Eckert, S., Krueger, K.A., *et al.* (1999). The effect of raloxifene on risk of breast cancer in postmenopausal women: results from the MORE randomized trial. Multiple Outcomes of Raloxifene Evaluation. *Journal of the American Medical Association*, **281**, 2189–97.

Emery, J., Watson, E., Rose, P. and Andermann, A. (1999). A systematic review of the literature exploring the role of primary care in genetic services. *Family Practice*, **16**, 426–45.

Fisher, B., Costantino, J.P., Wickerham, D.L., *et al.* (1998). Tamoxifen for prevention of breast cancer: report of the National Surgical Adjuvant Breast and Bowel Project P-1 Study. *Journal of the National Cancer Institute*, **90**, 1371–88.

Gapstur, S.M., Morrow, M. and Sellers, T.A. (1999). Hormone replacement therapy and risk of breast cancer with a favorable histology. *Journal of the American Medical Association*, **281**, 2091–7.

Grabrick, D.M., Hartmann, L.C., Cerhan, J.R., *et al.* (2000). Risk of breast cancer with oral contraceptive use in women with a family history of breast cancer. *Journal of the American Medical Association*, **284**, 1791–8.

Haber, D.A. (2002). Prophylactic oophorectomy to reduce the risk of ovarian and breast cancer in carriers of BRCA mutations. *New England Journal of Medicine*, **346**, 1660–1.

Hartmann, L.C., Schaid, D.J., Woods, J.E., *et al.* (1999). Efficacy of bilateral prophylactic mastectomy in women with a family history of breast cancer [see comments]. *New England Journal of Medicine*, **340**, 77–84.

Huang, Z., Hankinson, S.E., Colditz, G.A., *et al.* (1997). Dual effects of weight and weight gain on breast cancer risk. *Journal of the American Medical Association*, **278**, 1407–11.

Janne, P.A. and Mayer, R.J. (2000). Chemoprevention of colorectal cancer. *New England Journal of Medicine*, **342**, 1960–8.

Jarvinen, H.J., Aarnio, M., Mustonen, H., *et al.* (2000). Controlled 15-year trial on screening for colorectal cancer in families with hereditary nonpolyposis colorectal cancer. *Gastroenterology*, **118**, 829–34.

Kerlikowske, K., Carney, P.A., Geller, B., *et al.* (2000). Performance of screening mammography among women with and without a first-degree relative with breast cancer. *Annals of Internal Medicine*, **133**, 855–63.

Kuhl, C.K., Schmutzler, R.K., Leutner, C.C., *et al.* (2000). Breast MR imaging screening in 192 women proved or suspected to be carriers of a breast cancer susceptibility gene: preliminary results. *Radiology*, **215**, 267–79.

Levy Lahad, E., Catane, R., Eisenberg, S., *et al.* (1997). Founder *BRCA1* and *BRCA2* mutations in Ashkenazi Jews in Israel: frequency and differential penetrance in ovarian cancer and in breast-ovarian cancer families. *American Journal of Human Genetics*, **60**, 1059–67.

Lucassen, A., Watson, E. and Eccles, D. (2001). Evidence based case report: advice about mammography for a young woman with a family history of breast cancer. *British Medical Journal*, **322**, 1040–2.

Lynch, H.T. and Casey, M.J. (2001). Current status of prophylactic surgery for hereditary breast and gynecologic cancers. *Current Opinion in Obstetrics and Gynecology*, **13**, 25–30.

Meijers-Heijboer, H., van Geel, B., van Putten, W.L., *et al.* (2001). Breast cancer after prophylactic bilateral mastectomy in women with a *BRCA1* or *BRCA2* mutation. *New England Journal of Medicine*, **345**, 159–64.

Mettler, F.A., Upton, A.C., Kelsey, C.A., Ashby, R.N., Rosenberg, R.D. and Linver, M.N. (1996). Benefits versus risks from mammography: a critical reassessment [see comments]. *Cancer*, **77**, 903–9.

Narod, S.A., Risch, H., Moslehi, R., *et al.* (1998). Oral contraceptives and the risk of hereditary ovarian cancer. *New England Journal of Medicine*, **339**, 424–8.

Narod, S.A., Brunet, J.S., Ghadirian, P., *et al.* (2000). Tamoxifen and risk of contralateral breast cancer in *BRCA1* and *BRCA2* mutation carriers: a case-control study. Hereditary Breast Cancer Clinical Study Group. *Lancet*, **356**, 1876–81.

NHS Breast Screening Programme and Cancer Research Campaign. (1999). *Be breast aware.* Department of Health, London.

Powles, T., Eeles, R., Ashley, S., *et al.* (1998). Interim analysis of the incidence of breast cancer in the Royal Marsden Hospital tamoxifen randomised chemoprevention trial [see comments]. *Lancet,* **352**, 98–101.

Rebbeck, T.R. (2000). Prophylactic oophorectomy in *BRCA1* and *BRCA2* mutation carriers. *Journal of Clinical Oncology,* **18**, S100–3.

Smith-Warner, S.A., Spiegelman, D., Yaun, S.S., *et al.* (1998). Alcohol and breast cancer in women: a pooled analysis of cohort studies. *Journal of the American Medical Association,* **279**, 535–40.

Veronesi, U., Maisonneuve, P., Vsacchini, N. *et al.* (2002). Tamoxifen for breast cancer among hysterectomised women. *Lancet,* **359**, 1122–4.

Watson, E.K. and Lucassen, A. (1999). *Familial breast and ovarian cancer – a management guide for primary care.* (Part of information pack containing referral guidelines and patient information). Cancer Research Campaign, London.

Watson, P. and Lynch, H.T. (1994). The tumor spectrum in HNPCC. *Anticancer Research,* **14**, 1635–9.

# Chapter 15

# Eating disorders

## Deborah Waller and Christopher Fairburn

Eating disorders such as anorexia nervosa and bulimia nervosa are a common source of psychiatric and physical morbidity among young women in Western societies (van Hoeken *et al.* 1998). Eating disorders are often not detected and they have a reputation for being difficult to treat. The general practitioner (GP) is in a special position to offer help to sufferers and to intervene early in the development of their disorder. This chapter gives an overview of eating disorders and their management from a GP perspective, to help increase awareness and detection of eating problems and to outline evidence-based treatments for eating disorders, some of which are suitable for use in primary care.

## A typical day in the life of a 20-year-old student with bulimia nervosa

Wake up with splitting headache, parched mouth, feeling sick and bloated. Memories of last night's binge fill me with remorse: I MUST NOT EAT TODAY. I'm so weak and pathetic. I hate myself. Can't face getting up so stay in bed and miss my morning lecture. Feel guilty and anxious about this and my essay. Dizzy when I get up – drink two glasses of water. Weigh myself: 9 stone 2 pounds. Oh no – I've gained 2 pounds since yesterday. Feel TERRIBLE. NO FOOD TODAY. Put on baggy jumper and track suit bottoms to hide my disgusting thighs and stomach. Sit down at my desk to make notes for my essay. Drink another glass of water. Try to concentrate, but my mind keeps wandering back to thoughts of food. About 20 minutes pass – it's no good, I'll go out for a run. Force myself to run round the park five times. Chose a route back to my room which passes by a newsagent's. I don't think I'd con-sciously planned to go in, but as I approach the shop I feel an overwhelming need for something sweet and comforting. Buy 2 flapjacks, a packet of biscuits, 2 choco-late bars and a jar of peanut butter. Start eating as soon as I get out of the shop. The food tastes delicious and I feel strangely elated: a sense of escape and release of tension. Hurry back to my room where I gorge on the peanut butter straight from the jar – can't stop myself. When it's all finished I head for the toilet. Put my fingers down the back of my throat until I gag. It's disgusting, but so easy. Throw up repeat-edly until I've got rid of everything in my stomach. I look at my face in the mirror: listless, puffy eyes, fat, 'hamster' cheeks. Hate myself, feel so ashamed by my lack of willpower. I MUST NOT EAT AGAIN TODAY. Decide to go to the library to write my essay. Will allow myself a diet coke at 3 p.m. Find it very difficult to concentrate, make slow progress. As lunchtime approaches, I imagine my friends meeting at the canteen. Part of me would love to join them, but I certainly don't deserve to eat anything and it would be embarrassing to sit there while they eat. They might even suspect something. Force myself to read another page. Have diet coke as planned in library snack-bar. Feel an incredible urge to eat, but with a huge effort I return to the library and my books. The afternoon and evening stretch out before me. I ought to be writing my essay, but all I can think about is how fat and out of shape I am and how no one could possibly like me the way I look at the moment. Despite this, I keep dreaming about just the sort of foods I must not eat. It's mental torture. I'm worried about bingeing tonight. I know there's a party for first years in college and decide to go along. Feel nervous and awkward, avoid talking to anyone and have several glasses of wine in quick succession. There's a buffet meal but I know I must get out of there before I give in and eat anything. Hurry back to my room. All that alcohol – so many calories. Feel lonely and depressed. What can I do now? It's only 9 p.m. Weigh myself: 9 stone 1 pound. Good. At least I've lost a pound today despite the binge. If I could only lose a pound every day for the next two weeks . . . . Half-heartedly sit down at my desk, but can't get motivated. Feel tense and bored . . . . I check the communal fridge at the end of the corridor. Pinch a yoghurt, consoling myself that it can't be that fattening. Eat it in my room. Well, now I've broken my resolve I might as well give in and binge. I can vomit afterwards and get rid of the calories. Hurry out to the late night shop and buy a packet of cornflakes, 4 pints of milk, a pound of sugar, a loaf of bread, half a pound of margarine, a chocolate cake, a jar of strawberry jam, a family sized carton of ice cream, two doughnuts and a litre bottle of lemonade. I chose things I can eat quickly and easily. All things I wouldn't normally allow myself. As soon as I get back to my room I start. I eat rapidly, washing down the food with the lemonade. It's as if I'm in a trance. I start with the chocolate cake, then the ice cream. I mix margarine and sugar and eat until it's all gone. I have slice after slice of bread and jam, bowl after bowl of cornflakes with milk. I eat steadily until I'm so full it hurts. The whole binge takes 45 minutes. Afterwards my stomach feels as if it's going to burst and every breath is painful. Time to get rid of all this. I go to the bathroom – it's easy to throw up. I vomit and vomit until the chocolate mixture reappears – now I've brought back everything. I'm exhausted. I lie down. I know I will have put on weight. Desperation and self-disgust flow over me. I wish I were dead.

# Definitions

The term 'eating disorders' refers to anorexia nervosa and bulimia nervosa and the 'atypical eating disorders'. Their diagnostic criteria are listed in Box 15.1. Anorexia nervosa and bulimia nervosa have in common a characteristic overevaluation of shape and weight and most of their clinical features are secondary to this.

## Box 15.1 **Diagnostic criteria for eating disorders**

### Anorexia nervosa

- Characteristic overevaluation of shape and weight (generally characterized by an intense fear of weight gain and fatness, accompanied by the pursuit of weight loss and thinness)
- Active maintenance of an unduly low weight (BMI less than 17.5; or less than 85% of expected weight for age, height, and sex), achieved mainly by strict dieting and excessive exercising, and in a minority, self-induced vomiting
- Amenorrhoea for at least 3 months (if not on the contraceptive pill)

### Bulimia nervosa

- Characteristic overevaluation of shape and weight (as found in anorexia nervosa)
- Frequent binges (bulimic episodes)
- Extreme behaviour to prevent weight gain, such as self-induced vomiting, misuse of laxatives and diuretics, and strict dieting
- The binges and weight control behaviours occur, on average, at least twice a week for 3 months

Purging behaviour (vomiting or laxative/diuretic misuse) is not essential for the diagnosis as long as there is recurrent binge eating and some weight control behaviours to prevent weight gain.

### Atypical eating disorders

- Disorders that resemble anorexia nervosa or bulimia nervosa but do not meet their diagnostic criteria

## Definition of a binge

- Eating, in a discrete period of time (e.g. within a 2-hour period), an amount of food that is definitely larger than most people would eat in a similar period and under similar circumstances.
- A sense of lack of control during the episode (an aversive feeling that one cannot prevent the episode from starting or stop it once it has started).

## Prevalence and distribution

Cases of anorexia nervosa were described as long as 120 years ago, whereas bulimia nervosa is thought to have emerged as a common eating disorder only relatively recently. Fig 15.1 shows rates of referral to a leading eating disorder centre in Toronto since 1979. While the anorexia nervosa referral rates

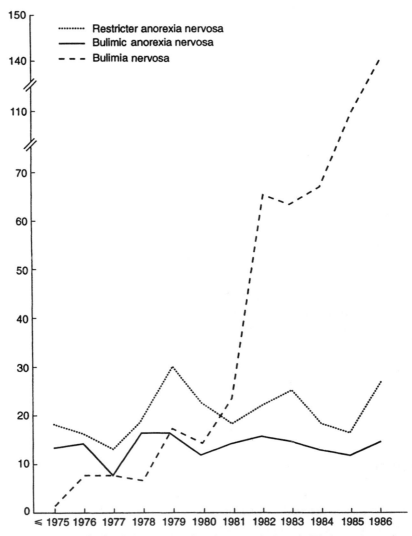

**Fig 15.1** Rates of referral to an eating disorder centre in Canada (Clarke Institute of Psychiatry and Toronto General Hospital). (Reproduced with permission from Garner, D.M. and Fairburn, C.G. (1998). Relationship between anorexia nervosa and bulimia nervosa: diagnostic implications. In Garner, D.M. and Garfinkel, P.E. (eds), *Diagnostic issues in anorexia nervosa and bulimia nervosa*, p. 60. Brunner/Mazel, New York).

have remained relatively constant, there has been a dramatic rise in the number of reported cases of bulimia nervosa. Similar trends have occurred in most Westernized countries.

Anorexia nervosa is largely confined to females aged between 10 and 30 and its prevalence among adolescent girls, the group most at risk, is 0.3% (van Hoeken *et al.* 1998). Fewer than 10% are male and the disorder is uncommon in non-whites. Bulimia nervosa is more common than anorexia nervosa and it affects a slightly older age group, most cases being in their twenties. The prevalence is about 1% among females aged 16–35. The disorder is rarely seen in males. Atypical eating disorders are thought to be more common, but little is known about their prevalence.

## Detection, assessment, and immediate management

GPs have difficulty detecting eating disorders. In the case of anorexia nervosa where weight loss is usually obvious, about 40% of cases are detected by GPs and 80% of these are referred on for specialist treatment. In bulimia nervosa, by contrast, only 10% of cases are detected by GPs and only half of these are referred for treatment (Hoek 1991). The atypical eating disorders comprise about 40% of patients seen by specialists.

The GP will often be the first professional to see a patient with an eating disorder. The doctor needs to be sensitive to any clues the patient might give alluding to an eating problem and to respond appropriately. Other members of the primary health care team may have a role in detection. Practice nurses often see patients for dietary advice and weight management, which puts them in a potentially good position to detect the minority of cases that co-occur with obesity. Health visitors have frequent contact with mothers, some of whom will have eating disorders.

### Why are so few people with eating disorders asking for help?

There are a number of reasons why women with eating disorders are reluctant to seek help.

◆ Chronic low self-esteem is very common: sufferers feel the disorder is self-inflicted and that they do not deserve help, or that it is not severe enough to warrant help.

◆ Feelings of shame and guilt often prevent people with binge eating problems from confiding in anyone.

- People often hope the problem will go away on its own (and in some cases it does).

- Many find it very difficult to tell doctors about their eating. They may have consulted with problems secondary to the eating disorder in the past and feel awkward about admitting to a problem that they had previously not disclosed.

- If they do tell the doctor they may come across obstructive attitudes, often because the GP does not know how to help. The GP may trivialize the problem or act inappropriately, e.g. hand over a diet sheet.

- They are often fearful that treatment will involve weight gain.

- In some cases, particularly with anorexia nervosa, the sufferer does not view the eating disorder as a problem and does not want to change.

## Presentation of anorexia nervosa

Few patients with anorexia nervosa present themselves for treatment. They typically come to see the GP reluctantly, accompanied by a concerned parent or friend. It is often difficult to establish a rapport with the patient who may make it clear at the outset that she does not want help and feels there is nothing wrong. If possible, the doctor should first see the patient alone to get her perspective and to try and win her confidence, and then see the inform-ant. Careful history-taking should make the diagnosis clear. The patient will have a highly restrictive eating pattern with avoidance of any foods viewed as 'fattening'. This is typically associated with the characteristic overevaluation of shape and weight in which there is an intense fear of weight gain and fatness together with a pursuit of weight loss and thinness. There may be over-exercising, self-induced vomiting, and the misuse of laxatives or diuretics. A minority have times when they lose control over their eating and overeat. Often this uncontrolled overeating (binge eating) does not involve the consumption of truly large amounts of food (subjective binge eating), but in some cases genuinely large quantities are eaten (objective or true binge eating). Depression and anxiety symptoms are often present and there is generally marked social withdrawal. Some patients present indirectly with features associated with anorexia nervosa rather than the disorder itself (e.g. gastrointestinal symptoms, amenorrhoea or infertility, or with depres-sive or obsessional features). In these cases, once the patient's low weight has been identified and recognized to be the result of their concerns about shape and weight, the diagnosis should be clear.

## Box 15.2 **Presentation of anorexia nervosa**

### Directly

- Cry for help
- Pushed into seeking help by relative/friend

### Indirectly

- Physical effects of starvation, e.g. feeling cold all the time, poor concentration, weakness, fatigue, early morning waking
- Gastrointestinal symptoms, e.g. constipation, abdominal pain
- Fluid retention, intermittent oedema
- Amenorrhoea, infertility
- Coexistent psychopathology, e.g. depression, anxiety, obsessional and compulsive symptoms

### Typical signs

- Emaciated: wearing layers of baggy clothing to conceal shape
- Bradycardia
- Resting and orthostatic hypotension
- Mottled, cold extremities
- Lanugo hair
- Yellow discoloration of palms and soles of feet (attributed to carotene pigmentation)
- Dry, scaly skin
- Sweet ketotic breath

## Presentation of bulimia nervosa

In bulimia nervosa there are repeated episodes of true binge eating accompanied by attitudes and behaviour similar to those seen in anorexia nervosa. The majority of patients vomit or take laxatives immediately after binge eating in an attempt to minimize the amount of food absorbed. Most are ashamed of their binge eating and keep it a secret, with the result that there is generally a substantial delay between the onset of the eating disorder and the seeking of help. Depressive symptoms are often a prominent feature, and some of these patients are prone to substance abuse (especially excessive drinking) and other impulsive behaviour including self-injury.

Patients with bulimia nervosa tend to present to the GP by themselves. Most complain of loss of control over eating, although they may present indirectly, complaining of features commonly associated with bulimia nervosa (e.g. depression, substance abuse, irritable bowel symptoms, or irregular periods). They are usually within the normal weight range for their height (BMI 20–25) and under these circumstances making the correct diagnosis can be difficult as there may be no pointers to the eating disorder.

## Box 15.3 **Presentation of bulimia nervosa**

### Directly

◆ Loss of control over eating: wanting help to stop binge eating/vomiting, but not usually to stop dieting

### Indirectly

◆ Requesting help with dieting (e.g. appetite suppressants or laxatives/diuretics)

◆ Gastrointestinal symptoms (e.g. irritable bowel symptoms, constipation, abdominal pain)

◆ Fluid retention with oedema of hands and less commonly feet, feeling bloated

◆ Menstrual irregularities/infertility

◆ Coexistent psychopathology, especially depression, anxiety, substance abuse, and other impulsive behaviours, including self-harm

◆ Fatigue, dizziness, syncope

◆ Tooth sensitivity

### Typical signs

◆ Puffy face due to parotid gland enlargement

◆ Calluses or abrasions on the dorsum of the hand – due to repeated stimulation of the gag reflex

◆ Dental enamel erosion due to recurrent vomiting

## Diagnosis, examination, and investigations

The diagnosis of an eating disorder is made by using the history and mental state examination to identify the characteristic features, not by ruling out all physical causes for weight loss or abnormal eating. No laboratory investigations are required to make the diagnosis and, unless there are positive reasons to suspect the presence of underlying physical disease, no tests are needed to exclude other medical disorders. Since these patients are highly sensitive about their bodies and being weighed, thought needs to be given as to whether they need to be physically examined. Physical examination does not contribute to the diagnosis other than by allowing calculation of the body mass index (BMI). On the other hand, it is indicated if the patient is possibly underweight or if medical complications are suspected.

By the end of the first consultation, the doctor should be in a position to make a preliminary diagnosis. In most cases, a further appointment should be arranged to complete the assessment. In a small minority, there may be need for urgent referral. The main indications are an extremely low weight, especially if there is also rapid weight loss (more than a kilogram a week), and severe depression with suicidal ideation. Symptoms suggestive of electrolyte disturbance or hypoglycaemia also necessitate prompt attention.

### Physical investigations

A wide variety of haematological and biochemical abnormalities may be present (see below), but few are of relevance to management and most will resolve with resumption of healthy eating habits and weight gain. Despite this, it is sometimes argued that in cases of anorexia nervosa a baseline full blood

---

### Box 15.4 **Recommended physical investigations**

**Anorexia nervosa**

- Routine full blood count and biochemical profile
- ECG if BMI <15 to look for QT prolongation
- Consider bone densitometry scan
- Urgent blood glucose and electrolytes if symptomatic (e.g. dizzy spells or syncope) or frequent vomiting or laxative misuse

**Bulimia nervosa**

- Electrolytes should be monitored if vomiting is frequent or there is severe misuse of laxatives or diuretics

count and biochemical profile should be obtained (Box 15.4). Irrespective of the eating disorder diagnosis, if medical complications are suspected, investigation is indicated.

## Features of anorexia nervosa

### Psychological problems

Women with anorexia nervosa have a 'morbid fear of fatness'. They feel fat even though they are emaciated. The psychological effects of starvation include depressed mood, irritability, poor concentration, loss of libido, preoccupation with food, obsessional rituals, and social withdrawal. These symptoms usually improve with weight regain and are resistant to treatment with antidepressant drugs.

### Gastrointestinal symptoms

Constipation, bloating, and abdominal pain are all common complaints, due partly to delay in gastric and whole gut transit times.

### Amenorrhoea and infertility

Amenorrhoea of at least 3 months' duration remains a mandatory diagnostic criterion for anorexia nervosa, although its utility is questioned. Prepubertal levels of LH and FSH lead to hypogonadotrophic hypogonadism. In prepubertal girls this may result in failure of breast development and growth retardation. Menses and secondary sexual characteristics return with weight restoration, though full potential height may not be achieved. Spontaneous return of menstruation occurs early in some patients but in others can be delayed for months after full weight restoration.

### Muscle weakness

Patients of very low weight may complain of tiredness and muscle weakness with particular difficulty climbing stairs. A specific myopathy primarily affecting the proximal muscles of the legs is now recognized. A useful test to reveal this problem is to ask the patient to squat down on her haunches and then rise again to an upright position without using her arms as levers. Inability to perform this 'squat test' is a sign of significant myopathy (McLoughlin *et al.* 1998). In this state, the patient is at significant risk of collapse.

### Cardiovascular symptoms

Sinus bradycardia, hypotension, and mottled, cold extremities are common and may be associated with dizziness and syncope. They reflect physiological adaptation to the starved state and do not require specific treatment. Cardiac conduction defects, especially prolongation of the QT interval, can occur, usually in patients with electrolyte imbalance. They are of concern since they have been linked with ventricular arrhythmias and sudden death. For this reason, a routine ECG is indicated in all patients with a BMI less than 15 and if conduction abnormalities are present, a cardiological opinion should be sought.

## Haematological features

A mild normochromic normocytic anaemia, mild leucopenia with relative lymphocytosis, low platelet count, and low ESR are common findings. These findings are due to bone marrow suppression secondary to starvation and do not respond to treatment with iron or vitamin supplements. They resolve spontaneously with weight gain. There is no increased susceptibility to infection.

## Thyroid function

T4 levels are in the low-normal range whereas T3 levels are depressed and TSH levels are normal. These changes are seen in other starvation states and are presumably a means of conserving energy. There may be clinical signs of hypothyroidism, with dry skin, hypothermia, bradycardia, constipation, and delayed relaxation of deep tendon reflexes. Treatment with thyroxine is not indicated.

## Hypercholesterolaemia

This is present in up to 50% of patients with anorexia nervosa and is thought to be clinically insignificant.

## Liver function tests

Low weight can, rarely, cause hepatic damage. However, abnormal liver function tests should always raise the possibility of co-morbid illness such as alcohol abuse.

## Blood glucose

Blood glucose may fall with low weight but is generally asymptomatic even in the 40–60 mg/dl range. It can be a bad prognostic sign in anorexia nervosa because it indicates depleted hepatic glycogen and glucose stores.

## Electrolyte disturbances

Most patients with anorexia nervosa have remarkably normal electrolytes, albumin, and protein levels. In the minority who frequently vomit or misuse laxatives/diuretics regularly, electrolyte disturbances may be present. Hypokalaemia is particularly worrying as this may, rarely, lead to serious cardiac arrhythmias.

## Peripheral oedema

Oedema may be a manifestation of fluid and electrolyte disturbance in anorexia nervosa. The mechanism is often unclear since oedema is a regular feature of malnutrition in general (famine oedema). It can complicate the management of anorexia nervosa by making the assessment of true body weight difficult. Acute oedema can also occur during the early stages of refeeding, particularly in patients who abuse laxatives. Patients often find this very distressing and they should be forewarned about it.

## Osteoporosis

Patients with anorexia nervosa of 6 months' duration or longer may have some degree of osteopenia and fractures have been reported in patients who have been amenorrhoeic for only a year. Osteoporosis and stunting of growth are serious and possibly irreversible consequences of the disorder. Adolescents with anorexia nervosa may fail to reach their potential peak bone density, putting them at increased risk of osteoporosis in later life. The pathogenesis of osteoporosis in anorexia nervosa is not completely understood and may result from a number of mechanisms, including oestrogen deficiency, raised cortisol levels, inadequate vitamin and calcium intake, and nutritional effects on bone formation (Zipfel *et al.* 2000). The degree of bone loss seen in anorexia nervosa is more severe than in other low oestrogen states. Recent studies have shown that in the majority of patients with anorexia nervosa, osteopenia is resistant to treatment with oestrogens (in the form of hormone replacement therapy or the contraceptive pill), in contrast to the situation in postmenopausal women.

The best treatment for these patients is refeeding to achieve a healthy weight and nutritional state and the resumption of regular menstruation. Calcium supplements (1000–1500 mg/day) are often recommended for females with anorexia nervosa with a daily multivitamin containing 400 IU of vitamin D. Antiresorptive treatments used to reduce bone loss in postmenopausal women, such as the bisphosphonates, are not generally recommended: they may be ineffective in patients with anorexia nervosa and their long-term side effects are unknown. Patients with a long-standing very low weight may benefit to some degree from hormone replacement therapy. The role of bone density scans is limited but they may motivate some patients to change their behaviour.

## Neurological problems

A number of studies using various imaging techniques have demonstrated changes in brain anatomy in anorexia nervosa (Ellison and Foong 1998). The most consistent findings are of apparent cerebral atrophy with ventricular enlargement and sulcal widening. Their clinical significance is uncertain.

Peripheral neuropathy may occur in anorexia nervosa and it is postulated that this may be the result of thiamine deficiency. Korsakoff's psychosis and Wernicke's encephalopathy have been reported only rarely in anorexia nervosa. An argument in favour of routine supplementation with thiamine in severe anorexia nervosa can be made as milder forms of cognitive impairment may be related to thiamine deficiency.

# Features of bulimia nervosa

## Psychological problems

Bulimia nervosa has a profound effect on people's psychological well-being and the vast majority of sufferers will have some symptoms of depression and anxiety. Low self-esteem and feelings of guilt, helplessness, failure, and self-loathing are extremely common. Some may feel desperate at times and are driven to attempting suicide. Others resort to self-inflicted injury (e.g. cutting their skin) as a way of releasing tension. In the majority of cases the depression is secondary to the loss of control over eating and resolves as the frequency of binge eating declines. It is therefore generally best to defer using antidepressant drugs. The alcohol and drug abuse that is seen among some patients who binge eat can sometimes be managed in tandem with the eating disorder but this requires specialist expertise.

## Gastrointestinal symptoms

Constipation is common due to dehydration and laxative misuse. Patients may also get intermittent abdominal pain. Rarely, chronic stimulant laxative misuse can cause permanent damage to colonic innervation.

## Menstrual disturbances

Menstrual irregularities are common: in a recent study of 173 women with bulimia nervosa, 58% reported irregular menses and 5% reported secondary amenorrhoea (Crow *et al.* 2002). The amenorrhoea appears to be related to the weight control behaviours rather than to loss of body fat. With recovery from the eating disorder, ovulation and menstruation return. Bulimia nervosa appears to have little impact on the later ability to achieve pregnancy.

### Fluid and electrolyte disturbances

Vomiting and laxative or diuretic misuse lead to fluid loss and dehydration. Most electrolyte disturbances are mild and asymptomatic. The commonest abnormalities are an elevated serum bicarbonate (metabolic alkalosis), hypokalaemia, and hyponatraemia. In patients taking large amounts of laxatives, there can be excessive loss of bicarbonate in the diarrhoea, leading to a metabolic acidosis. The symptoms of electrolyte imbalance are non-specific and vague, including thirst, dizziness, lethargy, fluid retention, muscle twitches, and spasms. Cardiac arrhythmias secondary to severe hypokalaemia are rare, but potentially dangerous. For this reason it is important to monitor electrolytes in these patients.

Treatment of metabolic alkalosis and hypokalaemia requires replacement of total body potassium. This can be difficult if there is coexisting dehydration causing hyperaldosteronism; hospital admission for intravenous saline infusion is very occasionally required. Some people who vomit or abuse laxatives over years tolerate a degree of hypokalaemia that would be alarming if discovered in others. For example, some patients with chronic bulimia nerovsa may have levels of serum potassium as low as 2.4 mmol for months without apparent adverse effects. Rapid intravenous correction of fluid and electrolyte imbalance in these patients can be hazardous. In these patients and in some milder cases of hypokalaemia, it may be more appropriate to prescribe oral potassium supplements in the short term. However, the emphasis should be on stopping the vomiting to allow the body's homeostatic mechanisms to correct the imbalance, rather than providing a long-term electrolyte replacement which could serve to reinforce the abnormal behaviour.

## Social circumstances

The patient's social circumstances should always be assessed. They may well be contributing to the persistence of the eating disorder and they may also be relevant to its treatment. Underweight patients tend to withdraw socially and become isolated, and among those patients still at home relationships within the family may be strained. Patients with bulimia nervosa tend to be less isolated, but relationship difficulties are common and may impinge on the eating disorder.

## Aetiology

### Cultural pressures

In Western societies today, thinness in women is seen as the ideal in terms of health, success, and sexual attractiveness. Women are encouraged by the media to pursue the perfect body through special diets and exercise programmes. Cosmetic surgery is available to improve appearance. The inference is that anybody can have the perfect shape if they exercise and restrict their food intake sufficiently. In fact, genetic factors play a large part in body shape and weight, and the body cannot be 'shaped' at will (Brownell 1991).

The exercise and weight loss needed to attain the aesthetic ideal are far in excess of what is recommended for healthy living. Models exercise as many as 35 hours a week in order to keep 'in shape'. It is not surprising that most women fail to achieve these goals; but many judge themselves unfavourably as a consequence. Adolescent girls are particularly susceptible to these pressures with lower self-esteem among girls who regard themselves as unattractive.

Despite the great pressure to diet, only a small proportion of women develop full eating disorders. Genetic, psychological, and family factors may all influence the development of an eating problem. There is evidence to suggest that eating disorders increase in prevalence in rapidly developing countries as they take on the cultural values of the West, and that when immigrants move from less industrialized to more industrialized countries they are more likely to develop eating disorders. Eating disorders are known to occur more frequently among people in certain occupations, e.g. ballet dancers, models, athletes, in which the need to conform to a certain body shape is heightened.

Eating disorders are far commoner in females than males (approximately 10 to 1). This sex difference can be explained by the disproportionate cultural pressure on women to be thin.

## Personality traits

Women with anorexia nervosa tend to be unusually compliant and conscientious as children. They are often shy and solitary, emotionally restrained and tend to be performance-orientated. These traits seem to be the precursors of low self-esteem and perfectionism seen in anorexia nervosa sufferers.

People with bulimia nervosa tend to be very similar to those with anorexia nervosa – indeed, about a quarter have had anorexia nervosa in the past. They too tend to have been self-critical and perfectionist as children. What differentiates them from future anorectics is the high frequency of childhood obesity, early menarche, and critical comments about shape, all of which are likely to sensitize them to their appearance. A small subgroup appear to be prone to misuse alcohol or drugs, and there is a raised rate of substance abuse in their families.

## Environmental and genetic factors

Several published studies have shown that eating disorders appear to run in families. This could be due to inherited factors and/or to environmental influences. Twin studies in which the concordance for eating disorders in monozygotic and dizygotic twin pairs are compared, have shown the concordance rates for both anorexia nervosa and bulimia nervosa to be substantially greater for the monozygotic twins (Kendler *et al.* 1991; Strober 1992), indicating that genetic factors contribute to aetiology. What is inherited is uncertain but it appears to be a vulnerability to all forms of eating disorder rather than specifically to anorexia nervosa or bulimia nervosa.

There is also evidence to suggest that mothers with eating disorders have an effect on their children's eating habits. In Stein's controlled study (Stein *et al.* 1994) of 1-year-old children of mothers with eating disorders, the mothers were observed to be more critical of their children and there was more conflict during meal times than in the controls. The mothers were more reluctant to let the infants feed themselves, concerned that the children would make a 'mess'. The children tended to weigh less than controls, and children's weight was inversely correlated to their mother's concern about her own body image. Pike and Rodin (1991) compared the mothers of daughters with disturbed eating with a control group. The mothers differed from controls in that they had more disturbed eating themselves, they thought their daughters should lose more weight, and they were more critical of their daughter's appearance.

## Psychiatric disorders within the family

There are now considerable data showing that relatives of patients with eating disorders have a higher incidence of clinical depression. The reason for this is unclear; the results of family co-morbidity studies have been inconsistent.

How genes may contribute to the development of eating disorders remains speculative, but possible explanations include their influence on personality traits and behaviour regulation.

# Course and outcome

### Anorexia nervosa

Follow-up data on patients with anorexia nervosa are largely limited to cases treated in highly specialist centres. Such data are subject to selection bias and should be interpreted with caution. The results of 68 outcome studies of 3104 patients showed that, on average, more than 40% of cases recover, one-third improve, and 20% have a chronic course (Steinhausen *et al.* 1991). The mortality rate of anorexia nervosa is amongst the highest for psychiatric disorder and around half of these deaths are from physical causes rather than suicide (Sullivan 1995). The standardized mortality ratio (over 6–12 years) is 9.5. Early age of onset (though not childhood onset), short duration of illness, and early treatment are good prognostic factors. Profound weight loss and long duration of illness carry a bad prognosis. It is difficult to give an individual patient an accurate prognosis.

## Bulimia nervosa

Bulimia nervosa tends to run a chronic course in the absence of treatment. With the most effective treatment, cognitive behaviour therapy, up to 50% make a full and apparently lasting recovery. The remainder range between much improved to not improved at all. It has proved impossible to identify reliable predictors of outcome although there is emerging evidence that premorbid obesity is associated with a worse long-term prognosis. Conversion to anorexia nervosa is unusual. The mortality rate does not appear to be raised.

# Management

## Education and engagement

This is an important initial step irrespective of the eating disorder diagnosis. In anorexia nervosa, patients need to accept that they have a recognized problem that requires professional help. This can takes some weeks and requires sensitivity on the part of the doctor. With all eating disorders, education serves to counter misconceptions about eating and weight as well as provide information about the eating disorder.

Education may be sufficient treatment in itself in helping some patients with milder binge eating problems. Olmsted and colleagues in Toronto (1991) studied the effectiveness of a group educational programme for women with bulimia nervosa, providing educational material and advice on how to overcome the disorder, but no personal guidance or support. The effects of the programme were compared with individual cognitive behaviour therapy (CBT). The two treatments were found to be equally effective, except for those people with more severe bulimia nervosa who did better with CBT.

Reliable educational information may be obtained from various sources including national eating disorder organizations, certain books for the general public and a number of websites (see section on useful information for patients at end of chapter). Indiscriminate recommendation of the Internet is not advisable as there are websites that actively promote eating disorders (Shafran 2001).

## Drug treatments

There is no current evidence to support the use of any drug for anorexia nervosa. In particular, trials of antipsychotic drugs, tricyclic antidepressant drugs, and of lithium have shown no clinically significant benefit in anorexia nervosa.

### Antidepressant drugs in bulimia nervosa

There is some evidence to support the use of antidepressant drugs in bulimia nervosa, though the longer-term benefit of these drugs has barely been studied. The available data suggest that non-compliance and relapse are common. A series of short-term, double-blind, placebo-controlled trials using a range of different antidepressant drugs, have shown that drugs are superior to placebo in terms of reduction of binge frequency (by 50–60% within a few weeks of starting treatment), and this is accompanied by a general improvement in mood and decreased preoccupation with shape and weight. The drug effect occurs irrespective of whether or not the patient is clinically depressed, and this suggests that antidepressant drugs may have a specific 'antibulimic' effect unrelated to their effect on mood. This finding is further supported by a study of almost 400 patients in which fluoxetine at a dose of 60 mg a day, but not at 20 mg a day, was superior to placebo in treating bulimia nervosa (Fluoxetine Bulimia Nervosa Collaboration Study Group 1992). The therapeutic dose for treating clinical depression is 20 mg, so this reinforces the idea of a separate antibulimic effect of fluoxetine, which is only apparent at high dose.

Psychological treatments are more effective in the treatment of bulimia nervosa than antidepressant medication. However, there may be a place for the concurrent use of antidepressants in patients who are failing to respond adequately to good psychological therapy, and in patients who have a severe depressive illness independent of the eating disorder. At present, fluoxetine at a dose of 60 mg daily is the drug of choice in these situations.

### Vitamin and mineral supplements

Many patients with anorexia nervosa worry about the effects of their illness on their long-term physical health. They may take vitamin and mineral

supplements in the hope that these will make up for any nutritional deficiencies. However, there is little evidence of vitamin deficiency in most cases.
Thiamine (vitamin B1) deficiency is perhaps the most relevant as this can
cause neurological and neuropsychiatric complications (see page 000).
Taking vitamin supplements in normal doses probably does no harm though
it should be emphasized that resumption of a healthy balanced diet remains
the best remedy. Calcium supplements with vitamin D are sometimes
recommended, though they will not prevent osteoporosis from developing
(see page 530).

## Treatment of anorexia nervosa

Anorexia nervosa is a serious, potentially life-threatening disorder and requires
effective intervention as early as possible in order to minimize psychological,
social, and physical repercussions. The younger the patient, the more pressing
the need. Family therapy, parental counselling, and individual therapy all have
their place and there may be a need for a period of in-patient treatment.
Treatment is likely to be prolonged and intensive and early referral for specialist help is generally indicated.

### The role of the GP

The GP has an important role in helping patients accept the need for specialist referral and is in a good position to provide ongoing support for the
family. Young patients (under 18 years) who are not severely underweight
and have a short history (less than a year) have a relatively good prognosis.
With this group it is reasonable to have a trial of management in primary
care so long as there are not major family tensions. Management involves
both the patient and the family, requiring a combination of education,
support, and common sense nutritional advice. It is important to reassure
parents that they are not to blame, since guilt is common and unhelpful.
Patients generally need to be seen weekly at first to maintain their motivation
and have their weight monitored. Only if there is definite progress (in terms
of weight regain) should this form of management be continued for longer
than a few months. Otherwise referral for specialist treatment is indicated.
Often there is a waiting list for such treatment, in which case the GP will
need to support the patient and family in the interim while monitoring the
patient's clinical state.

The GP will also have responsibility for patients who refuse treatment. With
patients whose clinical state is stable and not life threatening, the goal should
be to help them accept treatment while providing support. With patients

whose health is seriously compromised, specialist advice should be sought and the Mental Health Act may need to be invoked.

## Specialist treatments

Treatment may take place as an in-patient, a day patient, or an out-patient. As things stand, good research evidence is lacking on which to base treatment for anorexia nervosa. Recovery involves regaining a healthy weight and a pattern of eating to sustain it. There also needs to be a psychological change to address the specific psychopathology of the disorder. Thirdly, patients need to be able to get on with their life in a positive way once they have recovered to reduce the risk of relapse.

### In-patient treatment (Box 15.5)

In-patient treatment has huge cost implications and if weight is to be fully restored before discharge it may require an admission of many months. Compulsory admission should be avoided if at all possible. When a sufferer is severely ill physically, she may feel she has little choice other than admission. The best circumstances for in-patient treatment are where the patient is well-motivated to change but cannot manage it alone. The usual problem is that she cannot bring herself to eat enough to gain weight.

In the past, most in-patient regimes were based on a strict behavioural approach. Access to various rewarding experiences were contingent on regular eating and weight gain. In-patient regimes tend to be more lenient nowadays,

---

### Box 15.5 **Indications for in-patient treatment**

- Very low body weight, e.g. BMI <13.5, or if weight loss has been very rapid, e.g. >1 kg per week. (What counts as very low weight is to some degree a matter of judgement. A stable low weight is less worrying than a rapidly declining weight)

- Serious physical complications (e.g. severe electrolyte disturbances, hypoglycaemia,) or significant suicide risk

- The patient or her carers feel out of control and request admission. Admission can serve to separate patient from main carers, allowing problems to be tackled in a different way

- Lack of response to out-patient treatment

- Severe behavioural disturbance

the aim being to create a secure, supportive atmosphere with agreed rules and goals for recovery. A typical approach would be to fix a target weight corresponding to a BMI of 20 on admission. The patient agrees to eat regular meals (a normal mixed diet) and the diet is titrated to produce an average weight gain of about 1 kg per week. Initially, nasogastric feeding may be an option if there are problems with food ingestion. Once the target BMI has been achieved, there is a weight stabilization phase. The transition from in-patient to out-patient care can be stressful for many patients and continuity of care is important with regular follow-up sessions.

### Family therapy

There is evidence to support family therapy as an effective treatment for anorexia nervosa in adolescence (Dare *et al.* 1990). The Maudsley group has gone on to evaluate 'family counselling', where the patient and her family are seen separately rather than together. Preliminary results suggest that this new treatment is as effective as conventional family therapy (Dare and Eisler 1995).

Family therapy used to be based on the hypothesis that eating disorders originate from a specific pathological pattern of family structure and functioning, and that they should be treated by tackling these causative factors within the family. However, research data point away from a family aetiological model that puts the 'blame' very much with the family. Instead the differences between eating disorder families and control families appear to be more to do with the secondary pressures of severe or chronic illness within the family than with a primary distinctive dysfunctional family (Le Grange *et al.* 1992). This model may also be more helpful as it shifts the blame away from the family and enables all family members to consider themselves as a resource for effective treatment.

## Management of long-standing anorexia nervosa

The needs of patients with long-standing anorexia nervosa are often neglected. No patient should be written off as having no chance of recovery; however, some are unlikely to benefit from repeated attempts at weight restoration in hospital unless they decide themselves that they want to change. Chronic sufferers are likely to have significant associated problems, both physical and mental. It should be remembered that anorexia nervosa has a high mortality rate and half the deaths are due to suicide. These patients need a supportive, long-term relationship with a clinician; often the GP is in the best position to provide this. They may need encouragement to make the most of their life within the confines of their eating disorder.

## Treatment of bulimia nervosa

### Cognitive behaviour therapy (CBT)

Unlike the situation for anorexia nervosa, a number of psychotherapeutic treatments for bulimia nervosa have been evaluated and shown to be of benefit (Box 15.6). A specific variant of CBT for bulimia nervosa is now considered to be the 'gold standard' treatment for the disorder (Fairburn 1981). It has been evaluated in over 40 randomized controlled trials and shown to be more effective than a variety of other treatments, including antidepressant drugs, behavioural therapy, and supportive psychotherapy (Fairburn *et al.* 1992a; Wilson and Fairburn 1993). For at least two-thirds of patients, individual CBT produced a substantial improvement in the frequency of binge eating and purging, with a third to half of patients stopping

---

### Box 15.6 **The core elements of cognitive behaviour therapy**

**Stage One**

- Educating the patient about bulimia nervosa and explaining the cognitive rationale for the treatment
- Recording in detail all eating, vomiting, and laxative misuse at the time that it occurs, together with relevant thoughts and feelings
- Introducing a pattern of regular eating, thereby displacing many binges
- Using alternative behaviour to help resist urges to binge
- Educating patients about the ineffectiveness of strict dieting, self-induced vomiting and laxative misuse, and informing them about their adverse effects

**Stage Two**

- Introducing avoided foods into the diet and gradually eliminating other forms of strict dieting
- Addressing the overevaluation of shape and weight and its various expressions

**Stage Three**

- Planning for the future, including having realistic expectations and strategies for use should problems recur

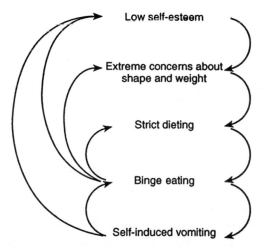

**Fig 15.2** Cognitive view of maintenance of bulimia nervosa.

binge eating altogether. Concerns about shape and weight are also reduced. Follow-up studies (up to 6 years post-treatment) suggest that changes are well maintained and that relapse is uncommon.

The treatment is based on a model of the maintenance of bulimia nervosa which proposes a series of interlocking vicious circles between low self-esteem, beliefs about the importance of body shape and weight, dieting, binge eating, and vomiting. The full treatment is described in detail in a therapist's manual (Fairburn *et al.* 1993a) and is delivered by a specialist therapist in about 15–20 50-minute sessions over 4–5 months.

## Interpersonal psychotherapy (IPT)

This is a form of short-term psychotherapy originally developed to treat depression (Klerman *et al.* 1984). It focuses on current interpersonal problems and does not attempt to tackle eating difficulties directly. There have been two studies to evaluate interpersonal psychotherapy for bulimia nervosa (Fairburn *et al.* 1993a, 1995; Agras *et al.* 1999). When compared with CBT, IPT was not as effective in the short term, but there were delayed benefits so that by 1- and 6-year follow-up IPT was found to be as effective as CBT. IPT may reap its effects by improving life circumstances, relationships, self esteem, and thereby the eating disorder.

## Treating bulimia nervosa and other binge eating problems in primary care

It has been estimated that up to 4% of young women in the UK have significant binge eating problems. Many of these women are not in treatment, and if more women did come forward for help the psychiatric services would not be able to cope with a problem on this scale. In any case, young people are often reluctant to see a psychiatrist because of the stigma attached. Full psychological treatment is costly and time-consuming. Treatment in primary care may be less threatening and easier in practical terms and therefore more attractive to women.

There is a mounting body of evidence that patients with binge eating problems may respond to simple self-help interventions suitable for delivery in primary care (Wilson *et al.* 2000). Several valuable self-help books have been published (see end of chapter for useful information for patients). They are now available as paperbacks for around £10 in most bookshops in the UK or via the Internet. All provide detailed, relevant information about eating disorders and their physical and psychological effects and two provide a highly structured, step-by-step treatment programme based on CBT.

The books may be used either by patients on their own (pure self-help) or with guidance from a non-specialist therapist such as the GP (guided self-help). If the GP is recommending that the patient treats herself, it is good practice to arrange a review appointment 2–4 weeks later to assess her compliance and progress. If she has not benefited by this time, she is unlikely to do so. The advantage of 'pure self-help' is that the sufferer can treat herself without involving anyone else, and this may appeal to her if she wants to keep her eating problem a secret. However, 'pure self-help' needs great motivation and commitment, and for many women the encouragement and support offered with 'guided self-help' improves compliance.

Guided self-help generally involves six to eight 20-minute sessions over 2–3 months, the first few being weekly. Again, if the patient has not responded by this point, she is unlikely to do so. The therapist needs to be familiar with the structure of the self-help book, but no specialist training is required and it can be provided by any interested member of the primary health care team (e.g. GP, practice nurse, health visitor, practice counsellor, or community dietitian). Each session has a similar format. The patient keeps detailed monitoring sheets (eating diaries, see Fig 15.3) and these are reviewed together during the sessions. Problems and possible solutions are discussed, drawing on the advice given in the programme. The therapist helps the patient to set the pace through the programme, provides praise and encouragement as the patient progresses, and helps with difficulties as they arise. The therapist may also need to keep the patient focused on the eating problem rather than being distracted by other difficulties. The sessions can be largely patient-led.

Some of the self-help books have been formally evaluated (Treasure *et al.* 1994; Cooper *et al.* 1996; Carter and Fairburn 1998; Wilson *et al.* 2000). The

Day... *Thursday*...... Date... *7th July*......

| Time | Food and drink consumed | Place | ★ | V/L | Context and comments |
|------|------------------------|-------|---|-----|---------------------|
| 7.45 | Black coffee<br>Yoghurt | kitchen | | | Didn't feel hungry but made myself eat this for breakfast as must keep to regular meal plan. |
| 11 am | Black coffee | office | | | |
| 1 pm | Rivita x2 with cottage cheese<br>Yoghurt<br>Black coffee | office | | | Ate lunch as planned. Pleased to be in control tempted to eat more – but resisted urge to go to canteen |
| 4.30 | Black tea<br>Apple | office | | | |
| 5.15 | Chocolate biscuits x3 | office | ★ | | friend offered me a biscuit – felt guilty as soon as I'd taken it. Then ate another 2 |
| 5.35 | Iced buns x2<br>Apple turnover | on the way home | ★<br>★ | | went into bakery<br>out of control |
| 5.50 | 2 bowls muesli with milk<br>6 slices bread/butter | kitchen | ★<br>★ | V | raided the cupboard as soon as I get home – couldn't stop.<br>HATE myself |
| 6.30 | | | | | went to gym to work out 11/2 hrs. |
| 9 pm | Baked potato<br>1/2 tin baked beans | kitchen | | | Ate supper with boyfriend. Cooked him cornish pastry as well. |
| 10 pm | 1 glass wine | pub | | | Refused peanuts when offered – good. |
| 11.30 | | | | | went to bed – fed up by binge, but pleased I managed to regain control after this. |

**Fig 15.3** A typical monitoring sheet for use in conjunction with overcoming binge eating. Asterisks signify eating viewed by the person as excessive. V/L means vomiting or laxative use.

evidence to date suggests that following a cognitive behavioural self-help programme can be helpful and is a useful first step in the management of binge eating problems. However, not all patients are suitable for this approach. Severe or complicated cases are unlikely to benefit and early referral is indicated (see Box 15.7).

## Treatment of atypical eating disorders

Although the atypical eating disorders are at least as common as anorexia nervosa and bulimia nervosa, there has been virtually no research on their

---

Box 15.7 **Indications for specialist referral for patients with binge eating problems**

- ◆ Low weight (BMI less than18)
- ◆ Alcohol or drug misuse
- ◆ Severe depressive symptoms
- ◆ Previous treatment failure
- ◆ High level of behavioural disturbance (frequent binge eating, vomiting or laxative misuse)

---

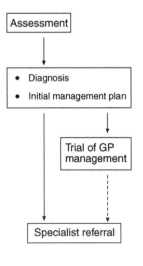

Assessment
- • History and mental state examination to establish diagnosis; and, if indicated, physical evaluation to assess medical complications

- • Diagnosis
- • Initial management plan
  - • AN, BN or an atypical eating disorder; or no eating disorder
  - • Specialist referral or trail of GP management

Trial of GP management
- • AN (young cases with a short history; not severely underweight) – education with nutritional advice; support for patient; involvement of family
- • BN (many cases) – guided or pure self-help
- • Atypical cases – manages as above if resemble AN or BN

Specialist referral
- • AN – refer most cases
- • BN – refer those with high frequence of binge eating or vomiting; low weight; severe depression or substance abuse; prior failure of specialist treatment; or failure of trial of GP management
- • Atypical cases – refer those not suitable for management in primary care, and those who do not benefit

**Fig 15.4** A management scheme for eating disorders.

treatment. Most can be viewed as variants of anorexia nervosa or bulimia nervosa and can be managed along similar lines (Fig 15.4). Thus patients who binge eat and are not underweight can be managed as if they have bulimia nervosa, whilst those who are underweight but are menstruating can be treated as if they have anorexia nervosa. Some atypical eating disorders defy classification in this way and their management is a matter of clinical judgement. If the disorder is severe, the patient should be referred for specialist treatment.

## Frequently asked questions

### Can you help me to stop bingeing?

Bear in mind that the sufferer may well have plucked up courage to come and see you for help and may be very ashamed of her binges. The GP needs to handle the consultation carefully to win her confidence, offering constructive help. The consultation should follow the model outlined below (see 10-minute consultation: binge eating).

### Can you help me to lose weight?

If the patient is not overweight, then this request should raise the possibility of an underlying eating disorder. A careful history should make the diagnosis clear. If the patient has anorexia nervosa, then clearly further weight loss is not in her best interests. If she has a binge eating problem, then attempts at dieting are likely to trigger further binges. In either case, she needs further assessment and to be offered help for her eating disorder.

### Will I ever be able to eat normally again? Now that I have recovered can I go on a diet?

This is a common question in people who have recovered from an eating disorder. Typically, whilst it is possible to eat a wide variety of normal foods without anxiety or restraint, most people are still very aware of what they eat and how potentially 'fattening' it is. Dieting is their Achilles' heel – if they attempt to diet, then there is a risk that the eating disorder will recur.

### Does dieting cause eating disorders?

It is clear that dieting precedes the development of anorexia nervosa and bulimia nervosa in young women, and epidemiological data support this. Patients with bulimia nervosa nearly always report that their binge eating first started when they were on a diet. Eating disorders are more common in occupations and sports where a low body weight is required. There is a correlation between cultural pressure to be thin and prevalence of eating disorders, both across and within ethnic groups.

Cultural pressures in the West are such that most young women diet at some time or other. Yet lifetime prevalence of bulimia nervosa is 1.5–2%. Some other factors must interact with dieting in susceptible subjects in order to precipitate eating disorders. Probable risk factors include certain personality traits (low self-esteem and perfectionism), vulnerability to obesity, genetic susceptibility, and family influences (see pages 533–4).

### Is binge eating an addiction?

Terms like 'compulsive overeating', 'food addicts', and 'carbohydrate craving' have become popular and suggest that binge eating is a form of addiction similar to alcohol or drug addiction. The self-help organization Overeaters Anonymous (OA) models its approach on Alcoholics Anonymous and believes that certain foods, such as sugar, have addictive potential in susceptible individuals. OA argues that the only way to deal with the addiction is by life-long avoidance of such 'toxic' foods.

In the case of bulimia nervosa, the sufferer is continually trying to restrict her food intake. Binge eating represents a loss of control and carries the risk of weight gain. By contrast, 'alcoholics' have no inherent drive to restrict alcohol intake. They show no fear of getting drunk and do not have equivalent cognitive characteristics, which interact in bulimia nervosa to maintain the disorder (see page 541). It follows that the treatment of alcohol and drug dependence is based on increasing self-restraint and abstinence, whereas the key to treating bulimia nervosa is stopping dieting (Vandereycken 1990).

## 10-Minute consultation: binge eating

A young woman has been binge eating for 6 months. She looks about normal weight, but she says she feels too fat. She is desperate for help to regain control of her eating.

### What issues you should cover

- *Ask about current methods of weight control.* Is she dieting at the moment? Does she make herself sick after eating? If so, how often? Does she take laxatives or diuretics to lose weight? How much exercise does she do? Is this extreme?

- *Ask about her attitude to her shape and weight.* Is she happy with her shape and weight? Would she like to be thinner? How important are her shape and weight to her? Is anything more important to her?

- *Ask her about her eating habits.* Does she have episodes when she loses control of her eating? What does she eat during a binge? Is it a true binge, i.e. eating, in a discrete period of time, an amount of food that is larger than most people would eat in a similar period under similar circumstances with a sense of lack of control during the episode. How often does she binge?

- *Weight.* Ask her what she weighs (less threatening in a first consultation than weighing her). Calculate her body mass index [weight (kg)/ (height (m)$^2$].

## What you should do

- You should now be able to determine the nature and severity of her eating problem and decide on management.

- If she has a binge eating problem (including bulimia nervosa), she may well respond to a self-help programme, and this can be supervised in primary care. In severe or complicated cases, self-help is unlikely to work. Early referral for more intensive treatment is advised for the following categories: very low weight (body mass index <18); previous treatment failure; alcohol or drug misuse; severe depression or marked suicidal ideation; and high level of behavioural disturbance.

- If self-help is appropriate, suggest she buys a self-help book that includes a treatment programme – available from most bookshops (or via the Internet or by telephone) for about £10. Show her a self-help book if you have one.

- Most books give detailed information about binge eating as well as a step-by-step treatment programme based on cognitive behaviour therapy. This therapy has been shown to be the most effective treatment available for bulimia nervosa in more than 40 randomized controlled trials. Programmes usually take about 12 weeks to complete and need motivation and commitment.

- If she wants to follow a self-help programme, offer to see her every 2 weeks for support and encouragement. Alternatively, this could be done by an interested practice nurse or counsellor, or you could simply arrange to see her again when she has completed the programme.

- Depressive symptoms may resolve without specific treatment as the eating disorder improves, but if they persist 3–4 weeks into the programme, consider prescribing antidepressant drugs and/or referring her to a specialist.

- Studies using written self-help material for the treatment of binge eating suggest that a third to a half of patients recover using this relatively simple and cost-effective intervention, though further research in primary care is needed. If self-help does not work, consider referring the patient to a specialist.

## Useful reading for patients

### Self-help books for binge eating problems

Cooper, P.J. (1995). *Bulimia nervosa and binge eating: a guide to recovery.* Robinson, London.

◆ very similar to 'Overcoming binge eating', but briefer

◆ may be an easier read for poor readers.

Fairburn, C.G. (1995). *Overcoming binge eating.* Guilford Press, New York.

◆ divided into two sections, education and self-help programme

◆ highlights much of the research to date and provides evidence to support the facts

◆ six-step self-help programme, highly structured, emphasis on completing each step before moving on

◆ user friendly both for patient and therapist: structured programme is easy to follow.

Schmidt, U. and Treasure, J. (1993). *Getting better bit(e) by bit(e).* Erlbaum, Hove.

◆ chapters can be read in any order to suit the individual

◆ motivational enhancement-based exercises to address ambivalence about change

◆ easy to read, cartoons and short chapters – not so daunting for poor readers

◆ lack of structure may provide an excuse not to work on problems.

### Educational material for anorexia nervosa sufferers

Bryant-Waugh, R. and Lask, B. (1999). *Eating disorders: a parents' guide.* Penguin, London.

Treasure, J. (1997). *Anorexia nervosa: a survival guide for families, friends and sufferers.* Psychology Press, Hove.

### Other recommended literature on dieting and eating disorders

Abraham, S. and Llewellyn-Jones, D. (1992). *Eating disorders: the facts*, 3rd edn. Oxford University Press, Oxford.

Burns, D.D. (1992). *Feeling good: the new mood therapy.* Avon, New York.

Orbach, S. (1978). *Fat is a feminist issue.* Paddington Press, London.

Rodin, J. (1992). *Body traps.* William Morrow and Company, New York.

# Recommended websites

- Eating Disorders Association: www.edauk.com
- Something Fishy: www.something-fishy.org

# References and further reading

Agras, W.S., Walsh, B.T., Wilson, G.T. and Fairburn, C.G. (1999). A multisite comparison of cognitive behaviour therapy (CBT) and interpersonal therapy (IPT) in the treatment of bulimia nervosa. Paper presented at 4th London International Conference on Eating Disorders, April 1999.

American Psychiatric Association (1994). *Diagnostic and statistical manual of mental disorders*, 4th edn. American Psychiatric Association, Washington, DC.

Brownell, K.D. (1991). Dieting and the search for the perfect body: where physiology and culture collide. *Behaviour Therapy*, **22**, 1–12.

Brownell, K.D. and Fairburn, C.F. (eds) (1995). *Eating disorders and obesity: a comprehensive handbook*. Guilford Press, New York.

Carter, J.C. and Fairburn, C.G. (1995). Treating binge eating problems in primary care. *Addictive Behaviors*, **20**, 765–72.

Carter, J.C. and Fairburn, C.G. (1998). Cognitive-behavioural self-help for binge eating disorder: a controlled effectiveness study. *Journal of Consulting and Clinical Psychology*, **66**, 616–23.

Cooper, P.J. (1995). *Bulimia nervosa and binge eating: a guide to recovery*. Robinson, London.

Cooper, P.J., Coker, S. and Fleming, C. (1996). An evaluation of the efficacy of cognitive behavioural self-help for bulimia nervosa. *Journal of Psychosomatic Research*, **40**, 281–7.

Cowen, P.J., Anderson, I.M. and Fairburn, C.G. (1992). Neurochemical effects of dieting: relevance to changes in eating and affective disorder. In: Anderson, G.H. and Kennedy, S.H. (eds), *The biology of feast and famine: relevance to eating disorders*. Academic Press, New York.

Crow, S.J., Thuras, P., Keel, P. and Mitchell, J. (2002). Long-term menstrual and reproductive function in patients with bulimia nervosa. *American Journal of Psychiatry*, **159**, 1048–50.

Dare, C. and Eisler, I. (1995). Family therapy. In: Garner, D.M and Garfinkel, P.E. (eds), *Handbook of treatment for eating disorders*, 2nd edn. Guilford Press, New York and London.

Dare, C., Eisler, I., Russell, G.F.M. and Szmukler, G.I. (1990). The clinical and theoretical impact of a controlled trial of family therapy in anorexia nervosa. *Journal of Marital and Family Therapy*, **16**, 39–57.

Ellison, Z.R. and Foong, J.(1998). Neuroimaging in eating disorders. In: Hoek, H.W., Treasure, J.L. and Katzman, M.A. (eds), *Neurobiology in the treatment of eating disorders*. John Wiley and Sons, Chichester and New York.

Fairburn, C.G. (1981). A cognitive behavioural approach to the management of bulimia. *Psychological Medicine*, **11**, 707–11.

Fairburn, C.G. (1995). *Overcoming binge eating.* Guilford Press, New York.

Fairburn, C.G. and Belgin, S.J. (1990). Studies of the epidemiology of bulimia nervosa. *American Journal of Psychiatry,* **147,** 401–8.

Fairburn, C.G. and Wilson, G.T. (eds) (1993). *Binge eating: nature, assessment and treatment.* Guilford Press, New York.

Fairburn, C.G., Agras, W.S. and Wilson, G.T.(1992a). The research on the treatment of bulimia nervosa: practical and theoretical implications. In: Anderson G.H. and Kennedy S.H. (eds), *The biology of feast and famine: relevance to eating disorders,* pp. 317–40. Academic Press, San Diego.

Fairburn, C.G., Belgin, S.J. and Davies, B. (1992b). Eating habits and disorders amongst young adult women: an interview-based study. Unpublished manuscript.

Fairburn, C.G., Jones, R., Peveler, R.C., Hope, R.A. and O'Connor, M. (1993a). Psychotherapy and bulimia nervosa: the longer-term effects of interpersonal psychotherapy, behaviour therapy and cognitive-behaviour therapy. *Archives of General Psychiatry,* **50,** 419–28.

Fairburn, C.G., Marcus, M.D. and Wilson, G.T. (1993b). Cognitive-behavioural therapy for binge eating and bulimia nervosa: a comprehensive treatment manual. In: Fairburn C.G.and Wilson G.T. (eds), *Binge eating: nature, assessment and treatment,* pp. 361–404. Guilford Press, New York.

Fairburn, C.G., Norman, P.A., Welch, S.L., O'Connor, M.E., Doll, H.E. and Peveler, R.C. (1995). A prospective study of outcome in bulimia nervosa and the long-term effects of three psychological treatments. *Archives of General Psychiatry,* **52,** 304–12.

Fluoxetine Bulimia Nervosa Collaboration Study Group (1992). Fluoxetine in the treatment of bulimia nervosa: a multicentre, placebo-controlled, double-blind trial. *Archives of Psychiatry,* **49,** 139–47.

Hoek, H.W. (1991). The incidence and prevalence of anorexia nervosa and bulimia nervosa in primary care. *Psychological Medicine,* **21,** 455–60.

Kendler, K.S., MacLean, C., Neale, M., Kessler, R., Heath, A. and Eaves, L. (1991). The genetic epidemiology of bulimia nervosa. *American Journal of Psychiatry,* **148,** 1627–37.

Klerman, G.L., Weissman, M.M., Rounsaville, B.J. and Chevron, E.S. (1984). *Interpersonal psychotherapy of depression.* Basic Books, New York.

Le Grange, D., Eisler, I., Dare, C. and Hodes, M. (1992). Family criticism and self-starvation: a study of expressed emotion. *Journal of Family Therapy,* **14,** 177–92.

Loeb, K.L., Wilson, G.T., Gilbert, J.S. and Labouvie, E. (2000). Guided and unguided self help for binge eating. *Behaviour Research and Therapy,* **38,** 259–72.

McLoughlin, D.M., Spargo, E., Wassif, W.S., *et al.* (1998). Structural and functional changes in skeletal muscle in anorexia nervosa. *Acta Neuropathologica,* **96,** 632–40.

Olmsted, M.P., Davis, R., Garner, D.M., Eagle, M., Rockert, W. and Irvine, M.J. (1991). Efficacy of a brief group psychoeducational intervention for bulimia nervosa. *Behaviour Research and Therapy,* **29,** 71–83.

Palmer, R. (2000). *Helping people with eating disorders. A clinical guide to assessment and treatment.* Wiley, Chichester.

Patton, G.C., Johnson-Sabine, E., Wood, K., Mann, A.H. and Wakeling, A. (1990). Abnormal eating attitudes in London schoolgirls – a prospective epidemiological study: outcome at twelve month follow-up. *Psychological Medicine,* **20,** 383–94.

Pike, K.M. and Rodin, J. (1991). Mothers, daughters and disordered eating. *Journal of Abnormal Psychology*, **100**, 198–204.

Russell, G.F.M. (1979). Bulimia nervosa: an ominous variant of anorexia nervosa. *Psychological Medicine*, **9**, 429–48.

Russell, J. (1995). Treating anorexia nervosa. *British Medical Journal*, **311**, 584.

Shafran, R. (2001). Eating disorders and the Internet. In: Fairburn, C.G. and Brownell, K.D. (eds), *Eating disorders and obesity: a comprehensive handbook*, 2nd edn. Guilford Press, New York.

Stein, A., Woolley, H., Cooper, S.D. and Fairburn, C.F. (1994). An observational study of mothers with eating disorders and their infants. *Journal of Child Psychology and Psychiatry*, **35**, 733–48.

Steinhausen, H.-C., Rauss-Mason, C. and Seidel, R. (1991). Follow up studies of anorexia nervosa: a review of four decades of outcome research. *Psychological Medicine*, **21**, 447–51.

Strober, M. (1992). Family-genetic studies. In: Halmi K. (ed.), *Psychology and treatment of anorexia nervosa and bulimia nervosa*, pp. 61–76. American Psychiatric Press, Washington, DC.

Sullivan, P.F. (1995). Mortality in anorexia nervosa. *American Journal of Psychiatry*, **152**, 1073–4.

Thiels, C., Schmidt, U., Treasure, J., Garthe, R. and Troop, N. (1998). Guided self-change for bulimia nervosa incorporating use of a self-care manual. *American Journal of Psychiatry*, **155**, 947–53.

Treasure, J., Schmidt, U., Troop, N., *et al.* (1994). First step in managing bulimia nervosa: controlled trial of a therapeutic manual. *British Medical Journal*, **308**, 686–9.

Treasure, J., Schmidt, U., Troop, N., Tiller, J., Todd, G. and Turnbull, S. (1996). Sequential treatment for bulimia nervosa incorporating a self-care manual. *British Journal of Psychiatry*, **168**, 94–8.

Turner, M. St J., Foggo, M., Bennie, J., Carroll, S., Dick, H. and Goodwin, G.M. (1991). Psychological, hormonal and biochemical changes following carbohydrate bingeing: a placebo-controlled trial in bulimia nervosa and matched controls. *Psychological Medicine*, **21**, 123–33.

van Hoeken, Lucas, A.R. and Hoek, H.W. (1988). Epidemiology. In: Hoek, H.W., Treasure, J.L. and Katzman, M.A. (eds), *Neurobiology in the treatment of eating disorders*, pp. 97–126. Chichester: Wiley.

Vandereycken, W. (1990). The addiction model in eating disorders: some critical remarks and a selected bibliography. *International Journal of Eating Disorders*, **9**, 95–101.

Wilson, G.T. and Fairburn, C.G. (1993). Cognitive treatments for eating disorders. *Journal of Consulting and Clinical Psychology*, **61**, 261–9.

Wilson, G.T., Vitousek, K.M. and Loeb, K.L. (2000). Stepped care treatment for eating disorders. *Journal of Consulting and Clinical Psychology*, **68**, 564–72.

Zipfel, S., Herzog, W., Beumont, P.J. and Russell, J. (2000). Osteoporosis. *European Eating Disorders Review*, **8**, 108–16

# Chapter 16

# Sexual problems

Margaret Denman

## The mind/body link

When considering sexual problems, it is impossible to make a distinction between the mind and the body. Are sexual desire and pleasure felt in the mind or the body? Likewise is sexual dysfunction in the mind or the body? It is impossible to distinguish in all but the most blatant cases of physical or hormonal dysfunction. Even in these situations there will also be an emotional component and the patient and her partner will have feelings about the difficulty. Likewise, if the initial problem is mental illness, then the manifestation may be a loss of physical function.

Much can be achieved with brief early interventions within the scope of most primary care workers, as well as doctors working in family planning, gynaecology, and genitourinary medicine clinics. Physical causes for a problem need to be eliminated by examination or investigation. There may be indications for referral for specific physical or hormonal treatments, particularly with male patients. Referral for specialist psychiatric help, relationship or psychosexual counselling may be needed after initial assessment if the problems are intransigent.

## Presentation and incidence of sexual problems

### Presentation

Some women will come into the surgery and announce directly that they have a sexual difficulty. Often presentation is more covert and patients will come with a 'calling card', not telling the doctor directly about the real reason for their attendance. Frequent attendees, those patients with thick case notes for no particular reason, and those with vague symptoms, may all be trying to pluck up the courage to tell the doctor or nurse their real difficulty and doctors need to be alerted to an underlying problem. Sexual difficulties may be announced with the 'hand on the door' after a patient has worked her way through a list of trivial symptoms. Consultations such as this are very difficult within the time constraints of the general practice consultation, but it is important that the problem is addressed immediately or a firm follow-up arranged. If this is not done, the 'moment' may be lost. It is also important at the outset to establish whether a patient wants treatment for her problem or whether she has been brought or sent by her partner. If the patient has been 'sent', the prognosis is much worse and she may not even want to engage in any therapy.

## Incidence

As with all human behaviour, sexual difficulty is hard to quantify. There have been many studies assessing the prevalence of sexual difficulty amongst groups attending specialist clinics, but it is difficult to estimate the number of women with a sexual difficulty in the general population. The significance of any dysfunction is also hard to measure. On the one hand, women will report sexual dissatisfaction even if the problem lies primarily with their partner. On the other hand, they may not want treatment for their own difficulty if they do not have a partner or if they have a low sex drive.

A recent study (Dunn *et al.* 1998) in four general practices in England published the results of a postal questionnaire sent to a study population of 4000 men and women. Responses were received from 979 women (with a mean age of 50); 41% of these women reported a current sexual problem. The most widely reported problems were vaginal dryness (186) and infrequent orgasm (166). Of the men, 34% also reported a sexual difficulty. In men the proportion with problems increased with age but there was no such trend with women. Of responders with a sexual problem, 52% said that they would like help with this but only 10% (50) of this group had received such help. There therefore does appear to be a large unmet need within the general practice population. Although doctors are quite used to talking about other intimate areas of life, they often find it difficult to discuss sex.

# What are sexual problems?

## Female problems

The diagnosis of a sexual problem can be difficult as there is often more than one component, e.g. dyspareunia due to a painful gynaecological condition may lead to loss of desire. Alternatively, lack of arousal may lead to lack of lubrication and subsequent superficial dyspareunia. A woman who has extreme vaginismus and in fact non-consummation of her relationship may have no loss of libido and may be orgasmic with non-penetrative sexual activities. Patients may not use medical words to describe their problems and professionals need to understand their complaints and be prepared to use non-medical language when discussing sexual matters.

It is important to establish when a problem started, i.e. is it primary or secondary. Although there is seldom time for a lengthy history, it is worth establishing if sexual function has been better in a previous relationship and why the woman has come to the doctor at this juncture, as these may be crucial factors in the diagnosis and treatment.

## Box 16.1 **Female sexual problems**

| Female sexual problem | Common patient complaint |
| --- | --- |
| Loss of libido | 'Don't feel like it. Gone off sex' |
| Vaginismus | 'There's a block. I'm too small' |
| Dyspareunia | 'It feels sore. It hurts inside' |
| Lack of arousal | 'I don't get turned on. I'm dry' |
| Anorgasmia | 'I can't come' |

## Male problems

Female sexual dysfunction cannot be studied without some understanding of male problems. A woman may complain of loss of libido or lack of orgasm when in fact the problem lies with her male partner. It may not be until close questioning that this is disclosed. Discussion as to what actually happens during sexual activity may elucidate matters. If the woman presents, she is 'the patient', i.e. she is the one complaining. Sometimes after a short time, it becomes obvious that the man may need to be seen himself, but work with the woman can be relayed back to her partner. This is especially relevant if the man refuses to attend, although this in itself is a poor prognostic factor.

## Box 16.2 **Male sexual problems**

| Male sexual problem | Common patient complaint |
| --- | --- |
| Loss of libido | 'Don't feel like it. Gone off sex' |
| Impotence | 'Can't get it up' |
| Premature ejaculation | 'I come too quickly' |
| Non-ejaculation | 'I can't come' |
| Pain on ejaculation | 'It hurts when I come' |
| Pain on penetration | 'It hurts when I go in' |

## Couple problems

Couple therapy is outside the remit of most general practitioners (GPs) and other doctors dealing with women's health in the clinic situation. It is very time consuming and needs specialist skills. Even if not seen, the other member of the couple must be considered and discussed. It may transpire that the problem is primarily within the relationship and referral to an agency such as Relate can then be suggested. If patients are seen as a couple, then observations of their behaviour towards each other in the consulting room can give useful hints regarding the source of the sexual difficulty. These observations can be related back to them.

If they present as a couple, they can be seen together, but often better work is done if they are separated. Once alone with the doctor, the patient can be completely honest and the therapeutic doctor/patient relationship can be employed. Treating both halves of a couple can be difficult if one partner divulges a secrets, e.g. that he is having an affair and has no sexual difficulty with his mistress. Confidentiality is of paramount importance.

## Homosexual problems

Doctors must remember that all patients are not heterosexual. Patients may find their sexuality difficult to disclose to their doctors, especially to their GPs whom they may have known for years. Discussion may be easier in the relative anonymity of the genitourinary clinic. The National Survey of Sexual Behaviour in Britain (Wellings *et al.* 1994a) published figures relating to the prevalence of homosexual activity in men and women between the ages of 16 and 59. This part of the study was done on face-to-face interview and completion of a booklet. Numbers amongst men and women admitting to some homosexual experience were higher in the subsidiary written questionnaires. Overall 6.1% of men and 3.4% of women admitted to having had some homosexual experience. Substantial proportions of those reporting same-sex partners also reported opposite sex partners.

Sexual difficulties in homosexuals may arise from the same fears and phobias, relationship difficulties, life changes, and physical problems as in heterosexuals (Crowley 2001). There are particular problems associated with the break-up of long-term same-sex relationships, which may have been kept secret from friends and family.

## Problems in people without partners

Not all patients with a sexual difficulty have a partner. They may not have a partner because of the problem or they may not wish to have a partner and can be treated as individuals. For example, the initial treatment of vaginismus by examination by the doctor, followed by self-examination and use of tampons, may allow a woman to embark on a relationship. Full success cannot be claimed until penetration is achieved, if this is the aim. Many fulfil their sexual needs by masturbation. Changes in desire or response may occur. This also constitutes a sexual difficulty, sometimes with as much distress for the man or woman as loss of function within a relationship. It is worthy of help and may, especially with men, give them confidence to seek a new partner.

## Causes of sexual problems

There are many causes of sexual difficulty. Whilst it is worth knowing about some of the predisposing factors, a preconceived idea about the aetiology may be misplaced. For example, one woman who had a traumatic delivery with a third-degree tear may find intercourse painful and lose her libido. She may have a residual misconception of damage after all has healed. Another patient with the same presentation may have lost her libido because her husband had an affair whilst she was pregnant. It is impossible with human behaviour to extrapolate from one person to the next. A GP may have previous knowledge of a patient and her family. This is often helpful, but can be a hindrance if it leads to a theory of 'causality'. Sometimes a patient will especially seek out a new doctor or locum in order to talk about what may seem to them to be an embarrassing problem. They may then return to their regular doctor when all is well. When a difficulty is resolved, they may not want to discuss it with the doctor and any enquiry will then seem prurient.

### First – do no harm

Even if all doctors are not equipped to treat sexual difficulties they can at least make sure that they do not produce iatrogenic problems. We need to be careful how we speak to patients. 'Throw away' remarks by careless professionals can be the seed that causes the growth of a fantasy in a patient's mind. Statements to women such as, 'You look tight', or 'Your vagina is loose', or 'You have a nasty erosion', can lead to fantasies about the body and its function. The way in which we examine women is important. Many women have been traumatized by rough speculum examinations, often done when younger, to achieve an unnecessary smear. They may develop fear of vaginal examinations that may spread to their sexual lives.

## Gynaecological problems predisposing to sexual difficulties

Gynaecological problems and interventions may also cause sexual and psycho-sexual difficulties. Dyspareunia may be a symptom of endometriosis, pelvic inflammatory disease, ovarian pathology and other non-gynaecological diseases such as irritable bowel syndrome (see Chapter 11). If no pathology is found and no pain elicited on vaginal examination, then the professional must look elsewhere for the aetiology. Sometimes a physical cause can lead to vagin-ismus even after the initial condition has resolved. Fear of pain can lead to muscle tension – vaginismus – which is itself painful, leading to the belief that there is still something wrong. A simple explanation of the chain of events combined with sensitive examination by the doctor and self-examination by the patient can help to break this vicious circle (Fig 16.1).

## Post-hysterectomy

We regularly ask patients about other aspects of their lifestyle such as exercise, sleep, or hobbies, but neglect to ask them about sex or warn them about the effects of our interventions. If sex has been satisfactory before hysterectomy, it will usually continue to be so afterwards, especially if a cause of discomfort or bleeding has been removed. In a prospective study, 1101 women who under-went hysterectomy were surveyed at 12 months and 24 months (Rhodes *et al.* 1999). The results showed that the percentage of women who engaged in sex-ual activity increased, the rate of dyspareunia and anorgasmia declined, libido increased, and fewer women reported vaginal dryness following hysterectomy.

After hysterectomy some women fantasize about the shape of their bodies and what has actually been removed. Poor knowledge of anatomy and the process of the surgery may lead to misunderstandings. Some women may think that the residual vagina is tight or small, whilst others may think that their vagina is voluminous, stretching up into the abdomen. It is worthwhile asking about sex at the 6-week postoperative check-up and performing an examina-tion if there is any problem. This is another situation in which the encourage-ment of self-examination can help dispel fantasies about the remaining anatomy. Women need to know that intercourse may feel different both for them and their partners, especially if the uterus was enlarged before surgery.

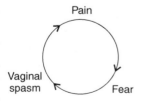

**Fig 16.1** The vicious circle of vaginismus.

Removal of the womb has an emotional component and some women may feel stripped of their femininity. There may be anger about the surgery and feelings that it was perhaps done without due discussion, especially if a woman, whatever her age or parity, has a deep-seated desire for more children. There may also be fears that the organs of sexual pleasure have been removed. Reassurance that this is not the case and that arousal and orgasm are still possible and permissible may be all that is necessary.

## Other gynaecological operations

Women may fear that they will not be able to have sexual intercourse after a vaginal repair. GPs need to establish whether the woman is still sexually active, even if she is very elderly, before referral for surgery, and the woman reassured that penetration will be possible postoperatively. If a woman has had repeated pelvic surgery, e.g. for endometriosis, there may be residual pain from adhesions. This may lead to dyspareunia and even to vaginismus (see Fig 16.1). Women who have been repeatedly examined by doctors may feel that their bodies are no longer their own. Residual pain may also be of an emotional nature and it may be difficult to enable the patient to make the mind/body link. Once again a sensitive genital examination and encouragement of self-examination, whilst being aware of the woman's feelings, are the keys to helping these patients.

Events such as termination of pregnancy, miscarriage, and colposcopy may have deep emotional significance and associated guilt. Relationships may be strained and there may be depression. All these emotional factors, plus the fact that women's bodies have been submitted to examination and manipulation, make these procedures potential danger zones for psychosexual problems.

### Case 1: fantasy of vaginal discharge

I saw Jennifer in my surgery during a routine evening appointment. She was 24 years old, wearing drab, unfashionable clothing. I had seen her before a few years ago when she had come for the oral contraceptive pill. She worked as a book-keeper.

Once in the consulting room she stared at the floor. I asked her what I could do for her. She told me how she had had a vaginal discharge for ages that would not go. I looked at her notes. Three swabs had been taken, all were clear. She had even been sent to the local clinic for sexually transmitted diseases and been given a clean bill of health. Finally, my partner had referred her to a gynaecologist. She had seen the gynaecologist and was on the waiting list for cryosurgery to her cervix. In the meantime she still had this 'awful' discharge, please could I help her. I was puzzled as she had seen the specialist and was due at the hospital soon.

'I had better examine you then,' I said.

She looked horrified but went behind the curtain. I followed to find that she had taken her things off but was lying on the couch with the blanket right up to her neck.

'This must be a horrible job for you doctor,' she said.

'I'm interested that you feel that about it,' I said.

As I went to examine her I could see the disgust on her face. There was no vaginismus and I easily passed a speculum. There was no more than the minimum of physiological discharge. There was a very small ectropion.

'Everything down there looks clean and healthy to me,' I said.

She looked sad and ashamed.

'You don't seem to like this part of yourself,' I said.

There was no answer. 'It must make sex difficult if you feel like this about your body.'

'You are right doctor, I can't have sex at all. I think my fiancé will leave me soon.'

At that point she burst into tears and, still sobbing, sat up clutching the couch blanket around her lower body. I perched on the edge of the couch still wearing my examination gloves. I did not want to lose this moment.

'When did this start?' I asked.

She calmed down and told me her story. 'Peter was my first proper boyfriend. We're planning to get married. I love him a lot and, although I thought it was wrong at first, we started to have sex together. It was great and we felt so close. I felt safe as I am on the pill. We were both virgins and we did not think that we would need to use condoms. My father would "kill me" if I got pregnant. My parents are very religious. When I came for a pill check-up, your nurse did a smear.'

Her lip started to tremble as she told me how the result had come back showing no abnormality apart from some candida on the slide. 'The letter that the nurse wrote to me said that I had an infection and that if I still had a discharge I must get it treated. I came to see another doctor who gave me a pessary but it did no good and I still had the discharge.'

I said, 'I am confused that an infection such as thrush can make you seem so disgusted with your body.'

Her demeanour changed and she looked angry. 'I want to know where I got it from,' she spat out. I must have got it from Peter as I have been with no-one else. He swears that he has not been unfaithful. I feel dirty and used. I can't let him near me. He refused to go to the clinic for a check-up as he said it wasn't his fault, and now I have got to have this operation.'

'You don't catch thrush *from* anyone,' I said quietly.

She sat bolt upright and looked me in the eye. 'What do you mean, you don't catch thrush from anyone?'

I explained to her the nature of the disease and she looked very thoughtful. 'How can I have been so ignorant?' she said.

She quickly put her things on and made to leave. There was a much lighter atmosphere in the room. I asked her to make another appointment to talk about the cryosurgery and she quickly left. The appointment had lasted about 15 minutes.

She came to see me again about 2 weeks later. She had changed her hairstyle and looked more grown up. I asked her how she was and she answered that she was much better. Sex was fine and she did not want to talk about it. She apologized for having been so stupid. She said she should have asked the other doctors about the transmission of thrush but felt too ashamed and embarrassed. She still had some discharge but agreed that she could live with it and asked me to cancel the surgery. I suggested that she did it by ringing the consultant's secretary. I did not suggest another appointment.

### Conclusion

What had happened in this consultation?

- I had stuck to the here and now, concentrating on the atmosphere in the room.
- I had reflected back to her the disgust with her body that she was emanating.
- The vaginal examination acted as a moment of truth when her defences were down and her real fears were addressed.
- I allowed her to regain control by cancelling her own appointment.
- Details of her newly improved sex life were not to be shared with the doctor as there was no longer a medical problem.
- She knows where I am if there are any future difficulties.

## Medical problems that may lead to sexual problems in women

General ill-health may lead to loss of libido. This is usually a secondary effect due to lack of well-being and discomfort. Diabetes seems to have an effect on all aspects of sexual function in women but is hard to separate direct effects from ones secondary to concurrent ill-health and distress regarding the disease. Neurological problems such as multiple sclerosis and spinal cord lesions will affect arousal and orgasm, although libido may be normal. Women with cardiovascular disease may fear recurrence of problems such as chest pain or stroke on exertion. Rarely, in conditions such as Addison's disease, there is a reduction in sex hormones that may lead to loss of desire.

Arthritis and back pain can interfere with movement. Advice regarding use of analgesia together with adoption of different positions for intercourse, often with judicial use of pillows, can be helpful. It is important that doctors appreciate that ill and old people may still have sexual desires and activity. Patients may not want to broach the subject and the doctor may also find it difficult. They may be looking for 'permission' from the practitioner to continue with some activity and confirmation that it is normal to still have sexual feelings.

The relationship between depression and loss of desire is complex. Someone may become depressed because of their psychosexual problem, especially if it is putting their relationship in jeopardy. Patients with loss of libido may seem depressed but on closer enquiry it will appear that other aspects of their life are fine. Conversely, depression can cause loss of libido and it is important not to embark on lengthy psychosexual counselling without establishing this. Some of the newer antidepressants, particularly the serotonin reuptake inhibitors, may cause difficulty in achieving arousal and orgasm and may reduce libido in men and women. Women may be prepared to put up with this side effect but become concerned if it is not explained to them that the effect is temporary.

Surgery, particularly disfiguring operations such as mastectomy, may have a severe detrimental effect on a woman's body image and subsequent sexual function. It may affect her partner and she may feel no longer desired. Women with stoma need special consideration but any surgical scarring can sometimes change the way a woman feels about herself and affect her body image. Doctors must get used to asking about resumption of sexual activity after traumatic illness and life events.

## Box 16.3 **Medical causes of male sexual dysfunction**

- Diabetes
- Cardiovascular disease
- Neurological disorders
- Prescription drugs
- Prostate disorders and surgery
- Conditions causing low testosterone
- Thyroid disease
- Any major illness
- Major surgery or trauma
- Psychiatric illness
- Drug or alcohol abuse

### Medical problems that may lead to sexual problems in men

Although this chapter is primarily about female sexual problems, these cannot be discussed fully without considering male problems (see Box 16.3). A woman may be the presenting patient whilst the primary problem is with her partner. This may be a covert presentation and it may take the doctor a while to get to the root of the problem.

# Age and stage

Women of any age can experience sexual difficulty but age and stage of life can predispose to particular problems.

### Adolescence

During adolescence there are rapid changes in body shape and hormonal levels. Girls are exposed to a wide variety of influences with sex being aired so much by the media. Magazines for teenagers are explicit, as are films and television. Peer pressure and pressure from boyfriends also play a part in the timing of a teenage girl's first sexual experiences. The National Survey of Sexual Attitudes and Lifestyles (Wellings *et al.* 1994b) interviewed men and women in 5-year age cohorts from ages 16 to 59. The reported median age of first intercourse decreased with age of responder. Thus the median age at which the youngest women in the sample experienced first sexual intercourse was 4 years earlier at 17, than that for those born 40 years earlier, when it was 21. The median ages for men were 17 and 20, respectively. There was also an increase in the numbers of both males and females who lost their virginity below the age of 16. The decline in the age of first sexual experience was greater than the decline in the age of menarche. The numbers confessing to first intercourse below the age of 16, particularly in the female group, were much lower in the groups from the Indian subcontinent than in any other ethnic minority. This may reflect religious and cultural influences.

Most people surveyed could easily remember the timing of their first intercourse. A survey of 7395 Scottish teenagers from a wide range of social groups with a mean age of 14 years 2 months found that 18% of boys and 15.4% of girls reported having had heterosexual intercourse. Many of the responders experienced regret. Thirty-two per cent of the girls and 27% of the boys thought that it had happened too early, whilst 13% and 5%, respectively, thought that it should not have happened at all. If there was any pressure surrounding the event, both sexes were more likely to report regret.

For girls, lack of prior planning with their partner was also significant (Wight *et al.* 2000).

The provision of contraception and advice regarding sexually transmitted infections is crucial in this age group. Confidentiality is a real issue for young people; teenagers living in rural areas may feel that a visit to the doctor's surgery for contraception will not go unnoticed. It is important that young people can get advice regarding sexual matters from other sources such as youth centres and schools. First sexual experiences can be traumatic and events surrounding them can leave indelible memories. Early fears and fantasies can often be expelled if nipped in the bud and it is important that medical professionals are aware that young people may be sexually active and may have problems. As with older age groups, there may be difficulty disclosing the problem directly. A non-questioning technique, noting the atmosphere in the room, may be helpful.

Particularly in the under 16s, there is the possibility that sexual activity may be abusive and gentle enquiry regarding the age of the partner and the enjoyment and willingness to partake in the activities described may be propitious.

## Case 2: anorgasmia

Stacey came to see me at an evening surgery. She was booked in as an urgent extra. I had seen her before a few times for contraceptive advice over the past 2 years She had needed postcoital contraception twice but was now established on depo progesterone. She had many boyfriends and we had talked a lot about condoms and sexually transmitted disease. Stacey was 17 years old but could pass for 21. She now attended the local college of further education. She slumped into the chair, looking glum. I noticed that she had even more studs in her ear lobes and caught a glimpse of one in her umbilicus as her skimpy tee shirt rose up. Her fringe was hanging over her face and she did not look her usual sexy, attractive, and confident self.

I asked her what I could do for her. In a wavering voice she said, 'I think that I have got a lump down below.'

'Well I had better take a look,' I said, directing her towards the couch. She slouched over to the couch and climbed up slowly pulling down her jeans but not taking them off. She looked ashamed and did not look me in the face. I carefully examined her vulva. It looked completely healthy. I told her so. She started to cry silently and suddenly looked younger than her years. I felt as if there was a child on the couch. There was a feeling of sadness and shame in the room.

'My boyfriend says that I am not normal! He says that I am not like other girls and that I must have something missing.' I said nothing, but allowed what seemed like a very long uncomfortable silence. I could see that she wanted to say something and gave her time to collect her thoughts and did not butt in with further questions or suggestions. In a wavering voice she said, 'I can't, you know, I can't come. I keep trying different boys to see if it makes a difference but however much I fancy them or get turned on I can't do it. With the others I faked it – I made the noises that they do in the films. But with Tony it is different –we love each other and I don't want to fake it with him. He's tried everything he can think of. We even got a book about sexual technique. He says that it is putting him off sex if I don't enjoy it. I am terrified that I will lose him.'

She sat up and pulled on her jeans. 'Well, everything looks all right physically,' I said. 'You have always seemed so laid back about sex on the surface. It seems that something about your body really upsets you. You seem ashamed. To have an orgasm you need to be able to feel relaxed and lose control.'

For the first time during that interview she looked me straight in the eye. 'Everything I tell you is confidential, right?' I nodded.

'I'm worried I'll wet myself if I come, if I lose control as you said.'

I said nothing but just looked puzzled. I sensed there was another secret.

I used to wet my bed until I was about 9. Once I did it on a Brownie camp – it was awful. I wouldn't stay the night with Tony even if we had the chance.

She got up and sat back on the chair. Regaining some of her usual confidence she said, 'Well, I feel better now I have told someone.'

We talked about the fact that it was unlikely that she would wet herself if she did have an orgasm and that maybe now that she has told one person it might be possible to discuss this with her boyfriend. She seemed hesitant about this but would give it some thought. She declined an invitation to come and see me again.

I did see her about 6 months later when she came in with a sore throat. She looked much less 'way out' in her style of dress and seemed more quietly confident. After we had discussed her throat infection, I tentatively asked her how things were otherwise. 'Oh that,' she said. 'It's fine. Not every time but sometimes it's great. I did tell him my secret. He kept on and on, asking me what you had said and eventually I told him. He said that I was stupid to worry about that and was glad that there was nothing wrong with me or him.'

### Conclusion

- I stuck with the 'here and now' of the consultation.

- I noticed that she was not her usual 'sexy' and 'cocky' self and reflected back to her that she seemed ashamed.

- I examined her and told her that physically she was normal. There was no lump – this was her calling card.

◆ I allowed a silence, enabling her to disclose her difficulty.

◆ Having excluded a physical cause and talked a bit about sexual technique, I explained that anorgasmia was often due to not being able to lose control. This freed her up to lose control in the consultation and gain insight into her problem.

## Pregnancy and childbirth

Pregnancy and childbirth produce physical, emotional, and social changes in women's lives and may also profoundly affect their partners, having a great influence on both general and sexual relationships. Whilst pregnant some women lose their libido and some men do not find their partner attractive. There may be fears relating to miscarriage early on and discomfort in the last trimester. After the trauma of childbirth, there may be additional physical or emotional problems. A woman may not like the changes in her body. Men who have watched their partner give birth may be overwhelmed by the changes that have taken place and the invasion of their partner's 'private areas' by others. Being a mother itself or having sex with someone who has become a mother may present a problem. There are the additional problems of tiredness and postnatal depression. On the other hand, there may be no problems at all.

In a study of 131 couples, 8 months following childbirth, 50% of first-time parents described their sex lives as 'poor' or 'not very good'. Twenty per cent said that they would like help for this. They also reported an associated increase in difficulties in their general relationship (Dixon *et al.* 2000). Health visitors and doctors in child health clinics are well placed to screen for these problems before they become too entrenched.

Vaginal examination is not done routinely at the 6-week postnatal check. In my experience, many women do have fears that their body has not returned to normal and concerns about stitches being too tight or too loose. Although no medical examination should be done routinely, careful enquiry at this stage can determine which women have fears about their anatomy, and could help to identify which women would benefit from a genital examination. The doctor can gently show the woman that her vagina is well healed and encourage self-examination. Some patients are actually seeking permission from the professional to resume sexual activity. This is also an important time to discuss contraception, which can be a lead into enquiry about resumption of sexual activity. Some may be simply seeking reassurance that it is fine not to feel like sex when exhausted and bursting with milk and that this is a normal reaction.

## The menopause

Midlife is a time of change for women. During the menopause there is a reduction in oestrogen and testosterone levels. The latter is more marked after an oophorectomy. It is thought that oestrogen may have a direct effect on libido and also on sexual arousal and lubrication. There is also the domino effect, which occurs when vasomotor symptoms induce tiredness and irritability with a secondary loss of desire. Periods may be erratic, frequent, and often heavy, which can also interfere with sexual function.

There are many conflicting studies on the value of hormone replacement therapy (HRT) in treating loss of libido in the menopausal woman. Some studies show that oestrogen replacement plus or minus additional testosterone improve libido, whilst others do not. Testosterone seems to be particularly helpful in castrated women. Some studies have shown that the addition of progesterone is detrimental to libido. Many studies have been small numbers and are inconclusive. A meta-analysis of sexuality and menopause research (Myers 1995) concluded that this was a difficult task to do because of the diffuse nature of the studies; the author concluded that hormones, both exogenous and endogenous, have some importance in peri-/postmenopausal sexuality. The most important factor is that the doctor considers each patient as an individual. If loss of libido coincides with the menopause and there are not other factors involved, a trial of HRT may be appropriate, especially if there are other indications.

Women who do not have HRT may develop atrophic vaginitis, vaginal dryness, and soreness. Urinary problems such as stress incontinence may also be a deterrent to sexual activity. Many women who do not want to take systemic oestrogen can use vaginal preparations to alleviate vaginal and urinary symptoms. As there is very little systemic absorption of milder topical oestrogens, these products may even be used in women with hormone-dependent cancers who have severe vaginal soreness following an iatrogenically produced menopause. There are also commercially available vaginal moisturizers and lubricants to help with intercourse.

Psychosexual problems are also common at the menopause. Some women may be delighted to be at the end of their reproductive lives with a cessation of periods, whilst others may mourn the loss of fertility and see it as the onset of old age. Intercourse can no longer be for reproduction. Some women may think that sex is no longer decent and may either seek the doctor's permission to continue or even to stop. Women may be experiencing the death or illness of their own parents for whom they may have to take on a caring role. Their children and grandchildren may be having difficulties and they may be trying to hold down a full-time job in the midst of this.

Partners may also have problems affecting their sexual function. Men may be made redundant or realize that they have not achieved their potential. They may also start to experience sexual dysfunction related to illness such as diabetes or heart disease. If a relationship has been stormy, these extra burdens can make it worse. All these confounding factors make it difficult to analyse the effects of hormones on sexual function at the menopause.

It may be easier for women to bring a sexual difficulty to the doctor under the guise of a menopausal problem than for either member of the partnership to come directly for help. Women who find it hard to talk to their own doctor about sexual matters may get themselves referred to a menopause clinic ostensibly to discuss a problem with HRT. It is important in these clinics, whether in hospital, community, or primary care setting – to ask women routinely about sexual problems. Women may be too embarrassed to mention their prolapse, their haemorrhoids, or their vulval eczema and there are often surprises on genital examination.

## Case 3: loss of libido

Sonia had been having problems with her HRT. She was now aged 45 and had two grown children. Five years ago she had had a hysterectomy and bilateral oophorectomy for endometriosis. Initially it was great, as she had no more pain. The hospital started her on HRT straight away and she never had any menopausal symptoms, but now she did not feel so good and wondered if she needed a higher dose of oestrogen. She was the manager of a small boutique and had a very exhausting job. I noted that she was on the maximum dose of oral medication and suggested that she tried patches to see if she felt any better. She was not clinically depressed, just tired. She seemed to be dull and lifeless in contrast to her highly fashionable clothes. She thanked me half-heartedly and left with a suggestion that I see her again in a couple of months.

Six weeks later she turned up again, clutching a piece cut out of a well-known magazine. 'I think this is what I need,' she said, handing me the cutting. It was an article about testosterone for female libido. 'I wonder why you think you need that,' I asked?

'I never feel like sex these days. I do it sometimes to please my husband, but I would not mind if I never did it again in my life.'

I asked her when this had started. Apparently sex had been good immediately after the hysterectomy when she had no pain or bleeding. Over the years she had felt less and less like it. She hardly ever got turned on. 'My poor husband has to work so hard. He thinks that I have gone off him, although I try to reassure him that this is not so.'

There was no problem in the relationship and no other major life changes. All this information was delivered in a lifeless monotone, which is typical of a consultation about loss of libido. I felt like her husband must feel; I was working very hard and getting nowhere.

'You seem very sad,' I said.

'It's as if all the feeling was removed with my womb,' she replied.

'Perhaps I should take a look,' I suggested, pointing towards the couch.

She looked a bit puzzled and climbed up, readily removing her beautiful underwear. 'How can you examine nothing,' she asked. As I went to look at the vulva she said, 'I've only felt half a woman since I had my hysterectomy. It's not that I want any more children but it makes me feel old to not have a womb and to have to take HRT. All my friends from the shop are much younger – I could never tell them that I had to take hormones. My husband is a few years younger than me and I feel that I can't keep up anymore.'

I quickly completed the vaginal examination and told her that everything was normal and healthy. She got dressed and sat down. We talked about the fact that the sensitive – erotic – areas are not removed by the surgery. We talked about what remained as opposed to what had been taken away. On a different level we discussed how she is still as much a woman despite not having a womb.

She gathered up her things and said, 'I had better go now doctor, I have taken up too much of your time.' At the door she said, 'I will come back when I need some more pills. I didn't start the patches. I don't want my friends to see them when I'm in the gym shower.' We had not discussed the testosterone.

She came back a couple of months later. She was much more buoyant with a spring in her step. Everything was fine and she did not want any change in her hormones. 'I have stopped feeling sorry for myself,' she said. 'You had better not examine me this time, I had a tattoo done a few weeks ago.'

### Conclusion

What had happened in the consultation?

- I neither dismissed her request for testosterone, nor agreed that it would be useful, without looking at the reason for her loss of libido.
- I had noted her sadness and fed this back to her.
- I had suggested an examination, although there was no immediate physical reason for this. It had enabled her to talk about her inner feelings.
- I paid tribute to her loss.

## Ageing

The media rarely portrays sexual activity between anyone who is not young, healthy, and beautiful and it may be hard for a young doctor to even imagine his or her octogenarian patients having a sex life. However, sexual activity may continue into old age in many couples. As divorce becomes commoner and marriage less of a precursor for sexual activity, there are increasing numbers of people in later years of life who are not with their life-long partners. Most studies show a steady decline in the frequency of sexual activity in both sexes with age. One survey showed that the reported frequency of heterosexual sex rose to a peak between the ages of 20–29 for women and 25–34 for men with a median rate of five times per month for each sex. Between the ages of 55–59 the median frequency was two for men with more than 50% of women in this age group reporting no sex in the last month. Over the age of 50, women are more likely than men not to have a partner (Wellings *et al.* 1994c).

Reduction in sexual activity with age may not be a problem if it is due to lack of desire and is mutual between a couple. It may be caused by physical problems affecting one member of a partnership. Patients often want to know what is normal and whether they should or should not be having sex at their age. The answer is that there is a whole range of 'normal activity' and it is what is right for them that is important.

Before treating one member of a partnership, find out the views of the other, especially when suggesting the physical and pharmacological treatments for physical erectile dysfunction that are now available. There is no point in enabling an elderly man to have an erection with a vacuum pump if his wife has severe atrophic vaginitis and osteoarthritis of the hip. There is no value in prescribing sildenafil if the female partner has no desire. Some women may have strong antipathy to what they might see as an artificially produced erection and for some men this is not the answer. On the other hand, some women may be delighted to become involved and will actually administer intracavernosal injections if their husbands have lost their dexterity. Even if both partners are not seen, their views must be discussed.

If there has been ill-health such as a heart attack or stroke, both members of the partnership may be frightened to initiate sex. The usual advice with heart disease is that intercourse should be safe if the patient can climb two flights of stairs without angina. If chest pain does occur during sexual activity then they should be advised to stop. The doctor is not always in a position to fix the problem and needs to acknowledge with the patient that a full sexual life is no longer possible.

## Terminal illness and bereavement

It may not seem decent for the doctor or the patient to discuss sex when someone is dying or bereaved. Seriously ill people or their partners may feel guilty about the persistence of their sexual desire, which may be increasingly difficult to fulfil as they become more infirm. Doctors may be in a position to enhance these precious last times by giving permission to continue with intercourse, reassuring them that sex will not do any harm. Physical treatments for erectile dysfunction can be employed. Women, who have vaginal dryness following chemotherapy, for example, can be given practical advice. Analgesics can be used prior to love-making. Privacy also becomes a problem as the dying are hospitalized and this may be a reason for weekends at home.

In four cases of terminal care within the community (Gilley 1998), the main carer was the patient's partner. Previous levels of physical intimacy account for differences in the ability or willingness to perform tasks for an invalid partner. At one extreme, a woman carer considered it a 'liberty' that her husband should ask her to brush his hair, whilst at the other extreme, a man was able to make sexual innuendoes when his wife handled his catheter.

After the death of a loved one, the loss of the sexual relationship may be an additional blow that is hard to discuss. The memory of a previous partner often presents a barrier to a new sexual relationship, as there may be feelings of guilt, especially if the death was relatively recent. Resumption of intercourse after a long time lapse may present physical problems in both men and women, and they may find this particularly hard to discuss with their GP.

## Special areas needing consideration

### Disability

It is beyond the remit of this book to discuss the technical details that can be employed when helping women or their partners with disability to enjoy their sexuality. There are many books written describing the physical needs and arrangements that can be made. These are discussed in the book *Sexuality and disability: a guide for everyday practice* (Cooper and Guillebaud 1999). It may be relatively straightforward to discuss adaptations and physical means of obtaining an erection or ways of dealing with a catheter, but it is much harder for the doctor or nurse to deal with the emotional aspects of a disabled person's sexual life and their feelings about their body. The patient's sense of exposure when their deformed or damaged body is revealed to their partner may be mirrored by a sense of shame apparent during a physical examination by the doctor. It is important to see the person with sexual desires rather than a patient with a deformity.

# Sexual abuse and rape

## The immediate problem

From time to time GPs will see women who have recently been raped. If they have not reported this to the police, they should be encouraged to do so. Even if they do not want to press charges, it is important that the forensic evidence is gathered as quickly as possible in case they change their minds. In most places this is now done in specialized 'rape suites' with sympathetic female policewomen and sensitive doctors. Women must be encouraged not to wash or change their clothes. They will have swabs taken from their mouth, vagina, and possibly rectum, depending on their statement. Samples of hair, blood, and nail scrapings may also be needed. All bruises and injuries will be recorded. A full screen for sexually transmitted diseases (STD) should be organized and postcoital contraception (PCC) provided if indicated.

Some women, fearing the humiliation and second assault of an examination will not wish to go to the police. There may be other reasons why they do not want to report the rape. If they cannot be persuaded to talk to the police, then the doctor can refer them to the rape crisis centre, where they will receive counselling and may be able to change their minds. It is important for the GP to arrange the STD screen and PCC if they are not going to be seen by the police doctor. Remember that these women may feel dirty, humiliated, shameful, and guilty about their rape. It is important that medical intervention does not exacerbate these negative feelings. A family doctor is well placed to help a woman through the aftermath of this type of trauma.

# The aftermath

All doctors and nurses working in the field of sexual problems will see women who have been abused as children or raped or assaulted as adults. This can have an extreme negative effect on subsequent sexual enjoyment and relationships. Patients may have told their story repeatedly or may be disclosing it for the first time. Even many years after an assault, women may still be left with the fear that they have been damaged. They may still feel dirty and feel that anyone can tell by looking at them that they have been violated. This may lead to difficulties with medical examinations as well as with sex, especially if any subsequent medical tests or court appearances were traumatic.

Sexual problems in women who had been abused as children can be treated by brief interpretive therapy (Vanhegan *et al.* 1997). Sexual problems in this group are not necessarily directly related to the abuse. The single most important factor in the severity of the sexual dysfunction is the quality of relationship that the woman has with her mother. A woman may be fine for a while in a good relationship until there is a major life change when, for example, the abuser dies or her own daughter reaches the age of her abuse. This may rekindle the problem.

# General management of psychosexual problems in primary care

All primary care doctors will come across patients with sexual and psychosexual problems. They need to decide whether to manage the patient themselves or whether they need to referral to a specialist is indicated. As yet drug treatment for female sexual dysfunction is still at the research stage.

## Facts to establish

- ◆ What is the diagnosis? (See Boxes 16.1 and 16.2.)
- ◆ Who is the patient and who is complaining – bear in mind that some women will present when the sexual difficulty is their husband's.
- ◆ Did the patient come on her own accord or was she sent? This is important as patients who have been 'sent' by their partner or someone else will have a poor prognosis.
- ◆ Why did the patient come now? The timing of their presentation can often throw light on the problem.
- ◆ When did the problem start? This is also a good indicator to the cause of the difficulty.
- ◆ What actually happens when they try to have sex?
- ◆ What does their partner feel about the problem and what is the nature of the relationship?

## Awareness of the doctor/patient relationship

Studying the doctor/patient relationship enables the doctor to throw light on the patient's problem. This has been demonstrated in the case histories earlier in the chapter. The feelings that are evoked in the consultation often echo those of the patient and may also throw light on the way that she behaves with her partner.

## Avoid routine questions

Although certain facts need to be established, it is important that a non-questioning technique is used and the patient's agenda addressed. Learn to tolerate silence in the consultation as this may allow the patient to disclose. It is important not to generalize or extrapolate from one patient to another. Every human being is an individual with different feelings.

## Interpretation

With practice the doctor can learn to reflect these feelings back to the patient. This will often help the patient to gain insight into the cause of the problem. This is demonstrated in the cases described. For example, you may notice that the patient is sad, angry, flirtatious, or childlike. Stick to the 'here and now' of the consultation and try not to digress into past history unless the patient takes you in that direction. This does not always take a long time and can be done in the context of the GP consultation. Comment if the patient keeps avoiding the subject in hand, as this may be relevant.

## The genital examination

The genital examination is very important. It is often a moment of truth when the real feelings are revealed. The doctor must notice whether the patient is nervous, tense, detached, or involved in the examination. These observations can also be reflected back to the patient. Even if a woman is complaining of loss of libido, it is worth doing a physical examination, as it may help the woman to talk (see case 3).

Avoid empty reassurance. This may not address the patient's fantasy about body changes. Pay tribute to these and do not dismiss them lightly. They must be explored. Self-examination is a useful tool. This can be done either in the surgery or as 'homework'.

## Deciding when to refer

Some doctors and nurses acquire skills that enable them to treat patients with sexual difficulties and work with them over several sessions. It is important to exclude any physical problems and to ensure that the patient is not depressed. If the problem is related to a gender issue or a disorder of sexual preference such as fetishism, a psychiatric opinion should be sought. If the problem seems to be mainly a relationship difficulty, then referral for counselling to an organization such as Relate may be helpful. The patients do not need to attend Relate as a couple if one member refuses. Trained sex therapists are also available at Relate and they are particularly good at treating couples. Most GPs have access to psychosexual counsellors who are trained either by the Institute of Psychosexual Medicine or trained in behavioural techniques, often by the British Association of Sexual and Relationship Therapists.

Bear in mind that the patient presenting in general practice has chosen to see a doctor and not a counsellor. She may not want to be referred on and may feel rejected. The doctor and nurse are in a privileged position as they can examine their patients. Most counsellors cannot do this. This may be very important in establishing the mind/body link.

## Training in psychosexual medicine

The Institute of Psychosexual Medicine (IPM) is a training organization for doctors from all specialties as long as they are able to examine patients; some groups also contain nurses. The teaching is done by case presentation at seminars. This training is particularly helpful for doctors in primary care who see patients in the course of their ordinary work and do not necessarily want to become specialists. The skills gained enable doctors and nurses to deal more effectively with psychosomatic illness in general – especially relating to the genital area. Other training is available via the British Association of Sexual and Relationship Therapists (BASRT). This is particularly useful for couple work and for doctors who want to specialize in this area of primarily behaviour therapy.

## Frequently asked questions

### Why don't I feel like making love?

There are a variety of reasons why women lose their libido. Very occasionally there may be a hormonal reason, e.g. at the menopause. A woman may lose her sex drive if she is ill, depressed, grieving, or if there is a particular stress in her life at that time. Commonly, loss of desire is due to a relationship difficulty.

### Why does there seem to be a blockage when we try to have intercourse?

Only extremely rarely is there an actual physical blockage. More commonly the block is due to the vaginal wall muscles going into spasm. This is known as vaginismus. This is usually due to a subconscious fear of penetration and damage that it might cause physically and emotions that it might unleash. The reason a woman feels like this are very complex and may be associated with her past.

### Why does it hurt when I have sex?

Vulval soreness may be caused by a skin problem, thrush, or oestrogen deficiency. Pain on intercourse deep inside the vagina may be due to a gynaecological problem. Irritable bowel syndrome and other conditions can also cause pain on intercourse. Pain can also be due to spasm of the vaginal muscles or it may have an underlying psychological cause and this must be considered if no physical cause is found.

### Why can't I have an orgasm?

This may be due to lack of foreplay and poor sexual technique. This can be discussed with your partner. On the other hand, it may be more deep seated and related to inability to 'let go' and more deep-seated sexual inhibition.

### Why does my partner lose his erection?

This may be due to a variety of problems such as physical illness and stress. It can also be due to problems in your relationship. If it is due to an emotional difficulty, it may be intermittent and improve with time or counselling. If it is due to a physical problem such as diabetes it is unlikely to improve spontaneously. There are now many drug and other treatments available.

## 10-Minute consultation on vaginismus

### A difficult smear

A young woman was asked to see her general practitioner by the practice nurse who had been unable to do her cervical smear. The patient was so tense that she could not insert the speculum. Her first baby had been born 6 months ago. The nurse asked her if sex had been difficult since the birth. The woman got very upset and confessed that it hurt so much that they had not tried lately.

### What issues should you cover?

- *Find out when the problem started.* The patient said that everything had been fine up until the birth. They had been able to have sex up until the last few weeks of the pregnancy. Before she had been pregnant it had also been good.
- *Find out what the patient thinks is the cause of the problem.* The patient said that she tore during the delivery and had lots of stitches. Although the midwife said that she had healed up it was still very sore and her husband thought that there was a blockage.
- *Find out about the relationship and what actually happened when she tried to make love.* She said that everything was fine in her relationship and the baby was thriving. She was not depressed and her son was sleeping through the night. Her partner was not 'pushing her' to have sex. He was very gentle and understanding, but it was getting very difficult now as she did not even want to cuddle him in case it led to intercourse. They were beginning to get irritable with each other.

◆ *Find out if she has fear of further pregnancy.* The patient was terrified of further pregnancy as the delivery had been so awful and her partner, who had been present at the birth, would not want to put her through that experience again. She was on the combined pill now that she had stopped breast-feeding and was not at all worried that she could fall pregnant.

### What should you do?

◆ Notice what is happening in the room between the doctor and the patient. Stick to the 'here and now' and avoid asking too many direct questions, especially about past history. Use open-ended statements as these will help to establish the patient's agenda in a short consultation.

◆ Be aware of the atmosphere during the examination and reflect this back to her. This patient looked terrified as she got on to the couch. She started to pull away as she was examined and the doctor offered to examine her gently with one finger only. She showed the doctor where she was sore and was surprised when the doctor touched her there and it did not hurt. The doctor noted some vaginismus and did not proceed to a full examination or speculum insertion. The smear-taking was deferred. There was no obvious physical abnormality and the doctor told her that everything had healed and looked healthy and normal.

◆ Encourage the patient to examine herself. This can be done in the consulting room if the patient is willing. This will help her to overcome any fantasy that she still has a painful area that has not healed. Suggest that she tries this at home.

◆ Discuss the mechanism of vaginismus with the patient. Explain that the fear of being hurt is causing her muscles to contract. It is the subsequent muscle spasm that feels painful. She may be able to feel this with her own finger if she contracts and relaxes her pelvic floor.

◆ Suggest that she could try sex gently with aid of a lubricant when she wants to but that she does not need to rush it.

◆ Arrange to see her again, but reassure her that it was not essential that the smear is done at the next consultation. Tell her that this could be left until she felt more confident.

## Useful addresses

Association of Psychosexual Nursing
PO Box 2762, London WIA 5HQ
   *Details on training for nurses.*

British Association of Sexual and Relationship Therapy (BASRT)
PO Box 13686, London SW20 9ZII.
Tel. 0208 543 2707
www.basrt.org.uk
  *Contact for advice on therapists and clinics in local areas.*

Institute of Psychosexual Medicine
12 Chandos St, London W1G 9DR
Tel: 020 7580 0631
e-mail: ipm@telinco.co.uk
www.ipm.org.uk
  *This can give advice regarding training seminars for doctors and suggest therapists and clinics in local areas.*

Relate
Herbert Gray College, Little Church St, Rugby, Warwickshire CV21 3AP
Tel: 01788 573241
e-mail: info@national.relate.org.uk
www.relate.org.uk
  *Relate now has trained sex therapists in most areas. Patients can self-refer.*

SPOD (Sexual Problems of the Disabled)
286 Campden Rd, London N7 0BJ
Tel: 020 7607 8851, Tuesday and Thursday 11 a.m.–2 p.m.
  *This association assists the sexual and personal relationships of people with disabilities. Leaflets are available.*

The Beaumont Trust – Charity for Support for Transvestites and Transsexuals
BM Charity, London WC1N 3XX
Tel: 0700 028 7878, Tuesday and Thursday 7.0–11.0 p.m.
For partners of transvestites and transsexuals – Tel: 01606 871 984

The London Friend Gay and Lesbian Help-line
86 Caledonian Rd, London N1
Tel: 020 7837 3337, 7.30–10 p.m. daily

# References

Cooper, E. and Guillebaud, J. (1999). *Sexuality and disability: a guide for everyday practice*. Radcliffe Medical Press, Oxford.

Crowley, T. (2001). Sexual problems when the partner is of the same gender. *Institute of Psychosexual Medicine Journal*, **26**, 12–17.

Dixon, M., Booth, N. and Powell, R. (2000). Sex and relationships following childbirth: a first report from general practice of 131 couples. *British Journal of General Practice*, **50**(452), 223–4.

Dunn, K.M., Croft, P.R. and Hackett, G.I. (1998). Sexual problems: a study of the prevalence and need for health care in the general population. *Family Practice*, **15**, 519–24.

Gilley, J. (1998). Intimacy and terminal care. *Journal of the Royal College of General Practitioners*, **38**, 121–2.

Myers, L.S. (1995). Methodological review and meta-analysis of sexuality and menopause research. *Neuroscience Biobehaviour Review*, **19**, 331–41.

Rhodes, J.C., Kjerulff, K.H., Langenberg, P.W., *et al.* (1999). Hysterectomy and sexual functioning. *Journal of the American Medical Association*, **282**(20), 1934–41.

Vanhegan, G., Tunnadine, P. and Kwantes, E. (1997). Treatment of problems in previously abused patients. *British Journal of Family Planning*, **22**(4), 191–3.

Wellings, K., Field. J., Johnson, A.M. and Wadsworth, J. (1994a). *Sexual behaviour in Britain*, pp. 178–229. Penguin, London.

Wellings, K., Field. J., Johnson, A.M. and Wadsworth, J. (1994b). *Sexual behaviour in Britain*, pp. 37–54. Penguin, London.

Wellings, K., Field. J., Johnson, A.M. and Wadsworth, J. (1994c). *Sexual behaviour in Britain*, pp. 137–9. Penguin, London.

Wight, D., Henderson, M., Raab, G., *et. al.* (2000). Extent of regretted sexual intercourse among young teenagers in Scotland: a cross sectional survey. *British Medical Journal*, **320**, 1243–4.

Chapter 17

# Domestic violence
## Iona Heath

## Definition

> That was my life. Getting hit, waiting to get hit, recovering; forgetting. Starting all over
> again. There was no time, a beginning or an end. I can't say how many times he beat
> me. It was one beating; it went on forever (Doyle 1996).

One in four women is hit by a current or former partner, at some time in her
life (Home Office Research Studies 1999). Pushing, shoving, and grabbing are
the most common forms of assault and reported in two-thirds of incidents.
Kicking, slapping, or punching are reported in almost half. Injuries result from
41% of incidents and women who experience a chronic pattern of violence are
particularly likely to have been injured in the most recent incident (58%).

> The term 'domestic violence' shall be understood to mean any violence between
> current or former partners in an intimate relationship, wherever and whenever the
> violence occurs. The violence may include physical, sexual, emotional or financial
> abuse (Home Office 1999).

This definition was formulated by the Home Office and has been used by all
police forces across England and Wales since April 1999. It has since been
adopted by the Department of Health (2000), with the qualification that:

> although domestic violence can take place in any intimate relationship, including gay
> and lesbian partnerships, and abuse of men by female partners does occur, the great
> majority of domestic violence, and the most severe and chronic incidents, are perpe-
> trated by men against women and their children.

## The scale and severity of domestic violence

The 1992 British Crime Survey showed that violence against women by partners, ex-partners, and relatives is the most common form of physical interpersonal crime (Mayhew *et al.* 1993). The total number of domestic assaults in the
12 months covered by the survey was estimated at just over 500 000. The 1996
British Crime Survey reported that 46% of all violent incidents against women

were domestic, and that four out of five incidents of domestic violence against women took place at home (Mirrlees-Black *et al.* 1996). Any woman is at risk of domestic violence, regardless of race, ethnic or religious group, class, age, sexuality, disability, or lifestyle (Women's Aid Federation of England 1992). Apart from the police and the military, the family is the most violent grouping and the home the most violent setting in society (Gelles and Straus 1979). Nor does the break-up of the family necessarily bring relief. Divorced and separated women risk violence as much as, and probably more than (Feldhaus *et al.* 1997), married women; once married, the risk of abuse falls significantly only for the widowed.

Domestic violence usually escalates in frequency and severity. By the time a woman's injuries are visible, violence may be a long-established pattern. On average, a woman will be assaulted by her partner or ex-partner 35 times before actually reporting it to the police (Yearnshire 1997). In a consecutive-sample survey study of 62 episodes of domestic assault to which police had been called, 68% involved weapons and 15% involved serious injury (Home Office Research and Statistics Department 1992). In 89% of episodes there had been previous assaults by the current assailant, 35% of them on a daily basis (Brookoff *et al.* 1997). For some women, the escalation is fatal. One in five of all murder victims is a woman killed by a partner or ex-partner; almost half of all murders of women are killings by a partner or ex-partner (30% of men charged with the murder of their spouse admit previously being violent, and 80% describe chronic marital problems, recent divorce, separation, or threats of separation) (Kay and Kent 1989).

## The nature of commonly inflicted injuries

Injuries resulting from domestic violence range from bruises, abrasions, cuts, fractures, and miscarriages to permanent injuries including damaged vision or hearing, and scars from burns, bites, or knife wounds (Council of Scientific Affairs 1992). Women suffering injury as a result of domestic violence are much more likely to have multiple injuries than those injured in accidents. Abused women are more likely to sustain injuries to the face, neck, breast, chest, and abdomen, as opposed to accident victims who are more likely to have injuries to the extremities.

Indeed, in one study, those injured as a result of domestic violence were 13 times more likely to have injuries to the breast, chest, or abdomen than those injured in accidents (Stark *et al.* 1979). One in four domestic violence incidents reported to police in the London Borough of Hackney involved serious injury such as strangulation, stabbing, fractures, or attempts to kill or set fire to the victim. One in ten abused women presenting to a GP surgery had been knocked unconscious and 7% had sustained fractures (Stanko *et al.* 1997). Domestic violence is often accompanied by sexual abuse and rape.

## The health consequences

Violence causes fear. Eighty per cent of women experiencing chronic domestic violence and 52% of women experiencing intermittent violence reported being very frightened during the incident (Home Office Research Studies 1999). Fear produces chronic stress and anxiety and these, added to the effects of physical injury, undermine the physical and mental health of women exposed to chronic violence. Chronic anxiety has an extremely pervasive, insidious, and destructive effect upon health through mechanisms that are more and more clearly understood (Wilkinson 2000). In crisis situations, the body triggers the 'fight or flight' response and mobilizes energy for muscular activity. More routine bodily functions such as tissue maintenance and repair, immunity, growth, digestion, and reproductive processes are run down. This adaptation appears to have developed to cope with short-term emergencies but in the long term, when anxiety and arousal are sustained over weeks or years, normal functions remain impaired, resulting in illness. It seems likely that such mechanisms underpin at least some of the association between multiple physical symptoms and exposure to domestic violence.

Women seem to be at particular risk during pregnancy with between 4% and 17% of women reporting abuse in the current pregnancy (Mezey and Bewley 1997). Violence is associated with increased rates of miscarriage, premature birth, low birth weight, fetal injury, and fetal death (Webster *et al.* 1996). There is a strong association between living in a physically abusive relationship and one or more episodes of pelvic inflammatory disease (Schei 1991), chronic pelvic pain, and a wide range of other gynaecological symptoms.

Finding oneself a repeated victim of someone else's violence is intensely demeaning and demoralizing. Victims tend to lose their self-esteem and begin to accept the counter-accusation that they themselves are somehow to blame (Harwin 1997).

> I said Make your own fuckin' tea. That was what happened. Exactly what happened. I provoked him. I always provoked him. I was always to blame. I should have kept my mouth shut. But that didn't work either. I could provoke him that way as well. Not talking. Talking. Looking at him. Not looking at him. Looking at him that way. Not looking at him that way. Looking and talking. Sitting, standing. Being in the room. Being.
>
> What happened?
>
> I don't know (Doyle 1996).

Evidence suggests that these processes take a profound toll on the psychological well-being of those who are subjected to repeated abuse. Women who have experienced domestic violence suffer a high incidence of psychiatric disorders, particularly depression, and various self-damaging behaviours including drug and alcohol abuse, suicide, and parasuicide. However, it is essential to understand that these present after the first exposure to violence and must therefore be viewed as consequences of the violence rather than causes of it, or even excuses for it. In Stark and Flitcraft's study, one in every four battered women attempted suicide at least once: one in seven abused alcohol and one in ten abused drugs. One in three were referred to emergency psychiatric services and one in seven were eventually institutionalized. The toll on these women's health is horrifying, yet these hugely damaging consequences can serve to distract attention from the underlying cause. The processes of medicalization focus attention on the consequences of violence rather than women's experience of the reality of the violence itself and the imperative for society to address the causes of this violence, rather than just patch up, more and more efficiently, the women who are exposed to it (Stark *et al.* 1979).

## A chronic, long-term condition

For less than 10% of abused women, domestic violence is an isolated event followed by effective resolution or permanent separation from the abuser. For the vast majority, domestic violence is endured as a chronic long-term condition that escalates over time. Hope that the violence will stop is very persistent and this probably explains the usually extended time which elapses between the start of the violence and the woman seeking help.

If she is to extract herself from an abusive situation, a woman must often pay a high price in terms of loneliness and, perhaps, disrupting her children's relationship with their father. The violent relationship may be the only intimate relationship that she has and this is a lot to lose. For many women, there is also an economic price to pay with the decision to leave a violent home bringing with it a substantial fall in income. Worse, a woman may have been threatened by her partner and may fear that she will be killed if she tries to leave. In these circumstances, staying may seem the only way to protect herself from something even worse (Women's Aid Federation of England 1992). All this helps to explain why so many women return again and again to face the risk of repeated violence to the amazement and sometimes the exasperation of the police, doctors, and others trying to help. Effective help must be directed towards enabling the woman to retake control of her own life, to offer her realistic choices while accepting that the decisions are hers alone and are always valid in her particular situation. No woman should be condemned for a decision to return to her abuser. It can take a very long time for a woman, demoralized by years of violence, to find the confidence and courage to choose a different life for herself and her children.

> The wonder is not that women find it hard to leave the scene of the violence but that so many find the courage to do so. It is often only when violence is directed at the children that women will summon up the courage to take a decision to do something about it and seek help (Victim Support 1992).

## The effects on children

The abuse of women and the abuse of children are intimately connected. In 90% of incidents of violence within families that include children, those children are in the same or the next room at the time (British Medical Association 1998). In a study of 62 episodes of domestic assault to which police had been called, 85% of assaults were directly witnessed by children (Brookoff *et al.* 1997).

> I was going nowhere, straight there. Trapped in a house that would never be mine. With a husband who fed on my pain. Watching my children going nowhere with me; the cruellest thing of the lot. No hope to give them. They saw him throw me across the kitchen. They saw him put a knife to my throat. Their father; my husband. (Doyle 1996)

The effect of this on the children can be imagined but is poorly documented. They may blame themselves for the violence or being unable to prevent it happening. They may try to intervene and be injured themselves. Refuge workers have noted a wide range of effects on children. These include confused and torn loyalties, lack of trust, unnaturally good behaviour, taking on the mother's role, guilt, isolation, shame, anger, lack of confidence, and fear of a repeat or return to violence (Gulbenkian Foundation Commission 1995).

Battered women are ten times more likely than non-battered women to report child abuse or to fear it (Stark *et al.* 1979). More than half of those men who use violence against their partners also abuse their children (Gayford 1975). Children whose mothers are battered are more than twice as likely to be physically abused as children whose mothers are not battered. In an American study, at least 45% of the mothers of abused children were found to be themselves battered, and these women had already presented an average of four injury episodes to the hospital. However, the battering clearly predated the child abuse, and the children of battered mothers are significantly more likely to be physically abused than neglected (Stark and Flitcraft 1988). Similar findings are now reported from the UK and the National Society for the Prevention of Cruelty to Children has found similar levels of domestic violence towards the mothers of children who are known to have been abused. In another UK study, 27% of abused mothers reported that their partners had also abused the children (NCH Action for Children 1994).

Despite these correlations, many general practitioners will have experience of women who have been held responsible, by social services departments, for their inability to protect their children from violence to which they are also being subjected.

> In contrast to battering, where sexist interpretations and practices confront a grass-roots political movement, in the child abuse field, stereotypic and patronizing imagery of women goes unchallenged. One result is that men are invisible. Another is that 'mothers' are held responsible for child abuse, even when the mother and child are being battered by an identifiable man. . . . – the best way to prevent child abuse is to protect women's physical integrity and support their empowerment. (Stark and Flitcraft 1988)

For just these reasons, the Statement of Aims and Principles of the Women's Aid Federation (England) defines domestic violence as 'the emotional, sexual or physical abuse of women and children in their homes by partners or known others, usually men'. Their explicit guiding principle is that the safety and empowerment of the non-abusing parent (usually the mother) is the most effective form of child protection.

## Male violence against women from ethnic minority communities

Women from ethnic minority communities face particular difficulties which include racism, language barriers, and worries about what will happen to their immigration status if they attempt to leave their violent partner. The enduring pervasiveness of racism within British society and the stereotyping of members of some communities means that black women may be very reluctant to call the police or involve them in any way, feeling that by doing so they are betraying their whole community. Some women may be subjected to enormous pressure from their extended families to stay with a violent partner because of the stigma that is attached to the breakdown of family structures. Some whose first language is not English may have insurmountable problems in communicating their predicament to professionals or agencies who might be able to offer help. Other women may fear deportation if they leave a violent partner within 12 months of coming to the UK (Women's Aid Federation of England 1992).

## Male violence against women with disabilities

In attempting to address the specific problem of male violence against women with disability, it is necessary to take into account the fact that all people with disability face a range of oppressive and discriminatory factors in their lives (Strathclyde Regional Council 1995). There is some evidence to suggest that disabled women are at increased risk of violence (Doucette 1986) and certainly the relatively increased dependency and isolation which so often accompanies disability can make it harder for disabled women to extricate themselves from violent situations. The abuser may be the woman's sole carer, and fears of continuing violence may be balanced by fears of being unable to cope alone, fears of becoming dependent on the inadequacies of statutory services, and, perhaps at worst, fears of being obliged to accept institutional care. Others, including relatives and friends, may be unwilling to accept that the partner who seems willingly to accept the additional burden of caring for a disabled partner, could be capable of violence. Health-care professionals should be aware that the confidentiality of a disabled person may be much more easily compromised because of the, sometimes accustomed, presence of a carer.

## Violence within other domestic relationships

Domestic violence is not exclusively male assault of women, although there is little doubt that this accounts for the major proportion of such violence, particularly violence that results in serious injury (Home Office Research Studies 1999). Even at the ultimate extreme of domestic violence, approximately 15 women in Britain kill their partners, as compared with 100 men (Home Office 1995). Significantly, there is a paradoxical gender bias in the response of the legal system, in that 40% of the women are convicted of murder, but only 25% of the men.

Very little is known about the extent of violence within other domestic relationships, and more research is needed into the extent and nature of violence directed against men by their women partners, violence directed against parents, particularly single mothers, by adolescent children, and violence within gay relationships, both male and female. While paying particular attention to the vulnerability of women and children, general practitioners need to retain an awareness of the potential for violence within any relationship, and the damaging health consequences of such violence.

> Domestic violence remains a major health issue affecting the lives of thousands of women and their families. The health community has a responsibility to intervene in this escalating spiral of violence which results ultimately in the homicide of many women and, indeed, of some men, when women kill in self-preservation and self-defence. (Edwards 1997)

## The role of general practice

General practice has enormous potential to offer help to women enduring domestic violence (Heath 1998). The general practice surgery is freely accessible to all and there is no stigma attached to a visit to the general practitioner, the practice nurse, or the health visitor, as there might be for a visit to the police domestic violence unit or the offices of the local social services department. Despite this, many general practitioners and other primary health-care professionals have been slow to exploit the potential of their situation.

> Although woman abuse is second only to male-male assault as a source of serious injury to adults, . . . clinicians rarely identify the problem, minimize its significance, inappropriately medicate and label abused women, provide them with perfunctory or punitive care, refer them for secondary psychosocial problems but not for protection from violence, and emphasize family maintenance and compliance with traditional role expectations rather than personal safety. (Stark and Flitcraft 1988)

In many cases of domestic violence, general practice is the first formal agency to which victims present for help. However, the possibility of violence is seldom raised directly (Pahl 1979; Mehta and Dandrea 1988), and it has been estimated that only a quarter of women seeking medical help actually disclose the fact that they have been beaten (Dobash and Dobash 1979). Many use the 'calling card' of an apparently unimportant physical symptom to test the attitudes and sensitivity of the doctor, and so beginning the processes of seeking help diffidently and indirectly. In the past, general practitioners have often failed to respond, accepting the 'calling card' at face value, because of lack of confidence in their ability to intervene effectively (Sugg and Inui 1992) and sharing the sense of helplessness of the victims in the face of society's apparent ambivalence (McWilliams and McKiernan 1993). Yet, the manner in which the general practitioner responds to a woman's first tentative attempt to seek help to change her situation can make an immense difference to that woman's life and those of her children (Richardson and Feder 1997).

## Consider the possibility

The possibility of domestic violence should be considered in *any* general practice consultation and particularly in the following situations:

- The patient reports past or present abuse.
- The patient presents with unexplained bruises, whiplash injuries consistent with shaking, areas of erythema consistent with slap injuries, lacerations, burns, or multiple injuries in various stages of healing.
- The patient has injuries to areas hidden by clothing which may be found inadvertently while, for example, doing a routine cervical smear (Mehta and Dandrea 1988).
- The patient has injuries to the face, chest, breast, and/or abdomen (Stark *et al.* 1979).

- The patient has symptoms or signs suggestive of sexual trauma.
- The extent or type of injury does not seem to match the explanation given by the patient.
- There is a substantial delay between the time of injury and the presentation for treatment.
- The patient describes an 'accident' in a hesitant, embarrassed, or evasive manner.
- Review of the medical record reveals that the patient has presented with repeated 'accidental' injuries.
- The patient presents repeatedly with physical symptoms for which no explanation can be found (Jaffe *et al.* 1986). This presentation may be particularly common among women whose first language is not English, and who therefore may find it difficult to express their feelings and suffering (Fenton and Sadiq 1993).
- The partner accompanies the patient, insists on staying close to her, and/or seems very attentive but is reluctant to allow her to speak for herself.
- The patient is pregnant (Mezey and Bewley 1997). Domestic violence often begins with the first pregnancy, and injuries are most commonly to the breasts or abdomen (Lent 1991).
- The patient has a history of miscarriage. Women experiencing domestic violence are 15 times more likely to have suffered a miscarriage (Stark and Flitcraft 1996).
- The patient or her partner has a history of psychiatric illness, or alcohol or drug dependence (Jaffe *et al.* 1986; Andrews and Brown 1988).
- The patient has a history of attempted suicide (Gayford 1975; Stark *et al.* 1979). In the USA, domestic violence accounts for one in four suicide attempts by women.
- The patient has a history of depression, anxiety, feeling unable to cope, social withdrawal, or an underlying sense of helplessness.
- There is a history of behaviour problems or unexplained injuries to children (Abrahams 1994).

## Ensure privacy and emphasize confidentiality

The family is meant to be a place of love, warmth, support, and intimacy. The difficulty of admitting that the family is also a source of violent abuse should never be underestimated. Many women will feel distressed and ashamed of their predicament, and it is essential that the patient feels that her account is respected and believed. If at all possible, the woman should be offered the chance to talk to a woman health-care professional if she prefers to do so. She should always be enabled to consult on her own, and she should be reminded that anything she chooses to talk about is confidential. The only exception to this will arise if the doctor becomes aware that a dependent child is also at risk (British Medical Association 1998; Wilson 1997).

The concept of medical confidentiality may be unfamiliar to many first-generation immigrant women and the protection it offers will need to be very carefully explained and emphasized. Provided the patient gives consent, the involvement of translators, advocacy workers, or ethnic community link-workers can be very helpful to both patient and doctor.

## Ask the question

This is more easily said than done; it is always difficult to confront a patient with the possibility that her injuries have been caused by domestic violence. Practitioners fear that the question will cause offence and jeopardize the mutual respect of the doctor/patient relationship. They also feel inadequate to deal with the problems presented, having neither sufficient time nor sufficient information at their disposal (Sugg and Inui 1992). Yet 'if you do not ask a direct question, you do not even have the possibility of a direct answer' (Stanko 1997), and the evidence suggests that women who are being subjected to violence want to be asked, and that women who are not, do not mind being asked (Friedman *et al.* 1992).

> I fell down the stairs again, I told her. Sorry.
>
> No questions asked. What about the burn on my hand? The missing hair? The teeth? I waited to be asked. Ask me. Ask me. Ask me. I'd tell her. I'd tell them everything. Look at the burn. Ask me about it. Ask. (Doyle 1996)

It is important to ask direct questions in a gentle, non-threatening and non-judgemental manner. Practitioners will need to try out various forms of words and identify those that feel most comfortable. Possibilities include:

- I have noticed you have a number of bruises. Could you tell me how they happened? Did someone hit you?
- Did someone at home do this to you? (Jones 1997)
- You seem frightened of your partner. Has he ever hurt you?
- Many patients tell me they have been hurt by someone close to them. Could this be happening to you?
- You mention your partner loses his temper with the children. Does he ever lose his temper with you? What happens when he loses his temper?

- Have you ever been in a relationship where you have been hit, punched, kicked, or hurt in any way? Are you in such a relationship now?
- You mentioned your partner uses drugs/alcohol. How does he act when drinking or on drugs?
- Does your partner sometimes try to put you down or control your actions?
- Sometimes, when others are overprotective and as jealous as you describe, they react strongly and use physical force. Is this happening in your situation?
- Your partner seems very concerned and anxious. That can mean he feels guilty. Did he hurt you?
- I notice that you have been drinking. Sometimes desperate situations demand desperate measures. Are you in a desperate situation?

In an American study of women using emergency departments, 27% had a history of physical or non-physical partner violence in the previous year. Of these, 70% were detected by the answers to any of the following three questions:

- Have you been hit, kicked, punched, or otherwise physically hurt by some-one in the past year? If so, by whom?
- Do you feel safe in your current relationship?
- Is there a partner from a previous relationship who is making you feel unsafe now?

In answer to any of the above questions, 25.5% reported having been physically hurt in the previous year, 19% by a current or past partner; 11.5% felt unsafe in their current relationship and 13% felt threatened by a partner from a previous relationship (Feldhaus *et al.* 1997).

> I'd get worked up waiting. I believed it was just a matter of luck. Maybe this time. A nurse would look at me and know. A doctor would look past his nose. He'd ask the question. He'd ask the right question and I'd answer it and it would be over. Charlo was always with me. He was always there. Behind the curtain was the only time I was alone. His shadow on the curtain. A few minutes. One question. One question. I'd answer; I'd tell them everything if they asked.
>
> Ask me. (Doyle 1996)

Many argue that all women presenting for health care should be asked routinely about their exposure to domestic violence, and that such an approach is justified by the estimated prevalence of domestic violence and by the toll it takes on the physical and psychological health of so many women (Jones 1997). This proposal may well prove to be appropriate in such settings as antenatal clinics, but it will be important to establish through systematic research that the intervention is effective before advocating its widespread introduction. It seems unlikely that routine screening questions will ever be appropriate in the very diverse setting of ordinary general practice consultations, where formulaic, protocol-driven approaches can so easily dominate the patient's own, often carefully planned agenda for the consultation. Nonetheless, it is essential that all practitioners retain a high index of suspicion within all consultations, and are prepared to act on those suspicions as soon as they arise.

## Examine

If there is any suggestion of physical injury, the patient should be carefully examined. Any examination should be both sensitive and thorough. The practitioner should bear in mind that the injuries characteristic of domestic violence are often to areas hidden by clothing, including the chest, breasts, abdomen, and perineum. It can be very easy to find an excuse, in the context of a busy surgery, not to examine a patient properly. Women from certain ethnic minority groups may be at particular risk of inadequate examination because of the excuse offered to the practitioner by the woman's apparent shyness and the sometimes unfamiliar nature of her clothing.

## Document

Accurate documentation of the patient's history and her injuries, at successive consultations over time, may provide cumulative evidence of abuse, and is essential for use as evidence in court, should the need arise. Proper records may also be needed to prove a right to rehousing.

The practitioner should make clear notes, which include the following:

- Any data from the previous medical record which is suggestive of prior abuse.
- The time, date, and place of, and any witnesses to the assault or accident.
- The whereabouts of any children at the time of the assault or accident.
- If the patient states that the injury was caused by abuse, preface the patient's explanation by writing: 'Patient states . . . .'
- Any subjective data that might be used against the patient should be avoided (for example, 'It was my fault he hit me because I didn't have the kids in bed on time.').
- If the patient denies being assaulted, write: 'The patient's explanation of the injuries is inconsistent with the physical findings' and/or 'The injuries are suggestive of battering.'
- Record the size, pattern, approximate age, description, and location of all the injuries. A record of 'multiple contusions and lacerations' will not convey

a clear picture to a judge or jury, but 'contusions and lacerations of the throat' will back up allegations of attempted strangling. If possible and appropriate, make a body map of the injuries, and include any signs of sexual abuse.

- Record any non-bodily evidence of abuse, such as torn clothing, or damage to the home if the patient is seen on a home visit.

## Photograph

Whenever possible, photographs should be taken of all patients with visible injuries. If the practitioner is not equipped to do this, the patient should be advised to have photographs taken by a professional photographer or at the police station.

## Assess present situation

The patient must be enabled and given time to tell her story.

> ... in order to understand the extent of the impact of violence on women, it is important not to pre-determine the meaning of the term. The starting point is to hear from women themselves and the meaning they attach to their experiences. (Lloyd, 1997)

It is important to gather as much information as possible and to try to include the following:

- any past history of abuse (including past and present physical, emotional and/or sexual abuse);
- any attempts the patient has made to remedy her situation (for example, through police, courts, separation, refuges, and so on);
- any sources of emotional support available to her;
- details of her current living situation. Is there some place, other than home, where she can go to recover, and take stock, if it is dangerous for her to return home?
- the degree of immediate danger to herself, her children and the professionals involved with her:
  (a) Is the abuser verbally threatening her?
  (b) Is the abuser frightening her friends and relatives?
  (c) Is the abuser threatening to use weapons?
  (d) Is the abuser intoxicated?
  (e) Does the abuser have a criminal record?
  (f) Are the children in danger? Where are they at the moment?
  (g) Is there any perceived threat to the professionals involved? Has the abuser any history of violence to those outside the home?

## Provide information

All general practitioners and other primary health-care professionals should assemble sufficient information about local resources and agencies, so that they are able and prepared to inform the woman's choice of action, both immediately and in the future:

+ Explain to the patient that violence in the home is as illegal as violence on the street and that she is the victim of a crime and has legal rights (Jones 1997).
+ Explain the physical and emotional consequences of chronic battering.
+ Provide written information (Osborne 1990) about:
  (a) legal options
  (b) help offered by:
     (i) police domestic violence units
     (ii) Women's Aid National Helpline (Tel: 08457 023468), women's aid refuges (Asian women's refuges and services available for women from other ethnic minorities can usually be contacted through Women's Aid)
     (iii) local authority social services departments
     (iv) local authority housing departments
     (v) Department of Social Security.
+ Offer help in making contact with other agencies.

The Department of Health has produced an extremely useful resource manual (Department of Health 2000).

## Devise a safety plan

In the context of a history of violence, often extending over many years, which erodes and destroys self-esteem, self-determination, and autonomy, it is essential to understand that effective help must be directed towards enabling the woman to retake control of her own life. The aim should be to offer her realistic choices, while accepting that the decisions are hers alone and are always valid in her particular situation. No patient should ever be pressurized into following any particular course of action. Her individual autonomy, self-esteem, and self-determination should be encouraged and respected. Even if the patient decides to return to the violent situation, she is not likely to forget the information and care given and, in time, this may help her to break out of the cycle of abuse. Beware of the danger of the needs of some ethnic minority patients being ignored under the guise of 'respect' for different cultures.

+ If she does not wish to return to the abuser, agree a plan of action and make an appropriate referral.

- If she chooses to return to the abuser, discuss (Pahl 1995):
  (a) a PROTECTION PLAN
    (i) When abuse is occurring, curl up into a ball to protect abdomen and head.
    (ii) Remove potential weapons from the home.
    (iii) Shout and scream loudly and continuously while being hit.
    (iv) If possible, arrange with a sympathetic neighbour that, if screams are heard, the neighbour will call 999.
    (v) Teach the children how to dial 999 if they feel unsafe.
  (b) an ESCAPE PLAN
    (i) Encourage her to plan ahead for what she will do the next time abuse occurs. Where will she go? How will she get there? What will she take?
    (ii) Give her the phone number of the local women's refuge.
    (iii) Advise her to keep some money and important financial and legal documents hidden in a safe place, in case of emergency.
- If children are likely to be at risk, consider referral to social services, if possible with the patient's consent.

Medicine and health care can never put right the causes or the effects of domestic violence. Yet there is much that can be done simply by recognizing the reality of a victim's situation, endurance and courage. This can be the beginning of helping to rebuild a woman's confidence and putting her in touch with agencies who can provide detailed advice, practical help, and refuge.

> ... the ability to imagine vividly ... another person's pain, to participate in it and then to ask about its significance, is a powerful way of learning what the human facts are and of acquiring a motivation to alter them. (Nussbaum 1995)

It seems safe to assume that roughly one in four women health professionals will have had direct experience of the pain of domestic violence. However, for the more fortunate, who must first understand if they are to offer help that is appropriate, sensitive, and effective, Roddy Doyle's imaginative achievement in *The woman who walked into doors* provides a model (Doyle 1996).

> The doctor never looked at me. He studied parts of me but he never saw all of me. He never looked at my eyes. Drink, he said to himself. I could see his nose moving, taking in the smell, deciding.

## Useful reading for patients

Department of Health (1999). *Domestic violence – break the chain*. HMSO, London.

## Acknowledgements

Parts of this chapter have been published previously in:

Heath I. (1998). *Domestic violence: the general practitioner's role.* Royal College of General Practitioners, London.

Amiel., S. and Heath, I. (Eds) (2003). *Family violence in primary care.* Oxford University Press, Oxford.

## References

Abrahams, C. (1994). *The hidden victims: children and domestic violence.* NCH Action for Children, London.

Andrews, B. and Brown, G.W. (1988). Marital violence in the community. *British Journal of Psychiatry,* **153**, 305–12.

British Medical Association (1998). *Domestic violence: a health care issue?,* pp. 32, 51–3. BMA, London.

Brookoff, D., O'Brien, K.K., Cook, C.S., Thompson, T.D. and Williams, C. (1997). Characteristics of participants in domestic violence: assessment at the scene of domestic assault. *Journal of American Medical Association,* **277**, 1369–73.

Council of Scientific Affairs (1992). Violence against women – relevance for medical practitioners. *Journal of the American Medical Association,* **267**, 3184–9.

Department of Health (2000). *Domestic violence: a resource manual for health care professionals.* Department of Health, London.

Dobash, R.E. and Dobash, R.P. (1979). *Violence against wives.* Free Press, New York.

Doucette, J. (1986). *Violent acts against disabled people.* Disabled Women's Network (DAWN), Toronto.

Doyle, R. (1996). *The woman who walked into doors.* Jonathan Cape, London.

Edwards, S.S.M. (1997). The law and domestic violence. In: Bewley, S., Friend, J. and Mezey, G. (eds), *Violence against women,* p. 105. Royal College of Obstetrics and Gynaecology Press, London.

Feldhaus, K.M., Koziol-McLain, J., Amsbury, H.L., *et al.* (1997). Accuracy of 3 brief screening questions for detecting partner violence in the emergency department. *Journal of the American Medical Association,* **277**, 1357–61.

Fenton, S. and Sadiq, A. (1993). *The sorrow in my heart . . . sixteen Asian women speak about depression.* Commission for Racial Equality, London.

Friedman, L.S., Samet, J.H., Roberts, M.S., Hudlin, M. and Hans, P. (1992). Inquiry about victimization experiences. A survey of patient preferences and physician practices. *Archives of Internal Medicine,* **152**, 1186–90.

Gayford, J.J. (1975). Wife battering: a preliminary survey of 100 cases. *British Medical Journal,* **1**, 194–7.

Gelles, R. and Straus, M. (1979). Violence in the American family. *Journal of Social Issues,* **35**(2), 15–39.

Gulbenkian Foundation Commission (1995). *Children and violence: report of the Commission on Children and Violence convened by the Gulbenkian Foundation,* pp. 162–6. Calouste Gulbenkian Foundation, London.

Harwin, N. (1997). Domestic violence: understanding women's experiences of abuse. In: Bewley, S., Friend, J. and Mezey, G. (eds), *Violence against women*, p. 63. Royal College of Obstetrics and Gynaecology Press, London.

Heath, I. (1998). *Domestic violence: the general practitioner's role*. Royal College of General Practitioners, London.

Home Office (1995). *Criminal statistics England and Wales*. HMSO, London.

Home Office (1999). *Domestic violence: break the chain*. Multi-agency guidance for addressing domestic violence. HMSO, London.

Home Office Research and Statistics Department (1992). *Criminal statistics*. Home Office, London.

Home Office Research Studies (1999). *Domestic violence: findings from a new British Crime Survey Self-completion Questionnaire*. HMSO, London.

Jaffe, P., Wolfe, D.A., Wilson, S., *et al.* (1986). Emotional and physical health problems of battered women. *Canadian Journal of Psychiatry*, **31**, 625–9.

Jones, R.F. III (1997). The abused woman. In: Bewley, S., Friend, J. and Mezey, G. (eds), *Violence against women*, pp. 76–82, 84. Royal College of Obstetrics and Gynaecology Press, London.

Kay, T. and Kent, J.H. (1989) Women victims of domestic violence. *British Medical Journal*, **299**, 1339.

Lent, B. (1991). *Reports on wife assault*. Ontario Medical Association Committee on Wife Assault, Canada.

Lloyd, S. (1997). Defining violence against women. In: Bewley, S., Friend, J. and Mezey, G. (eds), *Violence against women*, p. 8. Royal College of Obstetrics and Gynaecology Press, London.

Mayhew, P., Maung, N.A. and Mirrlees-Black, C. (1993). *The 1992 British Crime Survey*. HMSO, London.

McWilliams, M. and McKiernan, J. (1993). *Bringing it out in the open: domestic violence in Northern Ireland*. HMSO, Belfast.

Mehta, P. and Dandrea, L. (1988). The battered woman. *American Family Physician*, **37**, 193–9.

Mezey, G.C. and Bewley, S. (1997). Domestic violence and pregnancy. *British Medical Journal*, **314**, 1295.

Mirrlees-Black, C., Mayhew, P. and Percy, A. (1996). *The 1996 British Crime Survey: England and Wales*. HMSO, London.

NCH Action for Children (1994). *The hidden victims: children and domestic violence*. NCH Action for Children, London.

Nussbaum, M.C. (1995). *Poetic justice: the literary imagination and public life*. Beacon Press, Boston, MA.

Osborne, J. (1990). *Domestic violence fact pack*. HMSO, London.

Pahl, J. (1979). The general practitioner and the problems of battered women. *Journal of Medical Ethics*, **5**, 117–23.

Pahl, J. (1995). Health professionals and violence against women. In: Kingston, P. and Penhale, B. (eds), *Family violence and the caring professions*, p. 147. Macmillan Press, Basingstoke.

Richardson, J. and Feder, G. (1997). How can we help? – the role of general practice. In: Bewley, S., Friend, J. and Mezey, G. (eds), *Violence against women*, pp. 157–67. Royal College of Obstetrics and Gynaecology Press, London.

Schei, B. (1991). Physically abusive spouse – a risk factor of pelvic inflammatory disease? *Scandinavian Journal of Primary Care*, **9**, 41–5.

Stanko, E., Crisp, D., Hale, C. and Lucraft, H. (1997). *Counting the costs: estimating the impact of domestic violence in the London Borough of Hackney*. Hackney Safer Cities, London.

Stanko, E.A. (1997). Models of understanding violence against women. In: Bewley, S., Friend, J. and Mezey, G. (eds), *Violence against women*, pp. 291–301. Royal College of Obstetrics and Gynaecology Press, London.

Stark, E. and Flitcraft, A. (1988). Women and children at risk: a feminist perspective on child abuse. *International Journal of Health Services*, **18**, 97–118.

Stark, E. and Flitcraft, A. (1996). *Women at risk*. Sage, London.

Stark, E., Flitcraft, A. and Frazier, W. (1979). Medicine and patriarchal violence: the social construction of a 'private' event. *International Journal of Health Services*, **9**, 461–93.

Strathclyde Regional Council (1995). *Male violence against women with disability: a report for the Zero Tolerance Campaign*, Glasgow.

Sugg, N.K. and Inui, T. (1992). Primary care physicians' response to domestic violence. Opening Pandora's box. *Journal of the American Medical Association*, **267**, 3157–60.

Victim Support (1992). *Report of a National Inter-Agency Working Party on Domestic Violence*, Paragraph 1.10. Victim Support, London.

Webster, J., Chandler, J. and Battistutta, D. (1996) Pregnancy outcomes and health care use – effects of abuse. *American Journal of Obstetrics and Gynecology*, **174**, 760–7.

Wilkinson, R. (2000). *Mind the gap: hierarchies, health and human evolution*. Weidenfeld & Nicolson, London.

Wilson, P. (1997). Careless talk costs: the limits of confidentiality in histories of violence. In: Bewley, S., Friend, J. and Mezey, G. (eds), *Violence against women*, pp. 291–301. Royal College of Obstetrics and Gynaecology Press, London.

Women's Aid Federation of England (1992). Memorandum 22. In: *Domestic violence. Memoranda of evidence*. Home Affairs Committee, HMSO, London.

Yearnshire, S. (1997). Analysis of cohort. In: Bewley, S., Friend, J. and Mezey, G. (eds), *Violence against women*, p. 45. Royal College of Obstetrics and Gynaecology Press, London.

# Chapter 18

# Promoting the health of women in primary care

Sandra Nicholson and Yvonne Carter

## Introduction

A definition of women's health depends not only on the attitudes of health-care professionals but also on the perception and health beliefs of the women themselves. Healthy women are both physically and mentally well. This chapter is concerned with promoting the health of women in the UK, but the world-wide context of women's health, with for example unacceptably high maternal mortality rates and overt discrimination of women in developing countries, cannot be ignored and where appropriate is referred to. Indeed, all women have the right to 'the highest attainable standard of physical and mental health' (Beijing Platform for Action 1995).

Traditionally, health promotion consists of three parts: health education, prevention of ill-health and public health or social policy issues (Tannahill 1985). This chapter sets out each area for discussion and includes pertinent frequently asked questions (FAQs) that women may ask relevant to each section. The National Women's Health Information Center, run by the US Department of Health and Human Services, has a website (http://www.4woman.gov) which contains a FAQ section which was used to help devise some of these frequently asked questions.

The salient role of the primary health-care team in promoting the health of women and the possible barriers and difficulties in effectively achieving this aim are highlighted. The chapter closes with an illustration of a typical consultation dealing with issues of health promotion and recommended further information.

## The three main areas of health promotion

### Health education

Many valuable aspects of health promotion are concerned with ensuring women have enough readily understandable information to help them make their own informed choices about their lifestyles and the consequences that certain behaviours may have on their health. Primary health-care teams are ideally placed to discuss health education matters with women both opportunistically during consultations and at specific health-promotion sessions, such as well-women clinics. Information needs to be available in several different formats (verbal, written, such as patient leaflets and appropriate waiting room magazines) and also advice about how to contact self-help groups and reliable Internet sites. It is particularly helpful if the information disseminated by different sources and using varying styles cross-reference each other and that individual members of the primary health-care team reinforce each other's advice.

Areas of women's health education that are appropriately dealt with in primary care are outlined below. It is often more effective to discuss health-promotional matters with a woman in the context of her own individual health and personal risk. It is, for example, highly relevant to discuss a woman's smoking history at antenatal booking appointments or when she attends for contraceptive advice. Women also need to be informed about how best to use the health services available to them, such as access to emergency contraception. The specific role of the primary health-care team in health promotion is discussed later.

### Lifestyle advice

Many women eat above the recommended daily intakes of fat, exercise little, smoke, and manage their stress levels poorly. Lifestyle advice from health-care professionals can seem like an endless list of tedious 'do's and don'ts'. However, women often ask for advice as they are concerned about their appearance and so through these and other opportunistic consultations current evidence on what constitutes a healthy diet, appropriate exercise, and other health-promotion advice can be given.

### Diet

Obesity is increasing both in children and adults and gathering evidence highlights that obesity is a more serious risk factor for morbidity than previously thought. A large study that examined the effect of self-reported obesity, smoking, heavy drinking, and poverty on US adults concluded that obesity (BMI greater than 35) is more detrimental to health than the other risk factors. This study particularly considered a woman's risk of additional chronic medical conditions if she was overweight and found that obesity was associated with conditions such as hypertension, angina, gynaecological problems, and diabetes. The authors concluded that obesity is highly prevalent and, despite being associated with significant morbidity, does not receive appropriate attention either clinically or in public health policies (Sturm and Wells 2001).

Health-care professionals should actively seek opportunities to discuss diet with women who are overweight as their risk of hypertension, hypercholesterlaemia, and late-onset diabetes is increased and subsequently the rate of coronary heart disease. This is confirmed in a number of studies that have shown that coronary heart disease is associated with obesity, in both women and men. The Nurses' Health Study, a large prospective study of more than 120 000 American women, showed that overweight women were at two to three times the risk of coronary heart disease. This study similarly showed that women who maintain their ideal body weight have a 35–60% lower risk of myocardial infarction (Manson *et al.* 1990).

Women from lower social classes tend to eat diets with more saturated fat, less fresh fruit and vegetables, and they more frequently smoke, further increasing their risk of coronary heart disease. It can be particularly hard to promote healthy eating in low-income families whose access to a wide range of healthy foods may be limited. One study evaluated a community project which aimed to encourage low-income mothers to partake of a well-balanced diet that was affordable, tasty and easy to make. Following the sessions a reduction in consumption of full fat cheese, red meat, and cakes compared with an increase in low-fat spreads and fruit and vegetables was seen (Martin and Coe 1996). Coronary heart disease and its effect on women is specifically discussed in the section on illness prevention.

### Frequently asked questions (FAQs)
*So, what is a healthy diet?*

- A variety of foods should be eaten and lower fat options and healthy cooking methods, such as grilling instead of frying, should be used.
- Complex carbohydrates such as bread, rice, pasta, and potatoes. Try to eat wholemeal pasta, bread, and rice weekly.
- At least 5 portions of fruits and vegetables a day. This includes fresh, frozen, dried, and tinned varieties (fruit juice counts as one portion).
- Servings of low-fat dairy products a day. Use butter, margarine, and oils sparingly.
- Women, especially teenagers, should eat plenty of calcium-containing foods, such as dairy produce, green vegetables, and fortified breads and cereal. Calcium builds strong bones and reduces the risk of osteoporosis.
- Meat, fish, or other protein-rich foods such as beans and lentils, keeping to moderate amounts daily. Try to eat one portion of oily fish such as salmon once a week.
- Women need more iron than men, found again in fortified cereals and bread and red meat, due to the loss through menstruation and pregnancy.

*How can I lose weight?*

◆ Losing and maintaining weight loss is concerned with a gradual and permanent change in eating habits. This is helped by also increasing the amount of exercise you take.

◆ Fad and very low calorie diets are unlikely to be a long-term solution. Aim to lose weight slowly and make small easy changes to your diet first and then build on your success by attempting further changes.

◆ Do not underestimate the importance of small maintained changes such as reducing the amount of fat in your diet and be realistic about what you can change in any period of time, particularly if other life changes are occurring simultaneously.

◆ Eat regular meals, think before having seconds and try to avoid eating in between meals.

*Reducing the amount of fat*

◆ Use spreads on bread sparingly; try replacing with jam, marmite, or pickles.

◆ Use semi-skimmed or skimmed milk.

◆ Eat low-fat dairy produce, diet yoghurts, half-fat or cottage cheeses, replace cream with yoghurt or custard.

◆ Grill rather than fry and use small amounts of olive oil in cooking only when essential.

◆ Avoid processed meats such as mince and sausages which are very high in fat; try replacing with soya products or mixing meat and soya together.

◆ Remove fat and skin from meat before cooking.

### Exercise

Regular exercise helps to maintain weight, reduce stress, and is necessary for cardiovascular fitness. Weight-bearing exercise is particularly important to maintain skeletal strength. However, in a Health Education Authority study women were found not to consider lack of exercise as a significant risk factor for coronary heart disease (Sharp 1994). Many women do not enjoy playing sport and have little time or financial resource to join a gymnasium or exercise class. Lifestyles have become much more sedentary and working women may sit all day at a desk; in addition, much housework is now performed by labour-saving devices and people travel by car rather than walk. The UK National Fitness Survey in 1990 found that more than eight out of ten women exercised less than the minimum level indicated for beneficial health results.

Advice about exercise should be tailored to individual preferences and lifestyle. There is little point in advising a women who walks 3 miles to a cleaning job, which lasts 4 hours and entails cleaning ten floors including stairs, about gentle jogging. Similarly, whilst swimming is excellent all round exercise, it may be inappropriate to recommend it to women from ethnic minorities if there are no women-only facilities locally. Women who play sport, enjoy exercise classes, or dance should be supported, but all women should be encouraged to walk more and engage in some strenuous physical exercise regularly each week. Women who walk briskly for 1–3 hours a week were found to reduce their risk of having a coronary event by 30% in a study that specifically examined the relationship between exercise and coronary artery disease in women (Manson *et al.* 1999). A review paper examining over 50 studies that investigated the impact of exercise on preventing cardiovascular disease concluded that the risk was lower in physically active individuals (Miller *et al.* 1997).

## *FAQ:*

*What is the best form of exercise?*
Weight-bearing exercise, such as brisk walking and jogging, builds bone strength, helping to prevent osteoporosis. Aerobic exercise that makes the heart beat faster strengthens the heart and helps reduce heart disease. Swimming is a good all round exercise. For maximum effect, exercise should be taken at least twice a week for 30 minutes.

## Alcohol

There is less alcohol-related illness in women compared with men in the UK because in general women drink less alcohol than men. However, changes in lifestyle of young women in particular, adopting drinking patterns more akin to men's, have raised concerns that women's rates of alcohol-related illness may increase. Females metabolize alcohol more slowly and tissues may be more vulnerable to damage. Mortality from chronic liver disease increased threefold in women and increased alcohol consumption and binge drinking are of particular concern in younger women (Department of Health 2001). The health advice to women is clear that whilst moderate alcohol may be beneficial in terms of preventing coronary heart disease and cancers, regular heavy consumption is associated with hypertension, increased risk of cancers and liver cirrhosis, in a dose-dependent fashion (Department of Health 1995; Gronbaek *et al.* 2000). Recently, it has also been recommended that all alcohol should be avoided before and during pregnancy due to its effects on fetal brain development, although there is scant evidence that the occasional glass does any harm.

## *FAQs*

*Isn't alcohol good for you?*
Yes, depending on the volume and type consumed. In general, wine decreases mortality from all causes, particularly coronary artery disease. However, beer and spirits have less beneficial health effects and are associated with greater risks of cancer and mortality in excess.

*How much can I safely drink then?*

Unfortunately, most studies do not differentiate between women and men, but a large study that adjusted for gender comparing drinkers with non-drinkers concluded that:

◆ Light drinkers (1–7 drinks a week) of any alcohol has no detrimental effect on health.

◆ Moderate drinkers (8–21 drinks a week), particularly wine drinkers, reduce mortality from all causes, particularly their risk of coronary heart disease, by 32–49%.

◆ More than 22 drinks of beer or spirits is associated with increased mortality, a 63% increased risk of cancer specifically. This increased risk is reduced if wine is also consumed (Gronbaek *et al.* 2000).

It has been estimated that one in 12 women drink more than the recommended safe limits of alcohol consumption, which is no more than 14–21 units of alcohol per week or 3 units in any one day (Department of Health 1995). Gauging the amount of alcohol in drinks may be unreliable. One unit of alcohol corresponds to half a pint of beer, one glass of wine, or a single measure of spirits, but does not take into account stronger beers, lagers, and wines (with 12–14% alcohol) or the new alcoholic fruit-juice beverages (Drugs and Therapeutics Bulletin 2001).

Opportunities arise in primary care to advise women of the safe drinking levels (and to highlight that primary care is a safe and non-judgemental arena in which any concerns a woman may have about her drinking habits may be discussed confidentially). Members of the primary care team may be the first to be aware that there is a problem or potentially may be one. The team is also well situated to refer women for specialist help, and to promote Alcoholics Anonymous, should the need arise. Regular review, support, and short-term goals are helpful in assisting women to control their drinking.

The role of the practice nurse is particularly important in screening for alcohol misuse and in appropriate circumstances offering brief interventions. Brief interventions involve simple advice about the effects of harmful drinking and the need to cut down or stop drinking. Sessions may involve discussing results of blood tests, comparing drinking levels with the general population, simple condensed counselling, and/or practical help with reducing alcohol consumption. Studies have found that brief interventions may be as effective as longer assessments at reducing alcohol consumption (Drugs and Therapeutics Bulletin 2000). Practice nurses may be under-utilized in this area of health promotion but a need for further training has been highlighted. Specialist training aims to ensure that professionals take a careful alcohol history, know accurately the sensible drinking limits, are able to use screening tools to identify people struggling with their drinking, and know where and how to refer patients for further help (Owens *et al.* 2000).

*How can I screen for alcohol problems in primary care?*

Using the CAGE questionnaire (Box 18.1), MCV and GGT blood tests will detect about 75% of women with alcohol problems (WHO Collaborating Centre for Research and Training for Mental Health 1998).

---

### Box 18.1 **CAGE questionnaire**

- Have you ever felt you should **C**ut down on your drinking?
- Have people **A**nnoyed you by criticizing your drinking?
- Have you ever felt bad or **G**uilty about your drinking?
- Have you ever had a drink first thing in the morning (**E**ye-opener) to steady your nerves or get rid of a hangover?

(Ewing 1984)

---

### Smoking advice

More than half a million women are killed annually by smoking and, because some conditions may take years to develop, many countries have not yet experienced the full impact of smoking on women's health (Howell 1998). The number of women smoking has reduced, but the number of teenage women smoking now exceeds teenage men, and there is some evidence that these women will persist with smoking.

Smoking is a serious risk factor for cardiovascular disease, a variety of cancers, osteoporosis, and low birth weight babies. Most women are aware of the general health risks of smoking and the main role of primary care is to reinforce this with additional relevant information that particularly highlights an individual women's risk and seeks a potential opportunity to encourage quitting. Women are at higher risk of heart disease and stroke if they smoke and use oral contraceptives. Smokers should be encouraged to stop or reduce the number of cigarettes they smoke during pregnancy and women should be aware of the benefits of stopping before conception and the dangers of re-starting post-partum.

Studies have shown that gentle encouragement and limited counselling can have a beneficial effect on reducing smoking. Integrating smoking cessation into periconceptual care has been shown to be effective at reducing smoking in expectant mothers (Gonczi and Czeizel 1996). O'Connor *et al.* (1992) reported that 14% of women successfully gave up (shown by urinary cotinine levels) after attending a 20-minute smoking intervention session by a practice nurse.

Petersen *et al.* (1992) found in a randomized study of expectant mothers that 29% of those given self-help materials on smoking cessation managed to quit by 8 weeks post-partum compared with 10% who received the standard antenatal care. Similarly, smoking women attending cervical smear clinics can be offered contextual advice about the risks of smoking and cervical cancer and advised to give up.

Advice on strategies, support groups, nicotine replacement, and referral to smoking cessation clinics can be useful. A Cochrane Review of the use of nicotine replacement treatment (NRT) compared with placebo or no treatment in randomized trials reporting smoking cessation rates after 6 months showed that nicotine patches, rather than gum, almost doubled the number of people who quit (Silagy *et al.* 2001). Implementation of NHS plans to reduce smoking offers some areas of the UK additional funding and pilot schemes to practically help the least advantaged smokers to give up. Such schemes involve funding prescription of the first week of NRT for patients who meet the appropriate criteria and collaboration of pharmacies, primary care trusts, and primary care professionals to establish smoking cessation clinics (Department of Health 1998). The effectiveness of bupropion is presently being appraised by the National Institute for Clinical Excellence (NICE) and their report is due this year. Bupropion may serve as a useful adjunct, particularly in smokers who have failed to give up with NRT.

### FAQs
*I've tried to quit, but failed.*
- It's very common to take more than one attempt to finally give up but it's never too late to try. Often trying to give up with a friend, nicotine replacement, or bupropion may help you to be successful.
- The National Women's Health Information Center run by the US Department of Health and Human Services has a very wide-ranging and useful website (http://www.4woman.gov). Information and links to other sites to help you quit can be found there.

*What can I do to help me quit?*
- First, pick a date to quit. Quitting all at once is much more likely to succeed than trying to cut down gradually.
- Tell your family and friends about your plans to quit, and ask for their support. Then, before stopping, throw away all your cigarettes, don't keep any where you live.
- Before you stop smoking, think about the situations which make you want a cigarette. If you always smoke after a meal, plan what you'll do instead. If you smoke during certain tasks at work, figure out what can replace the cigarette.

+ Some people like to hold something in their hand in certain situations; substituting a pencil or pen can work for them.

+ Many feel comforted by having something in their mouth, sugar-free gum or candy, or carrot or celery sticks are good choices.

+ Some people use cigarettes to relax when they are stressed. Substituting walking, reading, or meditating can be a good alternative.

+ Many people need help to quit smoking. Help can come in several forms. Tell your doctor, who will advise about nicotine replacement therapy. Some general practices run smoking cessation clinics with specifically trained nursing staff. Being in a support programme makes it likelier you'll succeed.

## Dealing with teenagers

Fortunately teenagers are generally healthy, but sometimes their lifestyles can be imprudent; young women's attitudes are often akin to 'it won't happen to me'. By 1996, 33% of 15-year-old girls were classed as smokers, more than 40% of 16-year-olds reported weekly alcohol consumption at an average of 3.4 units and it is well recognized that the use of illegal drugs and solvents is rising, particularly in younger teenagers (Walker *et al.* 2000).

Risky behaviours should be openly discussed in the light of their possible consequences. It can be very helpful to discuss with teenagers possible reasons for engaging in activities that may damage their health (or barriers preventing them from adopting a healthier lifestyle). Smoking is a good example of this. Most people know the long-term risks of smoking, but young people do not think that they are presently at risk of lung cancer or heart disease whilst peer pressure to smoke may be high. Specific advice concerning the additional risk of thromboembolism with smoking and oral contraceptive pill use, discussed in context and relevant to young pill users, may be effective in reducing smoking.

A recent White Paper, 'Smoking Kills', prioritizes reducing smoking in young people in England by aiming to decrease the prevalence of smoking in children from 13 down to 9% by 2010 (Department of Health 1998). However, smoking uptake and continuation are complex behaviours and interventions are more likely to be successful if they are well coordinated, long term and combine local community action with mass media education campaigns. The importance of personal factors should not be forgotten and studies that have examined adolescents' personal competency skills and perceived benefits of smoking have found that smoking prevention programmes should highlight these areas (Epstein *et al.* 2000).

The UK has the highest rate of teenage pregnancy in Europe; 9.4/1000 women conceived before age 16 in England and Wales in 1996 (Office for

National Statistics 1998). The high levels of sexually transmitted infections among young people also indicate that present strategies to improve the sexual health of the country's youth is failing. A two-pronged approach is advocated that aims sexual health education at all young people but particularly those deemed at high risk. Studies have shown that the highest level of teenage births occur to the most socioeconomically disadvantaged women (Adler 1997). Unfortunately, there is little sound evidence that any current interventions effectively reduce teenage pregnancy or modify teenagers' sexual behaviour, as shown by a recent review of both observational and randomized studies (Guyatt *et al.* 2000).

Teenagers rarely receive health promotion advice from their physicians. Multiprofessional primary care consultations are good opportunities to target individuals in need of lifestyle advice. Concerns that teenagers would find surgery environments unfriendly, possibly unconfidential and disinterested in issues pertinent to themselves were not borne out by the high levels of satisfaction reported by teenagers who had been invited to a general practice consultation to deal with health behaviour advice. However, to maximize the impact of health education, primary care should work alongside schools, local government programmes, and family planning clinics (Walker *et al.* 2000).

## Prevention of ill-health

Women's health can be promoted by actively screening for conditions that adversely affect either the quality or length of women's lives. Specific cancers that affect women, breast and cervical, have established screening programmes in this country. Evaluation of ovarian cancer screening is awaited. Screening for other conditions, such as osteoporosis, urinary incontinence, and postnatal depression, all causes of significant morbidity in women, are not so well defined. These areas are discussed in other chapters. Inequalities in screening women compared with men for certain conditions, such as coronary heart disease, also need to be addressed and this is explored below.

### Coronary heart disease in women

Despite coronary heart disease being the leading cause of death in women, its prevention and treatment have not been optimum (Radley *et al.* 1998). The decline in mortality from cardiovascular disease in women has been slower than in men. The simplest explanation for these facts is that women have been treated as men, known as the Yentl complex (Healy 1991). The major trials concerning coronary heart disease all featured men, whose symptoms, test results, and pharmokinetics do not necessarily match those of women. This has led to women being underdiagnosed, under-referred, and perhaps inappropriately treated.

More worryingly, because women are not men, they may not be treated at all. Coronary heart disease is uncommon in younger women, certainly before the menopause, and so physicians and patients themselves may not consider the diagnosis (Lockyer 2000). Unfortunately, even when coronary heart disease has been confirmed, women are less likely to be offered surgical and pharmacological treatments than men. The national service framework for coronary heart disease, the government's plan to improve services throughout the UK, has been criticized for not specifically outlining how these gender differences should be addressed (White and Lockyer 2001).

Preceding discussion has emphasized the importance of giving healthy lifestyle advice to all women, but health education relating to coronary heart disease, that is to exercise regularly, maintain a normal weight, eat sensibly, and not to smoke, needs to be particularly targeted at women at risk. Premenopausal women are generally at low risk of coronary heart disease but women with a strong family history, diabetics, smokers, hypertensives, and those with dyslipidaemia need to be assessed. Relatives of patients who reported symptoms of coronary heart disease at an early age are particularly at risk. Diabetic women face the same magnitude of risk of coronary heart disease as men. Screening for these high-risk women is worthwhile and a history of gestational diabetes or family history of maturity-onset diabetes should be highlighted (Newnham and Silberberg 1997).

A 20–25% reduction in cardiovascular mortality in patients receiving exercise rehabilitation following myocardial infarction was reported by two meta-analyses examining 22 randomized trials. Eight trials reported improvements in heart failure and angina symptoms (Miller *et al.* 1997). Exercise therefore clearly has a role in not only preventing coronary heart disease but also helping patients recover from cardiovascular events and reducing further occurrences. However, it is difficult to isolate the effects of exercise on patients' health from other interventions, particularly as exercise may well reduce some of the other risk factors for coronary heart disease such as raised cholesterol levels.

Dietary advice, examples of which are discussed earlier in the chapter, conducted by specifically trained nurses can lead to a fall in coronary heart disease risk, which has been shown to be sustained in women (Imperial Cancer Research fund OXCHECK Study Group 1994). Antioxidant vitamins found in fruits and vegetables may have a role in decreasing atherosclerosis and thereby reducing coronary heart disease. However, the evidence is not conclusive. The consumption of low-dose aspirin has been shown to reduce the incidence of heart attack in both women and men diagnosed with coronary heart disease (Antiplatelet Trialists' Collaboration 1994). As yet, there is insufficient evidence to recommend taking aspirin in asymptomatic women, although the results from large-scale primary prevention trials in women are awaited.

Raised cholesterol levels are related to the development of coronary heart disease in women and men. Under the age of 50, women tend to have lower cholesterol levels than men, but after the menopause their HDL levels fall and their LDL levels rise, factors thought to increase the risk of heart disease. Lowering cholesterol levels in men is accepted as preventative. The incidence of major heart attacks in women with already existing coronary heart disease is reduced by lowering cholesterol levels (Miettinen *et al.* 1997). However, the effect of lowering cholesterol levels in healthy women is speculative. A trial examining the effect of lovastatin in people (15% women) with no demonstrable coronary disease and average blood cholesterol levels was stopped early after finding a 36% reduction in a combined fatal and non-fatal cardiac event. The limited trials looking at the specific effect of cholesterol-lowering drugs, such as statins, on women indicates that the therapeutic effect of the drugs is similar in women as men and that women do not suffer any additional or increased side effects from medication (Effective Health Care 1998).

Women who smoke more than 40 cigarettes a day increase their risk of coronary heart disease by 20-fold and even light smokers (1–4 cigarettes a day) have double the risk of coronary heart disease than non-smokers (Willett *et al.* 1987). The number of women that smoke is slowly declining but there are gender differences that need addressing such as the increased proportion of younger women who smoke and the fact that female smokers find it harder to quit (Reid 1995). Individual advice that can be given to smokers to help quitting has been discussed and further social policy avenues to discourage overall smoking are explored later.

It is thought that the hormonal changes associated with the menopause are responsible for the older woman's higher risk of coronary heart disease, a rise in blood pressure and changes in cholesterol levels being the principal causes of the increased risk. However, the role of hormone replacement therapy in the prevention and treatment of coronary heart disease remains controversial. Hormone replacement therapy may well help reduce a woman's risk by affecting lipid metabolism, but these effects seem to last only whilst taking medication. Women who had an early surgical menopause without oestrogen replacement have been found to have more than double the risk of coronary heart disease compared with premenopausal women of the same age. Subsequent evidence indicates that giving all postmenopausal women hormone replacement therapy to reduce their risk of coronary heart disease is not justified (Posthuma *et al.* 1994). A full discussion of hormone replacement therapy is found in Chapter 3.

## Maintaining the mental health of women

Women's mental health is greatly affected not only by their physical well-being but also their social structures, supporting relationships, self-esteem, and social roles. Women present more often than men to the primary health-care team with depression, the most common psychiatric complaint in women. Depression is twice as common in women as men and depressed patients use health services two to three times as often. It is therefore essential that depression is recognized and treated. Women also suffer from anxiety, phobias, obsessive–compulsive disorders and may self-harm. Any consultation dealing with these conditions needs to involve a detailed social assessment. Particular vigilance in detecting and treating postnatal depression not only helps the woman concerned, but also minimizes any cognitive effects on their children.

## Social policy

The health of women depends on good health services, both in terms of delivery and structure and also on their environment. Environmental issues are concerned with physical, social, and cultural paradigms and as such can be influenced by social policy. The effects the physical environment may have on women's health are enormous. Research on passive smoking and subsequent lobbying has decreased the number of workplaces where women, and their unborn children, are exposed to the effects of passive smoking. Restrictions on leaded fuels have reduced car emissions and hence air pollution, which is possibly associated with the rise in childhood asthma.

A combination of social policies can strongly affect women's health. Many environmental issues illustrate the overlap between promoting an individual woman's health and public health. A combined approach from policy makers, health-care professionals, educationalists, and the media is required if change is to be initiated and maintained (Barth 1994). Banning tobacco advertising, increasing taxation, restricting smoking areas, community education programmes as well as individual health promotion are hoped to reduce the number of women who smoke (Department of Health 1998). The recent introduction of emergency contraception available over the counter at selected pharmacies is yet to be fully evaluated but it is hoped that it will reduce the large number of unwanted teenage pregnancies in this country. The massive safe sex campaign in the early 1990s was a good example of media involvement in promoting a health message widely to the public.

Cultural aspects significantly affect women's health throughout the world. The inequalities that women face in many countries ensure that women's health will never be a priority. In this country there has been a shift away from addressing maternal mortality and infectious diseases, which were dramatically reduced in the last century, to the prevention and management of chronic disease and conditions that affect the ageing population of women. These major issues are cardiovascular disease, cancer, and osteoporosis (Freund and Battaglia 2000).

However, gender inequalities persist. Coronary heart disease screening clinics should not solely aim to reduce the risk in men. Health professionals, doctors, and, specifically, nurses involved in chronic disease management need to be trained to identify women at risk. The National Service Framework for coronary heart disease dictates that general practices undertake a risk assessment of adults to identify those most at risk of developing coronary heart disease. Unfortunately, how practices are to deal with gender differences is not specified. Community-based research needs to be conducted to address these issues and to establish appropriate guidelines on referral and treatment for women with established coronary heart disease.

Whilst applauding the advances in screening and management of women's conditions in the developed world, there is still a need to address the disparities in health outcome for women of low socioeconomic status. Women with low incomes still have poorer uptake of screening, diets of higher fat intake, more frequently smoke, and take less exercise. Hence women with low incomes and from ethnic minorities are more likely to have low birth weight babies, cervical cancer, and coronary heart disease. Improving access to screening may reduce some of the differences in the health outcomes of these women but further research is required and appropriate social policy to improve the lives of all women. Health centres that endeavour to provide a range of health and social services on one site may be successful in reaching some of these women.

Recent undergraduate medical curricula and GP vocational training schemes have included plans to cover topics such as domestic violence. This illustrates the broadening of the medical curriculum to encompass areas of interest particularly to women. Members of the primary health care team need to be specifically trained to facilitate health promotion in women (and work together in multidisciplinary teams), nurses often having advanced training and qualifications. Primary health-care professionals also need further training in mental health to enable them to cope with the increasing burden of mild to moderate psychological ill-health found in women in the community. Many UK undergraduate curricula have community-based components which encourage students to consider the advantages of working in a multidisciplinary team. Community-based obstetric and gynaecology modules also expose students to aspects of women's health that occur commonly, such as family planning and menopausal issues, and encourage students to examine the women's perspective on health matters (Nicholson *et al.* 2001).

## The role of the primary health-care team

General practices are often the first port of call in the UK for women with any health concern. It is therefore appropriate that primary health-care professionals are trained to deal with a wide range of conditions and also specifically when to refer to a specialist. Fragmentation of women's health services has largely been avoided in the UK due to the strength of primary care.

The diversity of the primary health-care team allows women a choice in practitioner, depending on their preference and also the nature of their complaint. Studies clearly show that women wish the opportunity to see a female practitioner for matters concerning sexual health, psychosocial issues, and intimate examinations. However, the most important factor for many women is whether they feel their general practitioner (GP) is 'approachable and understanding and who takes the time to listen to and communicate with patients' (Brooks and Phillips 1996). It has been well documented that patient satisfaction can affect compliance, clinical outcomes, and the take-up of screening and preventative health services (Phillips and Brooks 1998).

Although the primary health-care team may be diverse in terms of discipline, gender, age, and interests, it is cohesive in striving together to provide the best possible care for its patients. This is illustrated well by health needs, which are best met by a multidisciplinary team, such as antenatal care. The role of nurses within such a collaborative team is vital. Many women find that they can relate to, and therefore form better therapeutic relationships with, nursing staff. Nurses typically spend more time with patients and involve patients more fully in their care (Fisher 1995). This trust can be utilized to promote healthy lifestyle advice and to offer screening and counselling in a non-patronizing manner. Nursing has much to offer the primary health-care team. Nursing education has a broader aspect than many medical undergraduate curricula. Traditionally nursing has been patient-centred, concentrating on the caring aspect of medicine and effective communication skills, often being the women's advocate in health matters (Hoffman *et al.* 1997).

The primary health-care team can provide a comprehensive health-care system for women. However, some authorities believe that because primary care also treats women's families, men, and children, this causes a dilution of experience. Creating a multidisciplinary speciality that specifically focuses on women might enhance the care offered to women. Other concerns are that general practice clinics generally only provide medical screening and do not adequately deal with psychosocial matters. There are limited opportunities for women to receive counselling within the primary care setting and many women feel that insufficient time is available to discuss their problems in full. To address these issues, many general practices provide special clinics, with longer appointment times and female staff, to address the health-promotion needs of women. Some practices have set up specific facilities to meet the health-promotional needs of ethnic populations as pertaining to their practice area, e.g. the Bangladeshi women's group run by a practice in the east end of London (Gray and Livingstone 1998). Practice development plans need to reflect the educational needs of the whole primary care team and the services that each practice intends to provide for their patients. Establishing smoking cessation and coronary heart disease screening clinics entails further specialist training, particularly for practice nurses.

The primary care team plays an integral role in promoting and maintaining the health of women. It is imperative that all consultations dealing with women's health issues are woman-centred as this ensures that all aspects of the woman's problem, physical, psychological, and social, as seen by the woman herself, are covered. This process has evolved out of the philosophy behind women's health centres but the emphasis is on every personal interaction between professional and patient rather than the environment *per se* (Hoffman *et al.* 1997).

## 10-Minute consultation

Mrs White, a 47-year-old lawyer, books a 10-minute appointment with you to discuss her recent menstrual problems. She mentions that recently she has been gaining weight and her usual dieting has not helped. You have previously treated Mrs White for depression, and today she again appears low and tearful. She enquires whether you think HRT would help?

### What are the issues?

◆ Perimenopausal menstrual difficulties are common and usually easily treated. Mrs White's periods may be coming more frequently and lasting for longer, sometimes being very heavy. Alternatively, she may have started to miss periods and be concerned about this.

+ 'Period trouble' may have been used as a 'ticket' to legitimize her consultation, allowing her opportunity to discuss with you other concerns which she may feel do not warrant a doctor's appointment.

+ Health promotion and management of Mrs White's weight.

+ Exploration of Mrs White's mood. Her past history confirms that she previously required a course of antidepressants. Is there something in particular that has precipitated a recent onset of depression?

+ She furthers wishes to know your opinion on whether HRT will help. The most important question here is clarifying what Mrs White particularly wants help with and then in the context of her answer, discuss the possible benefits of taking HRT.

+ Time management is a serious problem with this scenario because many of the above issues may take a whole consultation and so what should be covered first and what can be deferred needs to be negotiated.

## What to do?

+ Take a comprehensive menstrual history, specifically highlighting any post-coital, intermenstrual, and postmenopausal bleeding. The possibility of fibroids, with symptoms of menorrhagia, should be considered.

+ Further assessment of her menstrual problems may involve a bimanual examination, haemoglobin measurement, pelvic ultrasound, and/or referral for specific gynaecological investigation, such as endometrial biopsy.

+ Advise appropriately on exercise, smoking, diet, alcohol, and stress management. Explain that following the menopause there is a shift in fat deposits from the lower to the central body, accounting for the change in body shape that many women find depressing. Regular exercise and a healthy, low-fat balanced diet, avoiding fad diets, will control body weight and enhance a woman's self-esteem (Deeks 2000).

+ Assess Mrs White for the symptoms of major depression: persistently low mood, early morning waking/sleep disturbance, poor concentration, poor appetite, and thoughts of suicide.

+ Ascertain whether there are any significant psychosocial issues that may be contributing to Mrs White's symptoms. Questions about her family and work situations may discover whether she is going through a change in social role with children leaving home or work difficulties.

◆ Enquire why HRT is an issue but time constraints mean that Mrs White needs to be invited to come back to see you or the nurse to fully discuss HRT. The possible benefits, reasons, and risks for HRT in Mrs White's individual case need to be covered. Mrs White needs to be examined and the different HRT preparations discussed if she decides to proceed. Patients often find it useful to read some further information before attending a second session specifically for HRT.

◆ Before ending the consultation, any questions Mrs White has should be dealt with and her understanding of the management plan checked and an appropriate follow-up appointment made.

## Recommendations and conclusions

Promoting women's health is a vast undertaking. It is a task that embodies more than those strategies already shown to be effective such as breast screening and smears. It must aim to ground itself in the unique physiology of women, appreciate the views of women about their health, and take into account the complex social parameters with which women live. The skill mix of the primary health-care team inevitably plays a central role in providing this woman-centred model of health that when fully developed will improve the health of women living not only in this country but also worldwide.

## Useful further information

The National Women's Health Information Center run by the US Department of Health and Human Services has a very wide-ranging and useful website (http://www.4woman.gov). The following information and further links to other sites can be derived from there.

### Smoking cessation

#### Can I find resources on the web to help me quit smoking?

The Internet can be an excellent way to locate resources on quitting smoking. As with all health-related information, search for information from reliable sources, which have been adequately researched. Be wary of 'individual' sites where the author may have a financial interest in the advice being given.

*http://www.lungusa.org/*

Provides information on stop smoking options, including an online 'Quit Smoking Action Plan' that uses a step-by-step approach to facilitate quitting.

*http://www.lungusa.org/tobacco/smkcessafac.html*

The Fact Sheet contains information on the following:

- Freedom from smoking: a self-help manual designed for smokers at different stages in the quitting process.
- 7 Steps to a smoke-free life: a book based on the Freedom from smoking programme, which can be purchased online or at local bookstores.
- A lifetime of freedom from smoking: a maintenance manual for the new ex-smoker.
- 'In Control' Freedom From Smoking Video Program: a video package, which includes the video cassette, viewer's guide, and audiocassette of relaxation techniques.
- Freedom From Smoking Cessation Clinics: 8-session group programme using positive behaviour change approach.
- Freedom from smoking audiotape – How To Quit Smoking: audiotape includes strategies for quitting, tools to deal with relapse, and relaxation exercises.
- Freedom From Smoking On-Line is an online version of Freedom From Smoking Cessation Clinics and can be found by returning to the American Lung Association main page and selecting 'programs and events', then selecting 'Freedom From Smoking' then selecting 'Freedom From Smoking On-line'.

*http://www.ash.org.uk*

This site includes information about the quit-smoking campaign with a resource guide and further links.

*http://www.eufic.org/gb/heal/heal.htm*

This is a useful website concerning diet and includes 10 healthy eating tips.

*http://www.alcoholconcern.org.uk*

Alcohol Concern believes it is essential that strategies are developed to tackle alcohol misuse in primary care and has developed a Primary Care Information Service.

### Health Development Agency website

The Health Development Agency's website (http://www.hda-online.org.uk) states that 'it is a special health authority, working to improve the health of people and communities in England, in particular, to reduce health inequalities'. It owns several websites of interest concerning health promotion.

# References

Adler, M. (1997). Sexual health – a Health of the Nation failure. *British Medical Journal*, **314**, 1743–7.

Antiplatelet Trialists' Collaboration (1994). Collaborative overview of randomised trials of antiplatelet therapy. 1: Prevention of death, myocardial infarction and stroke by prolonged antiplatelet therapy in various categories of patients. *British Medical Journal*, **308**, 81–106.

Barth, A. (1994). *Smoking: a review of effective interventions.* Anglia and Oxford Regional Health Authority, Cambridge.

Beijing Platform for Action (1995). Fourth World Conference on Women cited by Haslegrave, M. (1997). *Lancet*, **349**, 11–12.

Brooks, F. and Phillips, D. (1996). Do women want women health workers. *Journal of Advanced Nursing*, **23**, 1207–11.

Deeks, A. (2000). What are the emotional issues for women aged 40 and over? *Medical Journal of Australia*, **173**, S103–4.

Department of Health (1995). *Sensible drinking: the report of an inter-departmental working group.* HMSO, London.

Department of Health (1998). *Smoking kills. A White Paper on tobacco.* The Stationary Office, London.

Department of Health (2001). *Chief Medical Officer's Annual Report.* DoH, London.

Drugs and Therapeutics Bulletin (2000). Managing the heavy drinker in primary care. *Drugs and Therapeutics Bulletin*, **38**(8), 60–4.

Effective Health Care (1998). *Cholesterol and coronary heart disease: screening and treatment.* NHS Centre for Reviews and Dissemination, University of York.

Epstein, J., Griffin, K. and Botvin, G. (2000). A model of smoking among inner-city adolescents: the role of personal competence and perceived social benefits of smoking. *Preventive Medicine*, **31**(2 pt 1), 107–14.

Ewing, J. (1984). Detecting alcoholism. The CAGE questionnaire. *Journal of the American Medical Association*, **252**, 1905–7.

Fisher, S. (1995). *Nursing wounds: nurse practitioners, doctors, women patients, and the negotiation of meaning.* Rutgers University Press, New Brunswick, NJ.

Freund, K. and Battaglia, T. (2000). The two faces of health care for women. *Lancet*, **356**(Suppl), s66.

Gonczi, L. and Czeizel, A. (1996). Integrating smoking cessation into peri-conceptional care. [Letter] *Tobacco Control*, **5**, 160–1.

Gray, J. and Livingstone, A. (1998). Health promotion for Bangladeshi women in general practice must be appropriate. [Letter] *British Medical Journal*, **317**, 413.

Gronbaek, M., Becker, U., Johansen, D., *et al.* (2000). Type of alcohol consumed and mortality from all causes, coronary heart disease, and cancer. *Annals of Internal Medicine*, **133**, 411–19.

Guyatt, GH., DiCenso, A., Farewell, V., Willan, A. and Griffith, L. (2000). Randomised trials versus observational studies in adolescent pregnancy prevention. *Journal of Clinical Epidemiology*, **53**, 167–74.

Healy, B. (1991). The Yentl syndrome. *New England Journal of Medicine*, **325**, 274–6.

Hoffman, E., Maraldo, R., Coons, H. and Johnson, K. (1997). The women-centered health care team: integrating perspectives from managed care, women's health, and the health professional workforce. *Women's Health Issues*, **7**(6), 362–74.

Howell, F. (1998). Women and smoking. *Irish Medical Journal*, **91**, 15–16.

Imperial Cancer Research Fund OXCHECK Study Group. (1994). Effectiveness of health checks conducted by nurses in primary care: results of the OXCHECK study after one year. *British Medical Journal*, **308**, 308–12.

Lockyer, L. (2000). The experience of women in the diagnosis and treatment of coronary artery disease. PhD thesis, University of London, 240.

Manson, J., Stason, W., Willett, W., *et al.* (1990). A prospective study of obesity and risk of coronary artery disease in women. *New England Journal of Medicine*, **332**, 882–9.

Manson, J., Hu, F., Rich-Edwards, J., *et al.* (1999). A prospective study of walking as compared with vigorous exercise in the prevention of coronary artery disease in women. *New England Journal of Medicine*, **341**, 650–8.

Martin, B. and Coe, A. (1996). Changing dietary habits. *Community Nurse*, **2**(9), 60.

Miettinen, T., Pyorala, K., Olsson, A., *et al.* (1997). Cholesterol lowering in women and elderly patients with myocardial infarction or angina pectoris. Scandinavian Simvastatin Survival Study. *Circulation*, **96**, 4211–18.

Miller, T., Balady, G.J. and Fletcher, G.F. (1997). Exercise and its role in the prevention and rehabilitation of cardiovascular disease. *Annals of Behavioural Medicine*, **19**, 220–9.

Newnham, H. and Silberberg, J. (1997). Women's hearts are hard to break. *Lancet*, **349**, 13–15.

Nicholson, S., Osonnaya, C., Carter, Y., Savage, W., Hennessy, E. and Collinson, S. (2001). Designing a community-based fourth year obstetrics and gynaecology module: an example of innovative curriculum development. *Medical Education*, **35**, 398–403.

O'Connor, A., Davies, B., Dulberg, C., *et al.* (1992). Effectiveness of a pregnancy smoking cessation program. *Journal of Obstetric, Gynecologic and Neonatal Nursing*, **21**, 385–92.

Office for National Statistics (1998). *Population trends. Winter 1998*. HMSO, London.

Owens, L., Gilmore, I. and Pirmohamed, M. (2000). General practice nurses' knowledge of alcohol use and misuse: a questionnaire survey. *Alcohol and Alcoholism*, **35**, 259–62.

Petersen, L., Handel, J., Kotch, J., *et al.* (1992). Smoking reduction during pregnancy by a program of self-help and clinical support. *Obstetrics and Gynecology*, **79**, 924–30.

Phillips, D. and Brooks, F. (1998). Age differences in women's verdicts on the quality of primary health care services. *British Journal of General Practice*, **48**, 1151–4.

Posthuma, W., Westendorp, R. and Vandenbroucke, J. (1994). Cardioprotective effect of hormone replacement therapy in postmenopausal women: is the evidence biased? *British Medical Journal*, **308**, 1268–9.

Radley, A., Grove, A., Wright, S. and Thurston, H. (1998). Problems of women compared to those of men following myocardial infarction. *Coronary Health Care*, **2**, 202–9.

Reid, T. (1995). Coronary heart disease and the risk to women. *Nursing Times*, **91**(10), 27–9.

Sharp, I. (1994). *Coronary heart disease: are women special?* National Forum for Coronary Heart Disease Prevention, London.

Silagy, C., Lancaster, T., Stead, L., Mant, D. and Fowler, G. (2001). Nicotine replacement therapy for smoking cessation. *The Cochrane Library*, Issue 1. Update Software, Oxford.

Sturm, R. and Wells, K. (2001). Does obesity contribute as much to morbidity as poverty or smoking? *Public Health*, **115**, 229–35.

Tannahill, A. (1985). What is health promotion? *Health Education Journal*, **44**, 167–8.

Walker, Z., Oakley, J. and Townsend, J. (2000). Evaluating the impact of primary care consultations on teenage lifestyle: a pilot study. *Methods of Information in Medicine*, **39**, 260–6.

WHO Collaborating Centre for Research and Training for Mental Health (1998). Institute of Psychiatry, King's College, London.

White, A. and Lockyer, L. (2001). Tackling coronary heart disease. A gender sensitive approach is needed. *British Medical Journal*, **323**, 1016–17.

Willet, W., Green, A., Stampfer, M., *et al.* (1987). Relative and absolute excess risk of coronary heart disease among women who smoke cigarettes. *New England Journal of Medicine*, **317**, 1303–9.

## Chapter 19

# Complementary medicine and women's health*

## Christine A'Court, Chi Keong Ong, and Jacqueline Wootton

*An update of the original chapter by Christine A'Court, Jacqueline Wootton, Adriane Fugh-Berman, and Kim Jobst.

## Users of complementary medicine

### A consumer-led boom

According to recent surveys, up to one in four of the United Kingdom's general population over the age of 18 years report use of complementary medicine in the previous 12 months. This compares with one in seven in 1986 (Francis 1995; Dickinson 1996; Ernst and White 2000; Thomas *et al.* 2001; Ong *et al.* 2002; Ong and Banks 2003). Over a lifetime, it has been estimated that almost one-half (47%) of the UK population will have seen a complementary practitioner or purchased over-the-counter herbal or homeopathic remedies (Thomas *et al.* 2001; Ong *et al.* 2002).

In the UK, between 1993 and 1995, a 25% increase in sales of alternative medicines was noted (Mintel 1995). Expenditure has been estimated to be about £500 million a year for visits to complementary practitioners (Thomas *et al.* 2001) and the cost could be as much as £1.5 billion if over-the-counter purchases are included (Ernst and White 2000; Ong and Banks 2003). US expenditure on complementary medicine rose in 1990–97 from $13bn to $38bn a year, and twice as many consultations were with complementary medicine practitioners as with mainstream family doctors (Eisenberg *et al.* 1998). Australia has also witnessed an increase in usage, with four times as much public expenditure on complementary, as on conventional, medicines (MacLennan *et al.* 1996). The trend has been described as a consumer-led boom (Dickinson 1996). Poor outcomes from conventional care, especially in chronic conditions, may drive patients to seek alternatives (Murray and Sheperd 1993; Francis 1995). Use of complementary practitioners in the UK was found to be predicted by pain, disability due to physical health problems, and high levels of use of general practitioner services, amongst both those who report chronic illnesses and those who do not (Ong *et al.* 2002). However, patients are not always 'pushed' by dissatisfaction, they may also be 'pulled' by lifestyle and holistic beliefs towards alternatives (Francis 1995; Furnham and Vincent 1995; Dickinson 1996; Astin 1998). Recent work has also suggested that women are attracted to complementary therapies because of lifestyle reasons while men tended to utilize complementary medicine for health and illness purposes only.

Users of complementary medicine come from all socioeconomic groups, although in the UK the majority of users tend to be of higher educational level and social class (Fulder 1996). More recent work has confirmed that nearly eight out of ten users (78.3%) of complementary medicine practitioners' services were from a white collar background (Ong *et al.* 2002). In the UK, about two-thirds of all those reporting use of complementary medicine in 1999 were aged 35–64 (Ernst 2000; Ong and Banks 2003). Consultations with a practitioner

**Table 19.1** Consultations with complementary practitioners showing type of therapy and percentage of respondents for that therapy

| Practitioner | Percentage |
| --- | --- |
| Osteopath | 28 |
| Chiropractor | 17 |
| Homeopath | 16 |
| Acupuncturist | 12 |
| Aromatherapist | 12 |
| Reflexologist | 9 |
| Herbalist | 6 |
| Spiritual healer | 5 |
| Hypnotherapist | 4 |
| Alexander technique | 3 |
| Naturopath | 2 |
| Other practitioner | 5 |

Consumer Association Super Survey 1995, postal questionnaire with 8745 respondents. In the last 12 months 2724 (31%) had used a therapy.

**Table 19.2** Percentage of responders who consulted specified complementary medicine practitioners from the BBC Radio Five Telephone Survey 1999 (245 responders)

| Therapy | Percentage |
| --- | --- |
| Herbal medicine | 33.5 |
| Aromatherapy | 20.8 |
| Homeopathy | 17.1 |
| Acupuncture/acupressure/auricular therapy | 14.8 |
| Reflexology/shiatsu | 6.8 |
| Massage | 5.7 |
| Osteopathy | 3.7 |
| Bach flower | 2.9 |
| Chiropractic | 2.4 |
| Chinese medicine/T'ai chi | 3.2 |
| Yoga | 2.0 |
| Healing | 2.0 |
| Alexander technique | 1.2 |
| Hypnotherapy | 1.2 |
| Specified others | 11.7 |

were also highest in this age group (Ong *et al.* 2002). In the USA, high usage is seen in the wealthier white population, but is also characteristic of minority communities, reflecting their rich ethnic medical traditions (Wootton and Sparber 2001). In developing countries, 80% of the population still rely on traditional systems of medicine, including herbalism, spiritual healing, and acupuncture (Bodeker 1994).

The most popular and widely used methods on both sides of the Atlantic are: osteopathy, chiropractic, homeopathy, acupuncture, aromatherapy, reflexology, herbalism, healing, hypnotherapy, and naturopathy. Tables 19.1 and 19.2 suggest a change in predominant usage in the UK. In particular, comparison between early surveys of usage, and the most recent, admittedly small, BBC survey suggests the 'top two', osteopathy and chiropractic, may have been supplanted by herbalism, homeopathy, and aromatherapy or massage techniques (Ernst and White 2000; Thomas *et al.* 2001; Ong *et al.* 2002; Ong and Banks 2003). Use of osteopathic or chiropractic services may have been under-represented in the BBC survey. Alternatively, the increasing availability of herbal and homeopathic remedies in pharmacies and supermarkets, and the increase in availability of massage techniques and aromatherapy in leisure and beauty centres may have promoted consultation with the associated practitioners.

## Is there a philosophical divide between complementary and conventional medicine?

An early debate focused on whether various forms of unorthodox medicine are truly alternative or complementary to conventional medicine (Fulder 1996). Incorporating both views, the term CAM (complementary and alternative medicine) gained usage. It may yet be supplanted by the term 'integrated medicine' (or integrative medicine as used in the USA). *A British Medical Journal* editorial defined integrated medicine as, 'Practising medicine in a way that selectively incorporates elements of complementary and alternative medicine into comprehensive treatment plans, alongside solidly orthodox methods of diagnosis and treatment'. However, the same editorial recognized that, 'Integrated medicine has a larger meaning and mission, its focus being on health and healing rather than disease and treatment' (Rees and Weil 2001). In a second, even more provocative editorial, a different author argues that the enhancement of self-healing is an aim of complementary medicine which gets insufficient publicity, perhaps because it has been lost from much of conventional medicine (Reilly 2001). The therapeutic interaction between health professional and patient is something most should have experienced. Yet in an increasingly evidence-based and pressurized health-are system 'the human contribution is so undervalued it gets excluded from treatment protocols' (Reilly 2001). The current boom in complementary medicine should stimulate renewed interest in the healing as well as the helping power of compassion, holism, positive motivation, and enablement. Interestingly, the current message of the NHS Modernisation Agency is to put the patient's experience at the centre of all service planning and re-design. Embracing this basic tenet might help ensure that modern pressures and technological solutions do not push out older holistic values.

It is generally assumed that complementary medicine is based less on the scientific method than conventional medicine. Even this assumption is challenged by estimates of the evidence base for orthodox medical interventions, which range from 20% to 80% (Ellis *et al.* 1995; Gill *et al.* 1996). This chapter's authors hold the view that there is as great a need for evidence supporting the use of complementary medicine as there is for orthodox medicine. In this chapter we do not dwell further on these issues, but use the term complementary medicine to cover therapies which patients may choose to use in isolation, or as an adjunct to conventional medicine.

## Box 19.1 **Widely used complementary therapies**

### Acupuncture

Treatment by the insertion of fine, filiform needles at specific sites along lines of '$Qi$' (energy flow) called 'meridians' linking certain organs. Manipulation of the needle is believed to stimulate or dissipate unbalanced energy and so improve organ function.

### Aromatherapy

Massage, baths, compresses, and inhalations employing distilled or pressed aromatic ('essential') oils derived from plants, flowers, herbs, spices, and woods. Individual oils typically contain up to 100 different chemical compounds.

### Biofeedback

The use of equipment to monitor physiological signals and to bring involuntary processes under voluntary control.

### Chiropractic

Chiropractic postulates that various mechanical stresses (called 'subluxations') occur around intervertebral and other joints, and affect the functioning of the nervous system, and possibly other systems. These stresses may be the result of misuse of the skeleton – commonly bending and lifting, or prolonged adoption of poor postures at work, during recreation or sleep. Other causes include emotional stress and associated muscle spasm; trauma; or birth injury. Following diagnosis of the specific site of problems, manipulation of the spine and other joints is carried out.

### Healing

Transmission of psychic energy for therapeutic purposes.

### Herbalism

Use of whole plants, and in some cases minerals for therapeutic purposes.

### Homeopathy

Detailed history-taking evaluating multiple symptoms is followed by treatment of symptom complexes with a substance (the 'simillimum') creating near identical symptoms in a healthy person. Extreme dilutions are used (potentization), mixed in a proscribed way by violent agitation (succussion). In 'classical homeopathy', specific, tailored remedies are prescribed to

**Box 19.1** (*continued*)

an individual, in contrast to over-the-counter purchase of homeopathic remedies for common symptom complexes.

## Hypnotherapy

Based on the belief that the mind (conscious and unconscious) can influence organic diseases. After induction of a trance or deeply relaxed state, suggestions can be implanted. It aims to reduce general stress and unconscious disease-causing patterns, but sometimes selective suggestions may be made. Practised either in the presence of a therapist, or in absence (self-hypnosis). Hypnosis subjects can control blood supply, sensitivity to injury, and pain tolerance (Fulder 1996).

## Macrobiotic medicine

The macrobiotic philosophy attributes disease to heredity, climate, psychological states, behaviour, and an excessive intake of particularly 'yin' and/or 'yang' foods. Treatment emphasizes dietary manipulation, with reduction of intakes of excessively 'yin' foods such as sugar, food additives, tropical fruits, dairy products, refined flour, and commercial tea and coffee, and similar reduction of excessively 'yang' foods such as eggs, meat, salt, and salty varieties of cheese. The 'standard' macrobiotic diet, which is midway in the 'yin-yang' scale, is recommended to form the basis of any diet. It is based on grains, legumes, and forms of soy, with emphasis on root vegetables in patients who are too 'yin', and leafy vegetables in patients who are too 'yang'.

## Naturopathy

A system aiming to promote self-healing. Diagnosis employs a detailed interview concerning lifestyle, nutrition, bodily functions, and iris diagnosis (iridology). Treatment aims to eliminate toxins by dietary restriction or fasting, heat, internal or external hydrotherapy, exercise, manipulation, mud packs, and so on. Nutrition therapy, the dominant subspeciality within naturopathy, advocates a whole-food, high-fibre diet, preferably using food grown organically, and assumes that individual requirements vary according to genetic, physiological, and lifestyle influences. Some therapists advocate mega-vitamin and mineral supplements, whilst others adhere to the dietary approach.

## Osteopathy

Examination of musculoskeletal system, interpretation in terms of tension, adhesions, fibrosis, sprains, and circulatory stasis, then treatment by

## Box 19.1 (continued)

manipulation of soft tissues and joints. Many osteopaths believe this process affects not only the function of the musculoskeletal system, but also other organ systems.

### Reflexology

The application of manual pressure to 'reflex' points on the ears, hands, or feet that somatotopically correspond to specific areas of the body. Believed to reduce stagnation in the system and encourage the healing process.

### Relaxation and imagery

Assumes the mind can influence organic disease. Induction of states of deep relaxation and often guided visualization. In these states, suggestions can often be fully absorbed as effectively as in hypnotherapy.

### Traditional Chinese medicine

Holds that man is an indivisible combination of mind, body, and spirit. Disease may be a consequence of hereditary or environmental influences, and physical or psychological activity, any of which can interrupt the free flow of 'Qi' or energy. Therapy involves acupuncture, Oriental herbal medicine, diet, and psychophysical exercise such as T'ai-chi or Qigong designed to promote the free flow of Qi.

## Women as users of complementary medicine

Women's usage of complementary medicine is generally found to exceed that of men's (Fulder and Munro 1985; Thomas *et al.* 1991; Dickinson 1996). Women comprise more than two-thirds of the patients of alternative practitioners (Thomas *et al.* 1991; Vincent and Furnham 1996). Surveys carried out on general practice patient populations have found women to be nearly twice as likely as men to visit complementary medicine practitioners (Murray and Sheperd 1993; Thomas *et al.* 2001; Ong *et al.* 2002). The predominance of female usage may simply reflect the higher rates of consultation among women for medical care generally (Royal College of General Practitioners 1986). Prevalence of usage need not imply a difference in attitudes; earlier studies found no difference between men and women in attitudes to complementary medicine, or in reported satisfaction with the outcome of alternative care (Francis 1995; Vincent and Furnham 1996). A more recent study has suggested women are more likely than men to be satisfied with the outcome of either alternative or orthodox medicine (Ong and Banks 2003).

In two surveys, musculoskeletal symptoms, especially conditions such as back pain, were by far the most common presenting problem amongst patients attending osteopaths, chiropractors, naturopaths, and acupuncturists (Fulder 1996; Ong *et al.* 2002). Headaches, migraine, pain at other sites, anxiety, and depression also feature prominently in surveys confined to manipulative therapies. How often women turn to complementary therapy for specific 'women's problems' is more difficult to extract from the available data. While men often use massage, chiropractic, and osteopathy, women are more likely to consult herbalists and homeopaths (Murray and Sheperd 1993), or reflexologists and aromatherapists (Francis 1995). Women also favour a variety of lifestyle programmes, often used in combination. These include: dietary changes, mega-vitamin and mineral supplementation, relaxation and imagery, and various forms of exercise. It has been postulated that women appear to be attracted most to methods promoting general good health, whereas men tend to favour an emphasis on the management of an immediate condition (Dickinson 1996).

Recent work seems to bear out this postulate, demonstrating that lifestyle factors were primary motivators for the use of complementary medicine amongst women but not men (Ong *et al.* 2001). Thus, amongst *men*, only three factors were significant predictors of visits to complementary practitioners. The presence of long-standing illnesses was the best predictor, followed by taking exercise at least once a week for 30 minutes, and finally, higher socioeconomic class. Amongst *women*, long-standing illness and higher socioeconomic class were also strong predictors. However, lifestyle variables such as a desire for more exercise, worrying about the environment, being a non-smoker, and a desire to be involved in future NHS decision-making processes were also significant predictors of consultations with complementary practitioners.

Both men and women with cancer or AIDS frequently look to complementary therapy. While alternative 'cancer cures' may attract attention and controversy, complementary therapies are more likely to be used as an adjunct to conventional treatment for the relief of symptoms or side effects of treatment.

## Paying for complementary care inside and outside the NHS

Most people wanting complementary medicine have to pay for it at the point of contact. This situation discriminates against those who cannot afford it. On the other hand, the need for direct payment might in some cases contribute to the therapeutic effect, since patients may be more likely to feel the benefit of something actively sought out and directly paid for.

In the UK, regional differences in use of complementary therapies have been related to differences in amounts charged by practitioners (Fulder 1996).

Healing, which is often free, and other relatively inexpensive therapies like herbalism and hypnotherapy are used more in the north of the country whilst acupuncture, naturopathy, osteopathy, and chiropractic flourish in the more prosperous areas of the UK (Fulder 1996). In American society, high usage of some complementary therapies in low-income, minority ethnic groups reflects not only their cost but ethnic practice (Wootton and Sparber 2001).

A small Lancashire-based study asked users how the cost of therapies might influence their attendance. Seventy-four per cent of responders felt that cost would be an issue that affected their decision to have complementary treatment (Ong and Banks 2003). The majority of people were willing to pay a minimal amount, but most responders felt that £20 was more than they wanted to pay. Fees for an initial visit for complementary treatment are usually around £30–45, indicating that the Lancashire consumer desired prices for complementary medicine were unrealistic. The findings have also been used to suggest that the consumer might appreciate a subsidy of 33% to approximately 50%, if these therapies were made available on the NHS. However, the sheer volume of usage of complementary medicine is likely to make this proposition unattractive to the Treasury, as the figures below illustrate, unless savings in other areas were to ensue.

## Cost to consumers of using complementary medicine

Estimated annual expenditure on complementary medicine in the UK has increased from £580 million in 1998 (Thomas *et al.* 2001) to £1.47 billion in 1999 (Ernst and White 2000; Ong and Banks 2003).

The amount that individual consumers are prepared to pay can be gleaned from a variety of studies. In 1998, the mean annual expenditure on complementary medicine practitioners visits was estimated to be about £108 per user. In 1999, 60% of fees paid to complementary medicine practitioners came to £10 per month or less (Ernst and White 2000; Ong and Banks 2003).

## Cost to NHS of complementary medicine

The impact of devolution from health authorities to primary care trusts (PCTs) is having an uncertain effect on commissioning of complementary therapies by the NHS. Most published data comes from pre-PCT days. Thus, in 1995, only 6% of complementary therapy users were having their treatment paid through the NHS (Dickinson 1996). However, this low figure belied a considerable increase in availability within the NHS. Indeed, it was argued that complementary medicine was already an established part of the NHS (Smith 1996). A nationwide survey in 1995 found 60% of health authorities and 40% of general practitioners (GPs) were routinely purchasing complementary services. Most NHS referrals were for homeopathy or acupuncture. Fund-holding

GPs, in particular, were likely to commission complementary therapies, often provided within the health centre. Half of the commissioning GPs offered complementary treatments themselves (Thomas *et al.* 1995). One in 20 GPs employed a non-NHS therapist – often an osteopath. In 1996, out of the total NHS budget of £32 billion, an estimated £1 million was spent on complementary medicine. It was suggested that the perception of complementary medicine as low-tech, low-risk and relatively cheap was promoting its integration into NHS practice, despite the paucity of objective evidence of efficacy (Smith 1996). These comments, although apt, may have been founded on a vast underestimate of NHS spending on complementary medicine. A subsequent report, in 1998, estimated the NHS contribution to complementary medicine use to be £50–55 million (Thomas *et al.* 2001). The same report estimated that 79% of consultations were paid for directly by the patient, with the NHS providing an estimated 10% of the consultations.

### Sickness certification, insurance fees, and compensation

Non-registered medical practitioners can issue a sickness certificate. Many private medical insurance companies will reimburse the fees of registered (osteopaths and chiropractors) or medically qualified and well-established complementary practitioners, provided patients have been referred by a registered medical practitioner (Fulder 1996). Fees are being reimbursed by the Criminal Injuries Compensation Board and the Industrial Injuries Board (Fulder 1996). Some firms and trade unions now consistently reimburse the charges of osteopaths and chiropractors.

## Considerations for the referring or commissioning GP

### Professional liability

Complementary therapists in the UK enjoy a common law freedom to practise. In other countries, as in much of continental Europe and most states of the USA, only registered therapists are permitted to practise. Although at one time a doctor's association with unregistered practitioners was deemed serious professional misconduct, the General Medical Council (GMC) now recognizes the valuable role of alternative practitioners. The 1995 and 2001 updates of the GMC's professional guidance state that a GP can 'delegate medical care to nurses and other health care staff who are not registered medical practitioners' ... 'but you must be sure that the person to whom you delegate is competent to undertake the procedure or therapy involved' (GMC 1995, 2001). This is a tall order, given that few conventional doctors have an in-depth understanding of alternative therapies. Indeed, GPs recommend a complementary therapist in order to take advantage of an alternative paradigm. It has been argued that without GPs possessing the skills involved, the situation cannot properly be described as delegation (Stone 1996a, b). The GMC states that their guidance on this matter is under continuing review by the Standards Committee. Currently, 'referral' is not considered an appropriate term for a GP's recommendation to a patient to consult a complementary therapist; a GP is expected to have sufficient understanding of a complementary therapy to 'delegate' professional care, whilst retaining overall clinical responsibility. This is also the case in most states in the USA where most complementary therapists can only practice under medical supervision. When the GP cannot claim sufficient understanding of a therapy, the GMC view is that the GP runs the risk of not acting in the patients' best interests (GMC, personal communication). Use of a complementary therapist will often be in situations where the problem is chronic or intractable, or where a patient exercises choice. The GMC view is that any practitioners involved are responsible for their own actions, but since the GP retains overall clinical responsibility for a patient, he or she must throughout provide, or at least offer, a reasonable standard of care.

Doctors may hope that they will avoid professional and legal liability provided they recommend practitioners who are suitably qualified, or have statutory registration, as obtained in the UK by the osteopaths in 1993 and chiropractors in 1994. Although the standards imposed by various complementary professional bodies vary greatly, the GMC takes registration as a good indication of professional competence. In the absence of registration, the GMC view is that the GP should take reasonable steps to ensure the competence of individual alternative practitioners. (GMC, personal communication 1995).

## Legal liability

In the event of a mishap directly resulting from an alternative practitioner's intervention, UK medical defence bodies would, in general, resist any attempt to attribute liability to a GP. However, if the GP had referred the patient to a practitioner with a poor track record, then the GP might be deemed reckless, and liability might be shared (Medical Defence Union, personal communication). From the patient's point of view, the situation differs from that of referral to a specialist within the NHS (Stone 1996a). Although complementary therapists have a legal duty of care towards a patient, allegations of negligence may be hard to prove in the absence of nationally agreed standards of care. Moreover, many alternative therapists carry no indemnity insurance. The current unlicensed status of most herbal medicines in the UK protects the prescriber from legal liability, a situation potentially hazardous for patients

(De Smet 1995). However, the relatively low incidence of reported toxicity and side effects relative to the enormous sales of herbal products, and recent public resistance to European Union licensing proposals demonstrate the need for a separate herbal medicine licensing procedure, as in some other countries (Fulder 1996). In the meantime, the need for systematic safety monitoring is met in part by the recent extension of the Yellow Card scheme to include reporting of adverse reactions to unlicensed as well as licensed herbal medicines (Committee on Safety of Medicines/Medicines Control Agency 1996).

## Employment of complementary practitioners

If GPs themselves wish to employ complementary practitioners, they may be helped by guidelines from the West Yorkshire Health Authority, specifically drawn up to facilitate the employment of complementary therapists within the NHS. They emphasize the need to ensure that practitioners have appropriate qualifications, belong to a professional body complying with a defined code of ethics, and carry professional indemnity insurance (West Yorkshire Health Authority 1995). However, complementary practitioners have been cautioned against adoption of the conventional medical model of statutory regulation (Stone 1996b). It is argued they should continue developing their own standards of training, accreditation, voluntary self-regulation and thus professionalism, and avoid the philosophical and financial cost of an 'inappropriate statutory straitjacket.'

# Efficacy: source and nature of the evidence

To our knowledge, there has been no scientific evaluation of whole diagnostic and therapeutic systems such as those embodied in traditional Chinese medicine (TCM), macrobiotic medicine, naturopathy, or homeopathy. We have attempted to introduce and evaluate some studies applicable to the use of complementary medicine for women's health. In many cases we draw on studies that were not designed to investigate complementary medicine *per se*, but which are nonetheless relevant. Some of the more accessible evidence is concerned with nutritional aspects of complementary approaches. It should be noted that although dietary manipulation is central to macrobiotic therapy, it is only one of several elements dictated by, for instance, TCM, or naturopathy.

This review's layout mirrors the textbook's chapters. This single, problem-based approach to some degree runs counter to many alternative systems that emphasize that the significance of a symptom, such as dysmenorrhoea, or a disease such as breast cancer, may be apparent only when taken in the context of the whole person.

In pursuit of objectivity, this review draws whenever possible on the randomized control trial (RCT). However, much is recognized and written about the limitations of the RCT. Additional investigative approaches such as epidemiology, observational and case–control studies, the $n = 1$ trial, and experimental work are all needed to try and tease out the active, and the most potent ingredients of holistic health care. A survey carried out first with GP registrars, and then with dually qualified complementary and medical practitioners, has investigated what evidence they considered important before accepting that an alternative technique might benefit their patients. A controversial finding was that for the majority, the most important factor was personal experience of method use with patients, outweighing the importance of case–control or clinical trial evidence. This may indicate how strongly practitioners are influenced by their own, not necessarily representative, experience. Equally, it may show that practitioners modify the message they receive from scientific trials, which are seldom free from design or analytical flaws, according to their own experience. It also emerged that the practitioners' views concerning the nature of valid evidence were determined in part by age group and by their affiliation to either hospital, university, or primary care.

## Sources of information on complementary medicine

### Accessing the evidence

Clinical and experimental research relevant to complementary medicine is widely scattered in a number of databases world wide (see Directory of Databases, www.rosenthal.hs.columbia.edu/Databases.html). Several of the major biomedical bibliographic databases now contain significant numbers of citations on alternative medicine; both Medline and Embase (the European nearest equivalent to Medline) contain in the region of 270 000 references each, although with considerable overlap. Coverage in Medline has increased in recent years due to the policy of indexing the entire contents of journals, as opposed to the earlier policy of indexing only those articles that fitted pre-approved defined MeSH (Medical Subject Headings) categories. Accessibility has been further enhanced by the establishment of a Cochrane field of Complementary and Alternative Medicine since Medline personnel have agreed to include all RCTs identified by hand searches performed by the Cochrane initiative, irrespective of journal of origin.

There are approximately 55 serious journals, many with peer-reviewed research articles, in the field of complementary medicine. A comprehensive listing of these journals can be found at the Medbioworld website (http://www.medbioworld.com/med/journals/complementary.html). Two have been indexed in Medline since their start date in 1995, *Alternative Therapies in Health and Medicine* and the *Journal of Alternative and Complementary Medicine: Research on Paradigm, Practice, and Policy.* These newcomers to the serious biomedical research arena were reviewed in the *Journal of the American Medical Association* (Simpson and Bick 1996).

The Cochrane Collaboration is a worldwide consortium of researchers producing systematic reviews of medical research. A listing of review groups can be found at http://www.cochrane.org/cochrane/revabstr/mainindex.htm. The Cochrane Pregnancy and Childbirth Database includes some evaluations of complementary therapies. Other groups of potential interest to women's studies are breast cancer, fertility regulation, gynaecological cancer, menstrual disorders, and neonatal. New reviews are frequently updated at http://www.cochrane.org/cochrane/newreviews.htm, and many of them are relevant to women's health research. There is a Complementary Medicine Field that crosscuts the specific health issues of the review groups and a listing of CAM Reviews and Protocols can be accessed at the University of Maryland Complementary Medicine Program website (http://www.compmed.um mc.umaryland.edu/Compmed/Cochrane/Cochrane.htm). One anticipates expansion of the Cochrane resource as suitable studies are identified and reviewed.

A comprehensive list of UK organizations involved in specific forms of complementary medicine, and charitable organizations promoting research in this area is provided in a useful *Handbook of alternative and complementary medicine* (Fulder 1996). A worldwide listing of associations can be found on the Medbioworld web site at http://www.medbioworld.com/med/assoc/complementary.html.

## Websites for the consumer and professional

Further electronic resources are openly and publicly available on the World Wide Web. The most reliable sites are academic, non-commercial sites, which increasingly act as a necessary adjunct to library facilities for academics and professionals. Sites of particular interest for women's health and complementary medicine have been collected for the website of the R & H Rosenthal Center for Complementary Medicine at the Columbia University College of Physicians and Surgeons (http://www.rosenthal.hs.columbia.edu/Women.html). In addition, there are now 17 National Centers of Excellence in Women's Health nominated by the US Department of Health and Human Services (http://www.4woman.org/owh/index.htm).

The exponential growth of electronic information media coincides with both the development of health consumerism and the growing interest in complementary medicine. On the Internet, new health-care consumers are actively seeking and swapping information. Electronic access to full text articles, reviews, advice sheets, discussion groups, and increasing numbers of medical journals has enabled consumers as well as professionals to research the latest medical information, resulting in increasing patient sophistication. *CAM on PubMed*, developed jointly by the National Library of Medicine (NLM) and the National Center for Complementary and Alternative Medicine (NCCAM) (http://www.nlm.nih.gov/nccam/background.htm), has made it far easier to identify complementary medicine references. PubMed is the worldwide web interface to Medline, a free and searchable internet facility (search engine) for the general public and health professionals enabling access to over 11 million journal citations (abstracts only). If you wish to search *CAM on PubMed* through the NCCAM website, any search you perform will be automatically limited to CAM-related citations. Alternatively, if you access CAM directly through the PubMed website (www.pubmedcentral.nih.gov/), you will need to limit any searches to the CAM subset, which is easily achieved using the 'Limit' function. Own choice, and full text searching of the citations and abstracts throught PubMed affords yet more flexibility. In addition, the National library of Medicine is now refining the MeSH headings to include the full range of alternative and complementary medicine terms, and the Entrez database includes linkouts to the HerbMed database (http://www.herbmed.org) from the Alternative Medicine Foundation.

This new medium has proved particularly appropriate for those who seek to take control of their own health-care decisions in partnership with professionals. The 'downside' of all this is that GPs may be asked by patients about theories and products about which they know little. The GP must be aware that resources on the Web are heterogeneous and variable in quality, and that there is little to limit the making of extravagant claims and dissemination of promotional material. Guidelines on how to evaluate and selectively utilize promotional material are, however, available from the Rosenthal Directory of Databases (http://www.rosenthal.hs.columbia.edu/Databases.html), and the peer-reviewed journals of complementary medicine referred to earlier.

# Breast disorders

## Breast cancer: causation and prevention

### Influence of diet

Epidemiological studies show large differences between countries in the incidence of breast cancer. Race, lifestyle, and diet have all been implicated. Japan is reported to have the lowest risk of hormone-dependent cancers, and the importance of diet is suggested by the observation that following transition from a Japanese to a Western diet, the risk of breast cancer increases (Kolonel 1988; Adlercreutz et al. 1991; Lee et al. 1991) The diet recommended in macrobiotic medicine is very close to the traditional Japanese diet and, as with the traditional Chinese diet, and vegetarian or semi-vegetarian diets, carries with it a low risk of hormone-dependent cancers. These dietary groups are characterized by a lower prevalence of obesity and saturated fat intake, the former and possibly the latter being risk factors for breast cancer. A further factor that may afford protection to those in the low-risk groups is the intake of naturally occurring, oestradiol (E2)-like compounds of plant origin. These diphenolic phyto-oestrogens, which include the lignans and isoflavonoids, are converted by intestinal bacteria to biologically active compounds. Their effects in humans are those of a weak oestrogen with, in addition, proven antioxidant and antiproliferative activity (Knight and Eden 1996). The highest intakes of these compounds are found in countries or regions with a low cancer incidence.

Lignans are found in whole grain cereals, seeds, nuts, vegetables, legumes, and fruits. Isoflavonoids are less widely distributed, but occur in high concentrations in soyabean products, chick peas, and possibly other legumes. The consumption of soya products in some Japanese populations reaches 200 mg/day. Total isoflavone intake in Asia ranges between 25 and 45 mg/day, compared with an intake of less than 5 mg/day in Western countries (Knight and Eden 1996). Soya products contain differing amounts of phytoestrogens; tofu, for example, contains 10 times more phyto-oestrogens than soya drinks. Fermentation decreases the content but increases the bioavailability and excretion of isoflavones in soya (Hutchins et al. 1995b). In the macrobiotic medical system, great importance is attributed to a diet consisting of grains (50%), vegetables (20%), legumes (10%), fish, fruit, or nuts (10%), and seasoning with fermented soya products such as miso, tempeh or tamari (Kushi 1978).

Isoflavonoids and lignans have been shown to influence intracellular enzymes, protein synthesis, growth factor action, malignant cell proliferation, differentiation, and angiogenesis (Knight and Eden 1996). There is increasing interest in their possible role as natural cancer-protective compounds. They also influence sex hormone metabolism and biological activity. Fibre intake and phyto-oestrogen metabolite excretion show a positive correlation with the concentration of plasma sex-hormone-binding globulin and a negative correlation with plasma percentage of free oestradiol and free testosterone (Adlercreutz et al. 1987). In addition, being weak oestrogens, it has been hypothesized that phyto-oestrogen metabolites may have anti-oestrogen effects through competitive binding to oestrogen receptors. It is suggested that such a mechanism would attenuate the adverse consequences of obesity and might partly explain the low cancer incidence in Hispanic women (Horn 1995). A contrasting hypothesis is that dietary oestrogen intake might promote the growth of breast cancer cells, and antagonize the action of tamoxifen (Welshons *et al.* 1987). A study of Chinese women in Singapore found that soya product intake seemed to protect premenopausal women, but not post-menopausal women, from breast cancer (Lee *et al.* 1991).

There is considerable evidence that plasma levels and excretion of phyto-oestrogen metabolites is determined by dietary manipulation of the sort integral to many forms of complementary medicine. It can be shown under controlled dietary conditions that urinary lignan and isoflavonoid excretion changes in response to alterations in vegetable, fruit, and legume intake (Hutchins *et al.* 1995a). Following soyabean consumption, some isoflavonoids are secreted in amounts equivalent to classical oestrogens. When a total of 53 subjects adhering to macrobiotic or lactovegetarian diets were compared with those having an omnivorous diet, the excretion of phyto-oestrogen metabolites was eightfold higher in the macrobiotics, and twice as high in the lactovegetarians (Adlercreutz *et al.* 1986). The lowest levels of excretion were found in a group of post-menopausal breast cancer patients (Adlercreutz *et al.* 1986).

## Vitamins and cofactors

A prospective study of 89 494 nurses found a high intake of dietary vitamin A to be associated with a 16% reduction in risk of breast cancer (Hunter *et al.* 1993). No association was found between dietary vitamin C and E intake and risk of breast disease. Vitamin A supplements ($\geq$10 000 IU/day) appear to decrease the risk of breast cancer only in those with a low dietary intake ($<$6630 IU/day), in whom they reduced the incidence by a half. Vitamin C and E supplements, even at high dose and for long periods, appeared to have no effect on the incidence of breast cancer. Any conclusions concerning the possible beneficial effect of vitamin A must, in women of child-bearing age, be tempered by evidence concerning the teratogenic potential of high doses (see Fertility, below), and possible increased risk of osteoporosis (see Menopause, below). However, daily vitamin A intakes of $<$10 000 IU/day seem to carry no significant teratogenic risk, and carotenoids, which are vitamin A precursors, are not teratogenic (Smithells 1996).

The effect of $\beta$-carotene, the naturally occurring form of vitamin A in vegetables, has been examined not in relation to breast, but to cervical cancer. In a case–control study utilizing 191 pairs of women in Italy, women with the lowest intake of dietary $\beta$-carotene had a sixfold higher risk of developing invasive cervical cancer (La Vecchia *et al.* 1984). $\beta$-Carotene itself might only be a marker for other cancer-protective carotenoids as two lung cancer prophylaxis trials have shown no benefit, and even a possible risk associated with $\beta$-carotene supplements.

Vitamin E was found in the large multicentre 'HOPE' trial conducted in 9541 men and women to have a possible effect on the incidence of all cancers combined. Although this double-blind, randomized, controlled trial (DBRCT) has been completed and its results published, the vitamin E versus placebo arm has been extended for a further 2 years to investigate this possibility (HOPE 2000).

### Life events

The holistic view common to all complementary medicine holds that state of mind is linked with, and can be causally related to, disease. Some support for the holistic view comes from a well-designed, case–control study of 119 women under investigation for breast disease (Chen *et al.* 1995). Using predefined qualitative and quantitative definitions, details of 'life events and difficulties' experienced in the preceding 5 years were collected by researchers blinded to the results of breast biopsy. Severe life events were associated with a threefold increase in risk of breast cancer, and a 12-fold increase when adjustments were made for age, menopausal status, and other potential confounding factors.

### Exercise

A case–control study matched 545 women with breast cancer who had been diagnosed before age 40 with similar women without breast cancer (Bernstein *et al.* 1994). Women who had averaged 3.8 hours or more a week in physical exercise since puberty had a risk of breast cancer only 42% of that of inactive women.

## Breast cancer: palliation and prognosis

### Post-mastectomy pain and lymphoedema

A very small, randomized, controlled study suggests that topical capsaicin is helpful in neurogenic post-mastectomy pain syndrome (Watson and Evan 1992). Five of 13 patients receiving the capsaicin cream reported good to excellent results compared with only one of ten patients in the placebo group.

Secondary lymphoedema can be improved by massage. The efficacy of manual massage has been compared with that of pneumatic devices. In one study of 60 patients with post-mastectomy arm oedema, 12 manual lymphatic massage treatments over the course of a month resulted in a significant reduction in oedema lasting at least 3 months (Zanolla *et al.* 1984). A pneumatic device with constant pressure used for 6 hours a day was also effective, while a pneumatic device with variable pressure was ineffective. Patients might find a massage three times a week preferable to the wearing of a device for 6 hours a day, although both appear effective.

## Mood and pain in metastatic breast cancer

Few in the medical profession would disagree with any approach that improved mood and reduced pain in patients with breast cancer. Studies exist which suggest that the use of hypnotherapy, or relaxation and imagery, as an adjunct to routine oncological care, is associated with an improvement in general condition, and tolerance to chemotherapy (Spiegel and Bloom 1983; Bridge *et al.* 1988).

One study of 54 women with metastatic breast cancer compared the effect of group therapy with or without self-hypnosis training on mental suffering and pain sensation (Spiegel and Bloom 1983). Improvement was obtained in both treatment groups with the maximum effect seen in the group also learning self-hypnosis.

In another study, 154 breast cancer patients receiving therapy were randomized to three groups: one group received training in progressive muscle relaxation and deep breathing; another group added pleasant imagery to relaxation and deep breathing; whilst controls were encouraged to simply talk about themselves (Bridge *et al.* 1988). Before the trial began, women in all the groups scored similarly on validated measures of mood, depression, and anxiety. After 6 weeks, mood in the control group had deteriorated whilst mood in the intervention groups had improved, women in the relaxation and imagery group benefiting the most.

Many other supportive approaches might achieve the same laudable improvement in psychological parameters. A separate issue is whether this form of psychological therapy has any effect on disease outcome in terms of survival.

## Survival in metastatic breast cancer

It is claimed by some practitioners of complementary medicine and their patients that emotions and mental attitudes can influence disease prognosis. One group has examined the effect of altering patients' emotional state without attempting to change their expectations of survival and without employing any 'cancer-conquering' imagery (Spiegel *et al.* 1989). Psychologists used a programme of weekly support groups and self-hypnosis for pain, a programme which had earlier been shown to reduce anxiety, depression, and pain in women with metastatic breast cancer (Spiegel and Bloom 1983). The emphasis lay in encouraging patients to discuss the impact of cancer on their life, express their feelings, develop strategies for coping with the mental and physical distress, and counter the tendency to social isolation. In a prospective, randomized study of women with metastatic breast cancer receiving routine oncological care, the one-year psychological support programme appeared to double the length of survival (Spiegel *et al.* 1989). Fifty patients participated in the psychosocial intervention group while 36 acted as controls. Mean survival in the intervention group was 36.6 (SD 37.6) months compared with 18.9 (SD 10.8) months in the control group, a significant difference ($P < 0.0001$). It was concluded by the authors that the study bears out observational studies describing the apparent impact of social isolation versus support on disease outcome. Studies they quote report improved outcome in communities with good supportive networks, and in married women as compared with unmarried women. Accordingly, in their own study, unmarried women in the control group showed a survival disadvantage not shown by unmarried women in the intervention group (Spiegel *et al.* 1989).

Further studies, including some randomized controlled trials, suggest that hypnotherapy alone improves symptom control in, and outcome from, other types of cancer (Fulder 1996). It is difficult to separate the efficacy of hypnotherapy from relaxation and imagery or even concentrated psychological support, but the message emerges that these related 'mind/body' approaches help patients greatly.

It is suspected that the neuroendocrine and immune systems may be a major link between the psyche and course of cancer, with some experimental evidence. Thus, in 13 patients with stage 1 breast cancer, a combination of relaxation, guided imagery, and biofeedback had a measurable effect on the immune system, including an increase in natural killer cells and lymphocytes (Gruber *et al.* 1993).

A multimodality approach is that taken by the Bristol Cancer Help Centre (BCHC), which employs dietary manipulation, psychological techniques, and many forms of complementary medicine. A controversial case–control study published in 1990 suggested that patients attending the BCHC had poorer survival than selected controls (Bagenal *et al.* 1990). The study design and methods of analysis attracted much criticism and the consensus view is that the study was inconclusive.

## Mastalgia

Evening primrose oil (EPO), high in the essential fatty acids linoleic and γ-linoleic acid, may alleviate mastalgia. A retrospective study of 414 patients with either cyclical or non-cyclical mastalgia found EPO at 3 g/day (contains 240 g γ-linoleic acid) to be as effective as bromocriptine although less effective than danazol. The response rate for EPO was 58% in cyclical mastalgia and 38% in non-cyclical mastalgia. EPO was given initially for 6 months, and patients were counselled that it might take 4 months for EPO to exert an effect. EPO had fewer side effects than either drug (Gateley *et al.* 1992).

Cyclical mastalgia as part of the PMS syndrome was one of a cluster of symptoms helped by *Vitex agnus castus* extract 'ZE 440' in a number of open studies and in one recent DBRCT (see Premenstrual syndrome, below). Cyclical mastalgia in isolation has been evaluated in a DBRCT involving 100 women with cyclical mastalgia treated for three consecutive menstrual cycles (Halaska *et al.* 1998). Intensity of breast pain, as assessed by a visual analogue scale, diminished more quickly in women receiving *Vitex agnus castus* extract. The exact identity of the *Vitex agnus castus* extract used cannot be elucidated from the English abstract of this Czech publication. Exact specification of herbal remedies may be important as illustrated by the variation in essential oil composition of *Vitex agnus castus* extracts depending on the maturity of the fruit used, distillation period and extraction method (Sorensen and Katsiotis 2000).

# Contraception

## Natural family planning

The theory and applications of natural family planning are now well researched and validated. Symptothermal methods in menstruating women, and the lactational amenorrhoea technique in the post-partum period, provide a contraceptive option for the fully trained and highly motivated. These approaches enable some women to avoid exogenous forms of contraception, or can be combined with use of barrier contraceptives. This approach may be facilitated by the Persona™ device, which identifies fertile days by assay of urinary luteinizing hormone and oestrone-3-glucuronide, a metabolite of oestradiol.

Natural family planning is not 'owned' by any complementary medical discipline as such, but it often appeals to women who espouse a 'natural' ideology, and who are therefore reluctant to take hormones. The option should also be remembered when advising women with medical contraindications to hormonal contraception.

## Natural progesterone

Transdermal progesterone cream derived from wild yam root has been suggested as an alternative contraceptive by its chief proponent (Lee 1996). The transdermal route of administration, which avoids first-pass metabolism, is claimed to ensure efficacy at low concentrations, but this claim meets with considerable scepticism. Capsules containing natural progesterone can also be obtained and have been used for this purpose. Requests by women to their GPs, and electronic correspondence on the Internet, reflect the growth of interest in natural progesterone. Independent studies are needed (see also sections on premenstrual syndrome and the menopause).

# Infertility and early pregnancy loss

Many patients and practitioners share a suspicion that psychological stress compromises fertility. In couples struggling to conceive, any form of therapy, whether complementary or conventional, may have an anxiolytic effect. The opposite is also true, as many anxiety-filled IVF or GIFT patients will attest. There is a need to identify the impact of complementary therapies on fertility, the degree to which any apparent effect is related to psychological support, and whether there are other modes of action.

## Stress, anxiety, and fertility

One study has demonstrated an association between physiological and endocrine markers of stress and concurrent infertility (Harrison *et al.* 1986). Since a fertility problem undoubtedly causes anxiety, this study does not prove the hypothesis that stress may cause or exacerbate subfertility. The influence of behavioural therapy on conception rates has been examined in an uncontrolled study of couples with unexplained infertility (Domar *et al.* 1990). The study population was 54 women with a mean age of 34 years (range 25–42 years) and mean duration of infertility of 3.3 years. Following a mind/body programme held in a hospital department, 34% fell pregnant within 6 months. This compares with a conception rate of 18% in a separate longitudinal study of a comparable patient population (Domar *et al.* 1990). A controlled study is clearly required.

There are considerable data concerning the impact of orthodox social and psychological support in a different population; those women who had reached the first or second trimester of pregnancy, but in whom the fetus was judged to be at risk of having low birth weight. Studies in a total of 8000 women have been the subject of a recent systematic analysis, showing that in high-risk pregnancies, social support interventions had no effect on medical outcome (Hodnett 1995).

## Acupuncture

A comparison between auricular acupuncture and hormonal treatment has been carried out in 90 women with infertility associated with oligomenorrhoea or luteal insufficiency (Gerhard and Postneek 1992). The pregnancy rate of 22/45 achieved in the acupuncture group was similar to the rate of 20/45 in the hormone-treated group. Despite matching of age, duration of infertility, body mass index, previous pregnancies, menstrual cycle, and tubal patency, there was an imbalance between the two groups. Women in the acupuncture group had an excess of features such as adnexitis or reduced postcoital tests usually associated with a poorer outcome. Side effects were reported only in the hormone group. The prevalence of endometriosis was higher in the women in whom neither modality of treatment proved effective compared with successfully treated women. The lack of an untreated control group in this study limits the conclusions that can be drawn.

## Herbalism

In an uncontrolled study of 60 women with uncomplicated luteal phase insufficiency treated with traditional Chinese herbs, the pregnancy rate was 56% (Lian 1991). In a separate case report, use of the herbal medicine *Vitex agnus castus* was associated with symptoms suggestive of mild ovarian hyperstimulation syndrome (Cahill *et al.* 1994).

## Caffeine intake

Many forms of complementary medicine counsel against instant coffee or cola beverages as part of a general principle of avoiding processed foods. Most disciplines will allow, at least in some patients, a low intake of fresh coffee or tea, depending on the individual patient's health problems. No specific claims are made regarding the impact of caffeine intake on fertility. Indeed, more interest in this question has been shown by orthodox medical investigators. There are several studies concerning the effect of caffeine consumption on fertility or fecundity (time to conception). Their results are mixed but there is some support for a recommendation that women moderate their caffeine consumption.

Two studies which took account of caffeine from all sources suggested caffeine has a dose-dependent adverse effect on fecundity. For reference, 100 mg/day caffeine is equivalent to one cup coffee (and several varieties if tea) or one litre of cola. In the earliest study, a caffeine intake of more than 100 mg/day appeared to halve the chances of conception per cycle (Wilcox *et al.* 1988). The second study found an intake ranging between one cup of coffee/week to two cups/day had no effect on time to conceive (Joesoef *et al.* 1990). In a third study, the chances of conception per cycle were reduced by 10% with an intake of under 300 mg/day, and by 27% with an intake of over 300 mg/day. This study suggested a dose-dependent effect within the range of 1–300 mg/day (Hatch and Bracken 1993). A more recent study suggested a threshold of 300 mg/day, above which an adverse effect was seen (Stanton and Gray 1995). This and another (Alderete *et al.* 1995) study found the effect confined to non-smokers, smoking *per se* having a significant effect on conception rate, which may have been overriding. Confusingly, another study found the effect confined to smokers

(Olsen 1991). Further inconsistencies in the evidence exist, including a prospective study which found moderate levels of caffeine intake (400–700 mg/day) to be associated with higher fecundity than lower levels, and only those with an intake of over 700 mg/day to have reduced fecundity (Florack *et al.* 1994). This study found moderate smoking (1–10 cigarettes/day) to be associated with a higher level of fecundity than non-smoking, and found that, whilst alcohol had no effect on a woman's fecundity, for her partner more than 10 drinks/week had a beneficial effect compared with less than five drinks/week.

There is also some work concerning caffeine intake and fetal well-being. In pregnancy, coffee has a dose-dependent inverse effect on birth weight (Nehlig and Debry 1994), but only when intake levels are high (>7 cups/day). Moderate intake having no effect, it would seem reasonable for pregnant mothers to limit their intake to two to three cups per day. In this context it is interesting that many pregnant women lose the inclination to drink coffee, at least during the first trimester. Post-partum, caffeine stimulates breast milk production. However, it also enters breast milk, although measured quantities vary in different studies.

## Folic acid intake and homocysteine

A diet including regular green vegetable and fresh fruit consumption is central to many complementary philosophies. This advice is likely to be of particular importance to women hoping for a healthy pregnancy, since maternal folic acid administration is now known to reduce the incidence of neural tube defects (NTDs) in low- and high-risk pregnancies (MRC Vitamin Study Group 1991). Women planning a pregnancy are advised to consume more folate-rich foods, preferably raw, in addition to taking folic acid supplements.

The precise mechanism by which folic acid exerts its protective effect is unclear. However, it has become clear that both folic acid and vitamin B12 are necessary for the metabolism of homocysteine. Homocysteine levels are higher in women who have given birth to infants with NTDs than in control women with healthy offspring (Steegers-Theunissen *et al.* 1994). Increased levels are normalized by administration of folic acid or vitamin B12. Hyperhomocysteinaemia was also found in 21% of 102 women who had suffered at least two spontaneous early miscarriages (Wouters *et al.* 1993).

## Vitamin A in food and supplements

Vitamin A is an essential nutrient and the RDA of retinol for pregnant women is 2700 IU/day (800 μg/day). There is concern about potential teratogenicity of excess vitamin A when taken as a supplement or derived from food of animal origin. The concern stems from proven teratogenicity in animal studies, various case reports, and a controlled study in pregnant women, the conclusions of which have met with some criticism. The source of vitamin A is important; vegetables contain β-carotene, which appears to be safe, whilst animal sources contain retinol, the form known to be potentially teratogenic. There is good evidence that an intake of vitamin A of <10 000 IU is safe for the fetus. There is limited evidence in humans of teratogenicity associated with intakes of >25 000 IU/day (West Midlands Medicines Information Service 2002).

In general, it is difficult to exceed an intake of over 10 000 IU/day from food alone. However, an average portion of liver (especially lamb's liver) is likely to contain between 4 and 12 times the RDA for vitamin A. Other sources of vitamin A are full-fat dairy products and fatty fish. In order to maintain the safety margin, the DoH recommended in 1990 that liver consumption or fish-liver oils be avoided in early pregnancy. However, the bioavailability is much less than when retinol is ingested as a vitamin, and concern has been expressed that this warning may lead some women, especially those in low-income groups, to experience vitamin A deficiency in early pregnancy. In order to preserve vitamin A intake, one nutritionist has recommended an intake of 100 g (4 oz) liver per week (West Midlands Medicines Information Service 2002).

The current recommendation for women wishing to take vitamin supplements prior to and during pregnancy is to avoid doses of over 5000 IU/day (1650 μg/day). Manufacturers of prenatal vitamins limit the content to 5000 IU per dose and in many cases use β-carotene in preference to retinoids. An additional consideration is that long-term risk of osteoporosis in women seems to be increased by a retinol intake of more than 3000 μg/day (>10 125 IU/day).

## Fertility awareness

The well-validated concepts underlying natural family planning can also be used to improve fertility awareness. It provides a 'natural' approach, which is valued by couples, at least in the early stages of a fertility problem.

## Premenstrual syndrome

The severity of premenstrual syndrome (PMS) and ability to cope with it varies with patients' psychosocial situation. Any approach to management that includes reassurance and empathy is often successful. In 5–10% of patients, symptoms are severe enough to disrupt activities, work, or relationships, and further measures may be required. It has been the practice for some GPs to institute a trial of hormonal suppression of ovulation, or progesterone supplementation during the luteal phase. Outcomes are variable, and many women seek alternatives, usually vitamin B6 or evening primrose oil. The evidence concerning their efficacy is mixed, but this has not dissuaded GPs from suggesting their use as part of ortho-dox management of PMS (Chapter 2). New evidence concerning the herb *Vitex agnus castus* is likely to encourage its recommendation by GPs.

## Herbal medicine: *Vitex agnus castus*

*Vitex agnus castus*, or Chaste tree, is a herb traditionally used to treat PMS and menstrual disorders. The fruits contain iridoids and flavonoids, with effects described as similar to that of the corpus luteum. Thus it increases LH and inhibits FSH production, resulting in a lower oestrogen to progesterone ratio (Lewith 1996). Other possible mechanisms include its modulation of stress-induced dopamine secretion, or its interaction with endogenous opiods (Schellenberg 2001). An uncontrolled survey of *Vitex* use in 1542 women with PMS reported complete relief of symptoms in more than 90% of cases (Lewith 1996). Side effects were noted in 1–2% of recipients. Systematic evaluation of its efficacy has begun recently and includes a DBRCT in 170 women treated with a dry extract of *Vitex agnus castus* fruit (L extract Ze 440, one tablet daily) over three consecutive cycles (Schellenberg 2001). Improvement was reported in women's self-assessment of irritability, mood alteration, anger, headache, and breast fullness, whilst other symptoms such as bloating were unaffected. Responder rates (as defined by a 50% improvement or greater) were 52% and 24% for active and placebo groups, respectively. Mild adverse effects were reported equally in the two groups and none caused discontinuation of treatment.

## Evening primrose oil (EPO)

There is some evidence that EPO relieves cyclical mastalgia (see Breast disease, above). For the relief of other PMS symptoms, 3 g/day EPO was found in four small studies to be more effective than placebo (O'Brien 1993; Lewith 1996). It appeared that EPO was more effective for irritability and depression than for other PMS symptoms. As is often the case in this field, the studies were too small to have sufficient power to prove efficacy. A deficiency of omega-6 fatty acids of which EPO is a source, may cause abnormal sensitivity to prolactin, a putative cause of PMS (Lewith 1996).

## Vitamin B6

A variety of dietary supplements are often recommended for PMS, probably the best known of which is vitamin B6. Early evidence on which the high usage was based included two large placebo-controlled studies into the effect of vitamin B6 (50–200 mg daily), which found a response in 80% of recipients. In these studies the incidence of placebo-responders was also exceptionally high at 70%. Three smaller double-blind, crossover studies showing greater benefit in patients receiving vitamin B6 provided slightly more persuasive evidence (Lewith 1996).

A more recent systematic review identified nine published and no unpublished random, double-blind, placebo-controlled trials of which four were of sufficient quality to merit inclusion (Wyatt *et al.* 1999). These four trials involved a total of 541 patients treated with 50 mg or more of vitamin B6. The systematic review concluded that 100 mg (and possibly 50 mg) daily of vitamin B6 appeared significantly better than placebo for relieving overall premenstrual symptoms and in relieving depression associated with the premenstrual syndrome. The odds ratio relative to placebo for an improvement in overall premenstrual symptoms was 2.32 (95% CI 1.95–2.54). The odds ratio relative to placebo for an improvement in depressive symptoms was 1.69 (1.39–2.06). Confidence in these findings was limited by the overall poor methodology of the trials such as lack of clarity about coprescription of the oral contraceptive pill. However, those two trials that analysed separately women taking the oral contraceptive pill and those not taking the pill found no significant difference. All but one of the studies had low statistical power, leading to the all too familiar conclusion that a larger RCT was needed and justified.

In 1997, the UK Department of Health and Medical Control Agency published recommendations to restrict the dose of vitamin B6 available generally to 10 mg, and to limit the dose sold by a pharmacist to less than 50 mg. The recommended dietary allowance for vitamin B6 is around 2.0 mg/day, and deficiency of vitamin B6 is rare. Excessive ingestion (2000–6000 mg) of vitamin B6 causes peripheral neuropathy, and doses of 200 mg/day may cause similar, although probably reversible, effects. The more recent systematic review included analysis of side effects in all the trials identified, therefore covering 940 participants, and the use of doses up to 600 mg daily. It was in the one study using 600 mg/day that one patient reported tingling of the fingers. The low incidence of recognized side effects could have been due to the short duration of the trials (three to four cycles) or lack of assessment by a suitable qualified neurologist. Importantly, there was no apparent dose–response to the beneficial effects reported, which, combined with animal data concerning toxicity, makes the daily consumption of more than 100 mg inadvisable.

## Other dietary interventions

Other dietary interventions include supplementation with vitamins B6, A, E, or minerals such as magnesium or calcium. A review of clinical studies is available (Lewith 1996). These and further studies into vitamins A and E raise the possibility of differential effects on the various types of PMS, but none is conclusive. In one small, double-blind, placebo-controlled trial, oral magnesium supplements (360 mg/day, day 15 to onset of menstruation) were found to relieve premenstrual mood changes as well as menstrual migraine (see below) (Facchinetti *et al.*1991). Vitamin B6 supplementation at 100 mg twice daily is reported to normalize low erythrocyte magnesium levels in women with PMS (Lewith 1996). One reason why vitamin B6, magnesium, and calcium might be important is that they are all involved in neurotransmitter metabolism.

It has been observed that women with PMS have a significantly higher intake of refined carbohydrates than non-sufferers or patients with mild PMS (Abraham 1982; Goei *et al.* 1982). Refined sugar has been reported to increase the excretion of magnesium (Seelig 1971). There is a view, unsupported by any evidence, that PMS is in some way caused by hypoglycaemia, and can be combatted by the consumption of complex carbohydrates. Different diet theories stem from suggestions that diet has a measurable effect on serotonin and perhaps other neurotransmitter levels, a field ripe for further exploration.

## Natural progesterone

In the belief that PMS might be due to progesterone deficiency and relative oestrogen excess, natural progesterone derived from Mexican wild yam root has been administered as a transdermal cream in the latter third of the cycle (Lee 1996). Without any supporting data, the product is claimed to be effective and free from side effects. To date, no independent investigation of these claims appears to have been done, but women in the USA and UK have accessed a product, called Progest Cream™, for use in PMS and other conditions. Yam contains a plant sterol, diosgenin, said to be identical to human progesterone. This is in contrast to synthetic progestogens, which are chemically dissimilar to human progesterone, having been modified to promote oral absorption, delay metabolism, and to provide prolonged duration of action (and to be patentable). Independent validation of these claims is needed. (See also sections on contraception and the menopause.)

## Manipulative medicine

Osteopaths and chiropractors claim some success in treating PMS and menstrual disorders by means of spinal manipulation. The authors have not identified any clinical trials addressing these claims.

## Reflexology

In a randomized, controlled study of premenstrual symptoms treated with ear, hand, and foot reflexology, 35 women with PMS were assigned to weekly reflexology lasting 30 minutes for 8 weeks, or placebo reflexology (Oleson and

Flocco 1993). Somatic and psychological indicators of PMS, recorded daily by patients for 2 months prior to, during, and after the treatment showed a significant decrease in the reflexology group.

## Relaxation and imagery

A 5-month study of 46 women examined the effect on physical, emotional, and social indicators of three interventions (Goodale *et al.* 1990). The women were randomly assigned to a group learning to elicit the relaxation response, a reading group, or a group simply charting their symptoms. Improvements were noted in all three groups, with the greatest effect seen in the relaxation group. Regular elicitation of the relaxation response seems to be an effective treatment for physical and psychological symptoms, and was most effective for women with severe symptoms, in whom a 58% improvement was noted.

Another 6-month study in 30 women with regular menstrual cycles employed a 3-month run-in period and then 3 months of listening to an audio tape with progressive muscle relaxation exercise followed by guided imagery and a suggestive message focusing on lengthening the menstrual cycle and delaying the onset of menstrual bleeding (Groer and Ohnesorge 1993). Only 15 women completed the study, but in these, PMS symptoms were reduced and cycle length was significantly increased.

## Homeopathy

Classical homeopathy is often used for the many psychological and physical symptom complexes attributed to PMS, but no studies were found in our literature search.

# Menstrual problems

## Dysmenorrhoea

### Acupuncture

Acupuncture appears effective for menstrual cramps. In a one-year randomized controlled study of 43 women, subjects received either real acupuncture (at fixed, classical acupuncture points with no individual variation), sham acupuncture, extra consultations, or no intervention (Helms 1987). Ten of 11 in the true acupuncture group improved (defined by halving of the monthly pain score). Four of 11 in the sham acupuncture group improved, as did two of 11 in the group receiving extra consultations, and one out of the ten who received no intervention. During the 9 months after treatment, there was a 41% drop in analgesic usage for those receiving true acupuncture, whilst in the other groups analgesic usage increased or stayed the same.

### Manipulative medicine

A small dysmenorrhoea trial compared chiropractic manipulation in eight women with three controls (Thomason *et al.* 1979) Seven of the eight women treated twice weekly with manipulation experienced decreased pain and disability, compared with none of the controls. A trial conducted in 40 women with dysmenorrhoea compared chiropractic with intensive sham manipulation applied to 'incorrect' sites. Women in the two groups reported equal reductions in perceived menstrual stress, and equivalent reductions in plasma levels of prostaglandin F2a were observed (Kokjohn *et al.* 1992). This study suggests improvement with manual techniques but does not enable comparison with placebo.

## Migraines related to the menstrual cycle

Population studies find the prevalence of migraines to be 17% in women, compared with 6% in men, with a concentration of attacks between menarche and the menopause, suggesting a hormonal influence (MacGregor 1996a, b). This section is concerned not with non-migrainous headaches, which occur as part of PMS, or migraine caused or exacerbated by the oral contraceptive pill, but with two other distinct conditions; 'menstrual migraine' and 'menstrually related migraine' (MacGregor 1996b).

### 'Menstrual migraine'

A small proportion of female migraine sufferers have true 'menstrual migraine', attacks occurring regularly in the two days before and three days after the onset of menses, and at no other time (MacGregor 1996a). A pilot study carried out in migraine clinic attendees, using these strict criteria, found a prevalence of menstrual migraine of 7.2% (MacGregor *et al.* 1990). This condition has been linked with declining oestrogen levels and managed with some success by percutaneous or transdermal oestradiol supplementation, although such products are not yet licensed for this indication (MacGregor 1996a, b). Most women with menstrual migraine are 35–45 years of age (MacGregor 1996b) and therefore subject to the slow physiological decline in oestrogen levels occurring at this time. Given the proven oestrogenic content of soya and some other vegetable products (see above), one wonders whether diet has a role to play here. Another mechanism implicated in menstrual migraine is the secretion of prostaglandins from the myometrium into the systemic circulation during the luteal phase, with maximum entry during the first 48 hours of menstruation. There are double-blind, placebo-controlled studies showing that prostaglandin inhibitors effectively prevent menstrual migraine in some women and may be particularly useful if patients also experience dysmenorrhoea (MacGregor 1996b). This finding suggests that dietary manipulations able to influence prostaglandins might possibly help, but there seems to be little investigation in this area.

## Magnesium supplements

Women with menstrual migraine may be helped by oral magnesium supplements. A double-blind, placebo-controlled study of 20 women found a significant reduction of days with headaches (as well as other premenstrual complaints) in women taking magnesium at a dose of 360 mg/day, started on day 15 and continued until the next menses (Facchinetti *et al.* 1991). The effect lasted for some months beyond the time of supplementation. Intracellular magnesium levels were significantly lower in these migraine sufferers than in controls (Facchinetti *et al.* 1991). These findings, together with other studies concerning intra- and extracellular magnesium levels in migraine patients suggest that a lower migraine threshold may be related to magnesium deficiency.

## Menstrually related migraine

Thirty-five per cent of migraine clinic attendees have 'menstrually related migraine' (also known as 'premenstrual migraine'), which is thus more common than 'menstrual migraine' (MacGregor *et al.* 1990). The attack rate is increased in the luteal phase, with relief at the onset of menstruation (MacGregor 1996b). Although attacks can occur throughout the cycle, and may be triggered by well-known factors such as chocolate, soft cheeses, etc., the threshold for triggering seems to be lower in the luteal phase.

### Dietary restrictions

Approximately 25% of migraine sufferers believe that their attacks can be provoked by foodstuffs. Dietary changes can reduce the frequency of all types of migraine other than true menstrual migraine. An uncontrolled trial of 60 migraine patients given an elimination diet reported a dramatic improvement in symptoms: 85% became headache-free when 10 common foods were avoided (Grant 1979). The foods most commonly responsible were wheat, orange, eggs, tea, coffee, chocolate, milk, beef, corn, sugar, and yeast. Chocolate, caffeine, red wine, and mature cheese are well known triggers, but not other foods implicated in this study.

## Biofeedback

There are extensive data on the effectiveness of biofeedback for most types of migraine (Blanchard and Andrasik 1987). Using biofeedback, the patient learns how to increase hand temperature by dilating blood vessels in the hands, thus affecting blood flow to the head, which reduces the pain.

## Herbal medicine

There are clinical trials supporting the use of feverfew (*Tanacetum parthenium*) for migraine. In a randomized study of 17 patients whose normal practice was to eat feverfew leaves daily to prevent migraine, subjects randomized to placebo had a significant increase in the frequency and severity of migraines, while those in the feverfew group experienced no change (Johnson *et al.* 1985). This small study reveals only the effect of withdrawing feverfew from regular users.

In a larger, crossover trial, 76 migraine patients were given either one capsule of dried feverfew (equivalent to two medium-sized leaves) or placebo daily for 4 months, before crossover for a further 4 months (Murphy *et al.* 1988). In the 59 patients completing the trial, migraine attacks diminished during the months on feverfew. Patients with common migraine showed a 24% reduction in attack rate, and patients with classical migraine a 32% reduction. The severity of remaining attacks was reduced, although the duration of individual attacks remained the same.

Some migraine sufferers grow feverfew and eat a few leaves every day. In a small percentage of users, feverfew may cause mouth ulcers, swelling of the mouth, lips, or tongue, and loss of taste (Awang 1989). The herb is available in capsule form, which may reduce, but does not eliminate, these local adverse effects. Of note, in the crossover trial described above, more oral symptoms were reported by patients whilst taking placebo than whilst taking feverfew (Murphy *et al.* 1988).

## Homeopathy

Homeopathy may also help migraine. In a double-blind, placebo-controlled study of 60 migraine sufferers, individualized homeopathic prescriptions were given once every 2 weeks for 8 weeks (Brigo and Sepelloni 1991). In the placebo group, the attack rate dropped from 9.9 to 7.9 attacks per month after 2 months (the effect remained at follow-up 2 months after the study ended). In the treated group, the attack rate dropped from 10 to 3 per month by the end of the study, and at 2-month follow-up the rate was 1.8 per month. The intensity of attacks also decreased significantly in the treated group.

## Chiropractic

A randomized, controlled trial of 83 migraine sufferers compared a group receiving chiropractic manipulation with a group receiving cervical manipulation by a conventional practitioner, and a group taught head and shoulder exercises. All groups improved in the frequency, duration, or induced disability of migraine attacks. Although the severity of migraine was reduced more (by 40%) in those receiving chiropractic, compared with a 34% reduction in the exercise group, the difference was not statistically significant (Parker *et al.* 1978).

# Menopause

## Dietary supplements in the menopause

The temptation to try and resist ageing and illness with dietary supplements perhaps increases with advancing years. There are plenty of supplements to choose from, often accompanied by bold and unvalidated claims. Whilst supportive evidence is accruing in some areas, it should be noted that convenient extracts in the form of tablets or capsules do not necessarily contain the same bioactive constituents as the whole food (for example garlic or soya tablets, see below). Of perhaps greater concern, some concentrated supplements can contain harmful quantities of potent bioactive compounds (for example vitamin A supplements; see osteoporosis, below). Usage of soya products has grown to such an extent that they require separate coverage (see below).

## Osteoporosis

A calcium intake of 1500 mg/day can help retard osteoporosis, and calcium and vitamin D supplements have been shown to reduce hip and non-vertebral fractures. Where dietary intake may be inadequate (<400 mg/day), and sun exposure minimal, or in people at high risk of falls, such as in the elderly housebound or the institutionalized, supplements of calcium (1000 mg/day) and vitamin D (400–800 IU/day) are now recommended (Royal College of Physicians 1999). Calcium and vitamin D supplements should also be *minimum* therapy for the 0.5% population receiving long-term corticosteroids (prednisolone 7.5 mg/day or equivalent for 6 months or longer) or at increased risk of osteoporosis for other reasons. (National Osteoporosis Society 1998).

Whilst evidence of benefit is strong for the frail elderly, there is less evidence to support the widespread self-administration by healthy active women in postmenopausal years. Indeed, calcium supplements may not be as effective in bone protection as dairy products if protein intake is inadequate, but adequate intakes of the latter have fallen out of favour due to their atherogenic potential.

However, one trial has confirmed some benefit to supplementation in less frail populations: in an RCT of 389 men and women aged over 65 years and living at home, calcium and vitamin D supplementation was associated with a significant reduction in first non-vertebral fracture (Dawson-Hughes *et al.* 1997).

However, warning about a potential adverse effect of a different dietary supplement comes from the Nurses Health Study. This has recently reported that long-term high consumption of vitamin A of animal origin (high in retinol rather than the apparently harmless precursor β-carotene) may predispose to osteoporosis. The study showed a significant increase in low and moderate trauma fractures in women with high retinol intake (>3000 μg/day or >1010 IU/day) and a non-significant increase in women taking vitamin A supplements. The study suggests the need for re-evaluation of the retinol content of vitamin A supplements or fortified foods (Feskanich *et al.* 2001).

### Cardiovascular disease

The theory that antioxidants like vitamin E might help prevent coronary heart disease did initially seem to be borne out by the Nurses Health Trial. Women in the Nurses Health Trial taking vitamin E supplements for at least 2 years had a 41% reduction in ischaemic heart disease. Although 100 International Units (IU) is a modest amount for supplementation, it is difficult to obtain this quantity in food (Stampfer *et al.* 1993). The Nurses Health Trial is a case–control study and therefore the apparent benefit could be due to confounding, i.e. vitamin E supplement intake may be a marker of some other beneficial characteristic.

Accordingly, two recent large, randomized control trials seem to have ruled out the possibility that vitamin E supplements confer measurable protection against coronary heart disease. The HOPE trial, a study of people with, or at high risk of, cardiovascular disease, included an arm comparing people taking vitamin E (400 IU daily) with placebo (HOPE 2000). Vitamin E conferred no benefit on any cardiovascular outcome. Similarly, the Nurses Health Trial finding has not been supported by the recently completed British Heart Foundation Heart Protection Study carried out over 5 years in 20 000 patients with, or at increased risk of, occlusive cardiovascular disease. Patients were randomized to a statin, or daily multivitamin supplement containing vitamin E 600 IU, vitamin C 250 mg, and β-carotene 20 mg, or both, versus placebo. This study found no reduction in cardiovascular morbidity or mortality or incidence of various cancers ascribable to the multivitamin supplement.

### Dietary soya: beliefs and benefits

There are large international variations in the incidence of menopausal symptoms, osteoporosis and hip fractures, and cardiovascular disease. Lowest rates occur in Asian countries (as with breast cancer). The incidence of hot flushes, for instance, is 70–80% in Europe, 57% in Malaysia, 18% in China, and 14% in Singapore (Knight and Eden 1996). Race, body habitus, culture, lifestyle, and diet may all have a contributory influence, but the correlation with a high dietary consumption of soya products has stimulated investigation of the attributes of soya.

## Dietary soya and flushes

A randomized, double-blind, crossover trial in the USA investigating the effect of 20 g/day soya protein supplementation in 51 perimenopausal women found a significant reduction in perceived severity of vasomotor symptoms as well as cardiovascular benefits (Washburn *et al.* 1999). However, soya tablets taken for 5 weeks did not have the same efficacy when tested in a randomized, double-blind, crossover trial in 155 breast cancer survivors with hot flushes (Quella *et al.* 2000). This may illustrate important differences in the bioactivity of the whole food versus food supplements.

## Dietary soya and cardiovascular disease

A meta-analysis of 38 controlled trials found that consumption of soya protein reduced total cholesterol by an average of 9.3%, low density lipoprotein by 12.9%, and triglycerides by 10.5% (Anderson *et al.* 1995). There was an insignificant increase in high density lipoprotein. Substitution of soya protein for meat lowered cholesterol even when total fat and calorie intake remain the same. A similar impact on lipoproteins, together with a significant lowering of blood pressure as well as reduction in vasomotor symptoms, was found in a more recent trial (Washburn *et al.* 1999).

A crossover study in rhesus monkeys suggests that the beneficial constituents in soya protein are the alcohol-extractable components including the isoflavonic phyto-oestrogens (Anthony *et al.* 1996). Inclusion of phyto-oestrogen-intact soya protein in a moderately atherogenic diet has favourable effects on plasma lipid and lipoprotein concentrations. Soya subjected to removal of alcohol-extractable components had no such effect. The phyto-oestrogens had no adverse effects on the reproductive systems of either males or females, as evaluated by reproductive hormone concentrations and organ weights at necropsy.

## Dietary soya and atrophic vaginitis or recurrent urinary tract infection

Oestrogenization of vaginal epithelium in response to 6 weeks of dietary supplementation with soya flour and linseed has been demonstrated in a pilot study of 25 postmenopausal women (Wilcox *et al.* 1990). The postmenopausal increase in cystitis and vaginal infection has been attributed to the increase in vaginal pH and consequent colonization with pathogenic bacteria (Cardozo 1996). Oral oestrogen lowers vaginal pH, and topical oestriol reduces the incidence of urinary tract infections. Dietary phyto-oestrogens might therefore reduce the incidence of cystitis and vaginitis in postmenopausal women but this remains to be investigated.

## Natural progesterone creams

Skin creams containing 'natural progesterone' have been available in mainland Europe and the USA for around 20 years. They are not licensed in the UK but are available as Progest™ (to be phased out) or Pro-Juven™ creams from a distributor, Higher Nature, only by prescription on a named-patient basis. As few health authorities sanctioned these prescriptions, and only a limited number of GPs were prepared to issue them, women have also been obtaining related preparations by purchase abroad or by mail-order via the Internet (DTB 2001). (See also sections on contraception and premenstrual syndrome.)

### 'Natural' progesterone creams and bone density

The most vocal protagonist for the benefits of natural progesterone has been a US physician, John Lee, MD. One of the earliest and most controversial of his claims centred on use of natural progesterone cream, applied transdermally to cause a measurable increase in bone mineral density as assessed by dual photon densitometry (Lee 1996).The claim was said to be supported by a study which has been multiply published, but in inadequate detail (Fugh-Berman and Kronenberg 1996). The study was an unselected case series of 100 post-menopausal women, aged 38–83 years. Little objective evidence of osteoporosis was presented beyond the statement that 'the majority had already experienced height loss, some as much as five inches'. Bone densitometry in 63 of the women was reported to show an average increase in density of 15.4% over a 3-year period. In addition to treatment with natural progesterone cream, an unspecified number of women were taking oestrogen. Women were also advised to stop smoking, exercise three times weekly for 30 minutes, and take supplements of calcium, vitamins C and D, and β-carotene, all potential confounders.

Those criticisms apart, there is some support for Lee's claims that endogenous progesterone might be important in the maintenance of bone density. It is also apparent that not all synthetic progestogens share this property. There are progesterone receptors on bone and, *in vitro* at least, natural progesterone stimulates osteoblasts (DTB 2001). In a study of 66 premensopausal women, those with short luteal phases had decreased spinal bone density and loss of up to 2–4% of bone per year (Prior *et al.* 1990). Amenorrhoeic athletes given 10 mg medroxyprogesterone aetate (Provera) for 10 days a month show significant increases in trabecular bone (Prior *et al.* 1994). Lactation reduces bone density temporarily, and progestogen-only contraception seems to reduce post-partum bone loss (Caird *et al.* 1994).

To investigate the controversial claim that 'natural' progesterone creams enhance bone density, there is one fully published randomized, double-blind, placebo-controlled trial of 'natural' progesterone cream (20 mg daily) in 102 women within 5 years of the menopause. The women were instructed to also take a multivitamin supplement and 1200 mg calcium daily. This study showed at the end of one year's treatment no difference in bone density as assessed by dual energy x-ray absorptiometry (DEXA) bone scan of the hip and lumbar spine (Leonetti *et al.* 1999).

## 'Natural' progesterone creams and flushes

Oral natural progesterone capsules or skin cream have also been promoted, particularly in the USA, for vasomotor symptoms and vaginal dryness without, until recently, formal evidence of effectiveness.

In the one-year DBRCT study using 20 mg daily, described above, vasomotor symptoms improved in 86% (25 of 30) of women applying one-quarter of a teaspoon (20 g) daily of 'natural' progesterone cream compared with 19% (5 of 26) of women applying placebo cream ($P < 0.001$) (Leonetti *et al.* 1999). This promising, but limited, evidence, which suggests that natural progesterone creams do improve vasomotor symptoms, needs confirmation (DTB 2001).

## Natural progesterone cream-dosing, plasma concentration, and endometrial protection

There is variation in the concentration (1.5–3%), cost, dosing instructions (once or twice daily) and dose range (10–40 mg/day) for the various creams available (DTB 2001). It would seem that 20 mg daily improves vasomotor symptoms but has no effect on bone density, while the efficacy of higher doses had not been adequately evaluated.

Plasma concentration achieved by topical progesterone has been assessed in a double-blind, randomized, placebo-controlled crossover study of 20 women post-hysterectomy and with bilateral oophorectomy. The increase that topical progesterone (Pro-Gest 43.5 mg daily for 10 days) achieved in plasma concentration of progesterone was to a level of 2.9 nmol/l, which is only one-fifth of the median luteal level seen in women with normal menstrual cycles (DTB 2001). Prolonging the treatment to 6 weeks – as in an open randomized study in 24 postmenopausal women using 40 mg/day progesterone cream – increased the mean maximum serum progesterone level to 5.3 nmol/l (DTB 2001). These levels should be compared with normal levels in the follicular phases of below nmol/l, median luteal phase levels of 15 nmol/l and peak day 21 levels of around 35–45 nmol/l. Thus progesterone creams at the upper end of the recommended dose range achieve a real but limited increase in plasma progesterone levels, with a possible delay before peak levels are achieved.

It should be noted that natural progesterone creams cannot be depended upon to oppose the proliferative effect of oestrogen on the endometrium in women with an intact uterus. A randomized, double-blind, placebo-controlled study in 17 postmenopausal women using conventional oestrogen replacement therapy compared the effect on the endometrium of natural progesterone cream and dydrogesterone 10 mg. Endometrial biopsy performed once only between days 12 and 14 of the study showed proliferative changes in five of eight women using progesterone cream compared with two of nine women on dydrogesterone. Secretory transformation (a protective sign) was present in one of eight women using progesterone cream compared with four of nine women on dydrogesterone.

Occasional side effects such as acne, vaginal spotting, or bleeding are reported but apparently no severe side effects (DTB 2001).

## Other forms of hormone replacement: DHEA

A significant public health issue is raised by the increasing use of oral dehydroepiandrosterone (DHEA) in the USA, outside medical supervision, for its supposed anti-ageing effects. Clinical trials have begun and the first double-blind, placebo-controlled trial published involved 280 men and women and assessed the effect administration of 50 mg oral DHEA for 1 year. It appears to confirm restoration of premenopausal DHEA levels, increased oestradiol and testosterone levels, particularly in women, with accompanying improvement in skin condition, libido, and decreased bone turnover (Baulieu *et al.* 2000). There were no harmful consequences apparent after this year of treatment, but it is too early to recommend its use in primary care.

## Biofeedback

Women have been successfully trained to control their hot flushes using the techniques of biofeedback (Freedman and Woodward 1992). The impact on hot flushes is confirmed by skin conductance measurements. This control may be of value in women unwilling or unable to receive HRT, or who are receiving HRT but nonetheless experience occasional hot flushes.

## Manipulative medicine

One placebo-controlled trial suggested a form of osteopathy was helpful for menopausal symptoms (Lewith 1996).

## Ginseng

Ginseng is used most by the elderly and sales in the USA are increasing by more than 25% per year. The commonest belief is that it retards the ageing process and improves mental and physical performance. A systematic review of 16 RCTs demonstrated that most trials are in the young, and whilst some do address cognitive and physical performance, most address less common reasons for which ginseng is taken, such as immune modulation. Half show an effect and half do not, and some adverse events and drug interactions are reported (Vogler *et al.* 1999).

# Vaginal discharge and sexually transmitted infections

## AIDS

Available surveys suggest that usage of complementary medicine is even higher amongst AIDS patients than the general population. Of 287 patients questioned (67 women), 31% used complementary therapies (Bates *et al.* 1996). Other, smaller studies suggest higher usage. Nowhere is health consumerism better illustrated than in AIDS. The AIDS community has been highly vocal in demanding not just more from the research effort, but more information about alternative treatments. In the USA, buyers' clubs have been set up to help PWAs (persons with AIDS) obtain treatments which may be banned or difficult to obtain, such as marijuana for appetite stimulation and control of nausea. They have swapped information on nutritional manipulation and mega-vitamin and mineral supplementation to combat wasting syndrome. The reaction of the medical profession to these recommendations is often negative, with emphasis placed on the potential ill-effects of dietary supplements when taken in excess, or in combination with some prescribed drugs. Within the AIDS community, information is available concerning experimentation with herbs, natural hormones, and fungi believed to act as immune enhancers. There is also interest in a psychotropic drug called ibogaine, derived from the West African iboga plant and credited with the property of interrupting narcotic addiction when administered only once or twice a year, in contrast to the need for daily methadone administration. Massage, reflexology, and meditation are considered generally beneficial. AIDS activists claim, with some justification, that many of the recent improvements in life span and quality of life have been due more to community efforts than to biomedical research, facilitated by the rapid communication and feedback made possible by the Internet. One such source of information exchange used extensively is the Critical Path AIDS Project (http://www.critpath.org/critpath.htm).

## Candidiasis

This condition is sometimes diagnosed by patients attending complementary practitioners and is ascribed to diets high in carbohydrates, refined sugar, or yeast. It does not necessarily correspond to the vaginal, oral or visceral forms of *Candida* infection recognized by conventional medical science. No trials of the effect of dietary intervention on *Candida* infection have been conducted. Only two strands of evidence support a dietary approach: the first, the known predisposition of diabetics to *Candida* infection; the second, preliminary evidence that a proportion of women with recurrent, severe mucocutaneous *Candida* infection have undiagnosed coeliac disease, and following serological identification (using endomysial antibody), benefit from elimination of wheat and other gluten sources from the diet (personal communication, Dr G Bird).

## Urinary tract infection (UTI)

### Cranberry juice

Women suffering recurrent UTIs are in particular need of effective preventive measures and many women seek an alternative to antibiotics. High-risk groups include diaphragm users, sexually active, and elderly women. Cranberry juice is a folk remedy once widely used for both symptomatic relief and prevention. The first randomized, double-blind, placebo-controlled trial was carried out in 153 elderly women with a mean age of 78 years (Avorn *et al.* 1994). In a 6-month study, women were randomized to either 300 ml/day of a commercially available cranberry juice cocktail, or a placebo juice matched for taste, appearance, and vitamin C content. Those drinking cranberry juice showed a statistically significant halving of the number of urine specimens containing bacteriuria ($\geq 10^5$ c.f.u./ml) with pyuria. There was also a modest reduction in the frequency with which symptomatic UTI was diagnosed and antibiotics prescribed. Cranberry juice was more effective in treating than preventing bacteriuria and pyuria.

Possible mechanisms of action include urinary acidification, but consistent acidification may require consumption of up to 2000 ml/day. One study demonstrating the acidifying effect of cranberry juice on urine also showed that anticipated problems with increased number of bowel movements, weight gain, increased voiding frequency, did not occur (Kinney and Blount 1979). Recent interest has shifted to inhibition of bacterial adherence to bladder wall, or gut mucosa, with, in the latter case, a postulated reduction in gut bacterial load (Avorn *et al.* 1994). Two compounds in cranberry juice inhibit adherence (Zafriri *et al.* 1989): fructose, present in most fruit juices, and a non-dialysable polymeric compound isolated from cranberry and blueberry juice (both belonging to *Vaccinia* genus) but not from orange, grapefruit, pineapple, guava, or mango juice (Ofek *et al.* 1991). When a total of 77 clinical isolates of *Escherichia coli* were tested, cranberry juice inhibited adherence to uroepithelial cells by at least 75% in more than 60% of clinical isolates (Sobota 1984). Fifteen of 22 subjects showed significant anti-adherence activity in the urine 1–3 hours after drinking 15 ounces (430 ml) of cranberry cocktail. Together, these experimental studies implied the need for intake of perhaps six cups of juice a day (1 cup is 400–600 ml). Cranberry juice tablets are now commercially available but have not yet been evaluated in clinical trials.

A more recent RCT compared 50 ml daily of cranberry/lingonberry juice concentrate with 100 ml of lactobacillus concentrate 5 days per week, or no intervention, in 150 women aged 20–60 (mean age 30 years) (Kontiokari and Sundeqvist 2001). The cranberry/lingonberry juice halved the number of recurrent UTIs and produced a 20% reduction in absolute risk of recurrent infection The 50 ml cranberry concentrate contained 7.5 g cranberry and 1.7 g lingonberry, and was added to 200 ml water to make a drinkable preparation.

There are many reports of herbal medicines used for the treatment of UTI, and in some cases active ingredients with potent antimicrobial properties have been isolated. The paucity of data concerning safety constrains further discussion in this general overview.

# Urinary incontinence

## Pelvic floor exercises and biofeedback

For stress incontinence, pelvic floor exercises are now generally used as first-line treatment before surgery is considered, with significant improvements reported in between 42 and 52% of patients (Klarskov *et al.* 1986; Elia and Bergman 1993) (Chapter 8). In an uncontrolled study of 48 women, the combination of pelvic floor exercises with biofeedback was found to improve 62% of patients (McIntosh *et al.* 1993). Several small studies find biofeedback alone to be effective in the treatment of stress incontinence, with reported reductions in urinary loss of 80–90%. In a controlled study of 135 women, urinary losses were reduced by 54% in the pelvic floor exercise group, and reduced by 61% in the biofeedback group, whilst increased by 9% in the control group (Burns *et al.* 1993). Complete cure was reported by 16% in the pelvic exercise group, 23% of the biofeedback, and 3% of the control group. Pelvic floor exercises are part of many Yoga and Pilates exercises.

# Smoking cessation

## Acupuncture

Auricular acupuncture is one of the most widely used techniques for smoking cessation, and available studies suggest it is as effective as nicotine supplements or behaviour therapy. Cessation rates of 20–40% are reported for all these modalities. However, acupuncture, like other methods, suffers from a gradual decrease of therapeutic effect over time and a high relapse rate. Trials lacking follow-up are therefore of limited clinical significance. One-year success rates of only 8–10% have been reported for all three modalities in a comparative study of acupuncture, nicotine supplements, or placebo (Clavel-Chapelon *et al.* 1992). Hypnosis is commonly used to aid smoking cessation, but there is no evidence that it is superior to other approaches.

## Relaxation imagery

The high relapse rates and the fact that smokers identify stress as a major contributory factor highlight the need for smokers to develop additional long-term coping strategies and substitute behaviours. A randomized controlled trial carried out in 76 subjects who had completed a local smoking cessation programme compared the effect of a further 3 months of instruction in relaxation imagery in the experimental group, with regular meetings in the control group. The practice of relaxation imagery was associated with a reduction in perceived stress and prolongation of smoking abstinence (Wynd 1992).

# Anxiety and depression

## Anxiety

The anxiolytic effects of massage, aromatherapy, reflexology, meditation, relaxation, and imagery are widely assumed, and supporting evidence can be found (Fulder 1996). Virtually every other complementary approach has also been used in this context. Further research in the area of massage and aromatherapy is likely to be spearheaded by midwives and the nursing profession who have already studied its applications in childbirth, in cancer patients, and in the intensive care unit (Fulder 1996).

## Depression

Since up to 83% of patients report an increase in general well-being following consultation with a complementary therapist (Francis 1995), an improvement in mild depression might be anticipated, but awaits confirmation. One herbal preparation, St John's Wort (*Hypericum perforatum*) has proven efficacy in mild-to-moderate depression and an NHS prescription can now be issued, although depression is currently an unlicensed indication. Lack of guidance in the BNF regarding dosage reflects uncertainty stemming from different doses used in trials (200–1000 μg hypericin daily), and differing amounts of this active ingredient in various St John's Wort (SJW) or 'hypericum' preparations.

Two systematic reviews, the most recent of which included 27 RCTs (17 of which were placebo-controlled), have found extracts of St John's Wort to be more effective than placebo for treating mild-to-moderate depressive disorders (Linde *et al.* 1996; Linde 1998). No equivalent studies are available for severe depression. Median sample size in these trials was larger than the median sample size in trials comparing tricyclic antidepressants and selective serotonin re-uptake inhibitors. Comparison of hypericum with low doses of amitriptyline, imipramine, or maprotiline found no statistical difference in efficacy, and a lower incidence of side effects with hypericum. The most commonly reported side effects are dry mouth, gastrointestinal symptoms, allergic reaction, dizziness, confusion, tiredness/sedation, plus a few reports of photosensitivity reactions. Like synthetic antidepressants, hypericum extracts need 2–4 weeks to take effect.

Similar results were obtained in a more recent DBRCT of 324 patients with mild-to-moderate depression, in which a higher dose of imipramine (75 mg b.d.) was compared with 250 mg b.d. Hypericum extract ZE 117 (0.2% hypericin extracted in ethanol 50% w/w) (Woelk 2000). The hypericum extract was therapeutically equivalent but was better tolerated, with only 3% of hypericum-treated patients withdrawing due to adverse events compared with 16% imipramine-treated patients.

Extensive use of the herb in Germany has not resulted in published reports of toxicity due to SJW itself. However, increasing use in the UK resulted in recognition of important pharmacokinetic drug interactions. SJW interacts with drugs metabolized by the cytochrome P450 system or transported by P-glycoprotein so that their blood levels and hence efficacy is reduced. Because the level of active ingredients can vary between preparations of SJW, if patients switch between preparations, the degree of enzyme induction could change over time. A rise in blood levels of the drugs when SJW is discontinued can potentially lead to toxicity. Drugs affected in this way include oral contraceptives, warfarin, digoxin, theophylline, anticonvulsants, cyclosporin, HIV protease inhibitors and HIV non-nucleoside reverse transcriptase inhibitors.

In addition, SJW may increase serotonin levels through its weak monoamine oxidase inhibiting (MAOI) activity and serotonin re-uptake inhibition. Pharmacodynamic (additive or potentiating) interactions may therefore occur with selective serotonin re-uptake inhibitors and triptans used to treat migraine.

## Non-specific benefits of complementary medicine

Both critics and advocates of complementary medicine agree that complementary medicine produces an increase in well-being – a non-specific benefit – which will at the very least, help people deal psychologically with their specific physical illnesses (Francis 1995). That physical benefits may ensue from any therapeutic interaction between therapist and patient is the message of holism. The potential power of such an effect is apparent in conditions such as ischaemic heart disease, and perhaps breast cancer, where it is known that hopelessness accelerates disease and increases mortality (Everson *et al.* 1997; Reilly 2001).

## Conclusion

To quote a view expressed in *Stedman's medical dictionary*: 'the real value of homeopathy was to demonstrate the healing powers of nature, and the therapeutic virtue of placebos.' Arguably, all medicine, complementary or conventional, should, whenever possible, harness both these forces. Studies which suggest an effect exceeding that of placebo are appearing in many fields of complementary medicine, and future advances need to incorporate the best from all approaches to health and disease.

## References

Abraham, G. (1982). Nutritional factors in the aetiology of the premenstrual syndrome. *Journal of Reproductive Medicine,* **28**, 446–64.

Adlercreutz, H., Fotsis, T., Bannwart, C., *et al.* (1986). Determination of urinary lignans and phytoestrogen metabolites, potential antiestrogens and anticarcinogens, in urine of women on various habitual diets. *Journal of Steroid Biochemistry,* **25**(5B), 791–7.

Adlercreutz, H., Hockerstedt, K., Bannwart, C., *et al.* (1987). Effect of dietary components, including lignans and phytoestrogens, on enterohepatic circulation and liver metabolism of estrogens and on sex hormone binding globulin (SHBG). *Journal of Steroid Biochemistry,* **27**(4–6), 1135–44.

Adlercreutz, H., Honjo, H., Higashi, A., *et al.* (1991). Urinary excretion of lignans and isoflavonoid phytoestrogens in Japanese men and women consuming a traditional Japanese diet. *American Journal of Clinical Nutrition,* **54**, 1093–100.

Alderete, E., Eskenazi, B. and Sholtz, R. (1995). Effect of cigarette smoking and coffee drinking on time to conception. *Epidemiology,* **6**, 403–8.

Anderson, J., Johnstone, B. and Cook-Newell, M.E. (1995). Meta-analysis of the effect of soy protein intake on serum lipids. *New England Journal of Medicine,* **333**, 276–82.

Anthony, M.S., Clarkson, T.B., Hughes, C.L., Morgan, T.M., Burke, G.L. and Hughes, C.L. Jr (1996). Soybean isoflavones improve cardiovascular risk factors without affecting the reproductive system of peripubertal rhesus monkeys. *Journal of Nutrition*, **126**, 43–50.

Astin, J.A. (1998). Why patients use alternative medicine. Results of a national survey. *The Journal of the American medical Association*, **279**, 1548–53.

Avorn, J., Monane, M., Gurwitz, J.H., Glynn, R.J., Choodnovskiy, I. and Lipsitz, L.A. (1994). Reduction of bacteriuria and pyuria after ingestion of cranberry juice. *Journal of the American Medical Association*, **271**, 751–4.

Awang, D. (1989). Herbal medicine: feverfew. *Canadian Pharmacy Journal*, **122**, 266–70.

Bagenal, F.S., Easton, D.F., Harris, E., Chilvers, C.E. and McElwain, T.J. (1990). Survival of patients with breast cancer attending Bristol Cancer Help Centre [see comments]. *Lancet*, **336**, 606–10.

Baulieu, E.E., Thomas, G., Legrain, S., *et al.* (2000). Dehydroepiandrosterone (DHEA), DHEA sulfate, and aging: contribution of the DHEAge Study to a sociobiomedical issue. *Proceedings of the National Academy of Sciences of the United States of America*, **97**, 4279–84.

Bates, B., Kissinger, P. and Bessinger, R.E. (1996). Complementary therapy use amongst HIV infected patients. *AIDS Patient Care and STDs* Feb, 32–6.

Bernstein, L., Henderson, B., Hanisch, R., Sullivan-Halley, J. and Ross, R.K. (1994). Physical exercise and reduced risk of breast cancer in young women. *Journal of the National Cancer Institute*, **86**, 1403–8.

Blanchard, E. and Andrasik, F. (eds) (1987). Biofeedback treatment of patients with vascular headache. *Biofeedback: studies in clinical efficacy*. Plenum, New York.

Bodeker, G. (1994). *Traditional health knowledge and public policy*. UNESCO.

Bridge, L.R., Benson, P., Pietroni, P.C. and Priest, R.G. (1988). Relaxation and imagery in the treatment of breast cancer. *British Medical Journal*, **297**, 1169–72.

Brigo, B. and Sepelloni, G. (1991). Homeopathic treatment of migraines: a randomised double blind controlled study of sixty cases. *Berlin Journal on Research in Homeopathy*, **1**, 98–105.

Burns, P., Pranikoff, K., Nochajski, T.H., Hadley, E.C., Levy, K.J. and Ory, M.G. (1993). A comparison of the effectiveness of biofeedback and pelvic muscle exercise treatment of stress incontnence in older community-dwelling women. *Journal of Gerontology*, **48**, M167–74.

Cahill, D.J., Fox, R., Wardle, P.G. and Harlow, C.R. (1994). Multiple follicular development associated with herbal medicine. *Human Reproduction*, **9**, 1469–70.

Caird, L.E., Reid-Thomas, V., Hannan, W.J., Gow, S. and Glasier, A.F. (1994). Oral progestogen-only vontraception may protect against loss of bone mass in breast-feeding women. *Clinical Endocrinology*, **41**, 739–45.

Cardozo, L. (1996). Postmenopausal cystitis. *British Medical Journal*, **313**, 129.

Chen, C., David, A., Nunnerley, H., *et al.* (1995). Adverse life events and breast cancer: case control study. *British Medical Journal*, **311**, 1527–30.

Clavel-Chapelon, F., Paoletti, C. and Benhamou, S. (1992). A randomised 2 × 2 factorial design to evaluate different smoking cessation methods. *Revue d'Epidemiologie et de Sante Publique*, **40**, 187–90.

Committee on Safety of Medicines/Medicines Control Agency (1996). *Current Problems in Pharmacovigilance*, **22**, 10.

Dawson-Hughes, B., Harris, S.S., Krall, E.A. and Dallal, G.E. (1997). Effect of calcium and vitamin D supplementation on bone density in men and women 65 years of age and older. *New England Journal of Medicine*, **337**, 670–6.

De Smet, P. (1995). Should herbal medicine-like products be licensed as medicines? *British Medical Journal*, **310**, 1023–4.

Dickinson, D. (1996). The growth of complementary therapy. A consumer-led boom. In: Ernst, E. (ed.), *Complementary medicine: an objective appraisal.* Butterworth-Heinemann, Oxford.

Domar, A.D., Seibel, M.M. and Benson, H. (1990). The mind/body program for infertility: a new behavioral treatment approach for women with infertility [see comments]. *Fertility and Sterility*, **53**, 246–9.

DTB (2001). 'Natural' progesterone creams for postmenopausal women. *Drugs and Therapeutics Bulletin*, **39**(2), 10–11.

Eisenberg, D., Davis, R.B., Ettner, S.L., *et al.* (1998). Trends in alternative medicine use in the United States, 1990–1997: results of a follow-up national survey. *Journal of the American Medical Association*, **280**, 1569–75.

Elia, G. and Bergman, A. (1993). Pelvic muscle exercises: when do they work? *Obstetrics and Gynecology*, **81**, 283–6.

Ellis, J., Mulligan, I., Rowe, J. and Sackett, D.L. (1995). Inpatient general medicine is evidence based. *Lancet*, **346**, 407–10.

Ernst, E. and White, A. (2000). The BBC survey of complementary therapy use in the UK. *Complementary Therapies in Medicine*, **8**, 32–6.

Everson S., Kaplan, G., Goldberg, D.E., Salonen, R. and Salonen, J.T. (1997). Hopelessness and a 4-year progression of carotid atherosclerosis: the Kuopio ischemic heart disease risk factor study. *Arteriosclerosis, Thrombosis and Vascular Biology* **17**, 1490–5.

Facchinetti, F., Sances, G., Borella, P., Genazzani, A.R. and Nappi, G. (1991). Magnesium prophylaxis of menstrual migraine: effects on intracellular magnesium. *Headache*, **31**, 298–301.

Feskanich, D., Singh, V., Willett, W. C. and Colditz, G.A. (2002). Vitamin A intake and hip fractures among postmenopausal women. *Journal of the American Medical Association.* **287**, 47–54.

FIM (in press). Prince's Foundation for Integrated Medicine. FIM, London.

Florack, E.I., Zielhuis, G.A. and Rolland, R. (1994). Cigarette smoking, alcohol consumption, and caffeine intake and fecundability. *Preventive Medicine*, **23**, 175–80.

Francis, J. (1995). Report on Consumers' Association Members' usage of and satisfaction with Alternative Medicine Practitioners. Prepared for 'Which?' by Consumers Association Research Department and Survey Centre.

Freedman, R.R. and Woodward, S. (1992). Behavioral treatment of menopausal hot flushes: evaluation by ambulatory monitoring. *American Journal of Obstetrics and Gynecology*, **167**, 436–9.

Fugh-Berman, A. and Kronenberg, F. (1996). Natural hormones. In: *Herbalism and medicine.* Columbia University, College of Physicians and Surgeons, New York.

Fulder, S. (1996). *The handbook of complementary medicine.* OUP, Oxford.

Fulder, S. and Munro, R. (1985). Complementary medicine in the United Kingdom: patients, practitioners and consultations. *Lancet*, **2**, 542–5.

Furnham, A. and Vincent, C. (1995). The health beliefs and behaviours of three groups of complementary medicine and a general practice group of patients. *Journal of Alternative and Complementary Medicine*, **1**, 347–59.

The Heart Outcomes Prevention Evaluation Study Investigators (2000). Effects of an angiotensin converting enzyme inhibitor, Ramipril, on cardiovascular events in high risk patients. *New England Journal of Medicine*, **342**, 145–53.

Gateley, C.A., Miers, M., Mansel, R.E. and Hughes, L.E. (1992). Drug treatments for mastalgia: 17 years of experience in the Cardiff mastalgia clinic. *Journal of the Royal Society of Medicine*, **85**, 12–15.

Gerhard, I. and Postneek, F. (1992). Auricular acupuncture in the treatment of female infertility. *Gynecological Endocrinology*, **6**, 171–81.

Gill, P., Dowell, A.C., Neal, R.D., Smith, N., Heywood, P. and Wilson, A.E. (1996). Evidence based general practice: a retrospective study of interventions in one training practice. *British Medical Journal*, **312**, 819–21.

GMC (1995 and 2001). Delegating care to non-medical staff and students. *Duties of a Doctor. Guidance from the General Medical Council.* GMC, London.

Goei, G. *et al.* (1982). Dietary patterns of patients with premenstrual tension. *Journal of Applied Nutrition*, **34**, 4–11.

Goodale, I.L., Domar, A.D. and Benson, H. (1990). Alleviation of premenstrual syndrome symptoms with the relaxation response. *Obstetrics and Gynecology*, **75**, 649–55.

Grant, E.C. (1979). Food allergies and migraine. *Lancet*, **1**, 966–9.

Groer, M. and Ohnesorge, C. (1993). Menstrual-cycle lengthening and reduction in premenstrual distress through guided imagery. *Journal of Holistic Nursing*, **11**, 286–94.

Gruber, B.L., Hersh, S.P., Hall, N.R., *et al.* (1993). Immunological responses of breast cancer patients to behavioral interventions. *Biofeedback and Self-Regulation*, **18**, 1–22.

Halaska, M., Raus, K., Beles, P., Martan, A. and Paithner, K.G. (1998) Treatment of cyclical mastodynia using an extract of *Vitex agnus castus*: results of a double blind comparison with a placebo. *Ceskoslovenska Gynekologie* **63**, 388–92.

Harrison, R.F., O'Moore, R.R. and O'Moore, A.M. (1986). Stress and fertility: some modalities of investigation and treatment in couples with unexplained infertility in Dublin. *International Journal of Fertility*, **31**, 153–9.

Hatch, E. and Bracken, M. (1993). Association of delayed conception with caffeine consumption. *American Journal of Epidemiology*, **138**(12), 1082–92.

Helms, J.M. (1987). Acupuncture for the management of primary dysmenorrhea. *Obstetrics and Gynecology*, **69**(1), 51–6.

Hodnett, E. (1995). Support from caregivers during at-risk pregnancy. Pregnancy and Childbirth Module (1995, issue 2). Cochrane Database of Systematic Reviews. The Cochrane Collaboration.

Horn, R.P. (1995). Phytoestrogens, body composition, and breast cancer. *Cancer Causes and Control*, **6**, 567–73.

Hunter, D.J., Manson, J.E., Colditz, G.A., *et al.* (1993). A prospective study of the intake of vitamins C, E and A and the risk of breast cancer. *New England Journal of Medicine*, **329**, 234–40.

Hutchins, A.M., Lampe, J.W., Martini, M.C., Campbell, D.R. and Slavin, J.L. (1995a). Vegetables, fruits, and legumes: effect on urinary isoflavonoid phytoestrogen and lignan excretion. *Journal of the American Dietetic Association*, **95**(7), 769–74.

Hutchins, A.M., Slavin, J.L. and Lampe, J.W. (1995b). Urinary isoflavonoid phytoestrogen and lignan excretion after consumption of fermented and unfermented soy products. *Journal of the American Dietetic Association*, **95**(5), 545–51.

Joesoef, M.R., Beral, V., Rolfs, R.T., Aral, S.O. and Cramer, D.W. (1990). Are caffeinated beverages risk factors for delayed conception? [see comments]. *Lancet*, **335**, 136–7.

Johnson, E.S., Kadam, N.P., Hylands, D.M. and Hylands, P.J. (1985). Efficacy of fever-few as prophylactic treatment of migraine. *British Medical Journal*, **291**, 569–73.

Kinney, A.B. and Blount, M. (1979). Effect of cranberry juice on urinary pH. *Nursing Research*, **28**(5), 287–90.

Klarskov, P., Belving, D., Bischoff, N., *et al.* (1986). Pelvic floor exercises versus surgery for female stress incontinence. *Urologia Internationalis*, **41**, 129–32.

Knight, D. and Eden, J. (1996). A review of the clinical effects of phytoestrogens. *Obstetrics and Gynecology*, **87**, 897–904.

Kokjohn, K., Schmid, D.M., Triano, J.J. and Brennan, P.C. (1992). The effect of spinal manipulation on pain and prostaglandin levels in women with primary dysmenor-rhoea. *Journal of Manipulative and Physiological Therapeutics*, **15**, 279–85.

Kolonel, L. (1988). Variability in diet and its relation to risk in ethnic and migrant groups. *Basic Life Sciences*, **43**, 129–35.

Kontiokari, T. and Sundeqvist K. (2001). Randomised trial of cranberry-lingonberry juice and *Lactobacillus* GG drink for the prevention of urinary tract infections in women. *British Medical Journal*, **322**, 1571–3.

Kushi, M. (1978). *Natural healing through macrobiotics*. Japan Publications Inc, Tokyo.

La Vecchia, C., Franceschi, S., Decarli, A., *et al.* (1984). Dietary vitamin A and the risk of invasive cervical cancer. *International Journal of Cancer*, **34**, 319–22.

Lee, H.P., Gourley, L., Duffy, S.W., Esteve, J., Lee, J. and Day, N.E. (1991). Dietary effects on breast cancer in Singapore. *Lancet*, **337**, 1197–200.

Lee, J. (1996). *Natural progesterone. The multiple roles of a remarkable hormone*. Jon Carpenter, Chipping Norton.

Leonetti, H.B., Longo, S. and Anasti, J.N. (1999). Transdermal progesterone cream for vasomotor symptoms and postmenopausal bone loss. *Obstetrics and Gynecology*, **94**, 225–8.

Lewith, G. (1996). Premenstrual syndrome and the menopause. In: Lewith, G., Kenyon, J. and Lewis, P. (eds), *Complementary medicine. An integrated approach*. OUP, Oxford.

Lian, F. (1991). TCM treatment of luteal phase defect – an analysis of 60 cases. *Journal of Traditional Chinese Medicine*, **11**, 115–20.

Linde, K. and Mulrow, C.D. (1998). St John's Wort for depression (Cochrane Review) In: The Cochrane Library, Issue 1, Oxford: Update Software.

Linde, K., Ramirez, G., Mulrow, C.D., Pauls, A., Weidenhammer, W. and Melchart, D. (1996). St John's wort for depression – an overview and meta-analysis of randomised clinical trials. *British Medical Journal*, **313**, 253–8.

MacGregor, E. (1996a). 'Menstrual' migraine: towards a definition. *Cephalalgia* **16**, 11–21.

MacGregor, E. (1996b). Menstruation, sex hormones and migraine. *Clinics of North America*. W.B. Saunders, Philadelphia.

MacGregor, E.A., Chia, H., Vohrah, R.C. and Wilkinson, M. (1990). Migraine and menstruation: a pilot study. *Cephalalgia*, **10**, 305–10.

MacLennan, A., Wilson, D. and Taylor, A.W. (1996). Prevalence and cost of alternative medicine in Australia. *Lancet*, **347**, 569–72.

McIntosh, L.J., Frahm, J.D., Mallett, V.T. and Richardson, D.A. (1993). Pelvic floor rehabilitation in the treatment of incontinence. *Journal of Reproductive Medicine*, **38**(9), 662–5.

Mintel (1995). Sales of alternative medicine increase. *British Medical Journal*, **310**, 1624.

MRC Vitamin Study Group (1991). Prevention of neural tube defects: results of the Medical Research Council Study Group. *Lancet*, **238**, 131–7.

Murphy, J.J., Heptinstall, S. and Mitchell, J.R. (1988). Randomised double blind controlled trial of feverfew in migraine prevention. *Lancet*, **2**, 189–92.

Murray, J. and Sheperd, S. (1993). Alternative or additional medicine? An exploratory study in general practice. *Social Science and Medicine*, **37**, 983–8.

Nehlig, A. and Debry, G. (1994). Effects of coffee and caffeine on fertility, reproduction, lactation, and development. Review of human and animal data. *Journal de Gynecologie Obstetrique et Biologie de la Reproduction* **23**, 241–56.

National Osteoporosis Society (1998). Guidance on the prevention and management of corticosteroid induced osteoporosis. NOS, Bath, UK.

O'Brien, P. (1993). Helping women with premenstrual syndrome. *British Medical Journal*, **307**, 1471–5.

Ofek, I., Goldhar, J., Zafriri, D., Lis, H., Adar, R. and Sharon, N. (1991). Anti-*Escherichia* adhesin activity of cranberry and blueberry juices. *New England Journal of Medicine*, **324**, 1599.

Oleson, T. and Flocco, W. (1993). Randomized controlled study of premenstrual symptoms treated with ear, hand, and foot reflexology. *Obstetrics and Gynecology*, **82**, 906–11.

Olsen, J. (1991). Cigarette smoking, tea and coffee drinking, and subfecundity. *American Journal of Epidemiology*, **133**, 734–9.

Ong, C.K., Petersen, S., Bodeker, G. and Stewart-Brown, S. (2002). Health status of people using complementary and alternative medical practitioner services in 4 English counties. *American Journal of Public Health*, **92**, 1653–6.

Ong, C.K. and Banks, B. (2003). *Complementary Alternative medicine: the consumer perspective*. The Prince of Wales's Foundation for Integrated Health, London.

Ong, C.K., Petersen, S., Bodeker, G. and Stewart-Brown, S. (2001). The Use of Complementary and Alternative Medicine (CAM) in England: Lifestyle, gender and their impact on CAM Use. Internal Paper, Health Services Research Unit, Department of Public Health, University of Oxford.

Parker, G.B., Tupling, H. and Pryor, D.S. (1978). A controlled trial of cervical manipulation of migraine. *Australian and New Zealand Journal of Medicine*, **8**, 589–93.

Prior, J.J., Vigna, Y.M., Schechter, M.T. and Burgess, A.E. (1990). Spinal bone loss and ovulatory disturbances. *New England Journal of Medicine*, **323**, 1221–7.

Prior, J.J., Vigna, Y.M., Barr, S.I., Rexworthy, C. and Lentle, B.C. (1994). Cyclic medroxyprogesterone treatment increases bone density: a controlled trial in active women with menstrual cycle disturbances. *American Journal of Medicine*, **96**, 521–30.

Quella, S.K., Loprinzi, C.L., Barton, D.L., *et al.* (2000) Evaluation of soy phytoestrogens for the treatment of hot flashes in breast cancer survivors: a North Centre Cancer Treatment Trial. *Journal of Clinical Oncology*, **18**, 1068–74.

Rees, L. and Weil, A. (2001) Integrated medicine. *British Medical Journal*, **322**, 119–20.

Reilly, D. (2001). Enhancing human healing. *British Medical Journal*, **322**, 20–1.

Royal College of General Practitioners (1986). *Morbidity statistics from general practice – third national study*. HMSO, London.

Royal College of Physicians (1999). *Osteoporosis. Clinical guidelines for prevention and treatment*. RCP, London.

Schellenberg, R. (2001). Treatment for the premenstrual syndrome with agnus castus fruit extract: prospective, randomized, placebo controlled study. *British Medical Journal*, **322**, 134–7.

Seelig, N. (ed.) (1971). Human requirements of magnesium: factors that increase needs. Springer Verlag, Paris.

Simpson, R. and Bick, D. (1996). Alternative therapies. *Journal of the American Medical Association*, **275**, 1034–5.

Smith, I. (1996). More than pin money. *Health Service Journal*, **106**, 24–5.

Smithells, D. (1996). Vitamins in early pregnancy. *British Medical Journal*, **313**, 128–9.

Sobota, A.E. (1984). Inhibition of bacterial adherence by cranberry juice: potential use for the treatment of urinary tract infections. *Journal of Urology*, **131**, 1013–16.

Sorensen, J.M. and Katsiotis, S.T. (2000) Parameters influencing the yield and composition of the essential oil from Cretan *Vitex agnus castus* fruits. *Planta Medica*, **66**, 245–50.

Spiegel, D. and Bloom, J. (1983). Group therapy and self-hypnosis reduce metastatic breast carcinoma pain. *Psychosomatic Medicine*, **45**, 333–9.

Spiegel, D., Bloom, J., Kraemer, H.C. and Gottheil, E. (1989). Effect of psychosocial treatment on survival of patients with metastaic breast cancer. *Lancet*, **2**, 888–91.

Stampfer, M., Hennekens, C., Manson, J.E., Colditz, G.A., Rosner, B. and Willett, W.C. (1993). Vitamin E consumption and the risk of coronary disease in women. *New England Journal of Medicine*, **328**, 1444–9.

Stanton, C. and Gray, R. (1995). Effects of caffeine consumption on delayed conception. *American Journal of Epidemiology*, **142**, 1322–9.

Steegers-Theunissen, R.P., Boers, G.H., Trijbels, F.J., *et al.* (1994). Maternal hyperhomocysteinemia: a risk factor for neural-tube defects? *Metabolism*, **43**, 1475–80.

Stone, J. (1996a). Complements slip. *Health*, **26**, 7.

Stone, J. (1996b). Regulating complementary medicine. *British Medical Journal*, **312**, 1492–3.

Thomas, K., Carr, J., Westlake, L. and Williams, B.T. (1991). Use of non-orthodox and conventional health care in Great Britain. *British Medical Journal*, **26**, 207–10.

Thomas, K., Fall, M., *et al.* (1995). National survey of access to complementary health care via general practitioners. Sheffield Centre for Health and Related Research, Sheffield, University.

Thomas, K.J., Nicholl, J.P. and Coleman, P. (2001). Use and expenditure on complementary medicine in England: a population based survey. *Complementary Therapies in Medicine*, **9**, 2–11.

Thomason, P., Fisher, B., Carpenter, B. and Fike, G.L. (1979). Effectiveness of spinal manipulative therapy in treatment of primary dysmenorrhoea: a pilot study. *Journal of Manipulative and Physiological Therapeutics*, **2**, 140–5.

Vincent, C. and Furnham, A. (1996). Why do patients turn to complementary medicine? An empirical study. *British Journal of Clinical Psychology*, **35**, 37–48.

Vogler, B.K., Pittler, M.H. and Ernst, E. (1999) The efficacy of ginseng. A systematic review of randomised clinical trials. *European Journal of Clinical Pharmacology*, **55**, 567–75.

Washburn, S., Burke, G.L., Morgan, T. and Anthony, M. (1999). Effect of soy protein supplementation on serum lipoproteins, blood pressure, and menopausal symptoms in perimenopausal women [see comments]. *Menopause*, **6**, 7–13.

Watson, C. and Evan, R. (1992). The post mastectomy pain syndrome and topical capsaicin: a randomized trial. *Pain*, **51**, 372–9.

Welshons, W.V., Murphy, C.S., Koch, R., Calaf, G. and Jordan, V.C. (1987). Stimulation of breast cancer cells *in vitro* by the environmental estrogen enterolactone and the phytoestrogen equol. *Breast Cancer Research and Treatment*, **10**, 169–75.

West Yorkshire Health Authority (1995). *Guidelines for the employment of complementary therapists in the NHS.*

West Midlands Medicines Information service (2002). e-mail: druginfo@goodhot.wmids.nhs.uk.

Wilcox, A., Weinberg, C. and Baird, D. (1988). Caffeinated beverages and decreased fertility. *Lancet*, **2**, 1453–6.

Wilcox, G., Wahlqvist, M.L., Burger, H.G. and Medley, G. (1990). Oestrogenic effects of plant foods in post-menopausal women. *British Medical Journal*, **301**, 905–6.

Woelk, H. (2000) Comparison of St John's wort and imipramine for treating depression: randomized controlled trial. *British Medical Journal*, **321**, 536–9.

Wootton, J.C. and Sparber, A. (2001) Surveys of complementary and alternative 0medicine: part 1. General trends and demographic groups. *Journal of Alternative and Complementary Medicine*, **7**, 195–208.

Wouters, M.G., Boers, G.H., Blom, H.J., *et al.* (1993). Hyperhomocysteinemia: a risk factor in women with unexplained recurrent early pregnancy loss. *Fertility and Sterility*, **60**, 820–5.

Wyatt, K.M., Dimmock P.W., Jones, P.W. and Shaughn O'Brien, P.M. (1999). Efficacy of vitamin B-6 in the treatment of premenstrual syndrome: systematic review. *British Medical Journal*, **318**, 1375–81.

Wynd, C.A. (1992). Relaxation imagery used for stress reduction in the prevention of smoking relapse. *Journal of Advanced Nursing*, **17**, 294–302.

Zafriri, D., Ofek, I., Adar, R., Pocino, M. and Sharon, N. (1989). Inhibitory activity of cranberry juice on adherence of type 1 and type P fimbriated *Escherichia coli* to eucaryotic cells. *Antimicrobial Agents and Chemotherapy*, **33**, 92–8.

Zanolla, R. and Monzeglio, C., Balzarini, A. and Martino, G. (1984). Evaluation of the results of three different methods of postmastectomy lymphedema treatment. *Journal of Surgical Oncology*, **26**, 210–13.

# Index

abortion 229–61
  counselling 249
  legislation 230–5
    Abortion Act (1967) 233–5
    abortion laws outside England
      and Wales 233
  medical termination 241–4
  missed 288–9, 290
  patient information 255–61
    medically induced abortion
      255–6
    prostaglandin termination
      257–8
    surgical termination 259–61
  patients' questions 250–1
  risks of 245–6
  service issues 246–7
  statistics 235–41
    England and Wales and Scotland
      236–9
    international 236
    repeat terminations 239–41
  statutory ground for 231–2
  surgical termination 244–5
  terminology 229–30
  *see also* miscarriage
Abortion Act (1967) 231, 233–5
*Actinomyces*-like organisms 193
acupuncture 623
  dysmenorrhoea 647–8
  infertility 640–1
  smoking cessation 660
acute myocardial infarction 127
adolescents
  contraception 219
  health promotion 605–6
  sexual problems in 562–5

age
  and breast cancer risk 429
  and incidence of cystitis 309–10
  of menarche 32–4
  and sexual problems 568–9
  and use of IUDs 186
AIDS, complementary therapy 657
alcohol xix, 601–3
  and breast cancer 431
alendronate
  osteoporosis 93, 105
  side effects 96
ambulatory urodynamic monitoring 330
amenorrhoea 29–40
  anorexia nervosa 528
  assessment 30–1
  causes of 30, 32–40
    delayed menarche 32–4
    hyperprolactinaemia 35–6
    hypothalamic 34–5
    polycystic ovary syndrome 36–8
    premature menopause 39–40
  history and examination 31
  investigation 31–2
  weight-related 278–9
amoxicillin 363
ampicillin/amoxicillin 307
anastrozole 449–50
anorexia nervosa
  course and outcome 534–5
  diagnosis 521
  features 528–31
    amenorrhoea and infertility 528
    blood glucose 529
    cardiovascular symptoms 528–9
    electrolyte disturbances 529–30
    gastrointestinal symptoms 528

anorexia nervosa *(continued)*
    haematological features 529
    hypercholestrolaemia 529
    liver function tests 529
    muscle weakness 528
    neurological problems 531
    osteoporosis 530
    peripheral oedema 530
    psychological problems 528
    thyroid function 529
  investigations 527
  presentation 524–5
  treatment 537–9
    family therapy 539
    GP's role 537–8
    in-patient treatment 538–9
anti-phospholipid syndrome 133
antibiotics
  and combined pill 156
  cystitis 305–8
  *see also individual drugs*
anticonvulsants, and combined pill 156
antidepressants
  eating disorders 536
  premenstrual syndrome 60
antifibrinolytics 16
antisperm antibodies 275
anxiety xxi
  complementary therapy 660–1
anxiolytics, premenstrual syndrome 60
aromatase inhibitors 449–50
aromatherapy 623
artificial urinary sphincter 337
Asherman's syndrome 23, 32
aspiration curettage 13
assisted conception *see* in-vitro
    fertilization
ataxia telangiectasia 431
atrophic vaginitis 83–5
azoospermia 274

bacterial vaginosis 353, 358–9
  and adverse pregnancy outcome 358–9
  diagnosis 358, 364
  symptoms and signs 358
  treatment 358, 364
bacteriuria 297
  asymptomatic 298, 315
  relapse/reinfection 298–9
  significant 297–8, 314–15
  *see also* cystitis
basal cell carcinoma of vulva 389
binge eating *see* eating disorders
BiNovum 141
biofeedback 338, 623
  menopause 656
  menstrually related migraine 650
  urinary incontinence 659
black cohosh 81
bladder
  filling 326
  overactive *see* detrusor instability
  retraining 338
  voiding 326
  *see also* urinary incontinence
body mass index 278
  and menstruation 33
bone density 89–90
bone loss 86
bone markers 88
bone scans 88–9, 103–4
Bourne Judgement 230
Bowen's disease *see* vulval intraepithelial
    neoplasia
*BRAC* genes 490, 499, 502
  *see also* breast cancer
breakthrough bleeding 142, 144, 158
breast cancer 429–62
  adjuvant hormone therapy 448–50
    aromatase inhibitors 449–50
    ovarian ablation 50
    tamoxifen 448–9
  chemotherapy 445–8
    adverse effects 447–8
  and combined pill 121–5
    benign breast disease 124–5
    older women 124
    risk analysis 122, 123

complementary therapy 459, 633–8
  diet 633–5
  exercise 636
  life events 636
  metastatic cancer 637–8
  post-mastectomy pain and
    lymphoedema 636
  vitamins and cofactors 635–6
diagnosis 438–9
  clinical examination 438
  pathological diagnosis 438–9
  radiology 438
ductal carcinoma *in situ* 480, 483
familial *see* familial breast cancer
follow-up 450–1
genetic testing 432
medical emergencies 453–4
  brachial plexopathy 454
  cerebral or choroidal metastases 454
  immobility associated with pain 454
  spinal cord compression 453
  superior vena caval obstruction 454
  thromboembolic disease 454
non-invasive 437
patient information 461–2
prognosis 440–1
psychosocial aspects 454–6
radiotherapy 443–5
  side effects 444–5
recurrence and metastases 451–4
  chemotherapy 452
  endocrine therapy 452
  supportive care 452–3
  symptoms 453
risk factors 429–31
  age 429
  alcohol 431
  diet 431
  family history 431, 456–7
  geographical variation 429
  hormone replacement therapy
    97–9, 430, 435
  ionizing radiation 431
  menstrual cycle 429

oral contraceptive pill 430
  previous breast disease 429, 435
  reproductive factors 429
  weight 431
screening *see* breast screening
staging 439–40
surgery 441–3
  adverse effects of 443
  breast reconstruction 442–3
  silicone implants 443
under age 50 years 434
  breast self-examination 436–7
  interval of screening 434
  organization of 436
  potential adverse effects 435
  special groups 434–5
breast disorders 421–65
  benign 422–9
    management and referral 422–4
    symptoms 422, 423
  breast cancer *see* breast cancer
  complementary therapy 633–9
  infection 427–9
  lumps 424–5, 456
  mastalgia 423, 425–6
    complementary therapy 638–9
    treatment 425–6
  nipple discharge 426–7
  pain and nodularity 425–6, 456
breast screening 433–7, 476, 479–83
  age of women screened 482
  familial breast cancer 497–8
  frequency of 482
  NHS Breast Screening Programme
    433–7, 476, 479–80
  number of views taken 482
  outcome 480
  outcome of referrals 480–1
  over age 70 years 433–4
  potential effect on mortality 481–2
  results 478–80
  UK screening programme 433–7
breast self-examination 436–7
Brevinor 141

bromocriptine 63, 426
bulimia nervosa 519–20
  course and outcome 535
  diagnosis 521
  features 531–2
    fluid and electrolyte disturbances
      532
    gastrointestinal symptoms 531
    menstrual disturbances 531
    psychological problems 531
  investigation 527
  presentation 525–6
  social circumstances 532
  treatment 540–4
    cognitive behaviour therapy 540–1
    interpersonal psychotherapy 541
buserelin 418

caffeine, and infertility 641–2
calcium intake 91
cancer
  breast *see* breast cancer
  cervical 125
  colorectal 125
  endometrium 125
  familial *see* familial cancers
  ovary 100, 125
  vulva 377, 383, 388–9
cancer screening 466–88
  breast cancer 433–7, 476, 479–83
    outcome 480
    outcome of referrals 480–1
    potential effect of 481–2
    results 478–80
  cervical cancer 468–76, 477, 478
    liquid-based cytology 474
    outcome of referrals 471
    potential effect of 471–3
    results 470–1
  definitions 466–7
  ovarian cancer 483–5
  predictive value 467
  sensitivity 466–7
  specificity 467

*Candida albicans* 353, 356–8
  complementary therapy 640
  diagnosis 357, 364
  recurrent 357–8
  symptoms and signs 356–7
  treatment 357, 364
  vulva 391
capsaicin, and post-mastectomy
    pain 636
cardiovascular disease
  and combined pill 126–30
  dietary supplements 652
  risk factors 132
  soya consumption 653
β-carotene 635
cephalosporins 307
Cerazette 163, 167
cervical cancer
  carcinoma *in situ* 471–2
  cervical intraepithelial neoplasia
    (CIN) 468
  and combined pill 125
  invasive 472–3
  *see also* cervical screening
cervical cap 206–7
cervical screening 468–76, 477, 478
  dyskaryosis 468, 476
  liquid-based cytology 474
  outcome of referrals 471
  potential effect of 471–3
    invasive cancer 472–3
    mortality 473
    registration of carcinoma *in situ*
      471–2
  repeat tests 474–5
  results
    NHS Cervical Screening
      Programme 270
    smear tests 470–1, 477–8
childlessness 292–3
Chinese medicine 625
chiropractic 623
  menstrually related migraine 651
  premenstrual syndrome 65

*Chlamydia trachomatis* 115, 272, 317,
    353, 359–62
  diagnosis 361–2, 364
  and future pregnancy 371–2
  IUD-related 191–3
  prevalence 360
  screening 362
  symptoms and signs 361
  treatment 362, 364
  and urethral syndrome 299
choriocarcinoma, and combined
    pill 125
chronic pelvic pain 399–420
  causes 404–10
    endometriosis 404–5
    irritable bowel syndrome 406–7
    musculoskeletal and nerve-related
      pain 408–9
    ovarian remnant syndrome 407–8
    pelvic congestion syndrome 408
    pelvic inflammatory disease 405–6
    psychosocial factors 409–10
    trapped ovary syndrome 407–8
  epidemiology 399–400
  examination 403–4
  history 400–3
  laparoscopy 411–13
  referral to hospital 410–11
  treatment 413–19
Cilest 133–4, 142
ciprofloxacin 363
clam cystoplasty 341
clindamycin 358, 359
clomipramine 60
clonidine, for menopausal
    symptoms 81
clotrimazole 357
co-amoxiclav 307, 363
cofactors 635–6
cognitive behavioural therapy 57–9
coital incontinence 85
coitus interruptus, failure rate 117
colorectal cancer
  and combined pill 125

familial 506–10
and HRT 99
colposuspension 336
combined oral contraceptive pill 119–62
  benefits versus risks 119–21, 501
  cardiovascular disease 126–30
    acute myocardial infarction 127
    dose/type of hormone 127
    haemorrhagic stroke 127
    ischaemic stroke 127
    venous thromboembolism 127–9
  comparative risks 130
  congenital abnormalities and fertility
    159–60
  contraindications 136–40
    absolute 136–8
    intercurrent diseases 139–40
    relative 138–9
  drug interactions 155–9
    enzyme inducers 155, 158–9
  duration of use 160–1
  failure rate 116
  initial choice 140–3
  menorrhagia 19
  migraine 147–50
  patient information 161
  pill-free week 151–3
  premenstrual syndrome 61
  prescribing guidelines 130–6
  previous failure 154–5
  reasons to stop 150, 151
  second choice 143–5
  supervision and follow-up 145–7
  tricycle regimen 152
  tumours 121–6
    breast cancer 121–5
    cervical cancer 125
    choriocarcinoma 126
    colorectal cancer 126
    liver tumours 125
    ovarian and endometrial
      carcinoma 126
  vomiting and diarrhoea 153–4
  when to stop 215

complementary medicine 619–69
  applications
    AIDS 657
    anxiety and depression 660–1
    breast disorders 633–9
    candidiasis 640
    contraception 639
    infertility and early pregnancy
        loss 640–3
    menopause 651–7
    menstrual problems 647–51
    premenstrual syndrome 63–4,
        643–7
    smoking cessation 660
    urinary incontinence 659
    urinary tract infection 658–9
  efficacy 630–1
  legal liability 629–30
  non-specific benefits 662
  paying for 626–8
  professional liability 628–9
  relationship to conventional
        medicine 622
  sources of information 631–3
  therapies
    acupuncture 623, 640–1, 647–8, 660
    aromatherapy 623
    biofeedback 338, 623, 650, 656, 659
    chiropractic 65, 623, 651
    evening primrose oil 64, 638–9, 644
    ginseng 657
    healing 623
    herbalism 623
    homeopathy 623–4, 647
    hypnotherapy 624
    macrobiotics 624
    manipulative medicine 646, 648, 656
    naturopathy 624
    osteopathy 624–5
    reflexology 625, 646–7
    relaxation and imagery 625, 647, 660
    traditional Chinese medicine 625
  users 619–22
  women as users 625–6

condoms
  female 205–6
    failure rate 117
  male 205
    failure rate 117
contraception xviii–xix,
        112–228
  adolescents 219
  barrier methods 203–7
  choice of method 113–18
  current use 114
  eligibility 115, 118
  emergency see emergency
        contraception
  and intercurrent disease 219–20
  natural 639
  older women 213–14
  oral see oral contraception
  post-partum 216–18
  and sexual health 115
  trends in 113
  unlicensed indications 220
  user-failure rates 116–17
  when to stop 214–16
  see also individual methods
contraceptive implants 172–6
  advantages and indications 174
  contraindications 174–5
  efficacy 173
  mechanism of action 173
  side-effects 175–6
    altered bleeding pattern 175
    hypo-oestrogenism 175–6
    local adverse effects 176
    minor side effects 175
  timing of insertion 173–4
Conveen Continence Guard 333
coronary heart disease xviii
  and HRT 96–7
counselling
  abortion 249
  emergency contraception 180–1
  infertility 262–3
  IUD insertion 198

menorrhagia 24
  sterilization 211
couples, sexual problems 555
Cowden's syndrome 431
cranberry juice
  cystitis 304
  urinary tract infection 658–9
cryptorchidism 273
cyproterone acetate 134
cystitis 297–321
  causes 302–4
  in diabetes mellitus 309
  investigations 300–1
    leucocyte esterase and nitrite dip
      sticks 300
    mid-stream urine sample 300–1,
      315–16
  in pregnancy 308–9
  presentation 299–300
  treatment 304–8
    antibiotics 305–8
    cranberry juice 304
    self-help groups 305
  urinary catheters 311
  urinary tract calculi 309
  urogenital ageing 309–10
  when to treat 314
cystometry 329

danazol 418
  mastalgia 426
  menorrhagia 19–20
  premenstrual syndrome 62–3
  side effects 417
DDAVP 339, 340
dehydroepiandrosterone 656
dementia, and HRT 100
Depo-Provera 168–71
depression xxi
  complementary therapy 660–1
dermatitis, vulval 376, 385–6
detrusor instability 337–41
  biofeedback 338
  bladder retraining 338

drug therapy 339–40
electrical stimulation 338–9
neuromodulation 341
surgery 341
diabetes
  and bacteriuria 309
  and combined pill 139–40
Dianette 134, 142
diaphragm 206–7
  failure rate 117
diclofenac 15
dicyclomine 340
diet 598–600
  breast cancer 633–5
  menopause 651–2
  menstrually related migraine 649–50
dilation and curettage 12–13
domestic violence 579–96
  against women with disabilities
    584–5
  assessment of present situation 591
  confronting the patient 588–90
  consideration of possibility 586–7
  definition 579
  documentation 590–1
  effects on children 583–4
  ethnic minority communities 584
  examination 590
  health consequences 581–2
  as long-term condition 582–3
  nature of injuries 580–1
  photography 591
  privacy and confidentiality 587–8
  provision of information 592
  role of general practice in 585–93
  safety plan 592–3
  scale and severity 579–80
Down's syndrome 39
doxorubicin 447
doxycycline 362
drospirenone 135–6
dydrogesterone 418
dysaesthetic vulvodynia 391–2
dyskaryosis 468, 476

dysmenorrhoea 26–9
  assessment 27–8
  complementary therapy 647–8
    acupuncture 647–8
    manipulative medicine 648
  primary 26–7
  secondary 27
  treatment 28–9
dysuria 85

eating disorders 519–51
  aetiology 532–4
  cultural pressures 532–3
    environmental and genetic
      factors 534
    personality traits 533
    psychiatric disorders within
      family 534
  anorexia nervosa
    course and outcome 534–5
    features 528–31
    investigations 527
    presentation 524–5
    treatment 537–9
  assessment 523–32
  atypical 544–5
  bulimia nervosa 519–20
    course and outcome 535
    features 531–2
    investigation 527
    presentation 525–6
    treatment 540–4
  definitions 520–1
  detection 523–32
  diagnostic criteria 521
  management 535–45
    drug treatments 536–7
    education and engagement 535–6
    immediate 523–32
  patient information 548
  prevalence and distribution 522–3
ectopic pregnancy, and IUD use 194, 201
eczema, vulval 376, 386
egg donation 281–2

embryo cryopreservation 280–1
emergency contraception 176–82
  choice of method 176
  copper IUD 178–82
  hormone methods 176–8
endometrial biopsy 12–13
  interpretation of 13–14
endometrial cancer
  and combined pill 125
  and HRT 99
endometriosis 272
  and chronic pelvic pain 404–5
  treatment
    medical 415–19
    surgical 414–15
endometrium
  menorrhagia 11–12
  normal menstrual cycle 4–5
*Enterococcus* 306
environmental factors xix–xx
  eating disorders 534
epirubicin 447
epsilon-amino caproic acid 15
erythromycin 362
*Escherichia coli* 303, 305, 306
ethamsylate 15, 16
Eugynon 141
European Committee for Proprietary
    Medicinal Products 129
evening primrose oil
  mastalgia 638–9
  premenstrual syndrome 64, 644
EVRA 134
exemestane 449–50
exercise 91, 600–1
  and breast cancer risk 636
EZ-ON condom 205

familial breast cancer 494–505
  breast examination 498
  chemoprevention 499
  genetic testing 502–5
    diagnostic 503–4
    predictive 504–5

higher-risk women 495–505
hormonal therapy 501
lifestyle factors 502
low-risk (average) women 495
magnetic resonance imaging 499
mammographic screening 497–8
prophylactic surgery 500–1
risk assessment 497–503
*see also* breast cancer; breast disorders
familial cancers 489–518
decision for referral 492–4
dominant high-risk genes 490–1
family history 492, 493
primary care in 510–12
susceptibility to cancer 489–90
*see also individual types of cancer*
familial colorectal cancer 506–10
early detection 508–9
genetic testing 509–10
hereditary non-polyposis type 507
higher risk 508
lifestyle modification 509
low (average) risk 508
management 507–10
prophylactic surgery 510
familial ovarian cancer 505–6
Family Planning Association 112
female sexual problems 553–4
Femidom 205–6
Femodene 141
Femulen 163
fertile period 270
fertility awareness 208–9, 643
failure rate 117
fibroadenoma of breast 424–5
fibroids 24–6
Flexi-T-300 196
flucloxacillin 429
fluconazole 357, 391
flurbiprofen 15
folic acid 642

galactorrhoea 271, 427
galactosaemia 39

gallbladder disease, and HRT 101
gamete intrafallopian transfer
(GIFT) 287
gemeprost 241
genetic testing
breast cancer 432
familial breast cancer 502–5
familial colorectal cancer 509–10
genital examination 573
genital herpes *see* herpes virus
genital warts 365–6
genitourinary clinics 367–8
gestrinone 20, 418
Gillick competency 234
ginseng 657
gonadotropin-releasing hormone
analogues
menorrhagia 20
premenstrual syndrome 62
gonadotropin-releasing hormone
antagonists 417
gonorrhoea 353, 362–3, 364
Gorlin's syndromes 431
goserelin 418
Gynefix 196

*Haemophilus* spp. 353
haemorrhagic stroke 127
healing 623
health education 597–8
health fashions xxi–xxiii
health promotion 597–618
adolescents 605–6
health education 597–8
lifestyle advice 598–605
prevention of ill-health 606–9
coronary health disease 606–9
mental health 609
primary health-care team 611–12
social policy 609–11
herbalism 623
menstrually related migraine 650
hereditary non-polyposis colorectal
cancer 507

herpes simplex 391
herpes virus 353, 366, 369–70
HERS trial 97, 100, 101
historical aspects xvii–xviii
homeopathy 623–4
  menstrually related migraine 650
  premenstrual syndrome 647
homocysteine 642
homosexuals, sexual problems 555
hormone replacement therapy
    xxii, 75–80
  contraindications 80
  genital complaints 83–5
  headache 82
  and libido 85
  premenstrual syndrome 61–2
  prevention of chronic diseases 85–101
    breast cancer 97–9, 430, 501
    colon cancer 99
    coronary heart disease 96–7
    endometrial cancer 99
    gallbladder disease 101
    memory loss and dementia 100
    osteoporosis 85–96
    ovarian cancer 100
    venous thromboembolic disease
      100–1
  quality of life 82
  side effects 80
  types of 76–9
  urinary complaints 85
  weight gain 83
hormones
  contraception 176–8
    *see also* combined oral contraceptive
      pill; progestogen-only pill
  menstrual cycle 3–4
  premenstrual syndrome 61
  *see also* hormone replacement therapy
hot flushes 75
  non-hormone treatment 81
HRT *see* hormone replacement therapy
Human Fertilisation and Embryology
    Act (1990) 231

human papillomavirus 365–6, 473–4,
  476
hyperprolactinaemia 32, 35–6
hypertension, and combined pill 140
hypnotherapy 624
hypothalamic amenorrhoea 32, 34–5
hysterectomy
  menorrhagia 21–2
  premenstrual syndrome 21
hysteroscopy 14

ibuprofen 15, 16
ileocystoplasty 341
imipramine 339, 340
Implanon 172–6
in-vitro fertilization 280–8
  complications 285–6
  egg donation 281, 283
  embryo cryopreservation 280–1
  ethical issues 291–2
  gamete intrafallopian transfer
    (GIFT) 287
  high-order multiple pregnancy
    286–7
  indications for 281
  male factor infertility 283–5
  microassisted fertilization 283
  miscarriage after 287–8
  outcome of children 288
  ovarian hyperstimulation syndrome
    286
  success rates 285
  surrogacy 283
  technique 282–3
  zygote intrafallopian transfer
    (ZIFT) 287
incontinence *see* urinary incontinence
Infant Life Preservation Act (1929)
  230, 231
infection
  of breast 427–8
  IUD-related 190–3, 201
  urinary tract 308–9, 313
  *see also* bacteriuria

infertility 262–96
  antisperm antibodies 275
  and caffeine intake 641–2
  causes of 266
  complementary therapy 640–3
    acupuncture 640–1
    herbalism 641
  counselling 262–3
  initial consultation 269
  investigation in general practice
      266–75
  male factor 267, 283–5
  male partner investigation 273–4
  menstrual cycle assessment 269–71
  normal fertility 264–6
  patient autonomy 263–4
  pelvic assessment 271–3
  psychological morbidity 263
  sperm-mucus interaction 275
  treatment 275–80
    anovulation and PCOS 277–8
    premature ovarian failure 279–80
    superovulation and intrauterine
        insemination 280
    weight-related amenorrhoea 278–9
    see also in-vitro fertilization
information sources xxiii–xxiv
  abortion 255–61
  breast cancer 461–2
  complementary medicine 631–3
  domestic violence 592
  eating disorders 548
  menorrhagia 24
  oral contraception 161
  sexually transmitted diseases 372
injectable contraceptives 168–72
  contraindications 171
  indications 171
  monitoring and management 172
  overdue injections 172
  protocols 170
  side effects 169
International Planned Parenthood
    Federation 168

International Society for the Study
    of Vulval Disease 379
intrauterine device 182–203
  copper-bearing 182–99
    absolute contraindications 196–7
    advantages of 183
    adverse effects 186, 188
    choice of device 195–6
    counselling 198
    duration of use 194–5
    ectopic pregnancy 194
    effectiveness 183
    expulsion and perforation 188, 190
    in situ contraception 186
    infection 190–3
    influence of age 186
    insertion techniques 198–9
    lost threads 187, 188, 189
    mechanism of action 183, 186
    pain and bleeding 194
    relative contraindications 197–8
    routine follow-up 199
    timing of insertion 198
  emergency contraception 177, 178–82
    counselling and management
        180–1
    effectiveness 178–9
    indications and contraindications
        179
    special indications 181–2
  failure rate 116–17
  levonorgestrel-releasing (Mirena)
      199–203
    absolute contraindications 202–3
    clinical advantages and indications
        199–200
    ectopic pregnancy 201
    infection 201
    insertion of 203
    mechanisms 199
    menorrhagia 200–1
    problems and adverse effects 201–2
  problems and complications 184–5
intrauterine growth retardation 278

intrauterine insemination 280
ionizing radiation, and breast cancer 431
irritable bowel syndrome 406–7
ischaemic stroke 127
isoflavonoids 634
IUD *see* intrauterine device
IVF *see* in-vitro fertilization

Kallman's syndrome 35
*Klebsiella* spp. 302, 306

lactational amenorrhoea 217–18
laparoscopic colposuspension 336
laparoscopic ovarian diathermy 278
laparoscopy 272
   pelvic pain 411–13
letrazole 449–50
leucocyte esterase test 300
leuprorelin 418
Levonelle 176–8
   contraindications 178
   effectiveness 176, 178
   side effects 178
levonorgestrel
   combined pill 133
   emergency contraception 177
   Mirena IUD 199–203
Li-Fraumeni syndrome 431
libido, and HRT 85
lichen planus 376, 386–7
   clinical features 386–7
   treatment 387
lichen sclerosus 377, 382–5
   clinical features 384
   treatment 384–5
lichen simplex 376, 385
lifestyle xix–xx, 598–605
   alcohol xix, 431, 601–3
   diet 598–601, 633–5, 649–50, 651–2
   exercise 91, 600–1
   smoking xx, 603–5
lignans 634
lipoma of breast 422
liver tumours, and combined pill 125

Loestrin 141, 158
Logynon 141
Lynch syndrome 507

macrobiotics 624
magnesium supplements 649
male factor infertility 267, 283–5
male sexual problems 554–5, 561–2
mammography *see* breast screening
manipulative medicine
   dysmenorrhoea 648
   menopause 656
   premenstrual syndrome 646
Marvelon 141, 158
mastalgia 423, 425–6
   complementary therapy 638–9
   treatment 425–6
mechanical pelvic pain 408–9
meclofenamic acid 15
medroxyprogesterone 81, 418
mefenamic acid 15, 16
memory loss, and HRT 100
menarche 32–4
menopause xxi–xxii, 73–111
   complementary therapy 651–7
      biofeedback 656
      dietary soya 652–4
      dietary supplements 651–2
      ginseng 657
      manipulative medicine 656
      natural progesterone creams
         654–6
   definition of 73
   diagnosis 74
   hormone changes 74
   menstrual changes 75
   postmenopausal bleeding 42
   premature 32, 39–40
   sexual problems in 566–8
   symptoms 74–5
   vasomotor symptoms 75
      non-hormone treatment 81
   *see also* hormone replacement therapy;
      osteoporosis

menorrhagia 8–24
  assessment of menstrual blood loss
    8–9
  causes of 9
  counselling, information and patient
    preference 24
  drug therapy 15–20
    hormonal 17–20
    non-hormonal 15, 16–17
  endometrial assessment 11–12
  endometrial biopsy 12–14
  GP treatment or referral 14–15
  hysteroscopy 14
  investigations 11
  levonorgestrel-releasing IUD 200–1
  surgical treatment 21–4
    combined oophorectomy and
      hysterectomy 21–2
    endometrial ablation 23–4
    hysterectomy 21
    laparoscopic hysterectomy 22
  transvaginal ultrasound 12
  treatment failure 20
menstrual cycle 3–8
  blood loss 5–6
  and breast cancer risk 429
  cycle length and duration 6–8
  endocrine changes 3–4
  endometrial events 4–5
  in infertility 269–71
menstrual problems 2–3
  amenorrhoea 29–40
  colour and smell of menstrual
    blood 42
  complementary therapy 647–51
    dysmenorrhoea 647–8
    migraine 648–51
  dysmenorrhoea 26–9
  fibroids 24–6
  intermenstrual and postcoital
    bleeding 41–2
  irregular menstruation 41
  menorrhagia 8–24
  oligomenorrhoea 29–40

  postmenopausal bleeding 42
  prolonged menstruation 41
  scanty periods 40
menstruation 2
mental health problems xviii
Mercilon 141, 158
metronidazole 358, 359
microassisted fertilization 283
microepididymal sperm aspiration 283
Microgynon 141
Micronor 163
mid-stream urine sample 300–1,
    315, 328
mifepristone 241–4
migraine
  and combined pill 147–50
    absolute contraindications 149–50
    relative contraindications 150
  menstrual 648–9
  menstrually related 649–50
mineral supplements 64
Minulet 141
Mirena device 199–203, 216
miscarriage 288–91
  after IVF 287–8
  complementary therapy 640–3
  recurrent 289–90
  spontaneous 288–9
  threatened 290–1
mismatch repair genes 507
missed abortion 288–9, 290
morbidity xx–xxi

nafarelin 418
naproxen 15, 16
National Health Service Breast Screening
    Programme 433–7, 476, 479–80
National Health Service Cervical
    Screening Programme 468,
    470–1
natural family planning 639
naturopathy 624
*Neisseria gonorrhoeae* 353, 362–3
Neogest 163

nipple discharge 423, 426–7, 428
nipple retraction 423
nitrite dip stick test 300
nitrofurantoin 307
nocturia 85
non-steroidal anti-inflammatory
    drugs 15, 16–17
Nonoxinol 9 206
norelgestomin 134
norethisterone 418
norgestimate 133–4
Norgeston 163
Noriday 163
Norimin 141
Norinyl-1 141
Norplant 172
nortryptiline 60
Nova-T 380 195–6
nystatin 391

oestrogens
    atrophic vaginitis 83–5
    hormone replacement therapy 76–9
    menorrhagia 19
    osteoporosis 91–3, 104
    premenstrual syndrome 61–2
    see also combined oral contraceptive
        pill
Offences against the Person Act
    (1861) 230
oligospermia 275
oophorectomy
    menorrhagia 21
    premenstrual syndrome 21
oral contraception xxii–xxiii, 119–67
    combined pill see combined oral
        contraceptive pill
    progestogen-only pill see progestogen-
        only pill
orchidopexy 273
osteopathy 624–5
osteoporosis 85–96, 101–5
    anorexia nervosa 530
    bone loss 86

clinical diagnosis 87–90, 103
    bone density 89–90
    bone markers 88
    bone scans 88–9, 103–4
    medical examination 88
    medical history 87
    X-rays 88
dietary supplements 651–2
drugs causing 90
fracture risk 87
peak bone mass 86–7
prevention and treatment 91–6
    calcium 91
    exercise 91
    non-oestrogen medication 93–6
    oestrogen 91–3, 104
    vitamin D 91
risk factors 102–3
ovarian ablation 450
ovarian cancer
    and combined pill 125
    familial 505–6
    and HRT 100
ovarian hyperstimulation syndrome 286
ovarian remnant syndrome 407–8
ovarian screening 483–5, 506
overflow incontinence 341
Ovranette 141
Ovysmen 141
Oxford Collaborative Group on
    Hormonal Factors in Breast
    Cancer 97–9
oxybutinin 339, 340

pad test 329
Paget's disease of vulva 377, 389
parathyroid hormone, and osteoporosis
    94
paroxetine 81
PCOS see polycystic ovary syndrome
peak bone mass 86–7
pelvic assessment 271–3
pelvic congestion syndrome 408
pelvic floor exercises 334–5, 659

pelvic inflammatory disease 186, 190–3, 363, 365, 405–6
pelvic pain *see* chronic pelvic pain
PEPI trial 99
percutaneous epididymal aspiration 283–4
perimenopause 73, 74–5
PERSONA 210
phyto-oestrogens 81, 634
polycystic ovary syndrome 32, 36–8, 134
and infertility 277–8
post-micturition dribbling 327
postcoital bleeding 41–2
postmenopause 73
pregnancy xviii–xix
sexual problems in 565
urinary tract infection in 308–9
premature ovarian failure 279–80
premenstrual syndrome 46–72
causes of 52
complementary therapy 63–4, 643–7
chiropractic 65
evening primrose oil 644
herbal medicine 644
homeopathy 647
manipulative medicine 646
natural progesterone 646
nutritional supplements 64
reflexology 646–7
relaxation and imagery 647
vitamin B6 644–5
cultural aspects 53–4
definition 46–50
education, understanding and support 55
effects of 50–1
health status 55–6
history 53, 54
management 52–3
prevalence 50
social and relationship context 53
symptom diaries 48, 49, 54
those likely to experience 51–2

treatment
cognitive behavioural therapy 57–9
drug therapy 59–63
self-help measures 67
surgical 65
primary health-care team 611–12
Progestasert 201
progesterone
natural
contraception 639
menopause 654–6
premenstrual syndrome 646
premenstrual syndrome 63
progestogen-only pill 162–7
contraindications 164–6
efficacy 162–4
failure rate 117
indications 164
mechanism of action 162–4
problems and management 166–7
starting routines 166
when to stop 216
progestogens
menorrhagia 17–19
premenstrual syndrome 63
propantheline 340
propiverine 340
prostaglandin inhibitors 61
Protectaid 207
*Proteus* 302, 306
*Pseudomonas* 306
psoriasis, vulval 376, 386
pudendal nerve stimulation 332
pyelonephritis 298
pyridoxine 64

quinolone antibiotics 308

raloxifene
breast cancer prophylaxis 499
osteoporosis 93, 105
side effects 95
rape 571
after-effects of 571–2

reflexology 625, 646–7
relaxation and imagery 625, 647
  smoking cessation 660
risedronate 93, 105

sacral neuromodulation 341
St John's Wort 158
sebaceous cyst of breast 422, 424–5
selective serotonin re-uptake
      inhibitors 60
self-help xxiii–xxiv
  urinary tract infection 313
self-help groups 305
sertraline 81
sexual health promotion 368
sexual problems 552–78
  age and stage 562–70
    adolescence 562–5
    ageing 568–9
    menopause 566–8
    pregnancy and childbirth 565
    terminal illness and bereavement
        569–70
  causes of 556–62
    gynaecological problems 557
    medical problems 560–2
    post-hysterectomy 557–8
  couples 555
  disability 570
  female 553–4
  homosexuals 555
  incidence 553
  male 554
  management 572–4
    avoidance of routine questions
        572–3
    doctor/patient relationship 572
    facts to establish 572
    genital examination 573
    interpretation 573
    referral 573–4
  mind/body link 552
  people without partners 555–6
  presentation 552–3

and rape 571
training in psychosexual medicine 574
vaginismus 557, 575–6
sexually transmitted diseases xix, 356–70
  bacterial vaginosis 353, 358–9
  *Candida see Candida albicans*
  *Chlamydia see Chlamydia trachomatis*
  contact tracing 367
  genital warts 365–6
  genitourinary clinics 367
  gonorrhoea 353, 362–3, 364
  herpes virus 353, 366, 369–70
  patient information 372
  trichomoniasis 359, 364
  *see also* vaginal discharge
sickle-cell disorders, and combined
      pill 140
smoking xx, 603–5
smoking cessation 614–15
soya 652–4
  and atrophic vaginitis 653–4
  and cardiovascular disease 653
  and hot flushes 653
  and recurrent urinary tract infection
      653–4
sperm count 274
sperm-mucus interaction 275
spermicides 207–8
  failure rate 117
*Staphylococcus aureus* 353, 427
*Staphylococcus saprophyticus* 302, 306
statins 96
sterilization 210–11
  counselling 211
  decision-making 212–13
  efficacy 211
  failure rate 116
  long-term side effects 212
  potential reversibility 211–12
  tubal occlusion 213
  vasectomy 213
*Streptococcus milleri* 353
stress incontinence 85, 326
stress, and infertility 640

subarachnoid haemorrhage 127
suction termination 244–5
superovulation 280
surgical termination of pregnancy 244–5
surrogacy 283
Synphase 141
systemic lupus erythematosus 133

T-Safe 380 A 196
T-Safe Cu 380 195
tamoxifen 426, 437
    breast cancer 448–9, 457, 459, 499
teenagers *see* adolescents
tension-free vaginal tape 336–7
testicular feminization 32
testicular sperm aspiration 284
thrombophilia, acquired 133
tibolone
    menopausal symptoms 81
    osteoporosis 94
    premenstrual tension 63
    side effects 95
Tietze's syndrome 425
tolterodine 340
toxic shock syndrome 42–3
tranexamic acid 15
transvaginal ultrasound 12
trapped ovary syndrome 407–8
Tri-Minulet 142
Triadene 142
*Trichomonas vaginalis* 353, 359,
        364, 391
trichomoniasis 359
trimethoprim 306–7
Trinordiol 141
TriNovum 141
triptorelin 418
trospium chloride 339
tubal occlusion 213
Turner's syndrome 32, 39

unconscious incontinence 327
unwanted pregnancy *see* abortion
urethral bulking agents 336

urethral plugs 333–4
urethral pressure profilometry 330
urethral sphincter incompetence
        332–7
    devices 332–4
        electronic 332
        elevating 332–3
        occlusive 333–4
    pelvic floor exercises 334–5
    surgical treatment 335–7
        artificial urinary sphincter 337
        colposuspension 336
        laparoscopic colposuspension 336
        sling operation 336
        tension-free vaginal tape 336–7
        urethral bulking agents 336
urethral syndrome 299
    need to treat 316–18
urge incontinence 85, 327
urinary catheters 311
urinary incontinence 322–50
    classification 322–3
    complementary therapy 659
    examination 327–8
    history 323–7
        constitutional 323–4
        drug history 325
        general medical 324
        general pelvic 324–5
        social history 325
        specific bladder history 326
    investigations 328–31
        ambulatory urodynamic
            monitoring 330
        blood biochemistry 328
        cystometry 329
        mid-stream urine sample 328
        pad test 329
        urethral pressure profilometry 330
        urodynamic studies 328–9
        uroflowmetry 329
        Valsalva leak point pressure 330
        videocystourethrography 330–1
    prevalence 323

urinary incontinence *(continued)*
  symptoms 326–7
    continuous leakage 327
    post-micturition dribbling 327
    retention of urine 327
    stress incontinence 326
    unconscious incontinence 327
    urge incontinence 327
  treatment 331–42
    detrusor instability 337–41
    overflow incontinence 341
    urethral sphincter incompetence
      332–7
urinary retention 327
urinary tract calculi 309
urinary tract infection 85, 298
  complementary therapy 658–9
  continuous prophylaxis 313
  follow-up 301–2
  intermittent self-treatment 313
  postcoital prophylaxis 312–13
  premenopausal women 311–13
  risk factors 300
  *see also* cystitis
urodynamic studies 328–9
uroflowmetry 329
urogenital ageing 309–10

vaginal cones 334–5
vaginal discharge 351–73, 558–60
  causes of 353–4
  diagnosis 354–6
  infective causes *see* sexually
    transmitted diseases
  management 356
  prevalence 351–2
vaginismus 557, 575–6
Valsalva leak point pressure 330
vasectomy 213
venlafaxine 81
venous thromboembolic disease
  and combined pill 127–9
  and HRT 100–1
  risk factors 131

veralipride 81
videocystourethrography 330–1
vitamin A 635, 642–3
vitamin B6 644–5
vitamin C 635
vitamin D 91
vitamin E 635, 636
*Vitex agnus castus* 64
  infertility 641
  mastalgia 639
  premenstrual syndrome 644
vulval atrophy 376
vulval carcinoma 377, 383, 388–9
vulval dermatitis 376, 385–6
vulval disorders 374–98
  clinical features 375–7
  diseases 379–89
    neoplastic 383–9
    non-neoplastic 382–3
  normal vulva 374–5
  pain 389–93
    dysaesthetic vulvodynia 391–2
    infective causes 391
    vulval vestibulitis syndrome
      392–3
  psychological features 378
  vulva clinic 379
vulval eczema 376, 386
vulval intraepithelial neoplasia 377,
  387–8
vulval melanoma 389
vulval psoriasis 376, 386
vulval vestibulitis syndrome 392–3

weight, and breast cancer 431
weight loss 600
women doctors xxiv–xxv
women as patients xxiii
Women's Health Initiative 96, 97

Yasmin 133–4, 142

zygote intrafallopian transfer
  (ZIFT) 287